AUTOIMMUNITY

Genetic, Immunologic, Virologic, and Clinical Aspects

AUTOIMMUNITY
Genetic, Immunologic, Virologic, and Clinical Aspects

Edited by

NORMAN TALAL, M.D.

Department of Medicine
School of Medicine
University of California, San Francisco
and Clinical Immunology and Arthritis Section
Veterans Administration Hospital
San Francisco, California

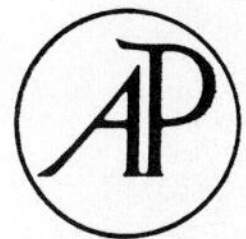

ACADEMIC PRESS New York San Francisco London 1977

A Subsidiary of Harcourt Brace Jovanovich, Publishers

ACADEMIC PRESS, INC.
111 Fifth Avenue, New York, New York 10003

United Kingdom Edition published by
ACADEMIC PRESS, INC. (LONDON) LTD.
24/28 Oval Road, London NW1

Library of Congress Cataloging in Publication Data

Main entry under title:

Autoimmunity : genetic, immunologic, virologic, and clinical aspects.

Includes bibliographies and index.
1. Autoimmune diseases. I. Talal, Norman. [DNLM: 1. Autoimmune diseases. WD300 T137a]
RC600.A85 616.9'78 77-74062
ISBN 0-12-682350-2

PRINTED IN THE UNITED STATES OF AMERICA

79 80 81 82 9 8 7 6 5 4 3 2

Contents

Chapter 6 Suppressor T Cell Dysfunction as a Possible Cause for Autoimmunity

RICHARD K. GERSHON

Chapter 7 Autoimmunity and Lymphoid Malignancy: Manifestations of Immunoregulatory Disequilibrium

NORMAN TALAL

Chapter 8 Thymic Hormones and Autoimmunity

J. F. BACH, M. A. BACH, C. CARNAUD, M. DARDENNE, AND J. C. MONIER

Chapter 9 Autoimmunity, Self-Recognition, and Blocking Factors

IRUN R. COHEN AND HARTMUT WEKERLE

Chapter 10 Self-Recognition: The Basic Principle in the Immune System

HEINZ KOHLER AND DONALD A. ROWLEY

Chapter 11 The Biology of Immune Complexes

ALAN O. HAAKENSTAD AND MART MANNIK

Part III VIRAL ASPECTS

Chapter 12 H-2 Restriction of Cell-Mediated Virus-Specific Immunity and Immunopathology: Self-Recognition, Altered Self, and Autoaggression

ROLF M. ZINKERNAGEL

Chapter 13 Viruses, Autoimmunity, and Murine Lymphoma

MAX R. PROFFITT, MARTIN S. HIRSCH, AND PAUL H. BLACK

Chapter 14 C-Type RNA Viruses and Autoimmune Disease

JAY A. LEVY

Part IV CLINICAL ASPECTS

Chapter 15 Infection and Autoimmunity

RALPH C. WILLIAMS, JR.

Chapter 16 Immunodeficiency Disorders and Autoimmunity

ARTHUR J. AMMANN

Chapter 17 Autoimmunity and Aging

F. M. BURNET

Chapter 18 Autoimmunity and Systemic Lupus Erythematosus

DAVID GLASS AND PETER H. SCHUR

Chapter 19 Rheumatoid Arthritis

NATHAN J. ZVAIFLER

Chapter 20 Cell-Surface Receptors and Autoimmune Responses

I. R. MACKAY AND P. R. CARNEGIE

Chapter 21 Autoantibodies to the Thyrotropin (TSH) Receptors on Thyroid Epithelium and Other Tissues

DEBORAH DONIACH AND NICHOLAS J. MARSHALL

Chapter 22 Autoimmune Neurological Disease: Experimental Animal Systems and Implications for Multiple Sclerosis

PHILIP Y. PATERSON

Chapter 23 Positive Autoimmunity

HANS WIGZELL

List of Contributors

Numbers in parentheses indicate the pages on which the authors' contributions begin.

A. C. ALLISON (91), Division of Cell Pathology, Clinical Research Centre, Medical Research Council, Harrow, Middlesex, England

ARTHUR J. AMMANN (479), Department of Pediatric Immunology, University of California, San Francisco, California

FRITZ H. BACH (1), Immunobiology Research Center and Departments of Medical Genetics and Surgery, The University of Wisconsin, Madison, Wisconsin

J. F. BACH (207), Inserm U25, Hospital Necker, Paris, Cedex, France

M. A. BACH (207), Inserm U25, Hospital Necker, Paris, Cedex, France

L. D. BACON (63), Department of Immunology and Microbiology, Wayne State University School of Medicine, Detroit, Michigan

P. E. BIGAZZI (63), Department of Pathology, University of Connecticut School of Medicine, Farmington, Connecticut

PAUL H. BLACK (385), Department of Medicine, Massachusetts General Hospital, and Harvard Medical School, Boston, Massachusetts

F. M. BURNET (513), Department of Microbiology, University of Melbourne, Parkville, Victoria, Australia

C. CARNAUD (207), Inserm U25, Hospital Necker, Paris, Cedex, France

P. R. CARNEGIE (597), Russell Grimwade School of Biochemistry, University of Melbourne, Parkville, Victoria, Australia

IRUN R. COHEN (231), Department of Cell Biology, The Weizmann Institute of Science, Rehovot, Israel

M. DARDENNE (207), Inserm U25, Hospital Necker, Paris, Cedex, France

DEBORAH DONIACH (621), Departments of Immunology and Nuclear Medicine, The Middlesex Hospital Medical School, London, England

P. ESQUIVEL* (63), Facultad de Medicina, Departamento de Medicina Experimental, Universidad Austral de Chile, Valdivia, Chile

* Present address: Universidad Austral de Chile, Valdivia, Chile.

RICHARD K. GERSHON (171), Department of Pathology, Yale University School of Medicine, New Haven, Connecticut

DAVID GLASS (531), Department of Medicine, Robert B. Brigham Hospital, Harvard Medical School, Boston, Massachusetts

ALAN O. HAAKENSTAD (277), Division of Rheumatology, Department of Medicine, University of Washington, Seattle, Washington

MARTIN S. HIRSCH (385), Department of Medicine, Massachusetts General Hospital, and Harvard Medical School, Boston, Massachusetts

HEINZ KOHLER (267), La Rabida-University of Chicago Institute, and Departments of Pathology and Biochemistry, University of Chicago, Chicago, Illinois

Y. M. KONG (63), Department of Immunology and Microbiology, Wayne State University School of Medicine, Detroit, Michigan

JAY A. LEVY (403), Department of Medicine and Cancer Research Institute, University of California, San Francisco, California

I. R. MACKAY (597), Clinical Research Unit, The Walter and Eliza Hall Institute of Medical Research, Royal Melbourne Hospital, Victoria, Australia

MART MANNIK (277), Division of Rheumatology, Department of Medicine, University of Washington, Seattle, Washington

NICHOLAS J. MARSHALL (621), Department of Nuclear Medicine, The Middlesex Hospital Medical School, London, England

J. C. MONIER (207), Hopital Edouard Herriot, Lyon, Cedex, France

PHILIP Y. PATERSON (643), Department of Microbiology-Immunology, The Medical and Dental Schools, Northwestern University, Chicago, Illinois

MAX R. PROFFITT (385), Department of Medicine, Massachusetts General Hospital, and Harvard Medical School, Boston, Massachusetts

N. R. ROSE (63), Department of Immunology and Microbiology, Wayne State University School of Medicine, Detroit, Michigan

DONALD R. ROWLEY (267), La Rabida-University of Chicago Institute, Chicago, Illinois

PETER H. SCHUR (531), Department of Medicine, Robert B. Brigham Hospital, Harvard Medical School, Boston, Massachusetts

R. S. SUNDICK (63), Department of Immunology and Microbiology, Wayne State University School of Medicine, Detroit, Michigan

NORMAN TALAL (183), Department of Medicine, School of Medicine, University of California, San Francisco, and Clinical Immunology and Arthritis Section, Veterans Administration Hospital, San Francisco, California

NOEL L. WARNER* (33), Genetics Unit, The Walter and Eliza Hall Institute of Medical Research, Melborne, Australia

WILLIAM O. WEIGLE (141), Department of Immunopathology, Scripps Clinic and Research Foundation, La Jolla, California

HARTMUT WERKERLE (231), Max-Planck-Institut für Immunbiologie, Freiburg, Germany

* Present address: Department of Pathology, University of New Mexico School of Medicine, Albuquerque, New Mexico.

HANS WIGZELL (693), Department of Immunology, Biomedical Center, Uppsala University, Uppsala, Sweden

RALPH C. WILLIAMS, JR. (457), Department of Internal Medicine, Bernalillo County Medical Center, University of New Mexico School of Medicine, Albuquerque, New Mexico

ROLF M. ZINKERNAGEL (363), Department of Immunopathology, Scripps Clinic and Research Foundation, La Jolla, California

NATHAN J. ZVAIFLER (569), Division of Rheumatology, Department of Medicine, University of California, San Diego, La Jolla, California

Preface

The pathogenesis of autoimmunity appears to involve genetic, immunologic, and viral factors interacting through complicated mechanisms still poorly understood. Recent evidence suggests that self-recognition of histocompatibility antigens may be a normal event in immune surveillance which promotes simultaneous recognition of viral or other new cell surface antigens. The "network theory" of immune regulation through idiotype recognition represents another physiological expression of autoimmunity which may have potential for immune tolerance and immunotherapy. The rapidly expanding area of autoimmunity directed against receptors for hormones and neurotransmitters opens the possibility that many presumed nonimmunologic diseases may actually have an underlying immune basis. The relationship between autoimmunity and malignant lymphoproliferation leads into the broad area of neoplasia and the normal control of cellular growth and differentiation.

Autoimmunity, then, is an important immunobiologic clue into the physiology and regulation of the immune system. At the same time, autoimmunity is an aspect of clinical medicine that is relevant to many afflictions involving several different organ systems. The task of editing a volume on autoimmunity becomes a challenge potentially as broad as immunology and medicine.

In selecting the contributors to this book, I hoped to create a compendium of fact and opinion that might state the problems and point out future directions in a way described so beautifully by George Santayana:

> Our knowledge is a torch of smokey pine which lights the path but one step ahead across a void of mystery and dread.

If successful, each chapter in this volume may serve as a torch illuminating a small area of the problem. Hopefully, the whole will be greater than the sum of its parts and the biologic mystery of autoimmunity will be found on and between these pages.

I am deeply grateful to the busy scientists and clinicians who found time to prepare these chapters, to Maurice Landy who suggested that I undertake this responsibility, and to the staff of Academic Press whose help has been invaluable. To the reader, I apologize not for what is on these pages, but for the many areas not included.

Norman Talal, M.D.

Part I

GENETIC ASPECTS

Chapter 1

The Major Histocompatibility Complex and Its Relationship to Autoimmune Disease

FRITZ H. BACH

Great interest has centered on investigations concerned with the major histocompatibility complex (MHC) in a number of species, including man. Most attention has focused on an understanding of the histocompatibility, or transplantation, antigens associated with the MHC. In fact, it was a study of these antigens that led to the definition of the MHC. More recent work has demonstrated the importance of various MHC genes in immune responsiveness (Ir genes) and in disease susceptibility as well. The exact mechanisms by which Ir genes function are not understood; we have even less insight into the reasons for the association between certain MHC genes and diseases. The basic observations have, however, proved useful and challenging in a variety of ways.

Our understanding of the importance of cellular immune reactions and various autoimmune phenomena is still embryonal. Some of the principles derived from studies in allograft immunity may either directly or with certain modifications be applicable to the cellular immune reactions involved in autoimmune processes. In addition, increased understanding of the target antigens that are involved in allograft immunity and in immunity across species may be directly applicable to autoimmune disease.

Since a discussion of histocompatibility genetics necessitates use of certain concepts and terms of general genetics, a brief section on basic genetics is included in this chapter.

I. BASIC GENETICS

In man there are 46 chromosomes made up of 23 pairs; 22 pairs are autosomes, and one pair consists of the sex chromosomes. Both an X chromosome inherited from the mother (included in the C group of chromosomes) and a Y chromosome inherited from the father are included. In any pair of chromosomes, one member of the pair is inherited from the father and one member from the mother. Two such chromosomes are called homologous chromosomes.

Chromosomes are homologous, that is, fit into a pair, because the genetic information on one of the two concerns itself with the same phenotypic traits as the genetic information on the other chromosome of the pair. For instance, one pair of homologous chromosomes contains the genetic information (genes) that determines the hemoglobin chains. On one member of the pair, a person can inherit the gene for Hb chain B, perhaps from the father, and, on the homologous chromosome, the gene for Hb chain S from the mother. The region on the chromosome (which is very small compared to the entire length of the chromosome) associated with a given trait is called a locus or location on the chromosome. The genetic material at this locus is referred to as a gene or allele. The latter term, allele, is used to refer to the alternate forms of a gene that can exist at a single locus. Thus, in the above example, the individual has a normal Hb B allele and a mutant S allele.

While one individual can have only two alleles at a given genetic locus, more than two alleles can exist in the population. An example of this is the ABO genetic system in which one individual can have the A allele from one parent and the B allele from the other parent. Such an individual would have blood type AB. However, another individual can have the O allele on both of his homologous chromosomes and, thus, have blood type O. These are three different alleles of the ABO locus. An individual who has the same gene at a given locus on the two homologous chromosomes is said to be homozygous at that locus; if there are different alleles on the homologous chromosomes, the individual is heterozygous. Polymorphism refers to the existence in the population of more than one allele at a given locus.

Let us consider first a single genetic locus in a mating in which the father and mother are both heterozygous for different alleles. The possible offspring of such a mating are depicted in Table I. If the two alleles of the father are called a and b, and those of the mother, c and d, then the four possible offspring are as shown. If a child inherits the a allele of the father, he can inherit either the c or the d allele of the mother, giving rise to the allelic combinations ac or ad. Similarly, the alleles b and c or b and d can be inherited. The inheritance of these alleles is random; thus, the four genotypes in the children should be present in equal numbers. No matter how many alleles there are at this one locus in the population, there can be only four alleles in the two parents, and, therefore, only four genotypes are possible for the children (barring mutation). Even with an infinite number of alleles in the population, a minimum of 25% of siblings are still identical for both homologous alleles at a given locus. The probability that one parent will be homozygous, while the other parent is heterozygous for two

TABLE I

Segregation of Parental Alleles at a Simple Genetic Locus[a]

Father			Mother
ab		×	cd
ac	ad	bc	bd
		Siblings	

[a] From F. H. Bach and M. L. Bach (1972).

TABLE II
Segregation of Parental Alleles at Two Independently Segregating Loci[a]

Mother (cd;yz)	Father (ab;wx)			
	aw	ax	bw	bx
cy	ac;wy	ac;xy	bc;wy	bc;xy
cz	ac;wz	ac;xz	bc;wz	bc;xz
dy	ad;wy	ad;xy	bd;wy	bd;xy
dz	ad;wz	ad;xz	bd;wz	bd;xz

[a] From Bach and Bach (1972).

other alleles, or that the parents, while both heterozygous, will share one allele increases as the number of alleles in the population decreases. In these two last-mentioned cases, there will be only two and three possible groups of sibling genotypes, respectively. The inheritance of alleles as discussed above is referred to as segregation.

If there are two separate loci, A and B, on different chromosomes, and if the parents are heterozygous for different alleles at each locus, another genetic principle can be demonstrated. If the alleles of the father are designated as a and b at the A locus and as w and x at the B locus, then the corresponding alleles of the mother can be designated c and d and y and z. Because the segregation of alleles at one locus has already been discussed, only siblings who inherit alleles a and c at locus A are now considered. Inheritance of alleles of locus B is independent of inheritance of locus A (independent assortment). Siblings with alleles ac can inherit either alleles wy, wz, xy, or xz. The possible combinations for segregation and independent assortment of the alleles at these two loci are shown in Table II. With two independently segregating loci, a minimum of 1 in 16 sibling pairs is identical for both loci.

If two loci are close together on a chromosome, each of the two homologous chromosomal segments (carrying two alleles—one from each locus) will usually segregate as a unit. Two such loci are linked.

During meiosis, homologous chromosomes pair prior to reduction of the number of chromosomes from 46 (the diploid number) to 23 (the haploid number). During this time, recombination can occur, resulting in an exchange or crossing-over of homologous regions of the paired chromosomes. After the recombinational event, the haploid set includes a new chromosome containing a part inherited from the father and a part inherited from the mother. The frequency of recombination between two linked loci is the fraction of gametes that contain alleles for these loci that had previously been on separate homologous chromosomes, indicating that a recombinational event has taken place. This recombination frequency is proportional to the genetic distance separating the loci. Two closely linked loci are usually inherited as a unit, i.e., the two alleles linked together normally segregate to the same gamete during meiosis. Two loci relatively far apart on the chromosome may show essentially independent assortment, segregating to the same gamete only 50% of the time.

A concept to which we shall want to return is that of genetic linkage disequilibrium. This term refers to the situation found with alleles of two closely linked loci. Given enough time in evolution, genetic theory would predict that alleles of two closely linked loci will be found together on the same chromosome (called a haplotype) with a frequency not significantly different from that determined by their two individual gene frequencies. For instance, if an allele of locus A is found with a frequency of 0.1 and an allele of closely linked locus B with a frequency of 0.1, one would predict that, given equilibrium, the two alleles would be found on the same haplotype (chromosome) with a frequency not significantly different from $0.1 \times 0.1 = 0.01$. If these two genes are found together with a frequency significantly exceeding 0.01, this increased frequency is referred to as linakge disequilibrium.

In the field of immunogenetics, there is a tendency to equate an "allele" with an "antigen." However, if an allele determines a polypeptide chain, and it is the polypeptide chain itself in its tertiary configuration that is the antigen(s), then complexity arises. An antigen, i.e., the moiety recognized by an antibody-combining site, may be a relatively small site on a molecule, so that even a relatively small polypeptide chain, when folded, can have many different antigenic sites. Thus, when the protein product of the allele in question is also the antigen, several different antigens may be associated with the product of that single allele. Therefore, two distinct (but not mutually exclusive) genetic models can be applied to systems in which several antigens are associated with a genetic region which is, for the most part, inherited as a unit. The first is the possibility of closely linked loci, each coding for separate polypeptide chains. The second is the above possibility of one genetic locus that codes for a single polypeptide that phenotypically expresses several distinct antigens.

As a general rule, in immunogenetic systems, both alleles at a given histocompatibility loci are phenotypically expressed (codominant). This is in contrast to genetic systems that show dominance, and to the production of immunoglobulins, where organismal expression is codominant, but, at the single cell level, only one allele is expressed (allelic exclusion).

II. MARKERS FOR MHC GENES

The fine dissection of H-2 and HLA has, in large measure, been accomplished by the use of *in vitro* techniques for the detection of phenotypic products of MHC genes. Before discussing the structure of the H-2 and HLA complexes, a consideration of the three *in vitro* test methods that are especially important is essential. In the first, antisera that are directed specifically at cell-surface antigens are employed to "define" certain MHC antigens in any individual. These methods for the most part involve mixing the cells with antibody and complement; if cell lysis takes place, the cell is said to have the antigen specified by that antiserum.

The second method, the mixed leukocyte culture (MLC) test (see Fig. 1), can be used as an *in vitro* model of the recognition phase of the reaction leading to rejection of a transplanted tissue (Bach *et al.*, 1976). Lymphocytes carry on their surfaces the antigens coded for by genes of the MHC. Lymphocytes can, thus, be used in mixed culture as both the "responding" cells that recognize foreign antigens and as the "stimulating" cells that carry these foreign antigens. In MLC tests, the lymphocytes are taken from the recipient and used as responding cells. They are mixed with lymphocytes of the donor, which are the stimulating cells.

Since one usually wants to ask how the lymphocytes of the recipient will respond to antigens of the potential donor, rather than the converse, a one-way MLC is performed in which the stimulating (donor) lymphocytes are

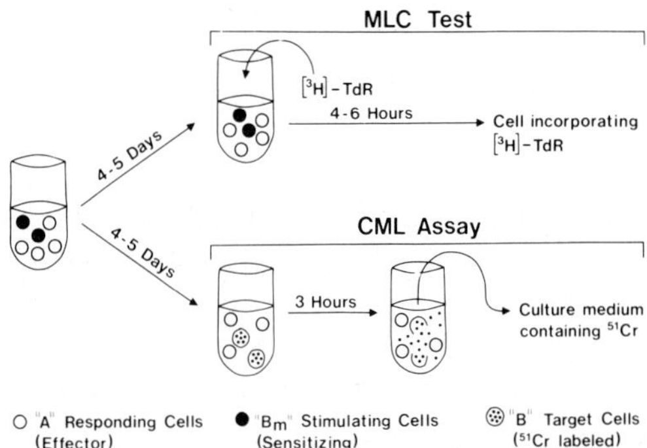

Fig. 1. Schematic representation of the MLC and CML tests. Cells differing for the major histocompatibility complex are mixed *in vitro*; for the MLC assay, proliferative activity is assayed after 4–5 days by measuring incorporation of radioactive thymidine. For the CML assay, the initial responding cells are tested for their cytotoxic capacity against radioactively labeled target cells. The amount of radioactive label released from the target cells by the effector cells is expressed as a percent CML. From Bach *et al.* (1976).

treated with mitomycin C or X-irradiation to prevent their proliferation and uptake of radioactive thymidine; this treatment still allows these cells to present their foreign antigens to the responding cells. When the stimulating cells are from an individual whose MHC is different from that of the responder, the untreated responder lymphocytes proliferate as they recognize foreign antigens on the treated stimulating cells. Response in MLC tests is measured by studying the incorporation of radioactive thymidine (^{3}H-TdR) into the proliferating cells in the MLC assay 4–6 days after the mixed culture is initiated. Representative data are given in Table III.

The third method is the cell-mediated lympholysis (CML) assay (see Fig. 1). For CML tests (Bach *et al.*, 1976), a mixed lymphocyte culture is set up, but, instead of assaying ^{3}H-TdR incorporation after several days of incubation, one assays for the production of "effector" lymphocytes—i.e., responder lymphocytes which have (during culture) acquired the ability to kill (lyse) target cells that carry the antigens of the stimulator. The responder cells are assayed for their ability to function as killer (effector) lymphocytes by testing their ability to cause release of radioactive sodium chromate (^{51}Cr) from ^{51}Cr-labeled target cells. The target cells are killed if they carry the same antigens as the original stimulating (sensitizing) cells. The amount of ^{51}Cr released into the medium is a quantitative assay for target cell lysis and is expressed as percent CML. Representative data for a CML experiment are also given in Table III.

In addition to these three *in vitro* methods, *in vivo* testing of an animal's ability to respond immunologically to well-defined antigens (Katz and Benacerraf, 1976) can be used to determine the genotype of the MHC-linked immune response or Ir loci. Animals can be classified as high or low responders on the basis of this procedure.

III. MHC LOCI

MHC loci and their products can be conveniently divided, on the basis of the above test procedures, into four groups. The first group, the SD (S determinant or serologically defined) antigens, are present on virtually all tissues of the body. Second, the Ia (immune response associated) antigens are also recognized serologically like the SD antigens but are present on only a limited number of tissues, including lymphocytes, macrophages, epidermal cells, and sperm. Third, the LD (L determinant or lymphocyte defined) antigens are recognized by responding lymphocytes in the mixed leukocyte culture test. Fourth, are the Ir (immune response) genes that control the ability of an animal to respond immunologically to a test antigen.

The designations SD, Ia, and LD are simply terms used to distinguish

TABLE III

Sample MLC[a]

Mixed culture	MLC assay: ^{3}H-TdR incorporated (cpm)
AA_m	383 ± 41
AB_m	371 ± 53
AC_m	34,844 ± 1,212
AD_m	82,569 ± 3,996

Sample CML results

Sensitizing MLC	CML target cell (%) A	CML target cell (%) D
AD_m	3.1 ± 2.4	78.5 ± 4.9
AA_m	2.0 ± 1.3	−1.3 ± 0.4

[a] Results are representative data from MLC and CML tests. The capital letters refer to individuals in a family; A and B are HLA-identical siblings and C and D are siblings that differ from A by one and two haplotypes, respectively. Subscript m refers to mitomycin C treatment of the stimulating cells for the MLC. Since A and B are HLA-identical, there is no stimulation in MLC (i.e., there is no excess thymidine incorporated after stimulation of A cells with those of B, as compared with the control culture AA_m). Individual C differs from A by one HLA chromosome; D differs from A by both HLA chromosomes. The counts per minute incorporated in the MLC assay reflect this quantitative difference in the two sibling pairs.

In CML tests, target cells are labeled with ^{51}Cr and tested as described in the text. Two control measurements are done. First, labeled target cells are incubated alone to assay how many counts per minute of ^{51}Cr are released spontaneously; second, labeled target cells are freeze-thawed several times to assay the maximum release possible. The percent CML is calculated as per the formula:

$$\frac{\text{Experimental release} - \text{spontaneous release}}{\text{Maximum release} - \text{spontaneous release}} \times 100$$

The experimental release refers to the counts per minute of ^{51}Cr released when the sensitized cells from the mixed leukocyte culture are mixed with the target cells. Standard deviations are given.

between MHC determinants that may have different biologic roles. Since the terminology for these antigenic systems and the loci coding for them are not the same in different species, the terms SD, Ia, and LD simplify discussion and comparison of what are presumably homologous systems in these species. In addition, within a species, the several genetically separable loci coding for antigens that all apparently subserve a single function can be conveniently referred to with a single term. The application of these terms should in no way imply a total restriction of function, e.g., that a function associated with LD cannot be associated with SD at all.

Schematic representations of the MHC's in mouse and man are given in Fig. 2. The H-2 complex in mouse is divided into five regions, K, I, S, G, and D, on the basis of marker loci for each region. The K and D regions have as their marker loci H-2K and H-2D, whose alleles control the H-2 SD antigens. The I region can be subdivided on the basis of different Ia determinants associated with each of three subregions: I-A, I-B, and I-C (Shreffler and David, 1975). Included in the I-A subregion are loci determining certain Ia antigens, immune response (Ir) genes, and the strongest H-2 LD locus (Lindahl and Bach, 1976). To date, these genes determining

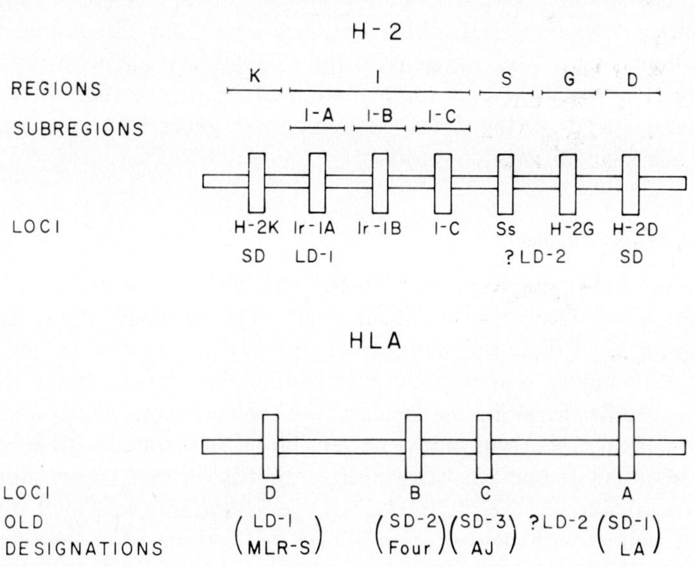

Fig. 2. Diagrammatic representation of the major histocompatibility complex in mouse and man. In mouse, the complex is divided into five regions with the I region subdivided into three subregions. Marker loci for each of the subregions are shown. The strongest LD locus is in the I-A subregion; a weaker LD locus may be present between Ss and H-2D. The H-2D and H-2K loci are the SD loci. A weak LD locus may be present between HLA-A and HLA-C in humans. From Bach *et al.* (1976).

Ia antigens, LD antigens, and those controlling immune response have not been genetically separated.

The marker locus for the S region is the Ss locus which codes for a serum protein that has been identified as the fourth component of the complement system (Klein, 1975). The marker locus for the G region is the H-2G locus; alleles of this locus code for cell-surface antigens found on red blood cells. The Ss and H-2G loci will not be further discussed.

The MHC in man is also well defined. The four loci of HLA that I shall discuss are called HLA-A, HLA-B, HLA-C, and HLA-D. In addition, there are many other loci that have now been found in the same linkage group. The genetics of the MHC in man has been recently reviewed (Bach and van Rood, 1976).

The phenotypic products of the MHC can be grouped into the four categories just listed. Whereas the SD and LD antigens are almost certainly homologous in these species [with extensive amino acid sequence homology existing for the SD antigens (Silver and Hood, 1976)], there is some question regarding the homology of the Ia antigens. The Ia antigens were first described in mouse. Although an apparently similar set of antigens has been described in rhesus monkey and man, the suggested homology is based largely on a similar tissue distribution and the linkage of genes coding for these antigens to the MHC. For the purposes of this discussion, I shall assume homology of the antigens in the two species, but with the appropriate reservations. There is some preliminary evidence that there are Ir genes associated with the MHC in man; these genes have not been well defined and have not been mapped.

A. The SD Antigens

The two SD loci in mouse, H-2K and H-2D, are separated by a recombinational frequency of about 0.005. The serology of the antigens coded by genes of these loci has been extensively investigated (Klein, 1975). The loci are highly polymorphic even within the inbred strains that are available. Studies in wild mice indicate that the number of alleles associated with each of these loci will indeed be very large. Associated with each allele of one SD locus is one "private" antigen that is, in most cases, unique to that allele, as well as several "public" antigens that are associated with that allele, as well as with several other alleles (both of the same and the other SD locus). The biochemical relationship of the private and public antigens is not well understood. A recent review of the genetic control of these antigens based on preliminary amino acid sequences that have been obtained in both mouse and man discusses this problem in some detail (Silver and Hood, 1976).

In man, there are three SD loci, HLA-A, -B, and -C. The A and B loci are separated by about 0.008 recombinational units (Kissmeyer-Nielsen, 1975). These loci are also highly polymorphic. Extensive studies have been done, not only on the serology of the HLA-A, -B, and -C loci, but also on the distribution of these antigens in different populations (Dausset and Colombani, 1973). Two SD loci have also been defined in both the rhesus monkey (Balner *et al.*, 1977) and the dog (van den Tweel *et al.*, 1974).

B. The LD Antigens

LD antigens are defined as those that lead to a proliferative response in the MLC test. There appear to be several loci in the H-2 complex that code for "LD-like" antigens (Dorf *et al.*, 1975b; Lindahl and Bach, 1976; Widmer *et al.*, 1973). The strongest of these is in the I-A subregion; however, there are also LD-like loci to the right of the I-A subregion. One of these has been placed between Ss and H-2D. Mice differing for only the K or the D region stimulate in MLC. Whether the stimulatory molecule in these cases is identical with the SD antigen or whether there are LD-like loci in the K and D region is not clearly established. We have recently discussed this topic in great detail (Bach *et al.*, 1976). Most important, however, is the finding that the strongest of the LD loci is genetically separable from the two SD loci.

A similar situation exists in man (Bach and van Rood, 1976) in that the genetic differences that led to MLC activation are determined by the HLA-D locus, which is approximately 1 recombinational unit distant from HLA-B. In studies of human families in which a recombinational event has taken place between HLA-B and HLA-D in one of the parents, MLC test results indicate that differences for the three SD loci lead to either no MLC activation or very weak MLC activation (see Fig. 3). As in the mouse, it is not clear in those cases whether the weak MLC activation is due to the SD antigens themselves or to a weak LD locus between HLA-A and HLA-C. An LD locus has been defined in both the rhesus monkey (Balner *et al.*, 1977) and the dog. (van den Tweel *et al.*, 1974).

C. Ia Antigens

The Ia antigens were first described in the mouse (Shreffler and David, 1975) and can be used to divide the I region into the three subregions, I-A, I-B, and I-C. These antigens are defined serologically but differ from the SD antigens in their tissue distribution and apparently in their function. The question of whether the "Ia-like" antigens recognized in the rhesus monkey

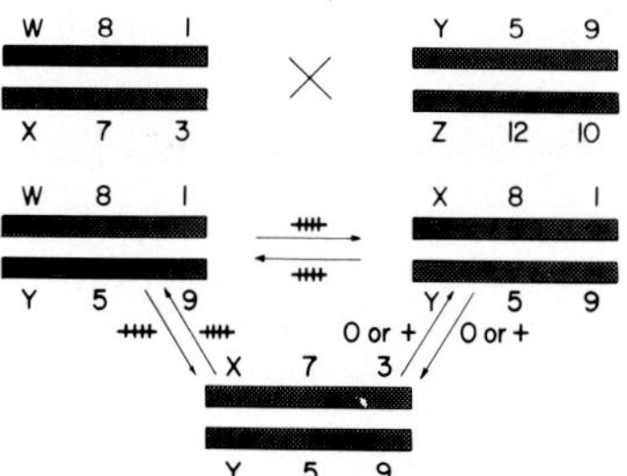

Fig. 3. Presumed major histocompatibility complex (MHC) chromosomes in a human family. The numbers refer to the HLA SD antigens of the A and B loci; the letters to presumed alleles of the D locus. The one parent carries a 1, 8 W and a 3, 7 X haplotype; the other parent a 9, 5 Y and 10, 12 Z haplotype. Two siblings who inherit the same HLA SD loci alleles, and, thus, the same HLA SD antigens, can differ for the D locus if a recombinational event in one of the parents occurs. In this particular case, a recombinational event in the first parent resulted in a 1, 8, X haplotype. These two siblings, thus, stimulate in MLC. The + signs refer to MLC stimulation in a quantitative sense.

(Balner *et al.*, 1977) and in man (Bach and van Rood, 1976) are homologous to the mouse Ia antigens has been discussed above.

D. Ir Genes

There are genes that control various parameters of the immune response that are linked to the MHC and others that are in different linkage groups. I shall discuss only the Ir genes of the MHC. This topic has been extensively studied (Katz and Benacerraf, 1976) and will not, in this article, get the emphasis it deserves in terms of its overall interest.

T lymphocytes include "helper" T cells and "killer" cells, usually referred to as cytotoxic T lymphocytes (CTLs) (Bach *et al.*, 1976). The helper T cells apparently function to facilitate antibody production by the B lymphocytes (T–B cell collaboration), as well as to optimize the development of effective cytotoxic T killer cells (T–T cell collaboration). T helper cells may function by secreting soluble molecules that help the cytotoxic T killer cell and the B lymphocyte to perform their effector functions. MHC Ir genes appear to control the ability of both T lymphocytes and B lymphocytes to perform their various functions, i.e., to respond immunologically (Katz and Benacerraf, 1976; Munro and Taussig, 1975). Most exciting is the series of recent findings concerning T–B collaboration that suggests the existence of two very closely linked MHC Ir genes that together control the ability of an animal to respond immunologically (Munro and Taussig, 1975).

IV. GENETIC CONTROL OF CML

Despite the findings that the MHC LD antigens are primarily responsible for activating the proliferative response in MLC, and that the killer lymphocytes active in CML are generated in a mixed culture, the prime target antigens recognized by the killer lymphocytes are not LD. Instead, the specific lytic effects are directed at either the MHC SD antigens themselves or at the products of genes very closely linked to those determining the SD antigens (Bach *et al.*, 1976). I shall, for simplicity, refer to the CML target as the SD antigens. This preeminent role of SD antigens in functioning as target antigens is true, not only in studies using different individuals of the same species (allogeneic combinations), but even when the mixed culture contains cells of individuals from two different species (xenogeneic combinations) (Lindahl and Bach, 1975).

These findings are most elegantly demonstrated in "three-cell" experiments (Bach *et al.*, 1976; Schendel and Bach, 1974) in which responding cells of one individual are simultaneously stimulated in mixed culture by mitomycin C-treated cells of two other individuals, one differing from the responding cells by LD and the second differing by SD antigens (see Table IV). The results demonstrate the epistatic interaction between the responses to the LD antigens and to the SD antigens in terms of leading to killer cell activity. Table IV summarizes results of studies in humans, using families containing members in whom recombinational events have occurred between HLA-B and HLA-D. Stimulation of the responding cells with lymphocytes from a family member with an MHC disparity at only the HLA-D locus results in marked MLC proliferation, but no killing against

TABLE IV

A "Three-Cell" Experiment for Generation of CML[a]

Sensitizing MLC	HLA difference between responding and stimulating cell	^{3}H-TdR incorporated	CML target cell (%)		
			A	B	C
AB_m	HLA-D	++++	–	–	–
AC_m	HLA-A, -B, and -C	– –	–	–	–
AB_mC_m	HLA-A, -B, -C, and -D	++++	–	–	++++

[a] Typical results of CML studies in a family in which a recombinational event has taken place. Siblings A and B are identical for the HLA-A, -B, and -C loci but differ for HLA-D. Siblings A and C differ for the three SD loci, HLA-A, -B, and -C but are identical for HLA-D. In the "three-cell" experiment, A is simultaneously stimulated with the cells of sibling B and the cells of sibling C. See text for discussion.

either the HLA-D antigens or against target cells carrying foreign HLA-A, -B, and -C antigens. Stimulation of the same responding cells with lymphocytes from a family member differing for the SD antigens of HLA-A, -B, and -C, but identical for the HLA-D locus, results in either no proliferative response or a very weak one. No cytotoxicity is generated against any target cell. Simultaneous stimulation of the same responding cells with both LD and SD differences (the three-cell experiment) results, not only in an MLC proliferative response, but also in the generation of strong killer cell activity which is directed specifically at target cells carrying the foreign SD antigen.

These results clearly demonstrate the different functions served by the LD and the SD antigens in stimulating the proliferative and cytotoxic responses, respectively. In addition, they demonstrate the phenomenon of LD–SD collaboration in which the presence of an LD difference in the stimulating mixture markedly enhances the development of cytotoxicity against the SD target even though neither the LD stimulus nor the SD stimulus by themselves generate cytotoxic cells against that target. This phenomenon is explained at the cellular level by the finding that two separate, functionally distinct subpopulations of T lymphocytes (the helper T cells and the killer T cells) respond to the LD and SD antigens, respectively. The T lymphocytes that respond to the LD antigens do not become killer cells but, rather, are the proliferating T helper cells. These helper cells somehow facilitate the response of the second subpopulation of T lymphocytes, the cytotoxic T lymphocytes or killer lymphocytes, against the SD antigens (Bach *et al.*, 1976). Although the findings in mouse are generally similar to those just depicted in man, there are certain interesting differences (Bach *et al.*, 1976).

V. TECHNIQUES FOR DETECTION OF MHC LD ANTIGENS

Whereas the definition of the MHC SD and Ia antigens has been relatively easy by the application of classical serologic techniques, the definition of the LD antigens as recognized in MLC has been much more difficult. In an MLC test, as illustrated in Table III, it is possible to determine if two individuals are identical for the LD antigens of the MHC or to what degree they differ by measuring the amount of thymidine incorporated by the cell mixture. However, MLC tests do not allow the identification of the LD antigens carried by any one individual. Toward this end, two approaches for defining LD antigens have recently evolved.

A. Homozygous Typing Cells

This approach entails the identification of individuals who are homozygous for at least the HLA-D locus (Bach and van Rood, 1976; Bradley *et al.*, 1972). Their cells [to be called homozygous typing cells (HTCs)] can then be used as stimulating cells in MLC to identify other cells that are either homozygous or heterozygous for the same HLA-D allele; such cells would not respond in MLC, since they would not see anything foreign on the HTC. One potential source of HTCs would be cells that are phenotypically homozygous for the HLA-B loci, since such cells may also be homozygous for the strong HLA-D alleles as a result of linkage disequilibrium. Alternatively, homozygous typing cells can be obtained from appropriate offspring of first cousin marriages. For what are probably technical reasons, one cannot necessarily equate the identical response of cells of two individuals to "typing cells" with MLC identity of those two individuals. The regular MLC test serves here as a "cross-matching" procedure to establish the degree of their similarity. Results of testing with HTCs are given in Table V.

Homozygous typing cells were used as part of the 1975 Histocompatibility Workshop (Kissmeyer-Nielsen, 1975). The results obtained showed that six different LD clusters [the determinant(s) associated with a single haplotype] (HLA-DW-1 through HLA-DW-6) could be identified by homozygous typing cells with at least two different typing cells identifying each LD cluster. These six clusters are listed in Table VI, together with the gene frequencies for the clusters. Two other potential clusters (LD 107 and LD 108) were less clearly identifiable.

The conclusion that a responding cell carries a given LD cluster is based on the relatively low or zero response of that cell to the appropriate homozygous typing cell (see Table V). In any given LD cluster, some typing cells give near identical results, while others show only a pattern of partial identity. A single HLA-D haplotype may code for more than one LD determinant and an HLA-D cluster defined by a homozygous typing cell may, thus, include several LD determinants.

B. Primed LD Typing (PLT)

An even more recent approach to identifying the LD antigens is the primed LD typing (PLT) test described in our laboratory. This test is based on the finding in mouse (Häyry *et al.*, 1973) that lymphocytes stimulated in an MLC and left for 10 days (beyond their peak proliferative activity) will give a very rapid and strong (secondary-type) proliferative response if restimulated with the cells of the original stimulating cell donor. We

(Sheehy *et al.*, 1975b) have used this technique to study the genetic control of antigens responsible for restimulation (see Table VII). The findings indicate that it is the HLA-D antigens that are primarily responsible for restimulation and that the SD antigens appear to be neither essential for, nor capable of, causing a secondary-type proliferative response. The secondary response can be assayed with radioactive thymidine within 24 hours and at an even earlier time with radioactive uridine (Sheehy *et al.*, 1975a).

TABLE V

Primary MLC with Homozygous Cells[a,b]

Responding cells	Stimulating cells: HB (DW-2/DW-2)	Stimulating cells: RR (DW-2/DW-2)
NK (DW-2 neg.)	42,030	21,057
BB (DW-2 neg.)	79,713	41,223
BKJ (DW-2 hetero.)	11,185	6,202
MT (DW-2 hetero.)	4,863	3,251
RR (DW-2 homo.)	1,073	364
HB (DW-2 homo.)	667	447

PLT-homozygous typing cell correlation

Restimulating cells	Responding PLT: $A(RR)_m$
A (DW-2 neg.)	588
BB (DW-2 neg.)	3,097
BKJ (DW-2 hetero.)	13,059
MT (DW-2 hetero.)	12,997
RR (DW-2 homo.)	20,778
KJ (DW-2 homo.)	21,110

[a] In the top part of Table V, responding cells are tested for their response to two homozygous typing cells defining the DW-2 cluster. The first two cells are DW-2 negative; the others are DW-2 heterozygous and DW-2 homozygous, respectively. In the second half of the table, a PLT cell was prepared in which the cells of an individual A_1 negative for DW-2 were used as the responding cells, and the homozygous typing cell (RR) was used as a sensitizing cell. The restimulating cells are as indicated in the table. In addition to differentiating between individuals who carry the DW-2 cluster and those who do not, a gene dosage effect appears to be detected in the PLT test, in that DW-2 heterozygous cells stimulate less than DW-2 homozygous cells.

[b] Reprinted by permission from F. H. Bach and J. J. van Rood (1976).

TABLE VI

Frequency of HLA-D Specificities[a]

HLA-D specificity group	Antigen frequency (%)	Gene frequency $(p)^b$	Most significant HLA-B association	Δ value
DW-1	19.3	0.102	BW-35 (W-5)	0.021
DW-2	15.2	0.078	B-7	0.031
DW-3	16.4	0.085	B-8	0.044
DW-4	15.6	0.082	BW-15	0.017
DW-5	14.6	0.075	BW-16	0.013
DW-6	10.5	0.054	—	—
"Blank"	—	0.524	—	—

[a] Frequencies for the six provisional HLA-D "clusters" calculated from the pooled data of the Sixth International Histocompatibility Workshop. The responses of 171 random white donors were available for analysis. A specificity was assigned to a responder if at least 50% of the typing cells belonging to a specific DW group elicited typing responses from the responder. DW-1–DW-6: provisional HLA-D specificities (clusters); blank: haplotypes that were not assigned a DW number. (Used with kind permission of authors and publisher from Throsby and Piazza, 1975. Munksgaard, Copenhagen).

[b] Gene frequency (p) calculated using the method of maximum likelihood.

The PLT test appears to measure the same factors that are measured by the homozygous typing cells in that PLT cells sensitized to a given LD cluster in a primary MLC are restimulated strongly by cells that carry that cluster (see Table V). A panel of different PLT cells can be used to type the lymphocytes of an individual for HLA-D. The PLT test may have certain practical advantages in that PLT cells can be generated against any LD haplotype, whereas homozygous typing cells may be difficult to find, especially for rare LD clusters.

VI. MODIFICATION OF THE SD ANTIGENS

Cytotoxic killer T lymphocytes can also be generated against antigens present on cells that have been infected with virus (see Chapter 12). Such killer lymphocytes apparently respond to the infected cell through recognition of a molecular "complex" between the new virally induced cell-surface antigen and the SD antigen of that cell. It is not clear whether such cells also present an LD-like stimulus. These findings, initially described by Zin-

TABLE VII

24-Hour PLT[a]

	c	d
F = ab	239	0(R)
M = cd	1863	361
C_1 = ac	1963	33
C_2 = bc	1807(S)[b]	−64
C_3 = ad	281	550
C_4 = bd	−8	455
C_5 = bd	0(R)[b]	437
C_6 = bd	39	565(S)
Bkgd.	364	638

[a] Two PLT cells were prepared within a family. The father was arbitrarily assigned haplotypes A and B and the mother haplotypes C and D. The segregation of the parental haplotypes to the children was determined by doing HLA SD typing. One PLT cell was prepared by stimulating the cells of child 5 with the cells of child 2. Since these two children shared the B haplotype inherited from the father, the cells of child 5 can recognize only the C haplotype on the cells of child 2. This PLT cell responds maximally only when restimulated with cells carrying the C haplotype. The other PLT cell defines the D haplotype in that father cells were sensitized to the cells of child 6. [Used with kind permission of authors and publishers from Sheehy *et al.* (1975), Munksgaard, Copenhagen.]

[b] Responder and stimulator for primary culture used to prepare PLT cell.

kernagel and Doherty (1977), are based on experiments such as that depicted in Table VIII. Cells of one mouse strain, A, can be sensitized to virally infected cells from the same strain (syngeneic cells) so that excellent killer activity will develop against virally infected target cells from strain A. If the target antigen were simply the virally induced antigen, then one might expect that lymphocytes of strain A would also kill target cells of other strains of mice (allogeneic cells) that have been infected with the same virus. This is true, however, only when these other mouse strains carry the same SD antigen(s) as the initial sensitizing cell.

The simplest explanation of these findings is that the virally induced antigen in some way complexes molecularly with the SD antigen and "modifies" it so that the killer lymphocytes recognize this complex of the "viral antigen–SD antigen." It must be noted that, in some cases, only the antigen of one SD locus can be successfully modified. For example, killing of allogeneic infected target cells may only take place if the allogeneic strain shares the H-2K antigen with the original sensitizing cell; sharing of the H-2D antigen is not sufficient. A similar H-2 SD region restriction on which allogeneic target cells will be killed has been noted in other experimental systems in which responding lymphocytes of one strain have been sensitized either to cells of the same strain whose surface has been chemically modified (Schmitt-Verhulst and Shearer, 1975) or to tumor cells from the same strain (Dorf *et al.*, 1976). The system has even been extended to the case where cells are "sensitized" in mixed culture against differences associated with genes segregating independently of the MHC; even here the killing will only take place if the target cell carries the same non-MHC differences plus the same H-2D region initially present on the stimulating (sensitizing) cell (Gordon *et al.*, 1975). It is not known in any of these experimental systems whether the SD antigens themselves or molecules coded by genes very closely linked to those determining the SD antigens function as targets for the killer T cells. However, the findings described above on the development of killer T cells against targets on cells of other individuals of the same species, against targets on cells of individuals of the same species, against targets on cells of individuals from other species, and against targets on virus-modified cells of the same strain all point very strongly to a unique role for the SD antigen as target molecules.

TABLE VIII

Modification of MHC SD Antigens[a]

Sensitizing MLC		Target cells infected with virus			
Responding cell	Sensitizing (stimulating) cells	Strain	H-2K antigens	H-2D antigens	CML
Strain A normal	Strain A virus infected	A	K^a	D^a	+++
		B	K^a	D^x	++
		C	K^b	D^b	–

[a] Lymphocytes of strain A sensitized to autologous cells infected with virus will kill target cells that (1) are infected with the same virus and (2) have either or both of the same SD antigens as strain A. See text for details. Target cells infected with the virus, but having different H-2 SD antigens, do not serve as good targets.

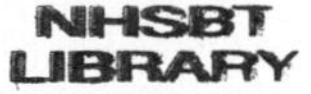

VII. *IN VIVO* ROLE OF MHC ANTIGENS

In the mouse, there are at least three different loci that lead to the rejection of skin and organ grafts (Klein *et al.*, 1974). These three loci are in the K, I, and D regions. The relevance of the *in vitro* phenomena discussed above (especially the LD–SD collaboration leading to the generation of more effective killing in CML) to the *in vivo* situation has been only recently addressed. At least in some *in vivo* transplantation models in mouse, stimulation of the recipient's immune system with an LD stimulus does potentiate the rate of rejection of an SD-different graft (Sollinger and Bach, 1976).

For kidney transplantation in man, matching donors and recipients for the LD and the SD antigens has been successful when the donors are identical to the recipients for the entire MHC. The prognosis of sibling kidney transplant grafts is greatly improved when the donor and recipient are matched for both SD and LD determinants. There is approximately 95% long-term survival of grafts in such situations. Success of bone marrow grafting is also, to a large extent, dependent on careful matching between siblings (Bach and van Rood, 1976).

The relative importance of the LD and SD antigens (which are the only antigens for which clinical testing is currently done) in predicting graft survival is somewhat controversial. It would appear that matching for the SD antigens (minimizing the number of SD antigens that the donor carries which are foreign to the recipient) is of relatively little, if any, value. Preliminary data suggest that matching for the LD antigens (requiring a reduced amount of stimulation in MLC between donor and recipient) improves graft survival. For bone marrow transplantation, it may be that the LD antigens are most important. These data must, however, be regarded as preliminary, and further studies are clearly needed. This area has been recently reviewed (Bach and van Rood, 1976).

VIII. DISEASE SUSCEPTIBILITY GENES

The demonstration by Lilly *et al.* (1964) that genes of the H-2 complex play a role in susceptibility to viral leukemogenesis broadened significantly the possible biologic importance of the MHC. Lilly (1973) found that certain loci of the H-2 complex affect the progression of both Gross and Friend virus associated diseases.

In these situations, there are several different genes (some segregating independently of H-2, while others are linked to H-2) which are important in the pathogenesis of the disease. In some cases, the factors segregating independently of H-2 behave as dominant genes in determining susceptibility; it has been suggested that these genes may function in controlling the ability of the virus to penetrate. The genes included within the H-2 complex determine resistance as dominant factors, and, therefore, in some cases influence the course of the disease. Resistance is manifested by a later age of onset in those animals that do contract the infection and a lower percentage of animals which succumb to the disease.

The H-2 complex genes that influence the progress of a virally induced leukemogeneic process have been mapped at the K end of H-2 and could be the same as the immune response genes. Based on the mouse model, one could assume that disease susceptibility in humans is under polygenic control, with the several genes involved possibly functioning at different levels in the pathogenesis of the disease.

The first demonstration that genes of the major histocompatibility complex may be associated with certain diseases in man was provided by Amiel in 1967 who found an increased frequency of HLA-4c in patients with Hodgkin's disease. This was confirmed by the extensive study of Forbes and Morris (1970) who suggested that the increased frequency of 4c was due almost entirely to an increased frequency of W-5, an antigen included within 4c. The "antigen" 4c in fact includes three cross-reacting antigens: HLA-5, W-5, and W-18.

Van der Does *et al.* confirmed some of a series of subsequent studies looking for associations between various HLA antigens and Hodgkin's disease (van der Does *et al.*, 1973). As a part of the Fifth International Histocompatibility Workshop (Dausset and Colombani, 1973), 11 different laboratories studied a total of 477 patients. These studies showed an increased frequency of HLA-1, HLA-8, and W-18, with only the last antigen known to belong to the 4c cross-reacting group (P. J. Morris *et al.*, 1973). In studying different populations, the general observation of an association between HLA and a given disease may be confirmed, but the association in different populations can be with different HLA SD antigens.

Since the initial study on Hodgkin's disease, a large number of diseases have been investigated for increased or decreased frequencies on various HLA SD antigens (McDevitt and Bodmer, 1974) These diseases have conveniently been classified by Morris (1974) into the lymphomas and leukemias (as typified by Hodgkin's disease), immunopathic diseases in which an autoimmune process may be involved in the pathogenesis, cancer other than lymphomas, and infectious diseases.

Some of the most reproducible associations have been found in the immunopathic diseases (Table IX) (McDevitt and Bodmer, 1974). Most frequently this has been with the HLA SD antigens 1 and 8 which are found in high linkage disequilibrium. In those cases where this was examined, the

TABLE IX

HLA and Disease Associations[a,b]

Disease	No. of Studies	HLA SD Antigen	Frequency in patients (%)	Frequency in controls (%)	Average relative risk	95% limits	Hetero-geneous	χ^2
Ankylosing spondylitis	5	B-27	90	7	141.0	80–249	No	290
Reiter's disease	3	B-27	76	6	46.6	23–94	No	116
Acute anterior uveitis	2	B-27	55	8	16.7	8–34	No	62
	6	B-13	18	4	5.0	4–7	Yes	120
Psoriasis	6	BW-17	29	8	5.0	4–6	No	143
	4	BW-16	15	5	2.9	2–5	No	19
Graves' disease	1	B-8	47	21	3.3	2–6	—	12
Coeliac disease	6	B-8	78	24	10.4	8–14	No	224
Dermatitis herpetiformis	3	B-8	62	27	4.5	3–8	No	35
Myasthenia gravis	5	B-8	52	24	4.6	3–6	No	103
Systemic lupus erythematosus	2	BW-15	33	8	5.1	2–11	No	17
Multiple sclerosis	4	A-3	36	25	1.7	1–2	No	23
		B-7	36	25	1.5	1–2	No	15
Acute lymphatic leukemia	7	A-2	63	37	1.7	1–2	Yes	15
	8	BW-35	25	16	1.6	1–2	Yes	14
Hodgkin's disease	7	A-1	39	32	1.3	1–2	No	7
	7	B-8	26	22	1.3	1–2	No	4
Chronic hepatitis	1	B-8	68	18	9.5	5–20	—	35
Ragweed hayfever, Ra5 sensitivity[c]	1	B-7	50	19	4.0	1–12	—	7
Ragweed fever, allergen E[d]	1	Multiple	—	—	—	—	—	—

[a] From McDevitt and Bodmer (1974).

[b] The relative risk is $pd(1\text{-}pc)/pc(1\text{-}pd)$ where pd = frequency in diseased and pc = frequency in controls. The averages, 95% limits, heterogeneity, and χ^2 are calculated using standard weighting procedures. The associations between the occurrence of a disease and the presence of a disease can be classified into three categories. In the first, the average relative risk is 4 or greater, the studies are, with rare exceptions, homogeneous and the χ^2 values overwhelming. In the second, the association is weak, the average risk is 2 or lower, and often the findings of different authors contradict each other. And in the last group (ragweed hayfever), there is no association with an HLA haplotype. (Reproduced with kind permission of authors and publisher from McDevitt and Bodmer, 1974.)

[c] Patients, Ra5 sensitive; controls, Ra5 insensitive.

[d] Family study.

excess of HLA-1 could be attributed to the linkage disequilibrium between 1 and 8. The diseases included in this category are active chronic hepatitis (Mackey and Morris, 1972), myasthenia gravis (Säfwenberg *et al.*, 1973, Fritze *et al.*, 1974; Feltkamp *et al.*, 1974), adult coeliac disease (Stokes *et al.*, 1972; Falchuk *et al.*, 1972; Albert *et al.*, 1972; van Hooff *et al.*, 1974) (which represents a hypersensitivity to gluten), childhood asthma (Thorsby *et al.*, 1971), and dermatitis herpetiformis (Katz *et al.*, 1972; White *et al.*, 1973; Gebhard *et al.*, 1973). In multiple sclerosis, to be discussed below with respect to the HLA LD specificities, an association has been reported with HLA-3 and HLA-7 (Jersild *et al.*, 1972, 1973b; Naito *et al.*, 1972; Bertams *et al.*, 1972).

It is with the infectious diseases, especially those which have occurred as major epidemics in history, where we might expect a strong association with the HLA SD antigens, if they play a role in disease susceptibility. The only suggestion for an association between HLA and the capacity to form antibodies against measles in healthy individuals is in a well controlled study of mono- and dizogotic twins performed by Haverkorn *et al.* (1975). Jersild *et al.* (1973a) have also observed such an association in patients with multiple sclerosis. In the case of an epidemic, if individuals with given HLA SD antigens are more susceptible to the disease, one would expect a decreased frequency of those antigens following the devastating results of the epidemic. One of the most interesting studies in this regard was done by Piazza *et al.* (1973) examining the HLA SD antigens in the highlands and lowlands of Sardinia. In the former area, malaria has essentially been nonexistent; in the latter area, malaria was, until recently, endemic. Two polymorphic traits, thalassemia and glucose-6-phosophate dehydrogenase deficiency, which are balanced polymorphisms maintained through the selective advantage of the heterozygote over the homozygote in resistance to plasmodial infection, have a much different frequency in the two areas. These authors found a highly significant difference in frequencies of HLA SD antigens of the HLA-B locus between inhabitants of the highlands and those of the lowlands, a difference which was not present for any other genetic markers examined including the HLA-A locus. This suggested that differential selection was responsible for these differences in HLA SD antigenic frequencies which could be directly associated with malaria. Morris and his collaborators (P. Morris *et al.*, 1973) have found a similar difference in the HLA antigens between the populations of New Guinea highlands and coastal areas, although, in that particular study, the findings were not as clear cut in the two populations.

Levine *et al.* (1972) have studied the association of ragweed hayfever and anti-ragweed reaginic (IgE) antibodies with HLA. In each of seven families, ragweed hypersensitivity and anti-ragweed reaginic antibodies were associated with a given HLA haplotype in first-degree relatives of the affected individual. Despite this association with HLA, the HLA SD antigens involved in the seven different families included in the study were not the same. This would suggest that a gene of the HLA chromosome, i.e., closely linked to the genes determining the HLA SD antigens, was associated with the hypersensitivity and controlled the immune response for that particular antigen, but that the gene was not identical with nor showed a very high linkage disequilibrium with the genes determining the HLA SD antigens. This study gave evidence for the existence of MHC-linked immune response genes in man (in analogy with mouse, monkey, and other species), and is consistent with the concept that the genes important in disease susceptibility are not necessarily the same as those determining the HLA SD antigens. Similar observations were made in a population study by Marsh *et al.* (1973).

A. Problems with Definition of Disease Susceptibility Genes

Despite the striking association between certain diseases listed in Table VIII and the frequency of given HLA SD antigens, association is usually not absolute. Obviously, there are a large number of reasons why this may be so. It is important for us to understand these reasons both to help evaluate the meaning of these associations and to allow us to improve our ability to find more significant associations if they do exist.

First, it should be realized that if the genes of the MHC which are associated in increased frequency with a given disease are not the HLA SD antigens themselves but, rather, genes linked to those determining the SD antigens, then the association depends on the linkage disequilibrium or interactions between the disease susceptibility genes and HLA SD genes. To the extent that linkage disequilibrium is not absolute, any association will be less than complete. In different populations, it is conceivable that the same gene is in disequilibrium with different HLA SD alleles, explaining the lack of association in the worldwide study of Hodgkin's disease mentioned above (van Rood, 1975).

Second, there is the problem of disease heterogeneity. To the extent that the diseases which we classify under one name are actually a collection of somewhat different entities, any strong association between a disease susceptibility gene of the MHC and one of these disease entities will be obscured by the fact that a second entity included within this same general category of disease may not be associated with the same disease susceptibility gene. We have already learned, in the studies looking for associations between the HLA SD antigens and disease, that in some cases diseases can be subdivided for instance on the basis of age (Fritze *et al.,* 1974) and the association between a given HLA SD antigen and the disease in one age group will be much stronger than the association between that antigen and individuals having that "same disease" in the second age group.

Third, the HLA SD antigens are, as has been discussed previously, still being subdivided and redefined as new sera become available. This serologic heterogeneity will lead to the same difficulties of finding significant associations as will disease heterogeneity.

Fourth, to the extent that genes segregating independently of HLA are important in the pathogenesis of a given disease process (as is true in mouse; see above), the genetic complexity of different individuals will influence our ability to find significant associations between one of the genes (that linked to HLA) and the disease itself.

Given these various considerations, it is remarkable, in a sense, that the significant associations discussed above have been found.

B. Disease Susceptibility Genes and Immune Response

One of the favored hypotheses to explain the association between given HLA haplotypes and diseases is to link the immune response (Ir) genes to the pathogenetic mechanisms underlying the disease in question. The association between the HLA SD antigens and a given disease would, thus, once again, be explained by linkage disequilibrium between the genes determining the SD antigens and the Ir genes. This seems a most likely explanation for a number of different entities, especially those in which immune phenomena are strongly implicated. The extremely high association between certain HLA SD antigens and given diseases, such as that found in ankylosing spondylitis (Brewerton *et al.*, 1973; Schlosstein *et al.*, 1973) may have other explanations, although a rather extreme form of linkage disequilibrium cannot be ruled out. The possibility that the SD antigens themselves, or phenotypic products of genes very closely linked to the SD antigens (thus, demonstrating very high linkage disequilibrium) will function as receptors for viruses or in other ways influence a disease process must be considered. The recent finding of a very high frequency of the antigen B-27 in ankylosing spondylitis in Japanese, despite the fact that B-27 is present in less than 1% of normal Japanese (Sonozaki *et al.*, 1975), is consistent with this suggestion. Thus, while we should perhaps focus our attention on the immune response genes because of the information currently available and for the reasons discussed below, we should not ignore the possibility that other mechanisms in which genes of this chromosomal region are involved may influence the pathogenesis of a disease or be otherwise significantly associated with a given disease.

As discussed in a previous section, in the mouse, the genes determining the LD antigens recognized in MLC are determined in the same region which includes the immune response genes, although at least in the monkey LD and Ir genes are genetically separable (Balner and van Vreeswijk, 1975; Dorf *et al.*, 1975a). To the extent that this close linkage between the LD locus and the Ir locus holds true in other species, it is reasonable to examine whether a more significant association can be demonstrated between certain LD alleles and given diseases. (One can make the assumption that if two genes are more closely linked in this region, then the linkage disequilibrium between them will be greater than between one of those genes and a gene further away on the same chromosome.)

The demonstration that there appears to be an increased frequency of HLA-3 and HLA-7 in patients with multiple sclerosis (Jersild *et al.*, 1972; Naito *et al.*, 1972; Bertams *et al.*, 1972) led to further studies using LD typing to see whether an association could be demonstrated between a given HLA LD allele and multiple sclerosis. The ensuing study (Jersild *et al.*, 1973a) demonstrated that, in fact, the association between multiple sclerosis and the LD allele is significantly greater than the association with HLA-3. Although these data should be considered preliminary, the further dissection of this complex and our ability at present to define certain HLA LD alleles offers promise that we may be able to demonstrate a greater number of more significant associations than only the HLA SD antigens.

IX. SUMMARY

This chapter has dealt with the present state of knowledge regarding the major histocompatibility complex as it relates to determination of transplantation antigens, immune responses, and disease susceptibility.

The extent to which the principles evolving from these studies, which have dealt primarily with problems of allograft immunity, can be extended to cellular immune reactions involved in autoimmunity, allergy, neoplasia, and other conditions must be verified. Whereas our understanding of the reasons for the disease associations is still very poor, our increasing ability to define MHC products will certainly be of help in this regard.

ACKNOWLEDGMENTS

This work is supported in part by NIH Grants AI-11576, AI-08439, CA-16836, and National Foundation–March of Dimes Grants CRBS 246 and 6-76-213. This is paper No. 2003 from the Laboratory of Genetics and paper No. 88 from the Immunobiology Research Center, The University of Wisconsin, Madison, Wisconsin 53706.

I would like to thank Ms. Nancy Van Der Puy for her patient and expert editorial assistance in the preparation of this manuscript.

REFERENCES

Albert, E. D., Harms, K., Wank, R., Steinbauer-Rosenthal, I., and Scholz, S. *Transplant. Proc.* **5,** 1785.

Amiel, J. L. (1967). *In* "Histocompatibility Testing 1967" (E. S. Curtoni *et al.*, eds.), p. 79. Munksgaard, Copenhagen.

Bach, F. H., and Bach, M. L. *In* "Clinical Immunobiology" (F. N. Bach and R. A. Good, eds.) Vol. 1, pp. 157–178. Academic Press, New York.

Bach, F. H., and van Rood, J. J. (1976). *N. Engl. J. Med.* **295,** 806.

Bach, F. H., Bach, M. L., and Sondel, P. M. (1976). *Nature* (*London*) **259,** 273.

Balner, H., and van Vreeswijk, W. (1975). *Transplant. Proc.* **7,** Suppl. 1, 13.

Balner, H., van Vreeswijk, W., and Roger, J. H. (1977). *Transplant. Rev.* (in press).

Bertams, J., Kuwert, E., and Liedtke, U. (1972). *Tissue Antigens* **2,** 405.

Bradley, B. A., Edwards, J. M., Dunn, D. C., and Calne, R. Y. (1972). *Nature* (*London*) *New Biol.* **240,** 54.

Brewerton, D. A., Caffrey, M., Hart, F. D., James, D. C. O., Nicholls, A., and Sturrock, R. D. (1973). *Lancet* **1,** 904.

Dausset, J., and Colombani, J., eds. (1973). "Histocompatibility Testing 1972." Munksgaard, Copenhagen.

Dorf, M. E., Balner, H., and Benacerraf, B. (1975a). *Transplant. Proc.* **7,** Suppl. 1, 21.

Dorf, M. E., Plate, J. M. D., Stimpfling, J. H., and Benacerraf, B. (1975b). *J. Immunol.* **114,** 602.

Dorf, M. E., Maurer, P. H., Merryman, C. F., and Benacerraf, B. (1976). *J. Exp. Med.* **143,** 889.

Falchuk, Z. M., Rogentine, G. N., and Strober, W. (1972). *J. Clin. Invest.* **51,** 1602.

Feltkamp, T. E. W., van den Berg-Loonen, P. M., Nijenhuis, L. E., Engelfriet, C. P., van Rossum, A. L., van Loghem, J. J., and Oosterhuis, H. J. G. H. (1974). *Br. Med. J.* **1,** 131.

Forbes, J. F., and Morris, P. J. (1970). *Lancet* **2,** 849.

Fritze, D., Herrman, C., Jr., Naeim, F., Smith, G. S., and Walford, R. L. (1974). *Lancet* **1,** 240.

Gebhard, R. L., Katz, S. I., Marks, J., Shuster, S., Trapani, R. J., Rogentine, G. N., and Strober, W. (1973). *Lancet* **2,** 760.

Gordon, R. D., Simpson, E., and Samelson, L. E. (1975). *J. Exp. Med.* **142,** 1108.

Haverkorn, M. J., Hofman, B., Masurel, N., and van Rood, J. J. (1975). *Transplant. Rev.* **22,** 120.

Häyry, P., Andersson, L. C., and Nordling, S. (1973). *Transplant. Proc.* **5,** 87.

Jersild, C., Svejgaard, A., and Fog, T. (1972). *Lancet* **1,** 1240.

Jersild, C., Ammitzbøll, T., Clausen, J., and Fog, T. (1973a). *Lancet* **1,** 151.

Jersild, C., Svejgaard, A., Fog, T., and Ammitzbøll, T. (1973b). *Tissue Antigens* **3,** 243.

Katz, D. H., and Benacerraf, B. (1976). "The Role of The Products of the Histocompatibility Gene Complex in Immune Responses." Academic Press, New York.

Katz, S. I., Falchuk, Z. M., Dahl, M. V., Rogentine, G. N., and Strober, W. (1972). *J. Clin. Invest.* **51,** 2977.

Kissmeyer-Nielsen, ed. (1975). "Histocompatibility Testing 1975." Munksgaard, Copenhagen.

Klein, J. (1975). "Biology of the Mouse Histocompatibility-2 Complex." Springer-Verlag, Berlin and New York.

Klein, J., Hauptfeld, V., and Hauptfeld, M. (1974). *Prog. Int. Congr. Immunol., 2nd, 1974* p. 197.

Levine, B. B., Stember, R. H., and Fotino, M. (1972). *Science* **178,** 1201.

Lilly, F. (1973). *In* "Genetic Control of Immune Responsiveness" (H. O. McDevitt and M. Landy, eds.), p. 273. Academic Press, New York.

Lilly, F., Boyse, E. A., and Old, L. J. (1964). *Lancet* **2,** 1207.

Lindahl, K. F., and Bach, F. H. (1975). *Nature* (*London*) **254,** 607.

Lindahl, K. F., and Bach, F. H. (1976). *J. Exp. Med.* **144,** 305.

McDevitt, H. O., and Bodmer, W. F. (1974). *Lancet* **1,** 1269.

Mackey, I. R., and Morris, P. J. (1972). *Lancet* **2,** 793.

Marsh, D. G., Bias, W. B., Hsu, S. H., and Goodfriend, L. (1973). *Science* **179,** 691.

Morris, P., Bashir, H., McGregor, A. A., *et al.* (1973). *In* "Histocompatibility Testing 1972" (J. Dausset and J. Colombani, eds.), p. 267. Munksgaard, Copenhagen.

Morris, P. J. (1974). *Contemp. Top. Immunobiol.* **3,** 141.

Morris, P. J., Lawler, S., and Oliver, R. T. (1973). *In* "Histocompatibility Testing 1972" (J. Dausset and J. Colombani, eds.), p. 669. Munksgaard, Copenhagen.

Munro, A. J., and Taussig, M. J. (1975). *Nature* (*London*) **256,**103.

Naito, S., Namerow, N., Mickey, M. R., and Terasaki, P. I. (1972). *Tissue Antigens* **2,** 1.

Piazza, A., Belvedere, M. C., Bernoco, D., *et al.* (1973). *In* "Histocompatibility Testing 1972" (J. Dausset and J. Colombani, eds.), p. 73. Munksgaard, Copenhagen.

Säfwenberg, J., Lindblom, J. B., and Osterman, P. O. (1973). *Tissue Antigens* **3,** 465.

Schendel, D. J., and Bach, F. H. (1974). *In* "Lymphocyte Recognition and Effector Mechanisms" (K. Lindahl-Kiessling and D. Osoba, eds.), p. 275. Academic Press, New York.

Schlosstein, L., Terasaki, P. I., Bluestone, R., and Pearson, C. M. (1973). *N. Engl. J. Med.* **288,** 704.

Schmitt-Verhulst, A. M., and Shearer, G. M. (1975). *J. Exp. Med.* **142,** 914.

Sheehy, M. J., Sondel, P. M., Bach, F. H., Sopori, M. L., and Bach, M. L. (1975a). *In* "Histocompatibility Testing 1975" (F. Kissmeyer-Nielsen, ed.), p. 569. Munksgaard, Copenhagen.

Sheehy, M. J., Sondel, P. M., Bach, M. L., Wank, R., and Bach, F. H. (1975b). *Science* **188,** 1308.

Shreffler, D. C., and David, D. S. (1975). *Adv. Immunol.* **20,** 125.

Silver, J., and Hood, L. (1976). *Contemp. Top. Mol. Immunol.* p. 35.

Sollinger, H. W., and Bach, F. H. (1976). *Nature* (*London*) **259,** 487.

Sonozaki, H., Seki, H., Chang, S., Okuyama, M., and Juji, T. (1975). *Tissue Antigens* **5,** 131.

Stokes, P. L., Asquith, P., Holmes, G. K. T., Mackintosh, P., and Cooke, W. T. (1972). *Lancet* **2,** 162.

Thorsby, E., and Piazza, A. (1975). *In* "Histocompatibility Testing 1975" (F. Kissmeyer-Nielsen, ed.), pp. 414–458. Munksgaard, Copenhagen.

Thorsby, E., Engeset, A., and Lie, S. O. (1971). *Tissue Antigens* **1,** 147.

van den Tweel, J. G., Vriesendorp, H. M., Termijtelen, A., Westbroek, D. L., Bach, M. L., and van Rood, J. J. (1974). *J. Exp. Med.* **140,** 825.

van der Does, J. A., Elkerbout, F., D'Amaro, J., van der Steen, G., van Loghem, E., MeergKhan, P., Bernini, L. F., van Leeuwen, A., and van Rood, J. J. (1973). *In* "Histocompatibility Testing 1972" (J. Dausset and J. Colombani, eds.), p. 579. Munksgaard, Copenhagen.

van Hooff, J. P., Pena, A. S., Hekkens, W. T. J. M., *et al.* (1974). *Proc. Int. Coeliac Symp., 2nd, 1974* p. 233.

van Rood, J. J. (1975). *Genetics* **79,** 277.

White, A. G., Barnetson, R. St. C., DaCosta, J. A. G., and McClelland, D. B. L. (1973). *Lancet* **1,** 108.

Widmer, M., Peck, A. B., and Bach, F. H. (1973). *Transplant. Proc.* **5,** 1501.

Zinkernagel, R. M., and Doherty, P. C. (1977). *Contemp. Top. Immunobiol.* (in press).

Chapter 2

Genetic Aspects of Autoimmune Disease in Animals

NOEL L. WARNER

I. INTRODUCTION

The pathogenesis of autoimmune disease is a complex process in which many factors have been implicated as playing essential roles. Among these are genetic, immunologic, viral, and various unidentified environmental factors. In both human autoimmune disease, and in many induced or spontaneous experimental animal models of autoimmunity, the role of genetic factors in determining both the incidence, onset, and nature of the autoimmune process is clearly evident. However, in most of these situations it has not been possible to assign this autoimmune predisposition to the action of a single genetic locus. Accordingly, analysis of the genetic control and mechanism of gene action in autoimmunity cannot be readily made without the availability of suitable inbred strains of animals, preferably involving congenic strains differing at defined genetic loci. The principal current information on the genetic basis of autoimmunity is, thus, derived from studies with the New Zealand mouse strains. The general nature of the autoimmune process occurring in different inbred and hybrid New Zealand strains is discussed elsewhere in this volume. This chapter will specifically concentrate on genetic studies of autoimmune disease in the New Zealand mice and, in a limited way, on other autoimmune systems where genetic influence has been shown to occur.

The New Zealand black mouse (NZB) and the hybrid of NZB with New Zealand white, (NZB $\times$ NZW)F_1, have generally been considered to be models for human autoimmune diseases, particularly systemic lupus erythematosus and autoimmune hemolytic anemia (Bielschowsky *et al.,* 1959; Holmes and Burnet, 1963; Howie and Helyer, 1968; Mellors, 1965; Talal, 1975). The expression of autoimmunity in these animals does not involve a single clone of autoantibody-producing cells. The mice develop LE cells, anti-nuclear antibodies to a variety of nucleic acid antigens, and a range of different anti-red cell antibodies associated with the autoimmune hemolytic anemia. They show generalized lymphocytic proliferation and infiltration in a variety of organ systems, and may develop a lethal immune complex glomerulonephritis. A listing of the pathological and immunologic changes that have been observed among the various New Zealand strains of mice is given in Table I. In attempting to determine the role of genetic factors in this variety of abnormal conditions, it is essential to separately determine whether specific genetic control is involved in each of the observed abnormalities. With this knowledge, it could then be questioned whether the various abnormalities have a common genetic basis. Accordingly, the first sections of this chapter will consider the major autoimmune manifestations of the New Zealand mice in terms of the number and nature of genetic controls operating, and will also consider evidence for a common or separate genetic basis of these different abnormalities.

In view of the current interest in the possible role of a failure of a regulatory mechanism to control autoimmune disease (Fudenberg, 1971; Allison, 1974; Talal, 1975), it is relevant to question whether this suppressor or regulatory control mechanism may itself be under genetic control, and lie at the basis of the genetic control in autoimmune disease. This, in turn, provokes a further question as to whether any genetically controlled events associated with autoimmune disease and expressed in cells of the lymphoid system might not be related to other known genetic systems controlling normal immunologic responses, such as the immune response genes associated with the major histocompatibility complex or with immunoglobulin allotypes

TABLE I

Principal Pathological and Immunologic Abnormalities Observed in New Zealand Mouse Strains

Condition	NZ strains reported to show condition	References[a]
Autoimmune hemolytic anemia	NZB, (NZB × NZC)F_1	(1, 2)
Immune complex glomerulonephritis	NZB, (NZB × NZW)F_1	(1, 3–5)
High incidence lymphoreticular malignancy	NZB, NZO, (NZB × NZW) F_1	(5–8)
Abnormality of response to extrinsic antigens *in vitro* or *in vivo*	NZB, NZC	(9, 10)
Abnormality of tolerance response to extrinsic antigens	NZB, NZW, (NZB × NZW)F_1	(9, 11, 12)
Pituitary tumors	NZY	(13)
Megacolon	NZY	(14)
Obesity	NZO	(15)
Hydronephrosis	NZC	(16)
Hematopoietic stem cell abnormalities	NZB, NZC	(17)
Chronic peptic ulcers	NZB	(18)

[a] A limited selection of references is given, and further references may be found in the text and in several review articles (Mellors, 1966; Howie and Helyer, 1968; Talal, 1975). Key to references: (1) reviewed by Howie and Helyer (1968); (2) Holmes and Burnet (1963); (3) Burnet and Holmes (1965a); (4) Lambert and Dixon (1968); (5) Mellors (1966); (6) East (1970); (7) Rappaport *et al.* (1971); (8) Sugai *et al.* (1973); (9) reviewed by Talal (1975), Talal and Steinberg (1974); (10) Herrod and Warner (1972); (11) Staples and Talal (1969); (12) Braverman and Slesenski (1970); (13) Bielschowsky *et al.* (1956); (14) Bielschowsky and Schofield (1962); (15) Bielschowsky and Bielschowsky (1956); (16) Warner (1971); (17) Warner and Moore (1971); (18) Wynn Williams *et al.* (1967).

(McDevitt and Landy, 1973). Available data on these aspects will also be considered.

II. GENETIC ANALYSIS OF AUTOIMMUNITY IN NZ MOUSE STRAINS

In considering the available data on genetic analysis of the various autoimmune manifestations in these inbred and hybrid mouse strains, it is appropriate to also review the origins of the different New Zealand mouse strains (Bielschowsky and Goodall, 1970).

In 1930, W. M. Hall brought a randomly bred mouse colony of various coat colors from the Imperial Cancer Research Fund Laboratories at Mill

Hill, London, to the University of Otago Medical School, Dunedin, New Zealand. In 1948, the Bielschowsky's selected several pairs of mice of similar coat color and commenced inbreeding on the basis of coat color selection. The original three pairs selected were agouti, tan, and chocolate. The NZO strain was derived from the pair of agouti mice inbred by brother/sister mating, with fixation of the agouti coat color. From F_{12} to F_{17}, selection for the obese character was made in the propagation of the strain. In the F_3 generation, descendants from these agouti mice included some offspring with black coats, and one pair of black littermates were selected to initiate the NZB line, which from F_{11} generation onward was observed to show hemolytic anemia (Bielschowsky *et al.*, 1959). The pair of tan mice gave rise to progeny with the piebald coat color, and at the F_4 generation a piebald brother/sister pair was available, and selection for piebald gave rise to the NZY strain. The original pair of chocolate colored mice led by brother/sister mating to the NZC strain. A further strain derived from the NZC line at F_7 was selected on the basis of sandy coats, but subsequently developed a very high incidence of cystic kidney and was discontinued at F_{32} (NZS strain). The NZX strain of mice originated from the cross between an NZC female and an NZY male, followed by brother/sister mating of the offspring. It is important to note, however, that the New Zealand white (NZW strain) were not derived during this same inbreeding series, but instead were developed by Hall, commencing in 1952, with mice from the original mixed colony from England. A series of other NZ strains have been mentioned at various points in the literature (Howie and Helyer, 1965), but a detailed report on the origin of these strains does not appear to be available. These strains include NZWA, NZCW, NZG, and NZF.

In relation to the general theme of this article, the major point to note is that all of the NZ strains were derived from a common random-bred colony, but were developed as independent lines and, in some instances, initiated at quite different times. The following consideration of various autoimmune manifestations in the NZ strains will now exclusively deal with genetic aspects and will not detail the natural history of the disorders, nor their pathological or immunologic manifestations. These aspects are considered elsewhere in this book, and have been previously reviewed (Mellors, 1966; Howie and Helyer, 1968; Talal, 1975; Talal and Steinberg, 1974).

A. Autoimmune Hemolytic Anemia

Analysis of the incidence of autoimmune hemolytic anemia in various hybrids, backcross, and intercross strain combinations involving NZB mice has clearly demonstrated the essential role of genetic factors in the pathogenesis of this syndrome. However, despite several investigations of this nature, the precise number of genes involved and their mechanism of action is still not clearly determined. The major problem in such an analysis is that the expression of autoimmune hemolytic anemia is not that of an "all-or-none" type. Thus, whereas the NZB parental strain shows an almost 100% incidence of Coombs'-positive hemolytic anemia at 12 months of age, and another normal parental strain may show 0% incidence, the F_1 hybrid between them does not usually show a 0, 50, or 100% incidence at this age, but, instead, frequently shows a steadily increasing incidence of a milder form of the disease from about 9 to 12 months of age onward. This general observation may indicate that a single dose of a particular gene permits an eventual later onset of the disease, whereas the double dose is associated with NZB inbred patterns of disease. With this reservation, analysis for incidence of Coombs' positivity at the age when most NZB mice have just converted, about 9–12 months, permits a reasonable determination of the number of genes involved in the full "NZB type" pattern of the disease.

1. NZ Inbred Strains

Many laboratories have demonstrated that virtually all inbred NZB mice eventually show Coombs'-positive hemolytic anemia (Bielschowsky *et al.*, 1959; Holmes and Burnet, 1963; Long *et al.*, 1963; Mellors, 1965; Holborow *et al.*, 1965; Braverman, 1968; Warner and Wistar, 1968; Costea *et al.*, 1970; Ghaffar and Playfair, 1971; Linder and Edgington, 1972; East and Harvey, 1971). This characteristic has persisted in all sublines of NZB mice carried by various laboratories around the world and indicates that genetic factors are of prime importance in the onset of this disease. The age of onset and total incidence of Coombs' positivity varies slightly in different reports, but this may only reflect sensitivity differences in the technique for detecting surface-bound immunoglobulin on erythrocytes. Some reports initially suggested that males had a slightly earlier onset of Coombs' positivity than females (Holmes and Burnet, 1963; Burnet and Holmes, 1965b), but these studies were with castrated males, and most subsequent studies with noncastrated males show a similar onset in male and female. At 6 months, approximately 50% of NZB mice are Coombs' positive, and by 10 months almost 100%. Once NZB mice develop Coombs'-positive reactions, they usually persist. The detection of hemolytic anemia in these mice has been shown by increased reticulocyte counts, reduced hematocrits, shortened red cell survival, erythrophagocytosis, splenomegaly, liver hemosiderosis, extra medullary hemopoiesis, and pigmented gallstones.

No other inbred NZ strain shows the NZB pattern of autoimmune hemolytic anemia. Of many NZC mice tested at various ages, none have been found to show Coombs' positivity (Warner, 1973), although this strain is particularly susceptible to the induction of anti-erythrocyte antibody production (Warner, 1973). Reports on the NZW strain have varied, although it is clear that they do not show the NZB pattern of disease. Several laboratories have reported a 0% incidence of Coombs'-positive tests in NZW mice, others have reported a low and transient incidence at around 1 year, but increasing to at least 50% in the second year (DeVries and Hijmans, 1967; Braverman, 1968; Hahn and Shulman, 1969; Ghaffar and Playfair, 1971). Similarly, NZY mice have only a very low incidence at 1 year, but later in life well over 50% become Coombs' positive (Helyer and Howie, 1961; Braverman, 1968).

Several studies have stressed a distinction between the Coombs'-positive state and full hemolytic anemia. Thus, in NZB mice, Coombs' positivity occurs well before the detection of other signs of hemolytic anemia, and the presence of the anti-erythrocyte autoantibody may not in itself be sufficient to account for other manifestations of hemolytic anemia, such as increased red cell destruction (Lindsey *et al.,* 1966; Braverman and Slesinski, 1968). Furthermore, in several of the non-NZB strains where transient Coombs' positivity or later onset occurs, it is in the total absence of any detectable hemolytic anemia (Braverman, 1968; Hahn and Shulman, 1969). Separate genetic factors may be operating to determine anti-erythrocyte autoantibody production and other manifestations of autoimmune hemolytic anemia. The full syndrome of autoimmune hemolytic anemia appears to be unique to the inbred NZB strain.

The nature of the autologous red cell antigens involved have been extensively studied in NZB mice, with a range of different antigenic determinants being detected (Long *et al.,* 1963; Holborow *et al.,* 1965; Costea *et al.,* 1970; Linder and Edgington, 1972; DeHeer and Edgington, 1975). It has been proposed that the autoantibody response is polyclonal and, therefore, contrary to the "forbidden clone" concept (Linder and Edgington, 1972). However, although analysis for immunoglobulin classes of autoantibodies (Table II) has shown that the anti-erythrocyte autoantibodies can be of several different immunoglobulin types (Warner and Wistar, 1968), allotypic analysis of the autoantibodies in heterozygous NZB mice has indicated that, in 34 of 35 mice studied, only one parental allele was expressed in the autoantibody population of any one mouse, with no preference for either parental allelic type being evident (Warner, 1974). These results, therefore, favor the concept of a monoclonal or restricted origin of the original autoantibody-producing cell population and do not indicate a role for allotype-linked immune response gene control in autoantibody production of this type.

2. *F_1 Hybrids of NZB with Other NZ Strains*

Variations have also been observed between the various NZ strains in the incidence and degree of anti-erythrocyte autoantibody production found in

TABLE II

Immunoglobulin Class of Red Cell Autoantibodies[a]

Strain	Age range (months)	Coombs' positive (%)		
		IgM	IgG1	IgG2
NZB	8–14	74 (54/73)	74 (51/69)	61 (43/70)
(NZB × NZC)F_1	8–16	75 (56/75)	67 (97/145)	21 (30/144)
(NZB × BALB/c)F_1	22–24	NT	63 (50/80)	3 (2/80)

[a] The values show the percent of mice giving positive direct Coombs' test with indicated anti-heavy chain reagents. Numbers in parentheses are the number of positive mice/total number tested. The majority of mice (over 60% of each group) were of an age close to the mean of the indicated range. NT, not tested.

the F_1 hybrids with NZB (Table III). The only hybrid that has been shown to develop a high early incidence of Coombs'-positive autoantibodies is the (NZB × NZC)F_1 hybrid. Virtually 100% of these mice are Coombs' positive by 1 year of age, and differ from the inbred NZB mouse only in general health and longer survival (Bielschowsky and Bielschowsky, 1964; Warner, 1973). Detailed analysis of other aspects of the hemolytic anemia of NZB mice however, have not, been investigated in this hybrid. Two other NZ strains, NZWA and NZCW, that have not been described in great detail, may be like NZC in this regard, in that the hybrid with NZB has an early and high incidence of Coombs'-positive autoantibodies (Howie and Helyer, 1965). Other NZ hybrids have been reported to show either virtually no incidence of Coombs' positivity, or a relatively low incidence and later onset as in (NZB × NZW)F_1, (NZB × NZG)F_1, and (NZB × NZY)F_1 (Helyer and Howie, 1961; Howie and Helyer, 1965; Burnet and Holmes, 1965b; DeVries and Hijmans, 1967; Hahn and Shulman, 1969; Ghaffar and Playfair, 1971). The incidence in these hybrids of NZ strains is not significantly different from many hybrids of NZB with other non-NZ strains (see Section II,A,3).

Within the NZ strains, it, therefore, seems that the NZC strain may be relatively unique, in that the genetic contribution from NZC either has relatively little modifying potential of the anti-erythrocyte autoantibody expression determined by NZB genes, or, that the NZC genome positively contributes genes required for the expression of Coombs'-positive autoantibodies (see Section II,A,4 and 5). However, as noted in Table II, the complete expression of all immunoglobulin classes in the anti-erythrocyte autoantibody response is not observed in the (NZB × NZC)F_1 hybrid.

TABLE III

Anti-erythrocyte Autoantibody Production in F_2 and Backcross Mice

Progeny mice	Incidence of Coombs' positivity (%)[a]	References[b]
NZB	100, 92, 85	(1, 6, 3)
(NZB × NZC)F_1	100, 90	(4, 2)
(NZB × NZW)F_1	66, 60, 22, 7	(5, 6, 7, 3)
(NZB × BALB/c)F_1	9, 9, 5	(3, 2, 8)
(NZB × C3H)F_1	10	(9)
(NZB × AKR)F_1	45	(10)
(NZB × NZC)F_2	74	(4)
(NZB × NZW)F_2	51, 9	(5, 3)
(NZB × BALB/c)F_2	15, 9	(8, 3)
(NZB × NZC)F_1 × NZB	28	(3)
(NZB × BALB/c)F_1 × NZB	30	(3)
(NZB × C3H)F_1 × NZB	60	(9)
(NZB × AKR)F_1 × NZB	70	(10)

[a] Values shown are for mice in the general age range of 10–14 months.

[b] References citations are in the same respective order on each line as the incidence values. Key to references is as follows: (1) Holmes and Burnet (1963); (2) Warner (1973); (3) Ghaffar and Playfair (1971); (4) Bielschowsky and Bielschowsky (1964); (5) Braverman (1968); (6) Burnet and Holmes (1965b); (7) Hahn and Shulman (1969); (8) East and Harvey (1971); (9) Holmes and Burnet (1964); (10) Holmes and Burnet (1966).

3. *F_1 Hybrids of NZB with Other Mouse Strains*

NZB hybrids have not been found to show either hemolytic anemia at any age, nor the nearly 100% incidence of Coombs' positivity at 12 months of age observed in the inbred NZB strain. However, many F_1 hybrid strain combinations do show a lower incidence of Coombs' positivity, increasing with age and often reaching around 50% or more by 18 months of age (Holmes and Burnet, 1964; 1966; Burnet and Holmes, 1965b; Ghaffar and Playfair, 1971; East and Harvey, 1971; Warner, 1973). At the age when NZB mice are virtually 100% Coombs' positive, i.e., 9–10 months, most NZB hybrids show only about 0–20% Coombs' positivity. In general, the responses are transient and weaker than in the inbred NZB strain. Mice are frequently observed at one time to be Coombs' positive, and the same mouse at a later stage may be Coombs' negative.

Autoantibody responses in the F_1 hybrids also differ from those of the inbred NZB in the expression of different immunoglobulin classes (Warner,

1974). Thus, whereas the IgM and IgG_1 classes of autoantibodies appear to predominate in all strains, only inbred NZB mice eventually develop a high incidence of autoantibodies of the IgG_2 class (Table II). Whether this reflects differences in T cell involvement in the response, macrophage activity in processing autoantigens, or a response to different autoantigenic determinants, remains to be elucidated.

4. *F_2 and Backcross Mice*

It is to be stressed that, at present, analysis of the number of genes involved in the development of autoimmune hemolytic anemia has only considered the production of Coombs'-positive anti-erythrocyte autoantibodies, not the full expression of clinical hemolytic anemia. Also, as noted earlier, such an analysis can only be made in terms of the early onset of Coombs' positivity, i.e., the development of the NZB type with 90–100% incidence by 9–12 months of life.

From the incidence of positive Coombs' tests in F_1 and F_2 hybrids of NZB with NZC (100 and 74%, respectively) Bielschowsky and Bielschowsky (1964) deduced that a single dominant gene was responsible for Coombs' positivity. Similarly, the data with (NZB × NZC)F_1 backcrosses to NZC (Warner, 1973), are consistent with a single dominant gene being involved. However, if a single dominant gene carried by the NZB mice was the *only* genetic factor involved in Coombs'-positive autoantibody expression, then all types of NZB F_1 hybrids would show Coombs' positivity. However, this is not so, and the data with the NZB and NZC combinations might, thus, be consistent with the concept of involvement of one dominant gene unique to NZB mice, with the NZC mice, as well as NZB mice, carrying a recessive gene also required for the expression of Coombs' positivity (Warner, 1973). In the data of Braverman (1968), a relatively high incidence of Coombs' positivity was also observed in the (NZB × NZW)F_1, and from the 50% incidence in F_2 mice, he also concluded that a dominant gene was involved in the anti-erythrocyte antibody production. A similar analysis by Ghaffar and Playfair (1971), however, suggested that recessive genes may be involved, as in several F_2 combinations, a strongly positive reaction was observed, whereas only weak responses (if any) were found in the F_1 hybrid. Similarly, East and Harvey (1971) observed a higher incidence of Coombs'-positive reactions in F_3 mice than in F_2 mice and, in turn, than in F_1 hybrids of the NZB and BALB/c strains. From the low frequency of strongly positive Coombs' tests in the progeny of the backcross to the non-NZB strain, Burnet and Holmes (1965b) concluded that some three to five genes might be involved. However, in view of the recognition of the role of the dominant gene in the NZC data, the overall progency data might be interpreted at present in one of two ways. One proposal (Warner, 1973) would be that two different genes are involved and essential for the full expression of the early onset and high incidence of Coombs'-positive autoantibody production. One of these genes acts in a dominant fashion and is unique to the NZB strain. The second gene is recessive and is present only in the NZB and NZC strains. The so-called dominant gene may actually function in terms of dosage effects; thus, a single gene might well be associated with the late positive Coombs' tests observed in many other NZ hybrids. The alternative explanation is to propose that the effect of the NZB dominant gene in determining the anti-erythrocyte autoantibody production can be modified to varying degrees by a second gene, thus reducing autoantibody production to erythrocytes. On this alternative, the gene carried by the NZC strain is relatively inefficient at modifying the effect of the dominant NZB gene, although some modification may be occurring as the intensity of Coombs'-positive tests is not as great in the F_1 with NZB as in inbred NZB mice, nor is the full expression of all IgG classes of autoantibodies observed (Table II). The modifying gene introduced by other non-NZ strains, is in general quite efficient at minimizing the effect of a single dose of the NZB dominant gene, although later in life this modifying effect has declined. This observation in itself might suggest that the cellular level of expression of the modifying gene is in a cell type that shows relative inactivity with advancing age. On this scheme, the NZW strain (and probably also NZY) may carry a modifying gene that, in concert with the NZB gene, results in a reduced incidence of anti-erythrocyte autoantibodies but also in the expression of other autoantibodies, primarily to nucleic acid components (Braverman, 1968; Ghaffer and Playfair, 1971).

This scheme is discussed again in Section II,B,3 in considering all types of autoimmune expression. The present data are, however, clearly indicative of a dominant gene action in autoantibody expression that can be modified by other gene expression. On such a concept, it is evidence that the identification of gene action in human autoimmune disease will be relatively difficult to define, although some associations may be evident (see Section IV).

5. *Linkage Studies*

One approach to resolve the issue of the number and interaction of genes in autoimmune disease pathogenesis is to attempt to detect linkage of these genes to other marker loci. As will be discussed later (Section IV), immune response genes (Ir) (McDevitt and Landy, 1973; Benacerraf and Katz, 1975) are of interest in this connection, although little direct data is available. Our present data with F_2 and backcross combinations of NZB and C57 strains do not indicate that either H-2 or allotype-linked genes are involved in autoimmune pathogenesis (Table IV). However, these data are preliminary, and a more complete analysis of autoimmune disease in H-2 and allotype congenic lines of NZB mice is currently in progress.

Analysis of Coombs' positivity in male and female NZB F_1 hybrid mice tends to suggest that either hormonal or sex chromosome factors are involved (Burnet and Holmes, 1965b). At present, all the available data favors the former alternative and does not suggest X chromosome associated genetic factors. Hormonal influence on the antibody response to nucleic acids in NZB/NZW F_1 mice is discussed in Chapter 7.

In various studies on F_2 and backcross mice, it has been stated that coat color is not associated with autoimmune expression. However, several different genetic loci are involved in determining mouse coat color, and the absence of apparent association of autoimmune incidence with coat color in some mouse strains does not necessarily imply a lack of linkage of the "autoimmune genes" with all coat color loci. In an intercross study (Warner and Moore, 1971) of (BALB/c × NZB)F_1 × (NZB × NZC)F_1

TABLE IV

Lack of Association of H-2 and Ig Type with Abnormalities of NZB Mice

	No. of mice of indicated genetic type with abnormality					
	H-2 type			Ig-1 type		
Abnormality	bd	bb	dd	be	bb	ee
Coombs' positivity						
OBS[a]	8	3	3	8	2	4
EXP[b]	7	3.5	3.5	7	3.5	3.5
Kidney disease						
OBS	14	4	2	12	4	4
EXP	10	4.8	5.2	10	4.8	5.2
Lymphoreticular tumors						
OBS	12	4	0	11	3	2
EXP	8	6	2	8	6	2

[a] OBS: Observed values show the number of mice of each genetic type with the indicated abnormality.

[b] EXP: Expected proportion of mice with particular abnormality if no association with H-2 or Ig-1 loci. These values are based on the number of F_2 or backcross mice involved in each grouping. Most groups contained approximately 80% (NZB × C57)F_2 and 10% each of the two backcross combinations. NZB are H-2^d, Ig-1^e, C57 are H-2^b, Ig-1^b.

hybrid mice, 44% of mice developed positive Coombs' tests by 12 months of age. Similar to the incidence of 50% expected from the incidence patterns in the parental and F_1 hybrid strains. However, of 52 progeny having chocolate coat color, only 23% were Coombs' positive, whereas 56% of black progeny were Coombs' positive. On the basis of this observation, it was considered that a "modifying" gene carried by NZC mice, might be linked to a gene determining the chocolate coat color. If a double dose of this gene could then be introduced into the NZB genome, the modifying effect on the development of anti-erythrocyte autoantibodies might be even more apparent. This has been attempted by developing a congenic line of NZB mice that carry the chocolate coat color gene. At the present stage, backcrossing of an initial (NZB × NZC)F_1 mouse to the NZB strain has proceeded for eight generations, selecting at each generation for mice carrying the chocolate coat color gene (these mice being detected by their ability to produce chocolate coat color mice on test mating with NZC mice). At the eighth backcross generation, two heterozygous mice were inbred, and the chocolate-colored progeny were brother/sister mated to establish an inbred line. Analysis of Coombs' positivity in these mice has now revealed a considerably lower incidence of anti-erythrocyte autoantibodies than in either inbred NZB or (NZB × NZC)F_1 hybrid mice (Table V). These data have yet to be validated by studies of inbred mice from later backcross generations, but, at present, they are strongly compatible with the view that the effect of the NZB gene determining anti-erythrocyte autoantibody production can be modified by another gene, which in NZC mice, is linked to a locus determining the chocolate coat color.

B. Immune Complex Glomerulonephritis

The second major autoimmune manifestation discovered in mice of the NZ strains was a lethal glomerulonephritis, analogous in many ways to human systemic lupus erythematosus. The initial report of positive LE cells and a renal pathology analogous to human lupus was made in F_1 hybrids of NZB and NZY (Helyer and Howie, 1961). Subsequently, similar findings were made with (NZB × NZW)F_1 hybrids (Helyer and Howie, 1963a; Burnet and Holmes, 1965a) and, to a lesser degree, in the inbred NZB strain (Holmes and Burnet, 1963; Helyer and Howie, 1963b; Mellors, 1965). Various laboratories have since confirmed these findings, with the main aspects of the lupus-type disease being a membranous glomerulonephritis (Holmes and Burnet, 1963; Helyer and Howie, 1963b; Hicks and Burnet, 1966; DeVries and Hijmans, 1967), immunoglobulin and complement fixation to glomerular capillary basement membranes (Mellors, 1965; DeVries and Hijmans, 1967; Lambert and Dixon, 1968), variable numbers of LE

TABLE V

Coombs'-Positive Reactions in Congenic NZB · ch Mice[a]

			Percent Coombs' positive[b]			
Strain	Sex	Age (months)	All positive grades	Strong reactions (3+, 4+)	Anti-Ig G_2	NZB · ch incidence (%)[c]
NZB · ch	M	8–9	13.5	5.7	NT	18
NZB	M	8–9	73.3	20.0	NT	
NZB · ch	M	12–15	25.9	14.8	13.3	29
NZB	M	11–14	89.6	48.3	50.0	
NZB · ch	F	8–9	55.8	8.8	NT	62
NZB	F	9	90.0	40.0	NT	
NZB · ch	F	12–15	66.7	40.7	25.0	70
NZB	F	11–14	95.0	80.0	70.0	

[a] NZB · ch mice are NZB · ch $N8F_2$.

[b] Percent of Coombs'-positive mice with polyvalent anti-Ig serum (containing anti-kappa chain antibodies). Positive reactions are scored of varying grades of positivity from weak (1+) to very strong (4+) (Long *et al.*, 1963). The IgG2 reactions are for positives of all grades.

[c] The values show the percent of NZB · ch Coombs'-positive mice relative to the age and sex matched NZB controls.

cells in blood (Helyer and Howie, 1963a; Norins and Holmes, 1964; Burnet and Holmes, 1965a), anti-nuclear factors, and anti-DNA antibodies (Norins and Holmes, 1964; Braverman, 1968; Steinberg *et al.*, 1969; Ghaffar and Playfair, 1971), and other secondary renal pathologic changes such as a necrotizing arteritis (Hicks, 1966).

The etiology of this lupus-like syndrome has been quite controversial, with particular attention being focused on a possible involvement of viruses, particularly C type viruses (Mellors *et al.*, 1969, 1971; Dixon *et al.*, 1974). Several different murine C type viruses and other viruses have been shown capable of causing the formation of anti-nuclear antibodies and an immune complex glomerulonephritis in various non-NZ mouse strains. These include MuLV Moloney (mentioned in Dixon *et al.*, 1974) FMR group viruses (Richer *et al.*, 1966; Branca *et al.*, 1971; Cannat and Varet, 1973), other MuLV agents (Oldstone *et al.*, 1972; Porter *et al.*, 1973) and even LCM and polyoma (Tonietti *et al.*, 1970). The relation of C type viruses and autoimmune disease is discussed in Chapter 14.

Despite the evidence implicating viruses in the pathogenesis of NZ mouse glomerulonepritis, the role of genetic factors must also be considered. Various studies have clearly indicated a crucial role of host genetic control in determining disease onset, incidence, and severity. Owing to considerable variations in the literature on the incidence of anti-nuclear antibodies in NZ mice, and to the possible role of environmental- or viral-associated factors (Friou and Teague, 1963) in determining their incidence, it is somewhat doubtful whether the number of genes involved in the development of these autoantibodies can be clearly defined. However, in several reasonably comprehensive studies (Braverman, 1968; Ghaffar and Playfair, 1971), clear evidence of a limited number of genetic factors has been shown.

1. NZ Inbred Strains

As for anti-erythrocyte autoantibodies, it is also necessary to consider the behavior of the different NZ inbred strains. Reports on anti-nuclear antibody incidence in NZB mice have varied considerably from almost 0 to 100% (Norins and Holmes, 1964; Mellors, 1965; Howie and Helyer, 1965; DeVries and Hijmans, 1967; Braverman, 1968; Hahn and Shulman, 1969; Steinberg *et al.*, 1969; Zeleznick *et al.*, 1969; Ghaffar and Playfair, 1971; Siegal *et al.*, 1972). This variation is in striking contrast to the consistency of incidence of anti-erythrocyte autoantibodies in NZB mice in different laboratories and clearly implicates other nongenetic factors in the anti-nuclear antibody production. Most laboratories report only a low incidence of LE cells in NZB mice (Helyer and Howie, 1963a; Burnet and Holmes, 1965a; Howie and Helyer, 1968), a low incidence of severe glomerulonephritis, but a high incidence of all grades of glomerulonephritis (Burnet and Holmes, 1965a; Mellors, 1965; Howie and Helyer, 1968; DeVries and Hijmans, 1967; Braverman, 1968).

Other inbred NZ strains have received relatively little attention in this regard (except for NZW). NZC mice have not been found to show any evidence of immune complex glomerulonephritis, although these mice have a high incidence of spontaneous hydronephrosis (Warner, 1971), which is under the control of a single autosomal recessive gene, unlinked to those genes controlling any other known abnormalities in these mice (Warner, 1971; Warner and Moore, 1971). The NZY strain has been shown to eventually develop a high incidence of antinuclear antibody and mild glomerulonephritis quite similar to the NZB strain (Braverman, 1968). Similarly, a high incidence of a mild glomerulonephritis has been found in inbred NZW mice (DeVries and Hijmans, 1967; Braverman, 1968; Hahn and Shulman, 1969), although most laboratories agree that this strain shows a low incidence of anti-nuclear antibodies (Braverman, 1968, Ghaffar and Playfair, 1971; Hahn and Shulman, 1969). Thus, in the inbred NZ strains, consistent association between clinical disease and serological findings is not observed. Furthermore, none of the inbred strains show the severity of the disease observed in the (NZB × NZY)F_1 or (NZB × NZW)F_1 (see next section).

2. *NZ Hybrids*

The majority of studies on the lupus model have used the (NZB × NZW)F_1 hybrid mouse. By all the parameters of this disease process listed above, this hybrid shows earlier onset, higher incidence, and more severe disease than either parental strain. This data would accordingly imply that a minimum of two genetic loci are involved in the pathogenesis of the severe form of this disease, with each parental strain contributing an effective allele at one of the genetic loci. The data also implies that either gene alone, particularly in a double dose, can result in a milder form of the disease. Studies of F_2 and backcross animals support this concept of a two-gene system, although considerable variation in severity of disease processes was observed (Braverman, 1968; Ghaffar and Playfair, 1971). The majority of animals show some degree of glomerulonephritis, although the incidence of severe disease closely followed that expected for a control by a dominant NZB-derived gene. Thus, backcrosses to NZB show a much higher incidence than do F_2 progeny, or backcrosses to NZW. The involvement of genes from NZW mice is further demonstrated by a comparison with disease incidence in F_1, F_2, and backcross mice of NZB with BALB/c (Ghaffar and Playfair, 1971), in which each respective comparison shows a lower incidence than in the progeny involving NZW parents [e.g., 52% Ig glomerular staining with NZB × (NZB × BALB/c)F_1, and 91% for NZB × (NZB × NZW)F_1].

The current data is generally compatible with the role of a dominant NZB-derived gene resulting in moderate autoimmune disease, the nature of which can be modified by other gene action. This conclusion is accordingly identical to one alternative reached in considering genetic control of anti-erythrocyte antibody production. Several authors have proposed that, although the character of the NZB autoimmune gene can be expressed in the heterozygous state, it is then that the modifying influences affect the type of autoantibody production that result (Howie and Helyer, 1965; Braverman, 1968; Ghaffar and Playfair, 1974). On this concept, it might, therefore, be questioned whether these modifying genetic factors are allelic or whether they represent multiple genetic loci. In this context, it is relevant to stress that, as noted earlier in this article, the derivation of the NZW strain, although from the same common random-bred stock, occurred independently from the derivation of NZB and NZC.

An approach to this general question is to determine possible negative or positive correlations between the different types of autoimmune disease.

This should ideally be made with hemolytic anemia and clinical renal disease; however, data is available only for the respective serological markers, and, although not conclusive, tends to point toward the action of independently segregating genes (Braverman, 1968; Ghaffar and Playfair, 1971).

3. *Proposed Genetic Model*

The case for an essential role of specific gene action in the pathogenesis of autoimmunity in NZ mice appears at present to be quite solid. It is not mutually exclusive of other etiologic agents, particularly virus action in the kidney disease. Although more than one specific gene must be involved, the number is probably quite small and may involve interactions between the effects of the various gene products. Although much of the genetic analysis rests on relatively "soft data," a provisional model of these genes might be proposed, if for no other reason, than to provide a focus for the design of suitable crosses to test for genetic interaction. Such a model does, however, indicate the complexities that might be encountered, to an even greater degree, in attempting to seek evidence of genetic involvement in the pathogenesis of human autoimmune disease.

The present model (Table VI) envisages a minimum of three loci.

i. Mutant gene A, when not suppressed or grossly modified in its action by the normal modifying gene M, results in generalized autoimmunity, involving various clones of autoantibody-producing cells, including anti-erythrocyte, nucleic acid, and probably other specificities. Thus, the inbred NZB mouse has hemolytic anemia and mild glomerulonephritis. The effect of gene A is not autoantigen specific but, in some manner, alters the balance of a regulatory mechanism.

ii. Mutant gene G is in some way specifically involved in provoking or predisposing to anti-nuclear antibody production and associated mild immune complex disease. Thus, the mild kidney disease of NZW is due to a different gene than the mild disease of NZB. NZC mice have neither mutant gene and show no autoimmunity.

iii. Three alleles are proposed for this modifying locus. The product of the normal allele M at this locus in some manner partially negates the effect of gene A. Thus, hybrids of NZB and normal mouse strains have only a single dose of gene A, which is also being considerably counteracted in its effect by gene M. In the (NZB $\times$ NZW)F_1 hybrid, a single dose of gene A also results in only moderate generalized autoimmunity such as anti-erythrocyte autoantibody, with the exception of autoantibody production under the influence of gene G as well as gene A. Hence, the combined action of A and G results in more severe kidney disease than in either parent. The allele

TABLE VI

Proposed Genetic Loci Involved in the Pathogenesis of Autoimmunity in NZ Mice[a]

	Proposed loci		
Strain	Autoimmunity (generalized)	Predisposition to anti-nuclear antibody	Modifying locus for autoimmunity
NZB	AA	gg	mm
NZW	aa	GG	MM
NZC	aa	gg	M^1M^1
"Normal" strains (wild type)	aa	gg	MM
(NZB × NZC)F_1	Aa	gg	M^1m
(NZB × NZW)F_1	Aa	Gg	Mm
(NZB × wild type)F_1	Aa	gg	Mm
NZB·ch N8	AA	gg	M^1M^1

[a] Mutant gene A is associated with generalized autoimmunity and is susceptible (in its effect) to inhibition by gene M. Mutant gene m is ineffective in inhibition, and M^1 is only weakly effective. Mutant gene G is specifically associated with immune complex kidney disease. In the presence of A, gene G has a greater effect on kidney disease. See text for full description. Note, data on immunologic tolerance (Section III,D) might suggest that genotype of NZW mice is AA/GG/MM.

possessed by NZW at the modifying locus cannot be determined and is not particularly relevant. Some data on Coombs' incidence (Ghaffar and Playfair, 1971) would suggest it is the normal M allele. NZB mice possess a defective allele m, which does not have any modifying or suppressive influence. NZC mice, however, have a third allele (M_1) that is weakly effective, and results in only a minimal suppression of the effect of gene A (in NZB × NZC)F_1 hybrids). However, when a double dose of this particular gene is introduced to NZB mice (as in NZB·ch N8 F_2 if it is assumed that M_1 is linked to a gene determining the chocolate coat color), the effect of the A mutant gene is more strikingly weakened in its effect.

This scheme is clearly quite provisional and is under further analysis with other strain combinations.

III. IMMUNE RESPONSIVENESS OF NZ MOUSE STRAINS

Given that the pathogenesis of NZ autoimmune disease involves the action of several specific genes, it is then appropriate to determine the possible cellular level of expression of these genetic effects. In view of current theories suggesting an abnormal regulation of immune responsiveness, it is relevant to examine NZ mice for their responsiveness to various extrinsic antigens, both *in vivo* and *in vitro,* particularly in terms of susceptibility to tolerance versus immunity. This discussion thus, is, divided into four aspects, considering separately the precursor cells of the immune system, responses *in vivo* and *in vitro,* and immunologic tolerance.

A. Hematopoietic Stem Cells

On the basis of several studies indicating a hyperresponsiveness of NZB mice to sheep erythrocytes (see next section) it was proposed (Morton and Siegel, 1969) that these animals might possess an elevated number of hematopoietic stem cells, and that an enhanced opportunity for the triggering of autoantibody formation might result from this increased availability of potentially responsive target cells. Inferential evidence for elevated stem cell numbers was then shown by the extremely high resistance of young NZB mice to the lethal effects of acute exposure to ionizing radiation (Morton and Siegel, 1971). Direct analysis for stem cell activity by the endogenous spleen colony-forming assay also revealed an elevated stem cell number in NZB mice (Warner and Moore, 1971). Elevated numbers of endogenous stem cells were also found in the NZC strain, but not in NZW or NZO mice. This abnormality was shown to be controlled by a single autosomal recessive gene that is not linked to coat color, agouti, H-2, or Ig-1 loci, nor to the gene controlling hydronephrosis in NZC mice. However, no evidence was found for a significant association between endogenous stem cell hyperactivity and autoimmune hemolytic anemia (Warner and Moore, 1971). At present it must, therefore, be concluded that NZB and NZC mice have derived from the original random colony, a common mutant gene affecting hematopoiesis that is not, involved however, in autoimmunity. NZC mice were also shown (Warner and Moore, 1971) to have a second genetically controlled defect involving the microenvironmental influence that controls the differentiation of transplanted stem cells. This defect was not found, however, in NZB mice.

B. Immune Response *in Vivo* to Extrinsic Antigens

Despite initial controversy, it is now clearly established that NZB mice produce excessive antibody responses to some, but not all, extrinsic antigens. This subject has been extensively reviewed elsewhere (Talal, 1975) and lists the original studies on this aspect. In this discussion, which emphasizes genetic aspects, a few points are relevant. Hyperresponsiveness is not restricted to a single antigen and is possibly reflected in a persistent elevated serum IgM level detected early in life (Warner and Wistar, 1968). However, this hyperresponsiveness does not persist throughout life, and aging NZB and (NZB × NZW)F_1 hybrid mice tend to be hyporesponsive (Diener, 1966; Salomon and Benveniste, 1969). Of particular relevance, however, is the finding that this hyperresponsiveness does not extend to all antigens (Cerottini *et al.*, 1969), and it was accordingly concluded that an important aspect concerning disease pathogenesis might be a hyperactivity to certain autoantigens. This aspect has been investigated both for anti-erythrocyte antibody production and for anti-nuclear antibodies.

Anti-nuclear antibodies can be readily induced in young (NZB × NZW)F_1 hybrids, long before the natural occurrence of such antibodies, using as immunogen heat-denatured DNA coupled to methylated BSA (Lambert and Dixon, 1970). Antibody responses were found in many strains, but the highest levels occurred in (NZB × NZW)F_1 hybrids. A genetic basis for this was found in studies of parental strains. Thus, whereas inbred NZB mice were poor responders, the inbred NZW strain was as good a responder as the (NZB × NZW)F_1 hybrid. These data therefore, are, compatible with the genetic model in Table VI and suggest that gene G is involved in a hyperresponse to nucleic acid antigens. However, in view of the marked heterogeneity of anti-viral and anti-host nucleic acid antibodies found in the spontaneous production of anti-nuclear antibodies (Talal *et al.*, 1971; Dixon *et al.*, 1974; Talal, 1975), the relevance of this experimentally demonstrated hyperreactivity of NZW mice to the natural disease process is still to clearly demonstrated.

Studies on the nature of the response to autologous (Linder and Edgington, 1972) and heterologous red cell antigens have also inferred that aberrant maturational characteristics of the response are found in NZB mice (DeHeer and Edgington, 1975). These data suggest either that a defect is intrinsic to the B lymphocytes to NZB mice or that a defect may operate at the level of macrophages, which play an important role in anti-erythrocyte antibody responses and which may influence affinity of the antibody responses. Evidence for a macrophage defect in NZB and NZC mice has been obtained and is discussed in Section III,C. The possible contribution from NZW mice of genetic factors predisposing to anti-nuclear antibody production is mirrored, to a certain extent, in the susceptibility of NZC mice to develop Coombs'-positive autoantibodies on immunization with heterologous mouse erythrocytes given in adjuvant (Warner, 1973). Although this response is not confined solely to the NZC strain, it may reflect a genetic contribution from NZC mice that is relevant to the high natural Coombs' incidence in the (NZB × NZC)F_1 hybrid.

It has been concluded (Talal, 1975) that the immunologic function of NZ mice is best characterized as an imbalance in which B cell activity tends to be excessive and T cell activity tends to be depressed. In considering levels of genetic control, it is, thus, likely that the B cell abnormalities could reflect either an inherent gene action expressed in B cells, or, be a reflection of a T cell-expressed gene that results in an imbalance in the T cell control of B cell activity (Hoffman, 1975). In view of the evidence for decreased suppressor T cell function in NZB mice (see Talal, 1975; and Chapter 7), it might be provisionally concluded that gene A (Table VI) is expressed in one of the cellular elements involved in the T cell-dependent suppressor regulatory mechanism (see Section III,D).

C. *In Vitro* Responsiveness

In striking contrast to the universal demonstration of NZB hyperresponsiveness *in vivo* to sheep erythrocyte antigens, *in vitro* initiated antibody responses to the same antigens are considerably depressed in NZB mice, relative to many other normal strains (Rollinghoff and Warner, 1973; McCombs *et al.*, 1974, 1975). Detailed analysis of the cellular basis of the immune depression in NZB mice has shown (McCombs *et al.*, 1974, 1975) a possible functional deficiency of splenic adherent cells from unprimed NZB mice. This deficiency may be limited to splenic adherent cells, i.e., to a subpopulation of macrophages. Hence, studies on the general phagocytic activity of NZB mice might not detect this functional deficiency in the particular subpopulation. Of the few studies reported on phagocytic activity of NZB-derived macrophages, most have shown elevated activity in terms of antigen clearance (Braverman and Slesinski, 1970; Thomas and Weir, 1972), although some data suggests that the cells from NZB mice are relatively unable to degrade the ingested antigen (Thomas and Weir, 1972). Two aspects of this problem are particularly relevant to genetic control of autoimmunity and concern whether genes A or m (Table VI) might be involved.

Is this functional defect under genetic control, and if so is it linked to any other abnormality of the NZ mice? In a series of recent studies, we have observed a similar functional deficiency in the spleen cells of young NZC mice (Herrod and Warner, 1972; Crewther *et al.*, 1977). Briefly summarized, the findings in NZC mice closely parallel those in NZB mice, and are as follows:

i. The *in vitro* response of NZC spleen cells to sheep erythrocytes, as measured by the generation of plaque-forming cells, is approximately 10% that of normal mouse spleen cells (Table VII).

TABLE VII

In Vitro Response of Spleen Cells to Sheep Erythrocytes[a]

Strain of spleen cells	No. of spleen cell pools tested	Plaque-forming cell response[b]	
		Mean PFC + SE	Control (%)
Normal[c]	22	2690 ± 580	100
NZC	13	260 ± 50	10
NZB	5	1212 ± 229	45
NZC F_1 hybrids[d]	23	750 ± 250	28

[a] Data from Crewther *et al.* (1977).

[b] Values show mean plaque-forming cells per culture. Normal spleen cell response is termed 100% for relative values.

[c] Normal strains include BALB/c, CBA, C3H, BRVR, and (NZB × C57BL)F_1 hybrids.

[d] NZC F_1 hybrids of NZC with NZB, CBA, and BRVR. (Values for all three hybrids were quite similar.)

ii. This defect is observed with several erythrocyte antigens, including sheep, horse, and donkey erythrocytes, although *in vitro* responses to DNP–flagellin and to allogeneic histocompatibility antigens are normal.

iii. Mitogen-induced T or B cell proliferative responses of NZC mice are either normal or slightly elevated, as compared to normal strains.

iv. The functional defect to sheep erythrocyte antigens can be considerably corrected by the addition of 2-mercaptoethanol to the *in vitro* culture.

v. Genetic analysis is still in progress, but current evidence shows that this defect is expressed in F_1 hybrids of NZC with normal strains (Table VII), but not to as great a degree as in the homozygous state. The data suggest that a single dose of this gene (if a single gene is involved) can have a definite effect.

In view of the uniqueness of the (NZB × NZC)F_1 hybrid regarding Coombs' incidence, it is essential to determine whether this *in vitro* functional defect of macrophages, common to NZB and NZC, might be involved in the autoantibody production, and, thus, indicate a possible macrophage level of expression of genes m and M^1.

Functional deficiencies in the activity of certain macrophage subpopulations may also have bearing on general regulation aspects of immune responses. In the above discussions, it has been inferred that gene A (Table VI) may be expressed in T cell-dependent suppression mechanisms. This need not imply a T cell expression of gene A, as it has been shown that an adherent, possibly non-T cell population, can play a cooperative role in suppression, in combination with T cell subpopulations (Basten *et al.*, 1975). Further analysis with these experimental systems, using defined NZB or NZC subpopulations, may assist in identifying the cellular level of action of these genes.

D. Immunologic Tolerance

If autoimmune disease basically represents a loss of tolerance to self-antigens, it might be expected that attempts to induce immunologic tolerance to extrinsic antigens would be relatively unsuccessful. Many laboratories have studied the susceptibility of NZB mice to tolerance induction with a range of antigens, and this subject is extensively reviewed elsewhere (Talal and Steinberg, 1974; Talal, 1975; Chapter 7). Several general conclusions relevant to genetic aspects might be stressed here. NZB mice older than 6 weeks are less susceptible to tolerance induction to several heterologous γ-globulins than normal mouse strains, although tolerance can be induced in these mice under certain conditions. The variability reported in the literature on susceptibility to tolerance induction (Weir *et al.*, 1968; Staples and Talal, 1969; Cerottini *et al.*, 1969; Braverman and Slesinski, 1970; Playfair, 1971; Talal, 1975; Warner, 1975) may be explained in terms of tolerance activation representing one side of a delicate balance between immunity and tolerance. Many factors relating to antigen presentation may alter the balance, thus producing tolerance in some studies and not in others. In general, susceptibility to tolerance at the B cell level appears to be quite normal in NZB mice (Purves and Playfair, 1973), and this relative resistance to tolerance in NZB mice may only involve tolerance induction where suppressor T cell activation is involved. This latter type includes tolerance to heterologous γ-globulin (Basten *et al.*, 1975), an antigen not grossly dissimilar from certain self-autoantigens. Hence, much of the current interest in NZB autoimmune pathogenesis centers on the evidence of a relative inefficiency of the T cell-dependent suppressor mechanism (Talal and Steinberg, 1974; Talal, 1975), and this, in turn, leads to the question of whether genetic controls operate in this system.

Several recent studies have demonstrated that the relative resistance to tolerance induction of certain mouse strains is under genetic control (Fujiwara and Cinader, 1974; Warner, 1975). NZB is not the only strain to show relative resistance to tolerance, as SJL and BALB/c (Staples and Talal, 1969; Staples *et al.*, 1970; Fujiwara and Cinader, 1974) are considerably more resistant to tolerance induction than many other normal mouse strains. It must be stressed again, however, that this is relative, not absolute, and can only be demonstrated under certain defined conditions of tolerance induction. Few data on this aspect are available on other inbred NZ strains. Under conditions where NZB mice are resistant to tolerance induction to human γ-globulin, NZC mice are readily made tolerant (S. Wallis and N. L. Warner, unpublished observations). However, NZW mice, like NZB, are resistant to tolerance induction (Braverman and Slesinski, 1970).

In attempting to analyze the number of possible genes involved in tolerance susceptibility, a similar problem is encountered as in genetic analysis of autoimmunity; namely, that only relative differences exist, not "all-or-none" situations. However, with the reservation that the conditions for inducing tolerance are critical, genetic analysis can be made, using a dose of deaggregated γ-globulin that distinguishes NZB (resistant) from normal strains (susceptible). Under these conditions, tolerance induction appears to involve the action of a single genetic locus (Fujiwara and Cinader, 1974; Warner, 1975). However, in one study, the trait for resistance to tolerance induction appeared to be dominant (Fujiwara and Cinader, 1974), whereas, in the other study, it seemed to be recessive (Warner, 1975; Wallis and Warner, 1977). Although further analysis is still proceeding, this again appears to be a situation where gene dose effects are involved, and, like the genetics of autoimmune disease, the influence of the NZB gene can be modified by genes from the other parent. An example of this is summarized in Table VIII. When the conditions of tolerogen treatment are such that NZB and the (NZB $\times$ NZW)F_1 hybrid are the only fully resistant strains (strong deaggregating conditions), SJL is partially resistant, whereas other strains including BALB/c, are rendered tolerant. A similar hierachy in tolerance susceptibility is observed in the F_1 hybrids. However, when tolerogen conditions are such that BALB/c is now partially resistant, the F_1 hybrids are now fully resistant. Thus, the apparent dominance of the trait for resistance to tolerance induction is only seen when acting in concert with genes from the other parental strain. It is yet to be determined whether independent loci are involved, or whether multiple alleles exist for this "tolerance resistance locus."

Linkage studies in this study have not shown a significant association to immunoglobulin allotype (Fujiwara and Cinader, 1974; S. Wallis and N. L. Warner, unpublished), to the C5 locus (Fujiwara and Cinader, 1974), or to the H-2 locus (S. Wallis and N. L. Warner, unpublished). However, if these studies on genetic control of the tolerance mechanism to extrinsic antigens represent the action of the same genes that are involved in autoimmunity, then linkage between these two phenomena should be shown, and investigations on this aspect are in progress. If such a linkage was found, it might suggest involvement of gene A (Table VI). However, in view of the

TABLE VIII

Tolerance Induction to Human γ-Globulin[a]

Strain	Tolerogen deaggregation[b]	Susceptibility to tolerance induction[c]
NZB	Strong	Fully resistant
SJL	Strong	Partially resistant
BALB/c	Strong	Susceptible
"Normal" (N)	Strong	Susceptible
(NZB × NZW)F_1	Strong	Fully resistant
(NZB × SJL)F_1	Strong	Predominantly resistant
(NZB × BALB/c)F_1	Strong	Partially resistant
(NZB × N)F_1	Strong	Susceptible
NZB	Moderate	Fully resistant
BALB/c	Moderate	Partially resistant
"Normal" (N)	Moderate	Susceptible
(NZB × BALB/c)F_1	Moderate	Fully resistant
(NZB × N)F_1	Moderate	Fully resistant

[a] Data of Wallis and Warner (1977).

[b] Human γ-globulin (HGG) preparations were deaggregated by ultracentrifugation for either 2.5 hours at 100,000 *g* (strong) or for 0.5 hours at 100,000 *g* (moderate). All test mice (2–3 months old) were then given 2.5 ng of deaggregated HGG and challenged 3 weeks later with 50 μg of HGG given in complete Freund's adjuvant. Control mice did not receive the first injection. All animals were subsequently bled and anti-HGG antibody levels determined by radioimmunoassay.

[c] The status of the mice given the tolerizing injection relative to controls is summarized. Fully resistant animals produced antibody levels similar to control (nontolerogen injected) mice. Susceptible animals were tolerized, and did not produce antibodies after challenge.

tolerance data with NZW and (NZB × NZW)F_1, it might also suggest that the NZW genotype is AA/GG/MM, with the potential effect of the A gene being normally countered by the M gene.

IV. GENETIC CONTROL IN OTHER AUTOIMMUNE DISEASES

Animal models of autoimmune disease include both those occurring spontaneously and those that are induced experimentally in recipients by the administration of autologous or heterologous tissue antigens. In the light of the extensive analysis of the mechanisms of immune response (Ir) gene control of "normal" antibody production and cellular immunity (McDevitt and Landy, 1973; Benacerraf and Katz, 1975; Shreffler and Chella, 1975; Klein,

1975), it must be determined whether immune responses to autoantigens may be subject to similar genetic controls (see Chapter 1). In the mouse, interest in the possible role of major histocompatibility-linked (MHC) Ir genes in disease susceptibility was initially based on studies of MHC control of susceptibility to Gross-virus-induced leukemogenesis (Lilly, 1968). Other studies have also shown MHC-linked control of susceptibility to LCM infection (Oldstone *et al.*, 1973), a disease process somewhat analogous to autoimmunity, in that a dominant controlled gene determines the ability of lymphocytes to respond to viral antigens and, thus, induce the disease. Similarly, in Marek's disease of chickens, the MHC (B locus) has been shown to control resistance to the disease (Stone *et al.*, 1970; Pazderka *et al.*, 1975). The pathogenesis of Marek's disease is complex and involves both a herpes-type virus and other, possibly immunologic factors. One concept of this disease (Rouse *et al.*, 1973; Rouse and Warner, 1974) is that (as in LCM infection) an autoimmune type of process may be involved, in which T lymphocytes are specifically reacting to cell-surface viral antigens. In susceptible lines of birds, a B locus-linked suppressor mechanism may fail to control T cell proliferation, resulting in either a chronic proliferative disease, or in frank T cell neoplasia. In view of the possible role of viral agents in "spontaneous" autoimmunity, these reports suggest a possible level of gene action and may parallel the responder status of NZW mice to nucleic acid antigens. This comparison would also predict that hyperresponsiveness to nucleic acid antigens in NZW mice might be MHC linked.

Evidence of genetic control in autoimmunity has not been limited to viral-associated or spontaneous conditions. A striking correlation has also been shown in mice between the MHC region and susceptibility to induced experimental autoimmune thyroiditis (Vladutin and Rose, 1971; Rose *et al.*, 1973), and to experimental autoimmune encephalomyelitis (Bernard, 1976). In this latter instance, disease susceptibility and cell-mediated responses to the relevant autoantigen were shown to be controlled by a gene located at the K end of the MHC, i.e., near the known Ir gene region. The studies on experimentally induced thyroiditis in mice are also comparable to the demonstration in chickens of a B locus (MHC) linkage (Rose *et al.*, 1973) for spontaneous thyroiditis, thus providing a genetic analogy between the spontaneous and induced autoimmune disease models.

Thus, from all types of animal models of autoimmune disease, evidence for the involvement of genetic factors in pathogenesis may be found. Does this also apply to autoimmunity in man? Clustering of certain autoimmune diseases and of associated autoantibodies has been observed within families, principally for diseases of thyroid gland and stomach (Doniach *et al.*, 1965). Several examples of concordance of autoimmune thyroid disease in monozygous twins have also been noted (Mitchell and Lawson, 1973), and similar clustering occurs for autoantibody activities and γ-globulin levels in association with Waldenström's macroglobulinemia (Seligman *et al.*, 1967). These associations may imply that these diseases involve a specific genetic defect, perhaps in relation to the regulation of immune tolerance to a limited group of autoantigens. In view of the experimental studies on Ir genes in animals, much of the current interest in relation to human autoimmune disease susceptibility has centered on possible HLA association. Considerable controversy is evident in this field and may only be resolved when the human Ir genes are better defined. Recent studies have suggested that the LD defined loci may be this equivalent, proposed to be called HL-B (Winchester *et al.*, 1975). Analysis of HLA or LD antigen frequencies in patients with autoimmune disease has shown an association for some, but not all, diseases, and this topic has been reviewed extensively elsewhere (Morris, 1974; Dausset *et al.*, 1974; Mackay *et al.*, 1976; and in Chapter 1). Although no significant deviation from the expected frequency of HLA antigens was found in patients with autoimmune hemolytic anemia or idiopathic thrombocytophenic purpura (Dausset and Hors, 1975), an increased frequency of HLA-8 has been found in myasthenia gravis, chronic autoimmune hepatitis (Mackay and Morris, 1972; Svejgaard *et al.*, 1975), idiopathic Addison's disease, juvenile diabetes, and Graves disease (Thomsen *et al.*, 1975; Whittingham *et al.*,1975a). The association with Addison's disease was more pronounced with the LD-8a determinant, consistent with the suggestion that this marker may be the Ir equivalent. However, despite the observation in both mice and chickens of an MHC association with thyroiditis, no HLA association with Hashimoto's disease was observed (Whittingham *et al.*, 1975b). It was also noted in this latter study, that where associations have been found to exist between autoimmunity and HLA, it does not necessarily involve a specific autoantibody, but rather the disease in general.

Thus, at the present time, the limited data on human autoimmunity might be considered to be consistent with the general concepts expressed earlier in this article (Section II,B,3), given that a noninbred population is at issue. By analogy, if random breeding were to be made with a combination of NZB, NZC, NZW, and normal mice, a low but significant incidence of autoimmunity would be expected, and would be of varying severity and involve different types of autoimmune expression. Some familial clustering would be evident, and linkage of certain autoimmune manifestations to the MHC might be found. However, to start with the progeny of such a random breeding would make the task of discerning a possible genetic control of autoimmunity a most formidable task. Such is the situation with human autoimmunity.

V. CONCLUSIONS

Analysis of the inheritance of autoimmune manifestations in various inbred and hybrid lines of mice has clearly demonstrated that specific genes play an essential role in the pathogenesis of the disease. Although several genes are involved in the overall pattern of disease, there is good evidence for a major role by a single dominant locus that predisposes to generalized autoimmunity. The nature of the autoimmune process will, however, be influenced by other genes that can have a modifying effect on the function of the dominant "autoimmune" gene. The incidence, onset, and severity of any one autoimmune process is, thus, in part a reflection of gene dosage of this autoimmune locus and of the degree to which its influence has been modified by other genes. In certain instances, specific immune response genes may also be involved in determining the response to a specific autoantigen, or possibly a related group of autoantigens, including endogenous leukemia viruses. The cellular level of specific gene action in autoimmunity has yet to be fully determined, and available evidence suggests that a major genetic influence is expressed in cell types involved in determining the balance of regulation between tolerance and immunity.

REFERENCES

Allison, A. C. (1974). *Contemp. Top. Immunobiol.* **3,** 227.

Basten, A., Miller, J. F. A. P., and Johnson, P. (1975). *Transplant. Rev.* **26,** 130.

Benacerraf, B., and Katz, D. (1975). "Immunogenetics and Immunodeficiency," p. 117. M. T. P. Press.

Bernard, C. (1976). *J. Immunogenet.* **3,** 263.

Bielschowsky, M., and Bielschowsky, F. (1956). *Aust. J. Exp. Biol. Med. Sci.* **34,** 181.

Bielschowsky, M., and Bielschowsky, F. (1964). *Aust. J. Exp. Biol. Med. Sci.* **42,** 561.

Bielschowsky, M., and Goodall, C. M. (1970). *Cancer Res.* **30,** 834.

Bielschowsky, M., and Schofield, G. C. (1962). *Aust. J. Exp. Biol. Med. Sci.* **40,** 395.

Bielschowsky, M., Bielschowsky, F., and Lindsay, D. (1956). *Br. J. Cancer* **10,** 688.

Bielschowsky, M., Helyer, B. J., and Howie, J. B. (1959). *Proc. Univ. Otago Med. Sch.* **37,** 9.

Branca, M., de Petris, S., Allison, A. C., Harvey, J. J., and Hirsch, M. S. (1971). *Clin. Exp. Immunol.* **9,** 1853.

Braverman, I. M. (1968). *J. Invest. Dermatol.* **50,** 483.

Braverman, I. M., and Slesinski, J. (1968). *J. Invest. Dermatol.* **51,** 274.

Braverman, I. M., and Slesinski, J. (1970). *J. Invest. Dermatol.* **55,** 317.
Burnet, F. M., and Holmes, M. C. (1965a). *Australas. Ann. Med.* **14,** 185.
Burnet, F. M., and Holmes, M. C. (1965b). *Nature* (*London*) **207,** 368.
Cannat, A., and Varet, B. (1973). *Immunol. Commun.* **2,** 527.
Cerottini, J.-C., Lambert, P. H., and Dixon, F. J. (1969). *J. Exp. Med.* **130,** 1093.
Costea, N., Yakulis, V., and Heller, P. (1970). *Blood* **35,** 583.
Crewther, P., Rollinghoff, M., Wallis, S., and Warner, N. L. (1977). In preparation.
Dausset, J., and Hors, J. (1975). *Transplant. Rev.* **22,** 44.
Daussett, J., Degos, L., and Hors, J. (1974). *Clin. Immunol. Immunopathol.* **3,** 127.
DeHeer, D. H., and Edgington, T. S. (1975). *Cell. Immunol.* **19,** 183.
DeVries, J. M., and Hijmans, W. (1967). *Immunology* **12,** 179.
Diener, E. (1966). *Int. Arch. Allergy Appl. Immunol.* **30,** 120.
Dixon, F., Croker, B., Del Villano, B., Jensen, F., and Lerner, R. (1974). *Prog. Immunol., Int. Congr. Immunol., 2nd, 1974* **5,** 49.
Doniach, D., Roitt, I. M., and Taylor, K. B. (1965). *Ann. N.Y. Acad. Sci.* **24,** 605.
East, J. (1970). *Prog. Exp. Tumor Res.* **13,** 84.
East, J., and Harvey, J. J. (1971). *Immunopathol., Int. Symp., 6th, 1970,* 1971.
Friou, G. J., and Teague, P. O. (1963). *J. Lab. Clin. Med.* **62,** 875.
Fudenberg, H. H. (1971). *Am. J. Med.* **51,** 295.
Fujiwara, M., and Cinader, B. (1974). *Cell Immunol.* **12,** 214.
Ghaffar, A., and Playfair, J. H. L. (1971). *Clin. Exp. Immunol.* **8,** 479.
Hahn, B. H., and Shulman, L. E. (1969). *Arthritis Rheum.* **12,** 355.
Helyer, B. J., and Howie, J. B. (1961). *Prov. Univ. Otago Med. Sch.* **39,** 3.
Helyer, B. J., and Howie, J. B. (1963a). *Nature* (*London*) **197,** 197.
Helyer, B. J., and Howie, J. B. (1963b). *Br. J. Haematol.* **9,** 119.
Herrod, H. G., and Warner, N. L. (1972). *Proc. Soc. Exp. Biol. Med.* **140,** 1254.
Hicks, J. D. (1966). *J. Pathol. Bacteriol.* **91,** 479.
Hicks, J. D., and Burnet, F. M. (1966). *J. Pathol. Bacteriol.* **91,** 467.
Hoffman, G. W. (1975). *Eur. J. Immunol.* **5,** 638.
Holborow, E. J., Barnes, R. D. S., and Tuffrey, M. (1965). *Nature* (*London*) **207,** 601.
Holmes, M. C., and Burnet, F. M. (1963). *Ann. Intern. Med.* **59,** 265.
Holmes, M. C., and Burnet, F. M. (1964). *Heredity* **19,** 419.
Holmes, M. C., and Burnet, F. M. (1966). *Aust. J. Exp. Biol. Med. Sci.* **44,** 235.
Howie, J. B., and Helyer, B. J. (1965). *Ann. N.Y. Acad. Sci.* **124,** 167.
Howie, J. B., and Helyer, B. J. (1968). *Adv. Immunol.* **9,** 215.
Klein, J. (1975). "Biology of the Mouse Histocompatibility-2 Complex." Springer-Verlag, Berlin and New York.
Lambert, P. M., and Dixon, F. J. (1968). *J. Exp. Med.* **127,** 507.
Lambert, P. H., and Dixon, F. J. (1970). *Clin. Exp. Immunol.* **6,** 829.
Lilly, F. (1968). *J. Exp. Med.* **127,** 465.
Linder, E., and Edgington, T. S. (1972). *J. Immunol.* **108,** 1615.
Lindsey, E. S., Donaldson, G. W., and Woodruff, M. F. A. (1966). *Clin. Exp. Immunol.* **1,** 85.

Long, G., Holmes, M. C., and Burnet, F. M. (1963). *Aust. J. Exp. Biol. Med. Sci.* **41,** 315.

McCombs, C., Hom, J., Talal, N., and Mishell, R. I. (1974). *J. Immunol.* **112,** 326.

McCombs, C., Hom, J., Talal, N., and Mishell, R. I. (1975). *J. Immunol.* **115,** 1695.

McDevitt, H. O., and Landy, M., eds. (1973). "Genetic Control of Immune Responsiveness." Academic Press, New York.

Mackay, I. R., and Morris, P. J. (1972). *Lancet* **2,** 793.

Mackay, I. R., Whittingham, S., and Tait, B. (1977). *Vox Sang.* **32,** 10.

Mellors, R. C. (1965). *J. Exp. Med.* **122,** 25.

Mellors, R. C. (1966). *Int. Rev. Exp. Pathol.* **5,** 217.

Mellors, R. C., Aoki, T., and Huebner, R. J. (1969). *J. Exp. Med.* **129,** 1045.

Mellors, R. C., Shirai, T., Aoki, T., Huebner, R. J., and Kruweyznski, K. (1971). *J. Exp. Med.* **133,** 113.

Mitchell, I., and Lawson, A. A. H. (1973). *Postgrad. Med. J.* **49,** 107.

Morris, P. J. (1974). *Contemp. Top. Immunobiol.* **3,** 141.

Morton, J. I., and Siegel, B. V. (1969). *J. Reticuloendothel. Soc.* **6,** 78.

Morton, J. I., and Siegel, B. V. (1971). *Proc. Natl. Acad. Sci. U.S.A.* **68,** 124.

Norins, L., and Holmes, M. C. (1964). *J. Immunol.* **93,** 148.

Oldstone, M. B. A., Tishon, T., Tonietti, G., and Dixon, F. J. (1972). *Clin. Immunol. Immunopathol.* **1,** 6.

Oldstone, M. B. A., Dixon, F. J., Mitchell, G. F., and McDevitt, H. O. (1973). *J. Exp. Med.* **137,** 1201.

Pazderka, F., Longenecker, B. M., Law, G. R. J., Stone, H. A., and Rush, R. F. (1975). *Immunogenetics* **2,** 93.

Playfair, J. H. L. (1971). *Immunology* **21,** 1037.

Porter, D. D., Porter, H. G., and Cox, N. A. (1973). *J. Immunol.* **111,** 1626.

Purves, E. C., and Playfair, J. H. L. (1973). *Clin. Exp. Immunol.* **15,** 113.

Rappaport, H., Bielschowsky, M., D'Ath, E. F., and Goodall, C. M. (1971). *Cancer Res.* **31,** 2047.

Richer, L., Tanaka, T., Sykes, B. A., Yumoto, T., Seman, G., Young, L., and Domchowski, L. (1966). *Natl. Cancer Inst., Monog.* **22,** 459.

Rollinghoff, M., and Warner, N. L. (1973). *Proc. Soc. Exp. Biol. Med.* **142,** 621.

Rose, N. R., Kite, J. H., Vlodutin, A. O., Tomazie, V. T., and Bacon, L. O. (1973). *Int. Arch. Allergy Appl. Immunol.* **45,** 138.

Rouse, B. T., and Warner, N. L. (1974). *J. Immunol.* **113,** 904.

Rouse, B. T., Wells, R. J. H., and Warner, N. L. (1973). *J. Immunol.* **110,** 534.

Salomon, J.-C., and Benveniste, J. (1969). *Clin. Exp. Immunol.* **4,** 213.

Seligman, M., Damon, F., Mihaesco, C., and Fudenberg, H. H. (1967). *Am. J. Med.* **43,** 66.

Shreffler, D. C., and Chella, D. S. (1975). *Adv. Immunol.* **20,** 125.

Siegel, B. V., Brown, M., and Morton, J. I. (1972). *Immunology* **22,** 457.

Staples, P. J., and Talal, N. (1969). *J. Exp. Med.* **129,** 123.

Staples, P. J., Steinberg, A. D., and Talal, N. (1970). *J. Exp. Med.* **131,** 1123.

Steinberg, A. D., Pincus, T., and Talal, N. (1969). *J. Immunol.* **102,** 788.
Stone, H. A., Rolly, E. A., Burmeister, B. R., and Coleman, T. H. (1970). *Poult. Sci.* **49,** 1441.
Sugai, S., Pillarisetty, R., and Talal, N. (1973). *J. Exp. Med.* **138,** 989.
Svejgaard, A., Platz, P., Ryder, L. P., Nelson, L. S., and Thomsen, M. (1975). *Transplant. Rev.* **22,** 3.
Talal, N. (1975). *Prog. Clin. Immunol.* **2,** 101.
Talal, N., and Steinberg, A. D. (1974). *Curr. Top. Microbiol. Immunol.* **64,** 79.
Talal, N., Steinberg, A. D., and Daley, G. G. (1971). *J. Clin. Invest.* **50,** 1248.
Thomas, H. I., and Weir, D. M. (1972). *Clin. Exp. Immunol.* **12,** 263.
Thomsen, M., Platz, P., Anderson, O. O., Christy, M., Lyngsoe, J., Nerup, J., Rasmussen, K., Ryder, L. P., Nielsen, L. S., and Svejgard, A. (1975). *Transplant. Rev.* **22,** 125.
Tonietti, G., Oldstone, M. B. A., and Dixon, F. J. (1970). *J. Exp. Med.* **132,** 89.
Vladutin, A. O., and Rose, N. R. (1971). *Science* **174,** 1137.
Wallis, S., and Warner, N. L. (1977). In preparation.
Warner, N. L. (1971). *Aust. J. Exp. Biol. Med. Sci.* **49,** 477.
Warner, N. L. (1973). *Clin. Immunol. Immunopathol.* **1,** 353.
Warner, N. L. (1974). *Clin. Immunol. Immunopathol.* **2,** 556.
Warner, N. L. (1975). *Immunogenetics* **2,** 1.
Warner, N. L., and Moore, M. A. S. (1971). *J. Exp. Med.* **134,** 313.
Warner, N. L., and Wistar, R. (1968). *J. Exp. Med.* **127,** 169.
Weir, D. M., McBride, W., and Naysmith, J. O. (1968). *Nature (London)* **219,** 1276.
Whittingham, S., Morris, P. J., and Martin, F.-I.R. (1975a). *Tissue Antigens* **6,** 23.
Whittingham, S., Youngchaiyud, U., Mackay, I. R., Buckley, J. D., and Morris, P. S. (1975b). *Clin. Exp. Immunol.* **19,** 289.
Winchester, R. J., Fu, S. M., Wernet, P., Kunhel, H. G., Dupont, B., and Jersila, C. (1975). *J. Exp. Med.* **141,** 924.
Wynn Williams, A., Howie, J. B. Helyer, B. J., and Simpson, L. O. (1967). *Aust. J. Exp. Biol. Med.* **45,** 105.
Zeleznick, L. D., Holm, M. S., and Barnett, E. V. (1969). *Proc. Soc. Exp. Biol. Med.* **131,** 716.

Chapter 3

Genetic Regulation in Autoimmune Thyroiditis

N. R. ROSE, L. D. BACON, R. S. SUNDICK, Y. M. KONG, P. ESQUIVEL, AND P. E. BIGAZZI

I. HUMAN THYROID DISEASE

A. Inheritance of Thyroid Autoimmunity

Scientific advances often follow the intuition of astute clinicians. Physicians caring for patients with thyroid disorders frequently commented that these diseases seem to "run in families" (Kitchin and Evans, 1960). Soon after the realization in the middle 1950's that some forms of thyroid disease are based on an autoimmune response, these clinical observations were affirmed in a more objective manner. Hall and his associates (1960) pointed out the marked familial clustering of thyroid disease. In certain family groups, they found a high incidence of the thyroid diseases such as chronic lymphocytic thyroiditis, primary adult myxedema, and thyrotoxicosis in close association with an autoimmune response. They proposed that there is a hereditary tendency to develop an autoimmune reaction to thyroid antigens.

Hall (1962) and Hall and Stanbury (1967) went further to point out that even clinically euthyroid relatives of patients with chronic thyroiditis, myxedema, or thyrotoxicosis due to Graves' disease have antibodies to thyroglobulin or other thyroid antigens much more frequently than age and sex-matched controls. Other clinicians were able to confirm Hall's figures (Bastenie and Ermans, 1972). However, this type of investigation is subject to several forms of statistical bias (Masi *et al.*, 1965). Roitt and Doniach (1967) critically evaluated their own earlier studies by eliminating any relatives who had clinically evident thyroid disease. They found that 45% of euthyroid female relatives of patients with thyroiditis or myxedema had one of the thyroid autoantibodies and 32% of euthyroid male relatives were positive. In contrast, controls matched for age and sex gave only 12–14% positive reactions. These carefully controlled seroepidemiologic studies clearly demonstrated that the predisposition to form autoantibodies to thyroid antigens is familial, even where no thyroid disease is evident.

B. Inheritance of Thyroid Defects

In some family groups, thyroid disorders that generally show no evidence of an autoimmune response, including simple and nodular goiters, are also associated with autoimmune thyroid disease (Kitchin and Evans, 1960). This observation suggests that individuals with various forms of thyroid disease share some fundamental hereditary defects in their thyroid glands.

C. Inheritance of Other Autoimmunities

Many physicians have noticed an extraordinarily high incidence of pernicious anemia and atrophic gastritis in patients who have autoimmune thyroid disease. Irvine (1965) and Ardeman *et al.* (1960) substantiated these clinical observations by demonstrating a significantly heightened incidence of antibodies to thyroid antigens in relatives of individuals with pernicious anemia or atrophic gastritis. Conversely, relatives of patients with thyroiditis or myxedema have gastric or intrinsic factor antibodies considerably more frequently than matched controls. Similar but more distant associations have been found with idiopathic adrenal insufficiency

(Addison's disease), idiopathic parathyroid failure, and the juvenile onset or insulin-dependent form of diabetes mellitus (Blizzard *et al.*, 1963; Fialkow, 1969; Bottazzo *et al.*, 1974; MacCuish *et al.*, 1974). Thyroid autoantibodies are also found in a certain proportion of patients with Sjögren's syndrome (Block *et al.*, 1965). These clinical observations suggest that individuals with one form of organ-specific autoimmunity are prone to develop another, distinct autoimmune response.

D. Genetic Predisposition

There are cogent reasons for suggesting that these associations are hereditary, rather than infectious or environmental (Fialkow, 1969). Several instances of thyroiditis have now been reported in identical twins, more than in nonidentical twins (Irvine *et al.*, 1961; Zaino and Guerra, 1964). Thyroid autoimmunity is extraordinarily frequent in patients with chromosomal aberrations, especially trisomy 21 (Downs' syndrome), as well as in the mothers of such patients (Fialkow *et al.*, 1971).

Although some measure of genetic determination can be assumed in the development of autoimmune thyroiditis and related diseases, it is likely that this control is complex. One element is probably some abnormality in the structure and function of the thyroid gland itself. A second factor seems to be a greater tendency toward the development of an autoimmune response to thyroglobulin. Finally, there appears to be a propensity to express a variety of unrelated organ-specific autoimmune reactions, especially those affecting different endocrine glands. Each of these genetic factors may occur separately or in association. The simultaneous occurrence of two or three abnormalities in the same individual probably gives the greatest probability of autoimmune thyroid disease.

It must be kept in mind that the expression of these genetic properties may be indirect. For example, a gene may code for heightened susceptibility to a virus that is harbored by the thyroid, producing thyroid damage. On the other hand, exaggerated susceptibility of the thymus to the toxic effects of certain drugs or infectious agents may be responsible for a loss of ability to suppress self-reactive lymphocytes.

Investigations of genetic regulation in human populations are necessarily difficult. Fortunately, several spontaneously developing hereditary forms of thyroiditis are now recognized in experimental animals (Bigazzi and Rose, 1975). For example, some colonies of dogs and monkeys develop thyroiditis with great frequency. But the two best studied models of genetically determined thyroiditis are in the Buffalo strain (BUF) rat and the obese strain (OS) chicken. In addition, it is possible to induce thyroiditis by immunization with thyroglobulin. While all animal species thus far studied are more or less susceptible to this experimental disease, genetic studies are more readily performed in the mouse and, to a lesser extent, in the rat.

II. EXPERIMENTALLY INDUCED THYROIDITIS

A. Mice

Lymphocytic thyroiditis can be induced in mice by injection of crude mouse thyroid extract or purified mouse thyroglobulin, provided that it is given with a suitable adjuvant. Autoantibodies to thyroglobulin can also be demonstrated in the immunized animals. When strains of inbred mice were compared for their responsiveness to mouse thyroglobulin, marked differences were observed (Rose *et al.*, 1971b). Some strains of mice began to produce antibody to thyroglobulin promptly after injection so that positive hemagglutination reactions were found within a week. Titers rose to high levels. Thyroid lesions were severe in these animals, with marked infiltration of their glands by lymphocytes and macrophages, sometimes virtually obliterating the normal thyroid structure. In other strains of mice, the onset of antibody production was later, and titers never reached the same elevated levels as good responder mice. Moreover, these strains developed little or no mononuclear cell invasion of the thyroid. No significant difference between good responder and poor responder strains of mice was found in the cell-mediated immune response as measured by the macrophage disappearance reaction (Tomazic and Rose, 1977).

1. Association with H-2

Most mouse strains can be classified as good responders to thyroglobulin with severe thyroid lesions or poor responders with little or no disease. A few strains of mice must be considered intermediate in susceptibility to thyroiditis. Collating mouse strains according to response to thyroglobulin reveals a close association with H-2 type (Vladutiu and Rose, 1971). For instance, all mouse strains with haplotype H-2^q, H-2^s, or H-2^k are good responders; mouse strains with haplotype H-2^b or H-2^d are uniformly poor responders (Table I). This consistency is all the more surprising when one realizes that the responders or nonresponders sharing the same H-2 haplotype often differ in most other genetic properties. The small number of strains considered intermediate responders, such as H-2^a, are recombinants of H-2^k and H-2^d.

Tests of H-2 congenic strains have clearly associated responsiveness to thyroglobulin with the H-2 complex (Table II). Mice of strain A.SW/J(H-2)^s respond to thyroglobulin as well as does another H-2^s strain, SJL/J, and

TABLE I

Response of Mice to Mouse Thyroid Extract[a]

H-2 type	No. strains tested	Pathology index[b] $x \pm SE$	Antibody titer[c] $x \pm SE$
k	9	3.23 ± 0.21	12.74 ± 0.61
s	3	3.43 ± 0.20	12.73 ± 0.93
q	3	3.03 ± 0.23	12.77 ± 0.90
a	3	2.27 ± 0.33	8.10 ± 0.77
b	6	0.45 ± 0.18	6.82 ± 0.73
d	3	0.47 ± 0.13	7.10 ± 0.60

[a] Modified from Vladutiu and Rose (1971).

[b] The pathology index is expressed as the mean of an arbitrary grading scale from 0 (no infiltration) to 4 (severe infiltration).

[c] The antibody response is expressed as the mean $\log_2$ titer in a tanned cell hemagglutination test using erythrocytes coated with mouse thyroid extract.

differed significantly from their A/WySn (H-2^a) parental line. Similarly, C_3H SW/J (H-2^b) mice showed a significantly lower response than C_3H/HeJ (H-2^k) mice, being indistinguishable from another H-2^b strain, $C_{57}BL$/6J. Seeking further evidence of H-2 linkage, in collaboration with Dr. D. Shreffler and Dr. C. David, we mated good-responder and poor-responder mice. Generally, the response of the F_1 hybrids was equivalent to the good-responder parent. In the F_2 generation, responsiveness to thyroglobulin segregated, and all good responders were of the good-responder parental H-

TABLE II

Response of Congenic Mice to Mouse Thyroid Extract[a]

Strain	H-2 type	Pathology index $\bar{x} \pm SE$	Antibody titer $\bar{x} \pm SE$
C57BL/6J	b	0.5 ± 0.2	7.3 ± 0.9
C3H·SW/J	b	0.3 ± 0.1	6.9 ± 0.5
C3H/HeJ	k	3.3 ± 0.1	11.5 ± 0.5
SJL/J	s	3.4 ± 0.2	12.5 ± 1.4
A·SW/J	s	3.3 ± 0.3	13.2 ± 1.1
A/Wy Sn	a	2.7 ± 0.3	6.9 ± 0.4

[a] Modified from Vladutiu and Rose (1971).

TABLE III

Response of H-2 Recombinant Mice to Murine Thyroglobulin[a]

Strain	H-2 region K I S D	Pathology index $\bar{x} \pm$ SD	Antibody titer $\bar{x} \pm$ SD
C3H	K K K K	3.30 ± 0.1	11.5 ± 0.5
B10·BR	K K K K	3.30 ± 0.2	12.4 ± 0.7
C57BL/10	D D D D	0.45 ± 0.3	7.0 ± 0.6
A·AL	K K K D	2.50 ± 0.7	11.0 ± 0.7
B10·A	K K D D	2.65 ± 0.6	10.5 ± 0.7
B10·A(2R)	K K D B	2.75 ± 0.6	11.0 ± 1.0
C3H·OL	D D K K	0.10 ± 0.1	9.8 ± 1.4
C3H·OH	D D D K	0.12 ± 0.1	9.6 ± 0.7
B10·A(5R)	B B D D	0.44 ± 0.2	8.4 ± 0.9

[a] Taken in part from Tomazic *et al.* (1974).

2 type, while poor-responder progeny possessed the H-2 type of their poor-responder progenitor, indicating that thyroglobulin responsiveness is very closely linked to H-2.

2. *Intra-H-2 Recombinants*

The experiments just described permit us to conclude that genetic control of response to thyroglobulin is governed mainly by one or more genes located adjacent to, or within, the H-2 complex of the mouse. Using intra-H-2 recombinants, more precise localization was determined (Table III). All strains with poor-responder (H-2^b or H-2^d) genes at the K or I regions were poor responders to thyroglobulin. On the other hand, recombinants with H-2^k genes at the K and I-A regions were intermediate or good responders. These results suggested that a major gene controlling thyroglobulin responsiveness is located close to the K end of the H-2 complex. It is very likely found in the I-A region. The experiments further suggest that responsiveness in recombinants having the H-2^k haplotype at the K or I end may be modified by additional genes that may be found in other regions of the H-2 complex or even elsewhere in the murine haplotype. Some of these modifying genes seem to be important in determining the severity of thyroid lesions.

3. *Antibody Response Versus Lesions*

In most of the experiments described above, there is a general correlation between the responsiveness of the strain of mice to thyroglobulin as measured by the titer of autoantibodies and the severity of thyroiditis. Careful study of H-2 recombinants, however, brought out the fact that these two manifestations of the autoimmune response are not invariably correlated (Table III). An example of the dissociation of antibody response and autoimmune lesions is clearly illustrated with studies of the BSVS and BRVR mice (Table IV). From an original population maintained at The Rockefeller University, these two strains were selected for resistance and susceptibility to bacterial and viral infection. The two strains now differ genetically in several respects. Both strains responded equally to thyroglobulin, as assessed by production of antibody (Rose *et al.,* 1973). However, BSVS mice developed severe disease, while BRVR animals had only mild lesions. When their H-2 haplotypes were determined by Dr. David, it was found that BRVR mice were H-2^k, thus representing an exception to the usual good-responder status of H-2^k mice. BSVS mice are H-2^{t5}, probably representing an H-2 recombinant with H-2^s at the K end and H-2^d at the D end. These results again suggest strongly that genes outside of the K or I region modify the immunologic response to thyroglobulin with regard to severity of disease. It is noteworthy that hybrids of BSVS and BRVR mice were intermediate in susceptibility to thyroiditis, rather than being good responders, perhaps suggesting genetically controlled suppressor effects.

4. *Cellular Basis of Genetic Control*

It was next established that responsiveness to thyroglobulin is dependent upon the presence of thymus-derived (T) cells. These experiments were carried out by immunization of mice depleted of T cells (called "B" mice) produced by adult thymectomy and lethal irradiation, followed by reconstitution with bone marrow cells treated with anti-θ-serum and complement (Vladutiu and Rose, 1975). Genetically athymic (nu/nu) mice were also tested and compared with heterozygous (+/nu) and thymus-grafted mice. In both types of T cell-deficient mice, the injection of mouse thyroglobulin

TABLE IV

Comparison of BSVS and BRVR Mice[a]

Strain	H-2 type	Pathology index $\bar{x} \pm$ SE	Antibody titer $\bar{x} \pm$ SE
BSVS	H-2^{t5}	3.6 ± 0.3	12.5 ± 1.0
BRVR	H-2^k	0.8 ± 0.3	11.8 ± 0.9
(BSVS × BRVR)F_1		2.5 ± 0.4	11.5 ± 0.9

[a] Modified from Rose *et al.* (1973).

TABLE V

Cellular Basis of Genetic Control[a]

Strain	Treatment[b] (or genotype)	Pathology index $\bar{x} \pm$ SD	Antibody titer $\bar{x} \pm$ SD
RF	None	3.7 ± 0.1	12.8 ± 1.1
	TxX + (RF) B cells	0.1 ± 0.1	1.5 ± 1.0
	TxX + (RF) B + (RF) T cells	3.3 ± 0.4	9.8 ± 0.9
BALB/c	None	0.5 ± 0.2	7.8 ± 0.3
	TxX + (BALB/c) B cells	Neg.	Neg.
	TxX + (BALB/c) B + (BALB/c) T cells	0.5 ± 0.3	6.8 ± 1.9
BALB/c	+/nu	1.0 ± 0.3	9.4 ± 0.4
	nu/nu	Neg.	Neg.
	nu/nu + thymus graft	0.5 ± 0.3	2.3 ± 1.5
(RF × BALB/c)F_1	None	3.6 ± 0.2	11.3 ± 0.2
BALB/c	TxX + (BALB/c) B + (BALB/c) T cells	0.5 ± 0.2	6.8 ± 1.9
	TxX + (F_1) B	Neg.	Neg.
	TxX + (F_1) B + (F_1) T cells	2.9 ± 0.4	7.7 ± 1.0
	TxX + (BALB/c) B cells + (F_1) T cells	3.3 ± 0.2	8.0 ± 0.8
	Sham TxX + (BALB/c) B cells + (F_1) T cells	0.6 ± 0.3	6.0 ± 0.7

[a] Modified from Vladutiu and Rose (1975).
[b] Tx, thymectomy; X, irradiation.

with complete Freund's adjuvant failed to elicit any immunologic response (Table V).

Experiments were then carried out to determine the cellular basis of genetic control, taking advantage of the fact that F_1 hybrid mice between RF and BALB/c strains are good responders. Poor responder (BALB/c) mice were thymectomized, lethally irradiated, and restored with good [RF × BALB/c (F_1)] or poor (BALB/c) responder bone marrow cells and good- or poor-responder thymus cells. Mice reconstituted with good- or poor-responder marrow cells, but given thymus cells from the good-responder donor, invariably developed high titers of antibody and severe disease. On the other hand, recipients of poor-responder thymus cells developed poor responses to thyroglobulin. These experiments point out that T lymphocytes principally determine the vigor of response to thyroglobulin in the mouse.

In these experiments, T cells promoted both antibody formation and production of lesions. There is substantial evidence that T cells also serve to suppress autoimmune disease in the mouse, since neonatal thymectomy induces thyroiditis in susceptible strains (Kojima *et al.,* 1976). It is noteworthy that sham-thymectomized, irradiated recipients of responder T cells do not develop severe lesions, even though they produce antibody nearly as well as thymectomized recipients.

5. *H-2-Associated Differences in Thyroglobulins*

In the experiments described previously, thyroid extracts of thyroglobulin were prepared from noninbred mice or from a pool of mice of many inbred strains. Thyroglobulin preparations from individual strains of inbred mice were also tested, and significant differences were found. Thyroglobulin from H-2^k mice elicited stronger responses in terms of antibody titers and severity of lesions in either good responder or poor responder strains of mice. Thyroid extracts or thyroglobulin from H-2^d mice consistently evoked weaker responses. The comparison was repeated using antigen from congenic mice. As shown in Table VI, H-2^k thyroglobulin elicited greater responses in both responder and nonresponder mice than did H-2^d thyroglobulin. The basis for this H-2-controlled difference in the antigenicity of different thyroglobulin is not yet apparent. Although purified thyroglobulin does not contain any of the serologically detected H-2 antigen, it is possible that the histocompatibility locus codes for some antigenic determinant found on the thyroglobulin molecule. It is intriguing to relate such an antigenic determinant to the Burnet-Fenner (1949) theory of self-markers, a long-neglected concept that may have some validity if we assume that control of self-recognition is the basic function of the major histocompatibility complex.

6. *Adjuvants in Good- and Poor-Responder Strains*

In all of the mouse strains tested, mouse thyroglobulin must be injected with an adjuvant to elicit any immunologic response. Foreign thyroglobu-

TABLE VI

Response to Different Thyroglobulins[a]

Thyroglobulin (H-2 type)	Recipient (H-2 type)	Pathology index $\bar{x} \pm$ SD	Antibody titer $\bar{x} \pm$ SD
B10·D2 (d)	B10·D2 (d)	0.5 ± 0.3	9.2 ± 1.1
	B10·BR (k)	2.6 ± 0.8	11.3 ± 1.1
B10·BR (k)	B10·D2 (d)	0.9 ± 0.3	11.3 ± 1.0
	B10·BR (k)	3.8 ± 0.2	12.0 ± 0.9

[a] Modified from Tomazic and Rose (1976).

lins, such as rat and human, evoke responses to the injected thyroglobulin, and a subpopulation of antibodies reactive with mouse thyroglobulin is also formed (Rose *et al.*, 1971b; Tomazic and Rose, 1975). In all instances tested, the differences in response to heterologous thyroglobulins coincided with good and poor responsiveness to mouse thyroglobulin (Tomazic and Rose, 1976). This result is rather surprising in view of the commonly held belief that the antigenicity of foreign thyroglobulins is due to the presence on these thyroglobulin molecules of exogenous determinants which activate T cells capable of cooperating with B cells reactive with murine thyroglobulin. If such were the case, it is difficult to understand why genetic differences in the immune response to foreign thyroglobulins parallel those to murine thyroglobulin.

In the previous experiments, complete Freund's adjuvant was always employed. Incomplete adjuvant also induced production of autoantibodies to thyroglobulin. Like those induced by the complete adjuvant method, the antibodies were mercapthoethanol resistant. Although the final titer of antibodies produced using incomplete adjuvant is often comparable in titer to those of mice given complete adjuvant, no lesions were seen in their thyroids.

Several other types of adjuvants have been tested with mouse thyroglobulin (Esquivel *et al.*, 1977). Polyadenylic–polyuridylic acid [poly(A:U)] is known to potentiate antibody response and prevent experimentally induced tolerance (Capanna and Kong, 1974; Johnson, 1976). Its site of action was shown to be the thymus and T lymphocytes. Bacterial lipopolysaccharides also serve as immunopotentiators and overcome acquired immunologic tolerance. The mitogenic action of lipopolysaccharide (LPS) in the mouse is on the B cell (Coutinho and Moller, 1975). Its major adjuvant action is also believed to be directed to the B cell, although there is evidence that it may act through T cells (Allison and Davies, 1971). These two adjuvants were compared, using a good-responder strain, B10.BR, and a congenic poor responder, B10.D2. With LPS, good-responder mice developed mercaptoethanol-resistant antibody in titers comparable to those found in similar animals injected with thyroglobulin plus complete Freund's adjuvant (CFA) (Table VII). The animals also developed disease which, after 49 days, was as severe as that found in animals injected with CFA. When poly(A:U) was used as adjuvant in good-responder mice, moderate titers of mercaptoethanol-resistant antibody to thyroglobulin were produced, and the animals had significantly less infiltration of their thyroids. In poor-responder mice, LPS also induced production of mercaptoethanol-resistant antibody in lower titers. These animals had no thyroid infiltration. Poly(A:U) was ineffective in inducing lesions in poor-responder mice and very little antibody was found in their sera.

TABLE VII

Comparison of Adjuvants in Good Responder and Poor Responder Congenic Mice

Strain	Treatment[a]	Pathology index $\bar{x} \pm$ SE	Antibody titer $\bar{x} \pm$ SE
	Tg (no adjuvant)	0.1 ± 0.0	0.0
B10·BR	Tg + poly(A:U)	0.4 ± 0.1	5.7 ± 1.5
(H-2^k)	Tg + LPS	2.3 ± 0.3	14.0 ± 0.7
	Tg + CFA	2.0 ± 0.6	13.6 ± 0.3
	Tg (no adjuvant)	0.05 ± 0.0	0.0
B10·D2	Tg + poly(A:U)	0.08 ± 0.04	1.0 ± 1.0
(H-2^d)	Tg + LPS	0.0 ± 0.0	8.0 ± 1.8
	Tg + CFA	0.06 ± 0.0	11.8 ± 1.0

[a] Tg, thyroglobulin; poly(A:U), polyadenylic–polyuridylic acid; LPS, lipopolysaccharide; CFA, complete Freund's adjuvant.

The effects obtained with poly(A:U) as adjuvant are consistent with its action on T cells. Thus, good-responder strains developed lesions, while poor responders did not. Poly(A:U) was relatively ineffective when T cells specific for thyroglobulin were ineffective, as in poor-responder mice. In the case of LPS adjuvant, the genetically determined differences between strains were also evident. If one assumes that LPS acts only upon the B cells, perhaps as a nonspecific "second signal," these T-cell-based differences between strains are difficult to explain. It seems more likely that LPS adjuvant acts also with help of the T cells. Experimental evidence to support this supposition has come from two additional experiments. First, LPS was found to be inoperative as an adjuvant when thyroglobulin was given to homozygous nude (nu/nu) mice, in contrast to control heterozygous (+/nu) litter mates (Esquivel *et al.*, 1977). Secondly, thymectomized, irradiated good-responder mice restored with syngeneic bone marrow cells alone showed no response to injections of thyroglobulin plus LPS in contrast to similar animals restored with both bone marrow and thymic cell suspensions (Table VIII). It is clear that self-reactive B cells were not triggered directly *in vivo* by a nonspecific mitogenic stimulus.

7. *IR–TG*

The ability of the mouse to respond to thyroglobulin is at least partially controlled by a major gene included in the H-2 complex. It is very likely an immune response (Ir) gene and may tentatively be called "Ir–Tg" (Tomazic *et al.*, 1974). What is at stake, however, is not just recognition of thyroglob-

TABLE VIII

Effect of Lipopolysaccharide (LPS) in Immune Response to Thyroglobulin in "B" Mice[a]

Cells transferred	Injected with	Pathology index $\bar{x} \pm$ SE	Antibody titer $\bar{x} \pm$ SE
Bone marrow	Tg + LPS	negative	negative
Bone marrow + thymus	Tg + LPS	1.1 ± 0.2	9.8 ± 2.2

[a] Adult good responder (B10·BR) mice were thymectomized, lethally irradiated (900 R), and reconstituted with bone marrow or with both bone marrow and thymus cells. Modified from Esquivel *et al.* (1977).

ulin per se, but the extent of lymphocytic infiltration of the thyroid gland, since all mice can be stimulated to develop autoantibodies to thyroglobulin. Some strains, in general those with slightly higher titers, develop thyroid lesions, while other strains, generally ones with lower titers, show minimal disease.

B. Rats

Further studies of the relationship of genetic control of antibody production and lesions have been performed in inbred rats (Rose, 1975b). Four strains of rats were employed, Ho (AgB-5), AO (AgB-2), DA (AgB-4), and Au (AgB-5). After injection with pooled rat thyroid extract plus CFA, AO rats developed high titers of antibody and extensive thyroid lesions (Table IX). Another strain, Au, also had high antibody titers, but showed only mild thyroid lesions, while strain DA rats had more severe disease with relatively low antibody titers. Ho rats had essentially no lesions and very low titers of antibody. These differences were not due to differences in anti-

TABLE IX

Response of Inbred Rats to Rat Thyroid Extract[a]

Strain	AgB type	Pathology index	Antibody titer
Ho	5	0.3	1.3
AO	2	2.0	10.3
DA	4	1.7	2.0
Au	5	0.7	7.0

[a] Modified from Rose (1975b).

genicity of rat thyroglobulin because antibodies in the disease-free strain, Ho, reacted with thyroglobulin of the same species. On the other hand, serological tests did reveal antigenic differences among rat thyroglobulins, somewhat similar to those previously described for mouse thyroglobulins. With regard to AgB type, both of the AgB-5 strains, Ho and Au, were poor responders in terms of thyroid infiltration, but Au rats had high antibody titers and Ho rats had low titers.

C. Relationship to Human Thyroid Disease

Taken together, these studies on experimentally induced thyroiditis in mice and rats suggest that the development of lesions is under control of an Ir gene, which is part of the major histocompatibility complex. Similar findings were recently reported in the guinea pig (Sharp *et al.*, 1976). By analogy, one can infer that some humans are good responders and others poor responders to certain determinants on human thyroglobulin. In man, this responsiveness may be controlled by a gene that is linked to the major histocompatibility region, HLA. In this respect, there are well-documented reports that patients with Graves' disease have a threefold greater incidence of HLA-B8 compared with matched controls (Grumet *et al.*, 1974). Graves' disease is believed to be part of the autoimmune constellation of thyroid diseases (see Chapter 21).

III. SPONTANEOUSLY APPEARING THYROIDITIS

A. BUF Rats

BUF (previously Buffalo) rats were established as a colony in 1931. They have been maintained by close inbreeding for over 70 generations. BUF rats are known to be relatively susceptible to a variety of tumors, either spontaneous or chemically induced. These tumors are common in endocrine organs, such as pituitary and adrenal glands. Thymic adenomas have been described in as many as 20% of older BUF rats. Glover and Reuber (1968) were the first to describe thyroiditis in BUF rats. Since the animals in this study had been given carbon tetrachloride, the disease was attributed to that treatment. Several carcinogenic agents, including methylcholanthrene, trypan blue, and dimethylbenzanthracene, were also found to be effective in producing thyroiditis in BUF rats. The spontaneous development of thyroiditis was first recognized by Hajdu and Rona (1969) and subsequently confirmed by Reuber (1970). Silverman and Rose (1971) described autoantibodies to thyroglobulin in affected BUF rats and suggested that the disease is autoimmune in origin. The incidence is related to age and sex. No spontaneous disease was found in animals younger than 3 months, and the incidence of thyroiditis rose to approximately 48% of BUF rats, 30 weeks of age. The disease incidence was lower in animals aged more than 60 weeks. Females were affected approximately three times more frequently than were males.

1. *Autoantibodies*

Circulating antibodies can be found in BUF rats at about the same time lesions are first observed. The antibodies are specific for thyroglobulin and react with antigen prepared from the same animal, demonstrating their autoantibody nature. Although tanned cell hemagglutination lends itself well to the demonstration of autoantibodies to thyroglobulin in experimentally immunized BUF rats, it is relatively poor for demonstrating antibodies in rats with spontaneous disease. This observation suggests that the antigenic determinants involved in eliciting spontaneous disease may differ from those involved in experimentally induced thyroiditis, even in inbred BUF rats. Thyroglobulin linked to red cells by means of chromic chloride (CCH) provides more positive reactions with sera of BUF rats with spontaneous disease. Indirect immunofluorescence (IIF) is also useful in demonstrating antibodies to thyroid in BUF rats. There is a close correlation between the occurrence of these antibodies and the appearance of lesions (Table X). Localization of fluorescence occurs in the colloid and not in the cytoplasm of the follicular epithelium, indicating that thyroglobulin, and not thyroid microsomal antigen, is responsible for the reaction. The

TABLE X

Relationship of Thyroid Pathology to Circulating Thyroid Antibodies in BUF Rats[a]

Age of rats (weeks)	Treatment	Thyroid pathology	Thyroid antibodies: IIF[b]	Thyroid antibodies: CCH[c]	Percent
> 52	None	+	2	5	26
		Neg.	1	4	4
		Neg.	Neg.	Neg.	70
18	Neonatal thymectomy	+	2	7	27
		Neg.	±	2	16
		Neg.	Neg.	Neg.	57

[a] Data from Noble *et al.* (1976).
[b] Mean scale.
[c] Mean titer ($\log_2$).

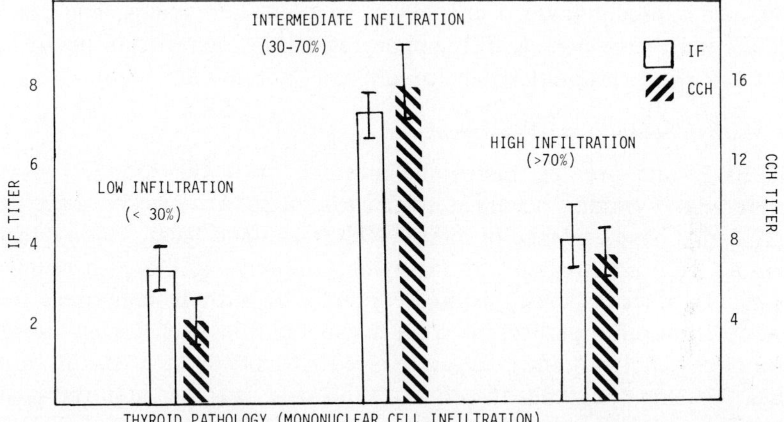

Fig. 1. Antibody production and thyroid pathology in BUF rats. IF, immunofluorescence; CCH, chromic chloride hemagglutination. Data from Noble *et al.* (1976).

titers of IIF and CCH antibodies show an interesting relationship with severity of disease (Fig. 1). Titers are lowest in animals with little mononuclear infiltration and highest in animals with intermediate degrees of infiltration. Rats with severe thyroiditis have lower titers than those with intermediate infiltration (Noble *et al.*, 1976). The most likely explanation for this finding is that animals with severe disease have less antigen available to maintain high levels of antibody production. It is also possible that the lower levels of detectable circulating antibody in severely diseased animals reflect the formation of circulating immune complexes.

Another striking contrast between experimentally induced thyroiditis in BUF rat and the spontaneous disease is the absence of positive delayed-type hypersensitivity skin reactions to thyroglobulin in spontaneous disease (Noble *et al.*, 1976).

2. *Lesions*

Histologically, the thyroid glands of normal BUF rats are characterized by relatively small thyroid follicles, bounded by high cuboidal epithelium and containing scanty colloid. The first changes of spontaneous thyroiditis are seen as perivascular cuffing by small lymphocytes. Later, dense collections of small and medium-sized lymphocytes with occasional germinal centers are found, sometimes destroying the normal architecture of large portions of the thyroid gland. No Hürthle cells are seen. In more mature lesions, macrophages are found in greater numbers, making up as much as 12% of cells teased from the diseased thyroid gland. Medium-sized lymphocytes predominate over smaller ones in later lesions, and plasma cells are more conspicuous. B lymphocytes can be identified in the thyroid infiltrates with appropriately labeled antisera (Noble *et al.,* 1976).

3. Methylcholanthrene Treatment

If BUF rats are fed methylcholanthrene or if the drug is injected parenterally, thyroiditis occurs at much earlier ages. At 12 weeks of age, 10% of BUF rats have evidence of disease (Silverman and Rose, 1975a). In 18-week-old BUF rats treated with methylcholanthrene, 42% show histological damage. In other respects, the disease induced by methylcholanthrene treatment does not differ perceptibly from the spontaneously occurring disorder. Since methylcholanthrene does not induce thyroiditis in other strains of rats tested, it seems likely that the effect of this drug is to heighten the genetic propensity of BUF rats to develop autoimmune thyroiditis.

4. Thymectomy

Neonatal thymectomy lowers the age of onset and increases the incidence of thyroiditis. Twenty percent of 8-week-old BUF rats that have been thymectomized at birth have histological evidence of disease and elevated titers of antibody in hemagglutination and immunofluorescence tests. At 12 weeks of age, 52% of animals are positive, but at 18 weeks, only 27% of neonatally thymectomized BUF rats have disease (Table X). Thymectomy performed 3 weeks after birth does not change the onset or incidence of thyroiditis (Silverman and Rose, 1975a).

Bucsi and Straussen (1972) found that neonatal thymectomy of rats prevented induction of experimental thyroiditis, although high titers of thyroid antibodies were present in both thymectomized and nonthymectomized rats. On the other hand, thymectomy at 5 weeks of age followed by sublethal radiation provoked thyroiditis in 60% of Wistar rats (Penhale *et al.,* 1973). The majority of these rats with severe disease were found to have low numbers of circulating T cells.

Since neonatal thymectomy increases the incidence of severe thyroiditis in BUF rats, studies were made of circulating lymphocytes. They indicate that BUF rats with thyroiditis are lymphopenic when compared with BUF rats that have not yet developed disease. The lymphopenia appears to be primarily a T cell deficiency and becomes more prominent in aging animals (Noble *et al.,* 1976).

Neonatal thymectomy cuts down thymic suppression so that about half of the animals eventually develop autoimmune thyroiditis (Rose, 1975a). However, if thymectomy is delayed, thymic-derived lymphocytes are peripheralized so that thymectomy has no observable effect. The most plausible interpretation of these results is that one population of thymus-derived lymphocytes acts to suppress the actions of thyroglobulin-reactive effector T lymphocytes in newborn BUF rats. During aging, thymic function diminishes, as reflected in lower circulating T cell levels and decreased suppression.

The role of methylcholanthrene in promoting thyroiditis of the genetically susceptible BUF rat is not known. Methylcholanthrene has a direct toxic effect on the thymus. Moreover, it was shown that methylcholanthrene-treated BUF rats have diminished T cell-mediated responsiveness to tuberculin, suggesting a functional decrease in thymic function (Silverman and Rose, 1974). The hypothesis was proposed, therefore, that premature cessation of thymus-dependent suppressor action in this inbred strain results from the thymotoxic action of the drug.

5. *Possible IR Genes*

The question arises of why BUF rats develop thyroiditis and not other manifestations of autoimmunity, for they are largely free of other autoantibodies and lymphocytic infiltration affecting other organs, including other endocrine glands. Studies on the experimental induction of thyroiditis in BUF rats indicate that they are extraordinarily susceptible to thyroglobulin-induced disease. They are, for example, the only strain of rat among those tested in which thyroiditis can be induced by use of incomplete Freund's adjuvant (Silverman and Rose, 1975b). It is probable, therefore, that these rats are genetically endowed with elevated responsiveness to thyroglobulin, as well as with diminished thymic suppressor function.

B. OS Chickens

Obese strain (OS) chickens were established by R. K. Cole (1966) of Cornell University by selective breeding of phenotypically hypothyroid chickens of the Cornell strain (CS). In 1956, Cole noted that about 1% of females in the CS, a population of white leghorns developed and maintained at Cornell since 1935, were grossly abnormal in appearance at 6–8 weeks of age. The females were smaller than normal and developed juvenile, long, downy feathers and large subcutaneous fat deposits. In 1956, selection was begun from this small group of affected females. Soon, males with similar pathological abnormalities were found and used for breeding. The incidence of disease increased rapidly until, by 1962, more than 80% of the isolated flock developed disease. At present, over 95% of OS offspring of both sexes spontaneously develop the obese phenotype (Rose *et al.*, 1976a; R. K. Cole, personal communication).

The abnormality of OS chickens is similar to that observed in thyroidectomized or hypophysectomized birds, suggesting that the disorder is due to thyroid deficiency (van Tienhoven and Cole, 1962). The disease can be partially prevented by treating birds with thyroid hormone. In fact, without such treatment, the fertility of the OS flock falls below levels feasible for maintenance. At 6–8 weeks of age OS thyroid glands are generally smaller than those of normal chickens. There is proliferation of the thyroid epithelial cells and invasion of the thyroid by mononuclear cells. Frequently, germinal center formation is evident. Antibodies specific for chicken thyroglobulin can be demonstrated in most diseased OS chickens over 4 weeks of age.

The bursa of Fabricius is necessary for the development of autoimmune thyroiditis in OS chickens (Cole *et al.*, 1968; Wick *et al.*, 1970a). Birds that have been surgically bursectomized at birth or have been chemically bursectomized by treatment with cyclophosphamide or testosterone developed only mild disease. However, serum alone generally cannot transfer the disease as will be discussed below. Frequently, newly hatched or 1-week-old chicks possess IgG antibody obtained through the yolk sac from the mother, and, yet, their thyroids are not infiltrated by lymphocytes.

1. The B Locus

The major histocompatibility complex of the chicken is the B locus. It codes for a surface alloantigen present on all nucleated cells, including red blood cells. Of 215 OS birds monitored at Cornell University, two B alleles, B^1 and B^4, predominated and were present in approximately equal frequency (Bacon *et al.*, 1973). A third allele, B^3, was observed rarely and only in a heterozygous state. The frequency of B^1 was similar in both OS and CS birds. The B^3 allele and another allele, B^2, were present in moderate frequency in CS, but B^4 is absent from the CS flock.

Once the B genotypes were determined in OS birds, studies were undertaken to determine its influence on the incidence of autoimmune thyroiditis. The first experiments were performed on offspring from $B^1B^4 \times B^1B^4$ matings (Table XI). The groups were bled periodically and classified according to the severity of disease. At all ages, the thyroids of B^1B^1 and B^1B^4 chickens had significantly greater lymphocytic infiltration than did thyroids of B^4B^4 birds. The hemagglutination titers to thyroglobulin were significantly higher in B^1B^1 and B^1B^4 birds. Clearly, genes within or closely linked to the B locus influenced the autoimmune response to thyroglobulin.

Additional studies were undertaken with (OS $\times$ CS) F_1 chickens of various B genotypes (Bacon, 1976). It was found that all offspring with the B^3 allele had relatively high titers of thyroglobulin antibody and severe disease (Fig. 2), regardless of whether the B^3 allele was present in a homozygous state or coupled with B^1, B^2, or B^4 allele. The results indicate that B^3 is associated with the most vigorous autoimmune response.

TABLE XI

Spontaneous Autoimmune Thyroiditis in OS Chickens of $B^1B^4 \times B^1B^4$ Mating (6 Weeks of Age)[a, b]

Genotype	No.	Pathology index $\bar{x} \pm$ SE	Antibody titer $\bar{x} \pm$ SE
B^1B^1	9	3.2 ± 0.3	5.3 ± 0.3
B^1B^4	8	2.6 ± 0.6	2.9 ± 0.5
B^4B^4	6	1.4 ± 0.3	Neg.

[a] Data taken from Bacon *et al.* (1974).
[b] Most of the birds were from one partially inbred family, OSA.

Chickens with the B^1 allele generally had moderate disease whether present homozygously or coupled with B^4. However, when the B^1 allele was present in the heterozygous state with B^2, no significant disease was found. These findings suggest that B^1 is associated with moderate disease, but its expression may be influenced by another B allele. B^2 may actually be associated with diminished responsiveness to thyroglobulin, perhaps due to suppression.

Other studies indicate that additional genetic factors influence the autoimmune response of OS chickens (Bacon *et al.*, 1974). B^4B^4 chickens obtained from partially inbred heterozygous B^1B^4 matings had only mild disease and low titers of antibody, as stated above. In contrast, some B^4B^4 chickens from homozygous (B^4B^4) OS parents had significantly higher pathological scores and antibody titers at 10 weeks of age. The B^4B^4 birds

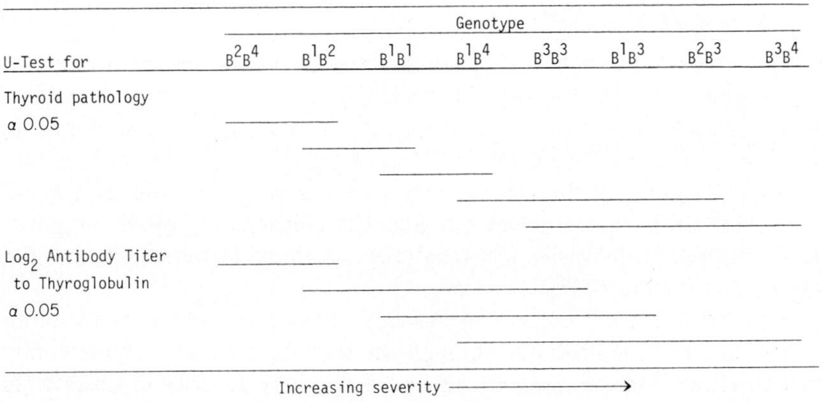

Genotype

U-Test for | B^2B^4 | B^1B^2 | B^1B^1 | B^1B^4 | B^3B^3 | B^1B^3 | B^2B^3 | B^3B^4

Thyroid pathology
α 0.05

Log_2 Antibody Titer
to Thyroglobulin
α 0.05

Increasing severity ⟶

Fig. 2. Thyroiditis in (OS × CS) F_1 chicks. α, level of significance. Genotypes linked by solid lines were not significantly different in response. Data from Bacon (1976).

with most marked pathological changes and elevated antibody titers were found principally in one of two hatch groups, suggesting a hatch effect (perhaps an infectious or environmental agent) on the expression of the B allele.

There are several possible mechanisms by which the B genotype may influence autoimmune thyroiditis. A likely possibility, based on studies in the mouse, is that an "Ir–Tg" gene is closely linked to, or part of, the B locus. The fine structure of the B locus has not yet been characterized in chickens, although genes controlling the immune response of several antigens have been linked to the B locus (Gunther *et al.*, 1974). Assuming that Ir genes are responsible for susceptibility to autoimmune thyroiditis, we propose that the B^3 allele determines high, B^1 moderate, and B^2 or B^4 low (or even suppressed) response to an antigenic determinant of thyroglobulin. We recognize the possibility that nonresponder birds might preferentially develop suppressor rather than effector T cells.

Other explanations for B-linked genetic control must also be considered. One possibility is heightened susceptibility to a viral or other infectious agent. Rather extensive studies have already been performed, attempting to isolate a virus from OS chickens. To date, these studies have not been rewarding (Ziegel *et al.*, 1970; Flanagan *et al.*, 1970). However, continued investigation is of the greatest importance.

Another possibility is that B-linked genes might influence the immunologic response in a nonspecific way. For example, proliferation of T lymphocytes during graft versus host reaction seems to be related to the B genotype (Longenecker *et al.*, 1972). B-linked genes may also influence the antigenicity of thyroglobulin or the integrity of the thyroid gland.

2. *Role of Thymus-Derived Cells*

The major histocompatibility locus of the chicken is one important factor in determining the severity of autoimmune disease. Still, it must be emphasized that parental CS chickens rarely develop autoimmune thyroiditis, even if they have the B^1B^1 genotype. The argument can be raised that the B' allele of the OS chicken differs from the B^1 alleles of the CS. However, we have compared OS and CS chickens in mixed lymphocyte reactions and graft versus host reactions and found no detectable difference (Jones and Bacon, 1977).

Additional genetic control of susceptibility of OS chickens to autoimmune thyroiditis is mediated through the thymus. Neonatal thymectomy of OS chickens leads to a significant increase in the severity of disease, as it does in spontaneous thyroiditis of the BUF rat (Wick *et al.*, 1970b; Welch *et al.*, 1973). Antibodies to thyroglobulin are not decreased by neonatal thymectomy, suggesting that a critical number of helper T cells have migrated from the thymus before the time of hatching. The principal action of the thymus during the early stages of disease must be to limit the immunologic response by suppression of effector cells (Rose, 1975a).

Assuming that the role of the thymus after hatching is primarily one of suppressing the disease, the question arises of how the thymus of OS chickens differs from that of CS birds. Indirect evidence is now available to support the hypothesis that the OS thymus releases effector T cells prematurely (or suppressor T cells relatively late) (Jakobisiak *et al.*, 1976). Intrastrain skin grafts were performed with (B^1B^1) OS and (B^1B^1) CS chickens so that rejection was due entirely to minor (non-B) histocompatibility antigens. As might be expected, neonatal thymectomy prolonged the survival of skin grafts on normal CS birds. In contrast, neonatal thymectomy of OS chickens had very little effect on skin graft survival. We interpret these experiments as suggesting that in normal chickens the thymus is responsible for generation of effector T cells which promote allograft rejection either directly or by cooperation with other cells. Neonatal thymectomy of CS chickens, therefore, reduces the number of effector cells. In OS chickens, on the other hand, effector cells leave the thymus prematurely and are located in peripheral lymphoid tissue so that thymectomy has no detectable effect. After being given X-irradiation at the time of neonatal thymectomy, both CS and OS chickens show a similar, modest prolongation of graft survival, probably because thymus-derived cells with an effector function have been reduced. Skin graft rejection due to weak histocompatibility antigens may be considered a model for autoimmune tissue destruction. It seems to depend upon the dynamic balance of effector and suppressor T cells.

3. *Role of Bursa-Derived Cells*

The role played by B cells in producing thyroiditis is not yet clarified. Cytotoxic antibody for thyroid cells grown in culture has not been demonstrated in the sera of OS chickens. In addition, passive transfer of high-titered antisera or even embryonic cross-circulation has been unsuccessful in transferring the disease from OS to CS chickens. On the other hand, it is possible to increase the severity of thyroiditis dramatically in B^4B^4 recipient chicks by injection of high-titered serum obtained from B^1B^1 donors (Jaroszewski *et al.*, 1977). These experiments suggest that thyroglobulin antiserum is able to affect thyroid glands only in genetically susceptible strains of chickens.

Recent experiments have suggested that B cells of CS chickens do not differ from those of OS birds (Polley and Bacon, 1976). F_1 hybrids of (B^1B^1) OS × (B^1B^1) CS were bursectomized by cyclophosphamide treatment. Full restoration of the antibody response comparable to that found in untreated

F_1 birds was achieved by restoration with either CS or OS bursal cells. Thus, bursal cells of CS are as effective as those from OS chickens in producing thyroid antibody if provided the appropriate thymic helper cells.

4. *Thyroid Defect*

The fact that passively transferred antibody can promote disease in OS and not CS chickens suggests that an abnormality in the thyroid glands of OS chickens may also be important in the production of autoimmune thyroiditis. This thyroid defect is probably controlled by genes not linked to the B locus. This is implied by the observation that (B^1B^1) CS birds seldom develop significant disease. Even after neonatal thymectomy, (B^1B^1) CS chickens only rarely develop thyroiditis and neonatally thymectomized (B^1B^1) CS chicks given repeated injections of an OS antiserum with a high titer of antibody to thyroglobulin failed to develop disease (Jaroszewski *et al.*, 1977). One explanation for these observations is that CS chickens do not have a thyroid defect which is present in OS birds.

Careful microscopic observation of the thyroid glands of newly hatched OS chicks reveals no morphological evidence of abnormality. However, when tested on the day of hatching, the thyroid glands of OS chickens incorporate significantly more ^{131}I than do thyroids of CS chickens (Sundick and Wick, 1974; Wick *et al.*, 1974). This effect is not related to thyroglobulin antibody transferred from the hen. As a further test, embryonic OS and control normal thyroid glands were cultured side by side on the chorioallantoic membrane of the normal chicken embryo (Sundick and Wick, 1976). Six days later, ^{131}I uptake of the two lobes was compared. The OS thyroids incorporated significantly more ^{131}I than the normal CS thyroid lobes. Increased ^{131}I uptake of OS glands, therefore, is due to an abnormality of the thyroid gland itself. In addition to the increased iodine uptake, the ratio of mono- to diiodotyrosine in the thyroid gland is significantly increased in OS chickens (Rose *et al.*, 1976a).

IV. CONCLUSIONS

Autoimmune thyroiditis in animals is a model for the study of the human disease, chronic lymphocytic thyroiditis. Based on experimental evidence, there is reason to believe that at least three genetically determined defects participate in triggering the autoimmune response. The first is the presence of a putative Ir gene within the major histocompatibility complex of the species. This gene predisposes directly or indirectly to an especially vigorous immune response to antigenic determinants of thyroglobulin. The second factor is diminished ability of the thymus or thymus-derived cells to prevent or suppress the autoimmune response. In this respect, a genetically determined thymic defect may be expressed in the ratio of suppressor to effector cells available in the periphery during embryonic development. Greater susceptibility to the thymotoxic actions of certain drugs (such as methylcholanthrene) may also be involved. Finally, there is substantial evidence for a genetic defect in the thyroid gland itself, marked by increased iodide uptake and an altered ratio of thyroid products. In the case of spontaneously arising thyroiditis, all three of these genetic defects may be required in varying degrees to initiate the autoimmune response. In experimentally induced thyroiditis, adjuvants may partly overcome the need for genetic predisposition. These experimental observations in mice, rats, and chickens provide a rationale for continued clinical and epidemiologic investigations of familial clustering of several different autoimmune thyroid diseases, nonimmune thyroid diseases, and other organ-specific autoimmune diseases.

ACKNOWLEDGMENTS

The experimental work described herein was supported by USPHS Grants CA 02357, CA 16426, and HD02841. P. Esquivel is on leave from Austral University of Chile, and is supported by Fogarty International Fellowship Award NIH TW 02220 02.

REFERENCES

Allison, A. C., and Davies, A. J. S. (1971). *Nature* (*London*) **233,** 330–332.

Ardeman, S., Chanarin, I., Krafchik, B., and Singer, W. (1960). *Q. J. Med.* **35,** 421–431.

Bacon, L. D. (1976). *Fed. Proc., Fed. Am. Soc. Exp. Biol.* **35,** 713.

Bacon, L. D., Kite, J. H., Jr., and Rose, N. R. (1973). *Transplantation* **16,** 591–598.

Bacon, L. D., Kite, J. H., Jr., and Rose, N. R. (1974). *Science* **186,** 274–275.

Bastenie, P. A., and Ermans, A. M., eds. (1972). "Thyroiditis and Thyroid Function." Pergamon, Oxford.

Bigazzi, P. E., and Rose, N. R. (1975). *Prog. Allergy* **19,** 245–274.

Blizzard, R. M., Tomasi, T. B., and Christy, N. P. (1963). *J. Clin. Endocrinol. Metab.* **23,** 1179–1180.

Block, K. J., Buchanan, W. W., Whol, M. J., and Bunim, J. J. (1965). *Medicine* (*Baltimore*) **44,** 187–231.

Bottazzo, G. F., Florin-Christensen, A., and Doniach, D. (1974). *Lancet* **2,** 1279–1283.

Bucsi, R. S., and Straussen, H. R. (1972). *Experientia* **28,** 194–195.

Burnet, F. M., and Fenner, F. (1949). "The Production of Antibodies." Macmillan, New York.

Capanna, S. L., and Kong, Y. M. (1974). *Immunology* **27,** 647–653.

Cole, R. K. (1966). *Genetics* **53,** 1021.

Cole, R. K., Kite, J. H., Jr., and Witebsky, E. (1968). *Science* **160,** 1357–1358.

Coutinho, A., and Moller, G. (1975). *Adv. Immunol.* **21,** 113–227.

Esquivel, P. S., Rose, N. R., and Kong, Y. M. (1977). *J. Exp. Med.* **145,** 1250–1263.

Fialkow, P. J. (1969). *Prog. Med. Genet.* **6,** 117–167.

Fialkow, P. J., Thuline, H. D., Hecht, F., and Bryant, J. (1971). *Am. J. Hum. Genet.* **23,** 67–86.

Flanagan, T. D., Barron, A. L., Kite, J. H., Jr., and Witebsky, E. (1970). *Avian Dis.* **14,** 613–616.

Glover, E. L., and Reuber, M. D. (1968). *Arch. Pathol.* **86,** 542–544.

Grumet, E. F., Payne, R. O., Konishi, J., and Kriss, J. R. (1974). *J. Clin. Exp. Metab.* **39,** 1115–1119.

Gunther, E., Balcarora, J., Hala, K., Rude, E., and Hraba, T. (1974). *Eur. J. Immunol.* **4,** 548–552.

Hajdu, A., and Rona, G. (1969). *Experientia* **25,** 1325–1327.

Hall, R. (1962). *N. Engl. J. Med.* **266,** 1204–1211.

Hall, R., and Stanbury, J. B. (1967). *Clin. Exp. Immunol.* **2,** 719–725.

Hall, R., Saxena, K. M., and Owen, S. G. (1960). *Lancet* **2,** 187–188.

Irvine, W. J. (1965). *N. Engl. J. Med.* **273,** 432–438.

Irvine, W. J., MacGregor, A. G., Stuart, A. E., and Hall, G. H. (1961). *Lancet* **2,** 850–853.

Jakobisiak, M., Sundick, R. S., Bacon, L. D., and Rose, N. R. (1976). *Proc. Natl. Acad. Sci. U.S.A.* **73,** 2877–2880.

Jaroszewski, J., Sundick, R. S., and Rose, N. R. (1977). Submitted for publication.

Johnson, A. G. (1976). *In* "Immune RNA" (E. P. Cohen, ed.), pp. 17–35. CRC Press, Cleveland, Ohio.

Jones, R. F., and Bacon, L. D. (1977). *Fed. Proc., Fed. Am. Soc. Exp. Biol.* **36,** 1191.

Kitchin, F. D., and Evans, W. H. (1960). *Br. Med. Bull.* **16,** 148–151.

Kojima, A., Tanaka, Y., Sakakura, T., and Nishizuka, A. (1976). *Lab Invest.* **6,** 550–557.

Longenecker, B. M., Pazderka, F., and Ruth, R. F. (1972). *Transplantation* **14,** 424–437.

MacCuish, A. C., Barnes, E. W., Irvine, W. J., and Duncan, L. J. P. (1974). *Lancet* **2,** 1529–1531.

Masi, A. T., Hartman, W. H., and Shulman, L. E. (1965). *J. Chronic Dis.* **18,** 1–22.

Noble, B., Yoshida, T., Rose, N. R., and Bigazzi, P. E. (1976). *J. Immunol.* **117,** 1447–1455.

Penhale, W. J., Farmer, A., McKenna, R. P., and Irvine, W. J. (1973). *Clin. Exp. Immunol.* **15,** 225–236.

Polley, C. R., and Bacon, L. D. (1976). *Poult. Sci.* **55,** 2081.

Reuber, M. D. (1970). *Arch. Environ. Health* **21,** 734–739.

Roitt, I. M., and Doniach, D. (1967). *Clin. Exp. Immunol.* **2,** 727–736.
Rose, N. R. (1975a). *Ann. N.Y. Acad. Sci.* **249,** 116–214.
Rose, N. R. (1975b). *Cell. Immunol.* **18,** 360–364.
Rose, N. R., Kite, J. H., Jr., Flanagan, T. D., and Witebsky, E. (1971a). *In* "Cellular Interactions in the Immune Response" (S. Cohen, G. Cudkowicz, and R. McCluskey, eds.), pp. 264–281. Karger, Basel.
Rose, N. R., Twarog, F. J., and Crowle, A. J. (1971b). *J. Immunol.* **106,** 698–704.
Rose, N. R., Vladutiu, A. O., David, C. S., and Shreffler, D. C. (1973). *Clin. Exp. Immunol.* **15,** 281–287.
Rose, N. R., Bacon, L. D., and Sundick, R. S. (1976a). *Transplant. Rev.* **31,** 264–285.
Rose, N. R., Bigazzi, P. E., and Noble, B. (1976b). *In* "The Reticuloendothelial System in Health and Disease" (H. Friedman *et al.,* eds.), pp. 209–216. Plenum Press, New York.
Sharp, G. C., Kyriaskos, M., and Braley-Mullen, H. (1976). *Immunogenetics* **3,** 205–208.
Silverman, D. A., and Rose, N. R. (1971). *Proc. Soc. Exp. Biol. Med.* **138,** 579–584.
Silverman, D. A., and Rose, N. R. (1974). *J. Natl. Cancer Inst.* **53,** 1721–1724.
Silverman, D. A., and Rose, N. R. (1975a). *J. Immunol.* **114,** 145–147.
Silverman, D. A., and Rose, N. R. (1975b). *J. Immunol.* **114,** 148–150.
Sundick, R. S., and Wick, G. (1974). *Clin. Exp. Immunol.* **18,** 127–139.
Sundick, R. S., and Wick, G. (1976). *J. Immunol.* **116,** 1319–1323.
Tomazic, V., and Rose, N. R. (1975). *Clin. Immunol. Immunopathol.* **4,** 511–518.
Tomazic, V., and Rose, N. R. (1977). *Eur. J. Immunol.* **7,** 40–43.
Tomazic, V., and Rose, N. R. (1976). *Immunology* **30,** 63–68.
Tomazic, V., Rose, N. R., and Shreffler, D. C. (1974). *J. Immunol.* **112,** 965–969.
van Tienhoven, A., and Cole, R. K. (1962). *Anat. Rec.* **142,** 111–121.
Vladutiu, A. O., and Rose, N. R. (1971). *Science* **174,** 1137–1139.
Vladutiu, A. O., and Rose, N. R. (1975). *Cell. Immunol.* **17,** 106–113.
Welch, P., Rose, N. R., and Kite, J. H., Jr. (1973). *J. Immunol.* **110,** 575–577.
Wick, G., Kite, J. H., Jr., Cole, R. K., and Witebsky, E. (1970a). *J. Immunol.* **104,** 45–53.
Wick, G., Kite, J. H., Jr., and Witebsky, E. (1970b). *J. Immunol.* **104,** 54–62.
Wick, G., Sundick, R. S., and Albini, B. (1974). *Clin. Immunol. Immunopathol.* **3,** 272–300.
Zaino, E. C., and Guerra, W. (1964). *Arch. Intern. Med.* **113,** 70–71.
Ziegel, R. F., Barron, A. L., Kite, J. H., Jr., and Witebsky, E. (1970). *Avian Dis.* **14,** 617–619.

Part II

Immunologic Aspects

Chapter 4

Autoimmune Diseases: Concepts of Pathogenesis and Control

A. C. ALLISON

I. INTRODUCTION

Among the fundamental observations and concepts on which was founded the science of immunology around the beginning of the twentieth century was the recognition that animals do not as a rule make antibodies against their own body constituents. In 1900, Ehrlich and Morgenroth described how they injected goats intraperitoneally with blood of other goats and looked for the development of lysins in the blood of the recipients. These lysins were regularly found and reacted with blood of many other goats but never with that of the recipients. Ehrlich recognized that "the organism has contrivances by means of which the immunity reaction, so easily produced by all kinds of cells, is prevented from reacting against the organism's own elements and so give rise to autotoxins. . . . Only when the internal regulating contrivances are no longer intact can great dangers arise."

The nature of the internal regulating contrivances remained without explanation until Burnet (1949), developing the clonal selection theory, proposed that the contact of antibody-forming cells with their respective antigens during fetal or early postnatal life leads to destruction or inactivation, with consequent elimination of the corresponding clones. In this way self-reactive clones are avoided unless they arise later in life by somatic mutation of lymphocytes. The progeny of such mutant cells, termed forbidden clones, give rise to self-reacting antibodies.

The clonal selection theory had wide appeal but was not easily reconciled with observations on the experimental induction of autoimmunity. In 1956, Witebsky and Rose found that rabbits immunized with extracts of rabbit thyroids in Freund's complete adjuvant develop antibodies against rabbit thyroglobulin and thyroiditis. Weigle (1961) showed that injections of thyroglobulins from other species in the absence of adjuvant elicit the formation of autoantibodies against thyroglobulin and thyroiditis. It was difficult to conceive why these simple immunization procedures should give rise through somatic mutation to clones of cells reacting with thyroid antigens.

It also became clear that fetal lambs and monkeys are able to respond immunologically to a variety of antigenic stimuli, including skin grafts (Silverstein *et al.*, 1964; Cotes *et al.*, 1966). Thus, the difference between immune responses in fetuses, newborns, and adults is quantitative rather than qualitative. Even in adult animals specific unresponsiveness to antigens, such as foreign serum albumin or γ-globulin, can be induced (Dresser and Mitchison, 1968). The denatured proteins are immunogenic, especially in the presence of adjuvant, whereas single large doses or repeated small doses of soluble, native antigen are tolerogenic; the animals so treated do not produce antibodies against these antigens when challenged with denatured antigens in the presence of adjuvant. These observations are taken as models of the unresponsiveness occurring in the course of ontogenic development.

This approach could be carried further when the distinction was made between B lymphocytes, which synthesize antibodies, and thymus-dependent (T) lymphocytes, which exert specific helper effects in the formation of most antibodies. Taylor (1969) showed, in mice injected with bovine serum albumin, and Chiller *et al.* (1970), in mice injected with human γ-globulin, that low doses of antigen induce unresponsiveness selectively in T lymphocytes, leaving the responses of B lymphocytes unimpaired, whereas high doses induce unresponsiveness in both T and B lymphocytes. However, even with high doses of antigen, the unresponsiveness of B lymphocytes is incomplete, and some antibody of low affinity can still be formed.

These results are relevant to self-tolerance, as pointed out independently by Allison (1971) and by Weigle (1971). Many antigens circulate in low doses, including thyroglobulin, polypeptide hormones and certain plasma membrane antigens. In these cases, only T lymphocytes may be tolerant, leaving B lymphocytes able to respond to autoantigens suitably presented to them with T lymphocyte help. Mechanisms allowing the requirement for specific T lymphocytes responding to autoantigens to be bypassed are discussed below. They include graft versus host reactions, bacterial and viral infections, treatment with certain drugs, and exposure of antigenic determinants by partial degradation of autoantigens. One prediction of this hypothesis is that B lymphocytes able to bind autoantigens will be present in normal individuals, and that elimination of these antigen-sensitive cells will prevent the formation of autoantibodies. These predictions have been confirmed by appropriate experiments.

Although it is now recognized that many antigens formerly thought to be segregated from immunocompetent cells, such as thyroglobulin, circulate in low dose, the possibility remains that there is effective segregation of some antigens from lymphocytes. Potential examples are organ-specific microsomal lipoprotein antigens, which are frequently involved in autoimmunity affecting endocrine glands, and the basic protein of myelin which is the principal antigen in autoimmune encephalomyelitis. If this view is correct, T lymphocytes able to respond to these antigens should be present in normal persons and experimental animals.

Tolerance of autoantigens based on selective unresponsiveness of T lymphocytes or seclusion is precarious, since it can readily be bypassed by infections and other events. It was, therefore, postulated by Allison *et al.* (1971) that an additional mechanism controlling autoimmunity is present: T lymphocytes which suppress autoimmune responses. Evidence which has accumulated in support of this interpretation is summarized below.

Autoimmune mechanisms have been implicated in a wide range of disorders, including Graves' disease, hypothyroidism, pernicious anemia, myasthenia gravis, glomerulonephritis, rheumatoid arthritis, pemphigus, and ulcerative colitis. However, identification of the specific roles played by immune processes in the pathogenesis of these diseases has proved difficult. Even in diseases which are unquestionably mediated by antibodies, such as autoimmune hemolytic anemias, pathogenetic mechanisms have not yet been completely defined. In experimental animals the relative roles of antibody-mediated, antibody-dependent cell-mediated, and T lymphocyte-mediated autoimmune reactions are not easily distinguished. The position is worse in humans, where the definition of lymphocyte subpopulations is less complete and where experiments such as transfer of autoimmune diseases by serum or syngeneic lymphoid cells are not feasible.

Indeed, the presence in human patients and experimental animals of so many autoantibodies is an embarrassment. Some of the autoantibodies are evidently not associated with any functional disorder, and, even when diseases are present, it is difficult to know whether the antibodies contribute to their pathogenesis or arise secondarily because of tissue damage. Nevertheless, there is now strong evidence that autoimmune reactions are responsible for certain diseases, including some that are common and important clinical problems. In many such diseases affected tissues show mononuclear infiltrates. This was formerly taken as indicating immune reactions mediated by T lymphocytes. The finding that lymphoid cells can damage target cells with which they are cultured was taken as proof that T lymphocytes are mediating the effect. It is now clear that neither interpretation is necessarily correct. T lymphocytes have many functions, including helper effects in antibody formation, so that their presence in tissue does not necessarily mean that they are cytotoxic. Antibody-dependent effector cells may be morphologically indistinguishable from lymphocytes and can, by collaborating with antibodies, damage target cells *in vivo* and *in vitro*. Moreover, other tests that have been widely used as indicative of T cell-mediated immunity (including inhibition of leukocyte migration and production of macrophage migration inhibition factor) are not specific for this cell type.

For all these reasons, it is necessary to examine critically each experimental model and supposed human autoimmune disease to assess whether autoimmune reactions play a part in the pathogenesis of the disease and, if so, by what mechanism. The second part of this chapter is a classification of these mechanisms, each illustrated by a few examples.

II. THE T LYMPHOCYTE BYPASS CONCEPT

As mentioned in the introduction, most autoantigens—such as thyroglobulin, protein hormones, and solubilized membrane antigens—circulate in what are, effectively, low doses. Prolonged exposure to these would be expected to produce selective unresponsiveness in T lymphocytes, leaving intact B lymphocytes able to bind autoantigens and be stimulated by autoantigens presented to them with appropriate T lymphocyte help (Fig. 1). Under these circumstances, the requirement for T lymphocytes responding to autoantigenic determinants can be bypassed. This concept overcomes difficulties inherent in the original clonal selection formulation and has become a widely accepted explanation for the development of autoimmunity. It is, therefore, worth considering how the concept could be tested because a hypothesis that is not refutable by experiment is of little value.

The first prediction is that B lymphocytes binding autoantigens will be present in normal humans and experimental animals. This was confirmed for thyroglobulin by Bankhurst *et al.* (1973), who found, in normal humans, lymphocytes that bound homologous thyroglobulin with reasonably high affinity. Such binding cells have been observed by others (see Calder and Irvine, 1975); their numbers are considerably increased in the thyroids, but not the peripheral blood, of patients with Hashimoto's thyroiditis. The presence in several mouse strains of lymphocytes binding the erythrocyte autoantigen X and other autoantigens is discussed by De Heer and Edgington (1976).

The second prediction is that most autoimmune diseases will be mediated by antibodies and not by sensitized T lymphocytes reacting with autoantigens. The representative list of pathogenetic mechanisms at the end of this chapter will show that this view is correct. Even diseases that were formerly thought to be cell-mediated, such as thyroiditis, almost certainly are

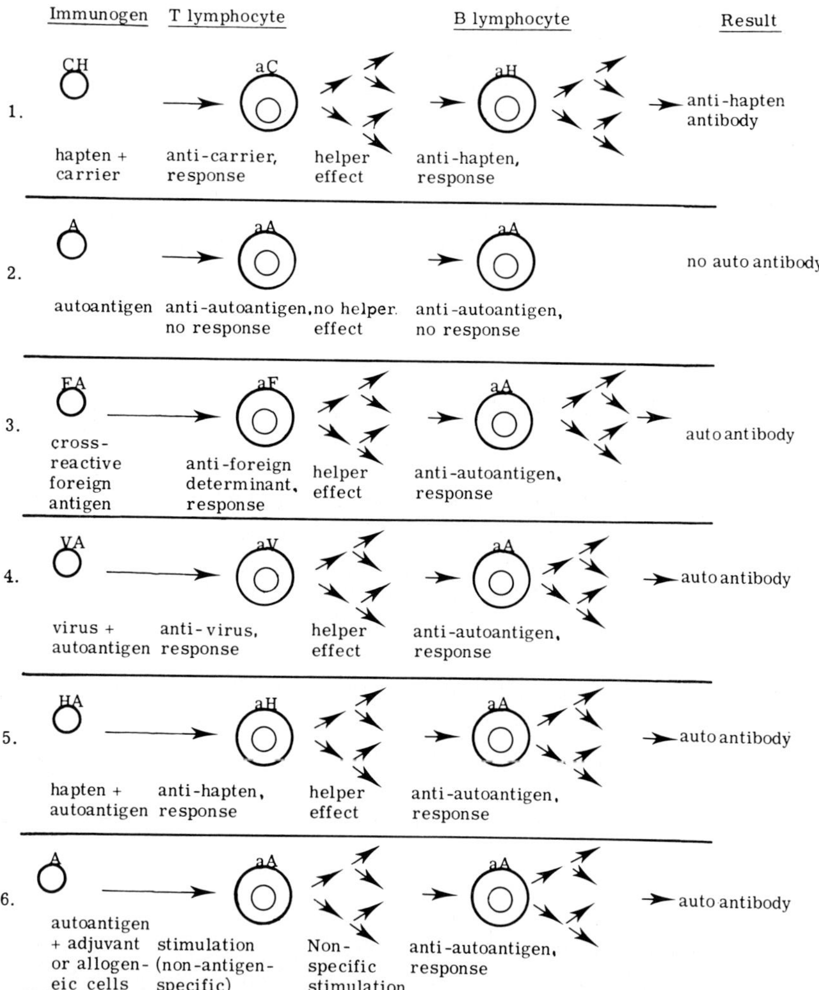

Fig. 1. Diagram of the relationships of T and B lymphocytes with different specificities in autoimmune responses.

not. The one exception is experimental allergic encephalomyelitis, where the balance of evidence still supports the view that it is cell mediated. Possibly T lymphocytes can react against determinants of autologous myelin basic protein. This situation requires further study; it may arise from the effective segregation of the antigen from immunocompetent cells, being, therefore, a special case. Because it is still widely believed that T lymphocytes are involved in the pathogenesis of autoimmune diseases, it is worth summarizing evidence that tests of leukocyte migration and macrophage migration inhibition, as well as cell and serum transfer experiments, are ambiguous.

The third prediction is that elimination of B lymphocytes binding autoantigens will prevent the formation of autoantibodies and autoimmune disease. This has been shown, with appropriate controls, for cells binding highly radioactive thyroglobulin in the mouse (Clagett and Weigle, 1974; Allison, 1974).

The fourth prediction is that T lymphocytes are required for the formation of autoantibodies and the development of thyroiditis. It is readily demonstrable that mice deprived of T lymphocytes produce only very low levels of antibody and no thyroiditis (see Allison, 1974).

The fifth prediction is that autoantigens forming immunogenic units with antigens able to stimulate T lymphocytes (helper determinants) should be able to elicit the production of autoantibodies. Among the helper determinants are drugs or small molecules, viral and bacterial antigens. Each of these will be considered in turn. It has long been held that modification of autoantigens could be involved in the pathogenesis of autoimmunity, and this interpretation has been supported by recent observations. Two relevant systems are outlined briefly.

The sixth prediction is that any procedure nonspecifically activating lymphocytes, such as the use of adjuvants or graft versus host reactions, should stimulate the formation of autoantibodies. The former needs no testing because it is the standard procedure by which autoimmune reactions are elicited experimentally. Evidence has accumulated showing that autoimmune reactions are often found in animals undergoing chronic graft versus host reactions.

A. Autoimmunity Following Administration of Drugs

Some autoimmune manifestations following drug administration are remarkably specific. Thus, in patients treated with α-methyldopa, Coombs'-positive autoimmune hemolytic anemias are not uncommon (Worlledge *et al.*, 1966). Often the autoantibody is IgG directed against the e antigen of the Rh series. The production of antinuclear factors and a syndrome like systemic lupus erythematosus is relatively frequent in patients treated with procaineamide (Dubois, 1969) and hydralazine (Alarçon-Segovia *et al.*, 1967). The latter has been reproduced in mice (Cannat and Seligmann, 1968). The simplest explanation is the coupling of the drug or a metabolite to an autoantigen; if host T lymphocytes can react against the antigenic determinants of the drug, autoantibodies could be formed through a helper effect (Fig. 1). Suitable experiments show that small molecules can function in this way as carriers. Rabbit thyroglobulin coupled with arsanilic and sulfanilic acids elicits the formation of autoantibodies in the rabbit, even in the absence of adjuvant (Weigle, 1965). Coupling of dinitrophenol (DNP) groups to myeloma proteins has been used to elicit the formation of anti-idiotypic antibodies in syngeneic mice sensitized to DNP (Iversen, 1970).

Evidence has been obtained for interactions of hydralazine with nucleoprotein (Tan, 1968), procaineamide with light-oxidized DNA (Blomgren *et al.*, 1972) and both drugs with DNA (Eldredge *et al.*, 1974). This was not found with several other drugs tested. The principle outlined above is illustrated by experiments of Yamashita *et al.* (1976). Mouse T lymphocytes were sensitized to *p*-aminobenzoic acid (PAB) by immunization with a hapten-isologous protein conjugate, and then the animals were challenged with PAB-conjugated isologous mouse erythrocytes. They developed Coombs'-positive hemolytic anemias. Evidence was presented that PAB-reactive helper T cells were essential for the production of autoantibodies.

In other cases, e.g., following administration of hydantoin in some patients, there is a generalized lymphoid hyperplasia and plasmacytosis, with a wide range of autoantibodies, with specificity for erythrocytes (Sayoc and Howland, 1974), nucleoprotein (MacKinney and Booker, 1972), and lymphocytes (Szegedi and Petranyi, 1972). In such cases, Gleichmann and Gleichmann (1976) suggest that hydantoin derivatives become attached to the surface of lymphoid cells and modify their major histocompatibility antigen complexes in such a way that autologous T lymphocytes recognize them as "foreign" and react to them. Thereafter, the sequence of events would be similar to that in the graft versus host reaction (see below). Since these mechanisms depend on the development of T lymphocytes recognizing antigenic determinants of the drug or altered host antigens, there is an analogy with contact hypersensitivity. Baumgarten and Geizy (1970) showed that delayed hypersensitivity can be induced in guinea pigs by dinitrophenylated lymphocytes. Asherson and Mayhew (1976) have presented evidence that reactivity to a contact sensitizer can be transferred by lymph node cells taken 18 hours after exposure to antigen. Plasma membranes were also immunogenic. Red cells and allogeneic lymphoid cells were ineffective.

Another remarkable situation is found in nitrofurantoin treatment, in which a variety of autoantibodies, including some with specificity for human serum albumin, are found (Teppo *et al.*, 1976). Tailing of albumin in immunoelectrophonetic strips occurred, because of the formation of complexes with polyclonal IgG autoantibodies. A lupuslike syndrome with pulmonary reactions has also been described in patients treated with nitrofurantoin. These patients show evidence of cell-mediated reactions to nitrofurantoin, but no antibody binding of the drug has ever been observed (Pearsall *et al.*, 1974), compatible with the drug functioning as a helper determinant.

B. Virus Infections

According to the schemes presented in Figs. 1 and 2, virus infections might be expected to elicit autoantibody formation in two ways. First, viral antigens and autoantigens may become associated to form immunogenic units. Viral antigens stimulating host T lymphocytes could then function as helper determinants, thereby favoring B lymphocyte responses to autoantigens. Second, some viruses such as the Epstein-Barr (EB) virus stimulate nonspecifically proliferation of and antibody formation by cells of the B lymphocyte lineage, and this could involve clones of cells reacting to autoantigens. At least two mechanisms are known by which viral and host antigens could form immunogenic units (Fig. 2). Host antigens, especially glycolipids, are incorporated into the envelopes of some viruses, and viral antigens frequently appear on the surface of infected host cells (see Burns and Allison, 1975). The viral antigens may form complexes with or modify histocompatibility antigens (Schrader *et al.*, 1975; Zinkernagel *et al.*, 1976) or other plasma membrane constituents, including the microfilament protein actin. Recent evidence suggests that virus infection can result in the appearance of histocompatibility antigens that are normally repressed in the host cells (Garrido *et al.*, 1976). The virus antigens, or modified, complexed or derepressed histocompatibility antigens, could be recognized by T lymphocytes. These could then exert a helper effect in autoantibody formation. Virus-coded polymerases can be immunogenic in animals, and these might function as helper determinants in the production of autoantibodies against nucleic acids.

Harboe and Haukenes (1966) found that chickens immunized with

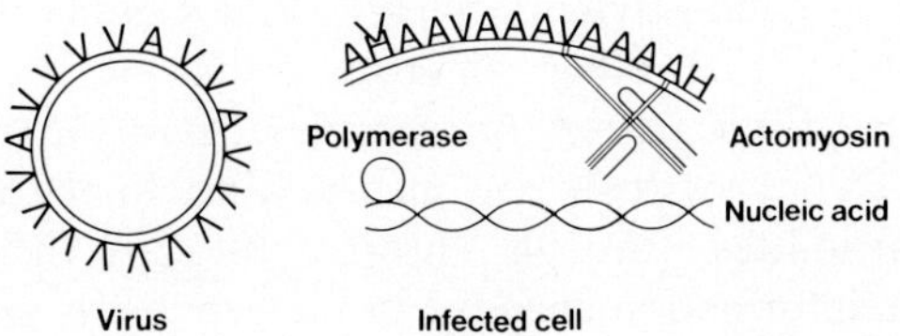

Fig. 2. How viral antigens (V) and autoantigens (A) can form immunogenic units. Autoantigens can become incorporated into viral envelopes, and viral antigens often appear on the surface of infected cells, perhaps forming complexes with histocompatibility antigens (H), or the actomyosin system. Viral polymerases are also immunogenic and complexed with nucleic acids.

influenza virus-containing antigen from the chorioallantoic cells in which it was cultured produce an autoantibody against the same antigen present in liver cells and bile. An analogous principle has been used by Lindenmann and Klein (1967) to increase immunity against tumor-specific antigens by immunizing mice with influenza virus grown in tumor cells.

The development of Coombs'-positive autoimmune hemolytic anemias in rats infected with Friend leukemogenic virus has been reported by Kuzumaki *et al.* (1974). Virus is seen to bud from the surface of erythrocytes, so the virus may provide helper determinants for formation of autoantibodies against erythrocytes. The depletion of T lymphocytes in the animals could lead to a decreased T suppressor cell activity: depression of helper function occurs only with profound T cell loss.

It has long been known that human infections with viruses, including influenza, measles, varicella, Coxsackie and *Herpes simplex* viruses, are sometimes followed by autoimmune manifestations, including antibody-mediated thrombocytopenia and positive Coombs' tests (see Dacie, 1963). The development of cold autoagglutinins often directed against the I blood group after *Mycoplasma pneumoniae* infection (Feizi *et al.*, 1969) may have a similar explanation.

Autoantibodies are more consistently seen in patients recovering from herpesvirus infections in which lymphocytes are target cells. Following infectious mononucleosis, many patients have in their sera autoantibodies, often reacting against several autoantigens. These include autoantibodies against nuclei (Kaplan and Tan, 1968), lymphocytes, and erythrocytes (Stites and Leikola, 1971) and smooth muscle (Holborow *et al.*, 1973). Similar autoantibodies are found after mononucleosis induced by cytomegalovirus (Andersen and Andersen, 1975).

In the examples so far considered, the distinction between antibodies against viral antigens and autoantibodies is readily made, although it can become blurred. For example, the EB virus genome is incorporated into the genome of some host cell B lymphocytes, so that it might be argued that the EB nuclear antigen and other antigens coded by the virus are now autoantigens. The distinction is further blurred in the case of oncornaviruses, where DNA proviruses are incorporated in the genome of every animal and transmitted through chromosomes to their progeny. The expression of the information encoded in the genome is under genetic control. For example, the G_{IX} antigen expressed on the thymocytes of certain mice is a type-specific constitutent of gp70, which forms the major envelope component of murine leukemia virus. This glycoprotein is a mendelian character expressed independently of virus production. Normally, mice do not produce antibody to G_{IX}, but certain hybrid mice produce large amounts of antibody spontaneously (Obata *et al.*, 1976). The authors suggest that two types of immunocompetent cells collaborate to produce the high antibody response.

These questions are relevant to the interpretation of the pathogenesis of disease in New Zealand mice. For example, in the diseased kidneys of NZB and B/W F_1 hybrid mice, immune complexes contain not only antibodies against nucleic acids but also two major viral proteins (gp69/71 and p30) of murine leukemogenic virus (Yoshiki *et al.*, 1974). Quantitative studies suggest that the expression of the viral envelope glycoprotein and the host immune response to it make a substantial contribution to the pathogenesis of the disease.

There has been much speculation about the possibility that an oncornavirus is involved in the pathogenesis of human systemic lupus erythematosus (SLE). The group antigen of oncornaviruses has been reported in the tissues of patients with SLE (Strand and August, 1974) and in the renal glomeruli of a patient dying of SLE (Mellors and Mellors, 1976). Further work is required to establish that oncornaviruses have a pathogenetic role in SLE.

The association of smooth muscle antibodies and mitochondrial antibodies in chronic active hepatitis and primary biliary cirrhosis is well known and of diagnostic importance. Evidence is accumulating that autoantibodies against a cytoplasmic liver-specific protein and liver cell-surface determinants are common in chronic active hepatitis and may play a pathogenic role (Hopf *et al.*, 1974; Eddleston and Williams, 1974). Because these antibodies are absorbed in the liver, they only occasionally enter the blood stream; they are demonstrated by immunofluorescence in biopsies. A widely held view is that the various autoantibodies are formed as a result of generalized stimulation of the immune system in hepatitis (reflected by hypergammaglobulinemia and high titers of antibodies against several viruses), perhaps following stimulation by products of intestinal bacteria; moreover, virus- or drug-induced damage to hepatocytes releases modified tissue constituents which can function as autoantigens. Eddleston and Williams (1974) have suggested that hepatitis B virus-specific determinants on the surface of infected hepatocytes can stimulate T lymphocytes to function as helpers in the formation of autoantibodies against cell-surface determinants. These could collaborate with K cells to damage liver cells in chronic active hepatitis. Evidence that the effector cells in this disease are K cells has recently been presented by Cochrane *et al.* (1975).

The role of helper effects in the development of autoantibodies to antigen F located inside liver cells of all mice tested, and in man, has been founded by Iverson and Lindenmann (1972). Mice make antibody to F if, and only if, they respond to a single cell-surface alloantigen which generates T cell help for the anti-F response.

C. Partial Degradation of Autoantigens

It has long been held that tissue damage might play a role in eliciting autoimmune reactions. Partial enzymic degradation can expose antigenic determinants that are not available in the native molecules, and these could react with T lymphocytes to induce autoimmunity. An example is the use of rabbit thyroglobulin digested by papain to immunize rabbits (Anderson and Rose, 1971). Intravenous injection of the cleavage products without adjuvant elicited the formation of autoantibodies against thyroglobulin and mononuclear infiltrates in the rabbit thyroid gland. Rabbit thyroglobulin digested with leukocyte proteinases is also able to elicit thyroiditis in rabbits (Weigle *et al.*, 1969).

Partially degraded collagen is likewise immunogenic in experimental animals (Steffen, 1969), and comparable changes may play a role in the pathogenesis of some autoimmune diseases. Denaturation of collagen frees the constituent α-chains which are then present as random coils. This exposes antigenic determinants not recognizable in the intact molecule. Some of these antigens are represented in several mammalian species and elicit cell-mediated immune responses (Adelmann *et al.*, 1972). These could serve as helper determinants in autoimmune reactions. In rheumatoid and other forms of arthritis, autoantibodies to native and denatured collagen are often found (Cracchiolo *et al.*, 1975).

Many bacterial, viral, and parasitic infections are associated with transient positive tests for antiglobulins of rheumatoid factor type (see Asherson, 1968). Among the underlying mechanisms are either partial degradation or alteration of immunoglobulin. Enzyme-treated γ-globulin is more immunogenic than native γ-globulin (Williams and Kunkel, 1963). In infections, immunoglobulins could be complexed to or altered by enzymes from microorganisms, but lysosomal hydrolases also can digest immunoglobulin (Menninger *et al.*, 1976). The formation of rheumatoid factor can be induced by the injection of antibody–antigen complexes into experimental animals (Aho and Wager, 1961). This may be due to the exposure of immunoglobulin determinants by complex formation. The spleens of normal, immunized mice contain many cells that make plaques in target layers consisting of their own erythrocytes pretreated with proteolytic enzymes. Cunningham (1976) reviews evidence that enzyme treatment reveals an autoantigen on the erythrocytes which is normally hidden.

D. Segregation of Antigens

It was formerly believed that many autoantigens are secluded from immunocompetent cells in the body. However, many antigens formerly thought to be secluded, such as thyroglobulin and protein hormones, are now known to circulate in small amounts (about 100 ng per ml in the case of thyroglobulin, Torrigiani *et al.*, 1969). Cell membrane constituents, such as major histocompatibility antigens, are likewise known to circulate in low doses.

However, there may well be effective segregation of some antigens in normal persons. For example, the lens is segregated from blood vessels and lymphatics, and its constituents do not normally elicit immune responses, as the acceptance of lens homografts shows. The basic protein of myelin may be effectively secluded from immunocompetent cells, which may explain the reaction of T lymphocytes against it in autoimmune encephalomyelitis. Some antigens are organ specific and insoluble in aqueous solvents. These include the organ-specific microsomal antigens of the thyroid, gastric parietal cells, and other cells (see Doniach, 1975). The antigens are lipoproteins which react in the same way to detergents and fixatives. There is no evidence that they pass into the immune system until the organs in question are damaged. Then both T and B lymphocytes could react against the antigen.

E. Graft Versus Host Reactions

The primary event in graft versus host (GVH) reactions is the response of donor T lymphocytes to the major histocompatibility complex on lymphoid and hemopoietic cells of the recipient. One result is stimulation of lymphocytes in the recipient manifested by lymphoreticular hyperplasia with germinal center enlargement and plasmacytosis. There is induction of proliferation in recipient B lymphocytes under the influence of a donor T lymphocyte signal (Cantor, 1972). According to the hypothesis presented above (Fig. 1), in a normal person, autoantibody formation does not occur because T lymphocytes are unable to react to autoantigens. However, when lymphocytes are nonspecifically stimulated, as in the GVH reaction, there is an "allogeneic effect" leading to the production of antibodies which normally require T lymphocyte help (see Katz, 1972). In this way, the need for carrier-specific T lymphocytes in the immune response can be bypassed. Hence, in GVH reactions the formation of autoantibodies would be expected.

The formation of antibodies reacting with host cells during GVH reactions had already been documented. Cock and Simonsen (1958) reported positive Coombs' tests in chickens that had been injected as embryos with allogeneic lymphocytes. Oliner *et al.* (1961) described Coombs'-positive hemolytic anemia in mice undergoing chronic GVH reactions. Boyse *et al.* (1970) reported that mice injected will allogeneic cells produce antibodies reacting with host thymocytes. In all of these cases, it was assumed that the reactions observed were due to alloantibodies produced by lymphocytes in the graft and not, therefore, true autoantibodies.

The prediction that autoantibodies would be formed in GVH reactions (Allison, 1971) was soon confirmed. Cannat and Varet (1973) and Fialkow *et al.* (1973) found that repeated injections of parental lymphocytes into F_1 mice rapidly induce the formation of antinuclear antibodies; the latter group used allotype markers to establish that these were produced by host and not donor B lymphocytes. The induction of Coombs'-positive autoimmune hemolytic anemias in mice undergoing GVH reactions has been studied in detail by Lindholm *et al.* (1973) and Gleichmann *et al.* (1976). These are induced more efficiently when F_1 mice are injected with parental cortisone-resistant thymocytes than with spleen cells. The antibodies eluted from the erythrocytes are of recipient allotype, are polyclonal, and react with erythrocytes of several mouse strains.

The mice undergoing GVH reactions also develop glomerulonephritis (Gleichmann *et al.*, 1976). A difference at the K end of the H-2 complex between donor and recipient was enough to initiate the nephritis. The kidneys were found to contain immune complexes of IgG antibody (a considerable fraction of host origin, as shown by allotype markers) and erythrocyte and lymphocyte surface antigens. Antibodies eluted from the glomerular complexes became attached to erythrocytes or lymphocytes; the cells could then be agglutinated by antiglobulin serum or lysed by antiglobulin serum and complement.

Hamsters undergoing systemic GVH reactions (with a major histocompatibility difference between recipient and donor) develop severe Coombs'-positive autoimmune hemolytic anemia (Streilein *et al.*, 1975). The question arises whether other manifestations of GVH reactions, including lymphocytolysis, rashes, and skin eruptions, also have an autoimmune basis, but there is no definitive evidence on this point at present.

F. Adjuvants and Bacterial Infections

On the model presented in Fig. 1, immunologic adjuvants that are polyclonal B lymphocyte activators (e.g., lipopolysaccharide or purified protein derivative of tuberculin) or nonspecific stimulators of T lymphocytes (e.g., Freund's complete adjuvant, see Allison, 1973) should induce autoimmune responses. Freund's complete adjuvant is widely used to induce experimental autoimmune diseases. Hammarström *et al.* (1976) have found, when bovine spleen cells are cultured with polyclonal B lymphocyte activators, large numbers of cells forming antibodies against autologous red cells, as well as other antigens. These results confirm that B lymphocytes are not normally tolerant to self-constituents. *Bordetella pertussis* and other bacteria and bacterial products also have adjuvant effects (see Asherson, 1968). Thus, bacterial infections, especially chronic infections with liberation of products with adjuvant activity, could produce polyclonal lymphocyte activation and autoimmunity.

Moreover, bacteria might provide helper determinants in several ways. One widely studied in rheumatic fever (see Zabriskie, 1976) is cross-reaction of some determinants with those of host tissues. Other determinants of the same molecules or complexes could be recognized by host T lymphocytes and, therefore, function as helper determinants. Bacterial glycolipids could become inserted into host cell membranes, and bacterial products such as tuberculin readily form complexes with host cell antigens.

Thus, chronic bacterial infections or repeated injections of bacteria or their products would lead to autoimmunity. The substantial evidence on this subject is so well known that there is no need to review it in detail (see Asherson, 1968, for earlier references). Among the examples that can be quoted are antibody to cardiolipin and cold autoantibodies to erythrocytes in syphilis, antibody to myocardial antigens in rheumatic fever, the production of antiglobulins in animals repeatedly inoculated with bacteria (Christian, 1963), autoantibodies to the lung in tuberculosis (Burrell, 1963), and various autoantibodies in leprosy (Bonomo *et al.*, 1965). Rabbits immunized with rabbit ribosomes developed autoantibodies to RNA (Panijel and Barbu, 1960).

G. Lymphocytotoxic Antibodies

It has been known for some time that patients with systemic lupus erythematosus (SLE) have in their sera antibodies which, in the presence of complement, lyse normal human lymphocytes (Mittal *et al.*, 1970; Terasaki *et al.*, 1970). A high incidence of such lymphocytotoxic antibodies has been found in the healthy relations of patients (consanguineous and nonconsanguineous), suggesting that a common environmental agent may be involved in their pathogenesis (De Horatius and Messner, 1975). In attempting to identify such an agent, analogies with experimental animals have been pursued. Aging New Zealand (NZB/W) mice, which develop a lupuslike syndrome, have in their sera antibodies which react with thymocytes and thymus-dependent T lymphocytes (Shirai *et al.*, 1973).

More recently, lymphocytotoxic antibodies have been described in the sera of patients with Crohn's disease and chronic ulcerative colitis. In both forms of chronic inflammatory disease of the bowel, the prevalence of lymphocytotoxic antibodies is about 40% (Korsmeyer *et al.*, 1974). Lymphocytotoxic antibodies have now been found in the relatives of patients with inflammatory bowel disease (Korsmeyer *et al.*, 1976). Of 90 relatives of 23 probands with the disease, 27 (30%) had lymphocytotoxic antibodies, whereas only 3 of 69 control family members (4%) had them. Of the 48 household contacts of the probands, 19 (40%) had antibodies, as compared with 8 of 42 nonhousehold contacts (19%). One-half of 16 spouses of probands were positive for antibody. The authors again suggest that the increased prevalence of lymphocytotoxic antibodies in family members of probands and its occurrence in household contacts (consanguineous and nonconsanguineous) may indicate exposure of probands and their family members to common environmental agents.

The possible involvement of a transmissible agent or agents has received some support from experiments in which homogenates of tissues from subjects with Crohn's disease have been inoculated into the footpads of CBA mice (Cave *et al.*, 1973) or into the ileum of New Zealand white rabbits (Taub *et al.*, 1974). Several of the recipient animals showed granulomatous changes with epithelioid cells and occasional giant cells. Mitchell *et al.* (1976) have serially transmitted the granulomatous lesions in mice, in some experiments using 0.2-μm membrane filtrates. This suggests that a virus, mycoplasma, or L form may be involved. Aronson *et al.* (1974) and Beeken *et al.* (1976) have recently reported the isolation of a small agent, probably a small RNA virus, from the tissues of patients with inflammatory bowel disease. However, another group of investigators failed to confirm the transmission in a different strain of mice (Bolten *et al.*, 1973). One interpretation of these findings is that the transmissible agent can reproduce the disease only in hosts with an appropriate genetic constitution. Inflammatory bowel disease is more common in the relatives of probands than in matched controls (Singer *et al.*, 1971).

Lymphocytotoxic antibodies in patients with SLE have been characterized (Winfield *et al.*, 1975). The requirement of a low temperature for reaction with cells suggested that they might not be monomeric IgG. Lymphocytotoxins have been found in fractions of high molecular weight IgG aggregates and in cold-reacting IgM fractions. There is no specificity for known lymphocyte surface antigens, including HLA. However, the lymphocytes of patients bearing lymphocytotoxins are less sensitive to their effects than are lymphocytes of normal subjects (Korsmeyer *et al.*, 1976).

Presumably, the formation of lymphocytotoxins is a manifestation of loss of tolerance to autoantigens, and possible underlying mechanisms have been discussed. One explanation is that viral antigens might form immunogenic units with plasma membrane antigens; the viral antigens would stimulate T lymphocytes, which would then exert helper effects, allowing autoantibody formation by B lymphocytes. Lymphocytotoxins are found in subjects recovering from infectious mononucleosis (Thomas, 1972) and after vacci-

nation with live rubella virus (Kreisler *et al.*, 1970). Not only are viral antigens expressed on the surfaces of infected lymphocytes; as discussed above, a genetically controlled differentiation antigen of murine thymocytes (G_{IX}) is the envelope glycoprotein of an oncornavirus. Virus-infected cells can express histocompatibility antigens that are normally repressed. All of these situations might result in the formation of autoantibodies against lymphocyte surface antigens. Other transmissible agents might have similar effects, e.g., endotoxins or other bacterial products that can function as adjuvants and thereby stimulate autoantibody formation.

There is not yet any evidence that cold-reactive lymphocytotoxins affect the functions of lymphocytes *in vivo.* Nevertheless, their presence in patients with SLE and inflammatory disease of the bowel, and in their relatives, can be taken as an indication of a disturbance in their immune system. Clearly, the search for transmissible agents, which in a high proportion of subjects induce the formation of lymphocytotoxins, and in a few genetically predisposed individuals contribute to the pathogenesis of SLE and chronic inflammatory disease of the bowel, should be pursued.

H. Leukocyte Migration and MIF Production

The most commonly used *in vitro* tests for cell-mediated immunity (CMI) are stimulation of ^{3}H-thymidine incorporation by cultured lymphoid cells in the presence of antigen and the release of migration-inhibition factor (MIF) by leukocytes in the presence of antigen. Two methods are used to detect the latter: the leukocyte migration inhibition test (Bendixen and Söberg, 1968), where addition of antigen to leukocytes inhibits their migration from a capillary tube, and the traditional MIF test, where lymphoid cells are cultured with antigen and the supernatants are then tested for inhibition of migration of macrophages (usually those recovered from the guinea pig peritoneal cavity).

Since these tests have been taken as evidence for CMI in various autoimmune diseases in humans and experimental animals, it is worth pointing out that all have limitations which must be recognized by those who use them. Increased ^{3}H-thymidine incorporation in the presence of antigen can occur in cultured B lymphocytes, as well as T lymphocytes. This is consistently found, for example, in animals previously exposed to viral antigens (Burns and Allison, 1976). Both purified human B lymphocytes and T lymphocytes, when suitably stimulated, can release MIF (Rocklin *et al.*, 1974). Although the leukocyte migration test can be due to lymphocytes able to form E rosettes, and, therefore, presumably T lymphocytes (Frimmel, 1975), inhibition of leukocyte migration can be due to other mechanisms. Packalen and Wasserman (1971) showed that when normal guinea pig buffy coat leukocytes are passively sensitized with the γ_2-fraction of serum from guinea pigs immunized with thyroglobulin in Freund's complete adjuvant, their migration was inhibited if thyroglobulin was added to the culture medium. Further evidence that cytophilic and other antibodies can result in leukocyte migration inhibition is discussed by Brostoff (1974). Similarly, the migration of normal guinea pig macrophages after passive sensitization with antibody can be inhibited by antigen (Amos *et al.*, 1967). It has also been shown that soluble immune complexes can inhibit leukocyte and macrophage migration (Spitler *et al.*, 1969; Eibl and Sitko, 1972; Kotkes and Pick, 1974).

As an illustration of the application of these methods to human autoimmunity, several studies reporting inhibition of migration of leukocytes from patients with Hashimoto's disease when incubated with thyroid microsomal and other antigens can be quoted (see Calder and Irvine, 1975, for references). These have been taken as evidence of release of MIF by T lymphocytes specifically sensitized to thyroid autoantigens. However, the observations are open to other interpretations.

I. Ambiguities in Transfer Experiments

The traditional method for distinguishing between antibody-mediated and cell-mediated reactions is transfer. If the effects are produced by transfer of serum-containing antibody from one individual to another, it is antibody mediated. If the effect cannot be transferred by serum antibody, but is transferred by immune cells, the conclusion is drawn that it is cell mediated. For many practical purposes, this is correct, but rigid adherence to these criteria have caused some authorities to conclude that certain autoimmune diseases are cell-mediated on the basis of unsatisfactory evidence. Obviously, cell transfer is ambiguous because the transferred cells could produce antibodies in recipients.

For many years, autoimmune thyroiditis could not be transferred by serum. Later, serum transfer, under certain conditions (early sera from thyroidectomized donors), was successful (Nakamura and Weigle, 1969). More recently, the kinetics of induction of autoimmune thyroiditis have been investigated in detail, using a Jerne-type assay for cells producing autoantibodies to thyroglobulin (Clinton and Weigle, 1972). The cells initially proliferate in the spleen, migrate through the blood stream, and are finally concentrated in the thyroid. Most of the autoantibodies formed in the thyroid are absorbed there, so that the concentration in the peripheral blood is relatively low. This explains the earlier failures of transmission. Transfers of autoimmune thyroiditis have now been achieved in several species (see below).

Autoimmune glomerulonephritis due to antibodies reacting with glomerular basement membrane antigen be transferred by antibodies eluted from the glomerular immune complexes. Because of absorption of the autoantibodies to the kidneys, they cannot be demonstrated in the serum unless the animals are nephrectomized (Lerner and Dixon, 1966).

Thus, all transfer experiments must be interpreted with caution. For example, it is conceivable that in allergic encephalomyelitis, autoantibodies reacting with brain constituents could play a role, being absorbed by the diseased nervous tissue so that the autoantibodies do not escape into the serum. However, evidence in support of the view that cell-mediated immunopathology plays a major part in the pathogenesis of this disease is discussed below.

III. THE CONCEPT OF T LYMPHOCYTE SUPPRESSION OF AUTOIMMUNITY

For a long time is was widely thought that T lymphocytes have two functions: as effectors in cell-mediated immunity and as helpers in antibody formation. In 1971, evidence from several sources combined to suggest that T lymphocytes can also suppress immune responses. Allison *et al.* (1971) presented evidence that T lymphocytes can inhibit autoimmune responses in New Zealand mice (NZB), and suggested that they might provide a general mechanism for preventing or delaying autoimmune responses. The existence of T lymphocytes suppressing immune responses is now supported by an enormous mass of experimental observations (see Chapter 6). Evidence has accumulated that the populations of T lymphocytes with suppressor and helper effects are distinct. Even the data on autoimmunity are too extensive to review in this chapter. Two models will suffice to illustrate the role of T lymphocytes in suppressing autoimmune reactions: the development of autoimmune disease in New Zealand mice and of autoimmune thyroiditis in various experimental animals.

Allison *et al.* (1971) summarized experiments on NZB mice, which develop a Coombs'-positive hemolytic anemia from about the age of 4 months. If spleen cells are transferred from old to young NZB mice, about one-half of the recipients show positive Coombs' tests, which usually disappear in a few weeks. If the recipients are given anti-lymphocytic globulin (ALG), more develop positive Coombs' tests, and these remain positive usually until the death of the animals. The simplest explanation of these observations is that T lymphocytes in the young animals exert an inhibitory influence on B lymphocytes from the old animals that are producing autoantibodies against erythrocytes. In keeping with this interpretation, repeated transfers of thymus cells from young NZB mice to ageing NZB mice markedly delays the onset of autoimmune hemolytic anemia (Allison, 1974; Gershwin and Steinberg, 1975).

Tests for several T lymphocyte-mediated functions show age-related changes. The T lymphocytes of young NZB mice are resistant to the development of immunologic tolerance (Jacobs *et al.*, 1971). NZB mice aged 2–3 mo have a selective defect of T cell suppressor activity, as shown in terms of antibody formation to pneumococcus polysaccharide type III and polyinosinic acid–polycytidylic acid (Chused *et al.*, 1973; Barthold *et al.*, 1973; Kysela and Steinberg, 1973). Later there is a defect in helper T cell activity responses to T lymphocyte mitogens and capacity to induce graft versus host reactions (Cantor *et al.*, 1970). Bach *et al.* (1973) showed that, in NZB mice older than 2 months, thymosin-like activity in the serum of NZB mice is very low. Dauphinee *et al;* (1974) showed that NZB mice injected repeatedly with thymosin preparations do not show the usual deterioration in T lymphocyte responses to mitogens. The concept that an endocrine disturbance may contribute to autoimmune and lymphoproliferative disease in NZB mice and possibly in humans is discussed in Chapter 1. Thymectomy in male B/W mice 2–3 days after birth markedly augments the production of both IgG and IgM antibodies to DNA (Talal, 1976). An increase in IgM antibodies to RNA was observed in both males and females. These results suggest that thymectomy eliminates suppressor cells, which exert their effect without influencing the switch from IgM to IgG.

Another strain of mice (Swan) develop anti-nuclear antibodies, immunoglobulin deposits in renal glomeruli, and autoantibody against lymphocytes, together with an early decrease in the concentration of thymosinlike activity in the serum and T lymphocyte functions (Monier and Septjian, 1975). The spontaneous development of autoimmune manifestations in congenitally thymus-deprived nude mice (Morse *et al.*, 1974) is a further argument in support of the interpretation that T lymphocytes in intact animals normally limit autoimmune reactions. The nude mice had higher titers of anti-DNA antibodies than littermates or thymus-grafted nudes, and only the former had deposits of IgM and IgG in the renal glomeruli.

Thymectomy also increases the incidence of erythrocyte-specific anti-nuclear factors in obese strain (OS) and normal white leghorn chickens (Albini and Wick, 1973). Thorough studies have been made of the role of the thymus in controlling the thyroid autoimmunity, which is a feature of OS chickens. Chickens are convenient experimental animals, since it is possible selectively to deplete B lymphocyte functions by bursectomy and T lymphocyte functions by thymectomy. Hormonal bursectomy by injection of androgen into obese chick embryos or surgical bursectomy *in ovo* abolished or markedly reduced the autoimmune thyroiditis characteristic of

this strain; very few of the bursectomized chickens showed circulating antibodies to thyroglobulin (Wick *et al.*, 1970a). Reconstitution of the bursectomized, irradiated chickens with autologous bursa cells completely restored the thyroiditis (Nilsson and Rose, 1972). In contrast, thymectomy of newly hatched obese chickens accelerated and aggravated the lymphoid infiltration of the thyroid and raised the incidence of birds with antibodies to thyroglobulin (Wick *et al.*, 1970b). Whole body X-irradiation after hatching also resulted in the development of more severe disease (Wick *et al.*, 1970c): T suppressor effects are more radiosensitive than helper effects (see below).

Penhale and his colleagues (1973) showed that depletion of T lymphocytes in rats leads to the spontaneous development of autoimmune thyroiditis, having many features in common with the human disease. The rat thyroiditis is chronic, histologically resembles clinical throiditis, and is associated with high titers of antibodies to thyroglobulin but not antibodies to thyroxin. The experiments were conducted in Wistar rats, which do not normally show thyroiditis. When they were depleted of T lymphocytes by thymectomy 3 weeks after birth, followed by repeated sublethal irradiation (4×200 R) and examined 2 months later, 60% of animals had developed thyroiditis. This treatment resulted in a marked depletion but not an absolute deficit of T lymphocytes. Since suppressor T lymphocytes are radiosensitive, whereas T lymphocyte helper effects are relatively radioresistant (Kapp *et al.*, 1974; Kölsch *et al.*, 1975), it is reasonable to postulate that the thymectomized, irradiated animals have a considerable depletion of suppressor T lymphocytes in the presence of enough helper T cells to cooperate in autoantibody formation. Further depletion of T lymphocytes in thymectomized rats by repeated administration of antilymphocytic serum resulted in less thyroiditis. Irradiation of the thyroid gland alone did not produce thyroiditis. The development of thyroiditis could be prevented by inoculating the rats with 10^8 syngeneic lymphocytes 14 days after irradiation; the active cells were destroyed by an antiserum reacting selectively with T lymphocytes (Penhale *et al.*, 1975). In another laboratory, it has been found that rats of the Buffalo strain spontaneously develop autoimmune thyroiditis, and the incidence is considerably raised by neonatal thymectomy (Silverman and Rose, 1974). Other reports confirm that neonatal thymectomy accelerates and increases the severity of autoimmune thyroiditis in rats (Busci and Strausser, 1972) and mice (Nishizuka *et al.*, 1973).

Since the regimes used to deplete rats and chickens of T lymphocytes markedly depress cell-mediated immune responses and yet predispose animals to the spontaneous development of thyroiditis resembling the human disease, it is very unlikely that T cell-mediated immune responses are playing a major pathogenetic role. The correlation of autoimmune disease with the presence of autoantibodies and the suppression of the disease in chickens by bursectomy are strong arguments that antibodies are important in pathogenesis, probably by collaborating with nonspecific effector cells as described below.

Cunningham (1976) has recently discussed experimental work showing active suppression of a natural autoimmune response to internal red cell antigen in normal mice. The major evidence for suppressor control is that antibody is made at a fairly steady rate, which is not influenced by injecting more antigen and that injection of antilymphocytic serum induces a large temporary rise in the number of autoantibody-secreting cells. Cunningham also discusses arguments why tolerance to many self-components maintained by active suppressor mechanisms overcomes difficulties posed by the deletion theoy of self-tolerance.

A. Affinity of Autoantibodies for Antigens

Discussion of the cellular mechanisms initiating immune responses, on the one hand, and unresponsiveness, on the other, is beyond the scope of this chapter. However, some discussion of affinity and avidity is necessary in any consideration of autoimmunity. Affinity refers to the intrinsic association constant between an antibody-combining site and the corresponding univalent antigenic determinant, whereas avidity is a measure of the overall combining power between antibody molecules and multideterminant antigens. For each determinant, there is a population of antibody molecules of varying affinity. The same considerations apply to receptors for antigen on the surface of immunocompetent cells, which in the case of B lymphocytes are antibodies with properties closely resembling those of antibodies secreted by the same cells. On theoretical grounds, it would be predicted that low concentrations of antigen would stimulate high-affinity cells preferentially, while higher concentrations of cells would also stimulate cells with receptors having lower affinity for antigens (Fig. 3). Moreover, specific unresponsiveness would be more readily induced in high- than in low-affinity cells.

Following the induction of partial tolerance in newborn rabbits with a DNP–bovine γ-globulin conjugate, there is marked reduction in the affinity of DNP antibodies elicited by challenging the animals as adults (Theis and Siskind, 1968). An analogous reduction of avidity occurs during neonatally induced tolerance to bovine serum albumin in rabbits. During spontaneous recovery of responsiveness, the antibody formed is initially of low avidity, and it slowly increases in avidity (Dowden and Sercarz, 1968). Preferential suppression of high-affinity or high-avidity antibody is also found with tolerance to haptens or proteins induced in adult rats and mice (Bell, 1973; Davnie *et al.*, 1972). *In vitro* studies have confirmed that precursors of high-affinity antibody-forming cells are preferentially eliminated following induction of tolerance by bovine serum albumin or DNP (Anderson and Wigzell, 1971; Davie *et al.*, 1972). When antigen is administered in Freund's complete adjuvant or in other effective adjuvants, antibody-formation, rather than tolerance induction, in high-affinity cells is favored, so that the overall antibody affinity as well as the amount of antibody formed is high (Siskind, 1974). This is one reason why the use of adjuvants may favor the development of autoimmune disease. Steward (1976) has presented evidence that some mice tend to produce antibodies of relatively high affinity, irrespective of the antigen used, whereas others produce antibodies of lower affinity.

These observations are relevant to autoimmunity for two reasons. First, they concern tolerance to autoantigens, which is likely to be more complete for cells with high-affinity receptors than for cells with low-affinity receptors. Since phenomena, such as agglutination and complement-dependent or cell-dependent lysis, require antibodies with reasonably high-affinity; low-affinity antibodies would have no clinical significance and would escape detection except under special conditions. Formation of low-affinity antibodies can however, be detrimental. Immune complexes with antibodies of low affinity are not eliminated from the circulation by the mononuclear phagocyte system, so that they have a tendency to accumulate in the renal

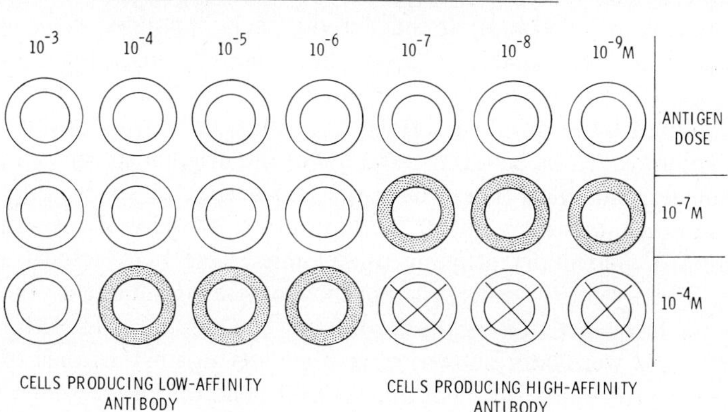

Fig. 3. Diagrams to illustrate the effects of different concentrations of antigens on lymphocytes with receptors varying in affinity for antigen. Low doses of antigen will stimulate only cells with high-affinity receptors (stippled). High doses of antigen will induce unresponsiveness in cells with high-affinity receptors (X) but will stimulate cells with low-affinity receptors.

glomeruli and blood vessel walls, with resultant immunopathological damage (see Steward, 1976). Steward reports that, in New Zealand mice, females consistently show a low avidity of antibody for DNA and in males the avidity falls after 5 months of age, with the interpretation that low-avidity antibodies may be involved in the pathogenesis of the lupuslike syndrome in these mice. In a small number of patients with systemic lupus erythematosus with renal disease, antibodies against DNA tended to have lower avidities than those without. These observations are difficult to interpret because of the possibility of selective elimination of antibodies of higher avidities from the circulation, but they do suggest that not only levels of autoantibodies but also their quality must be considered in relation to the mechanisms by which they arise and produce disease.

B. Natural Cytotoxic Cells

During the past few years, studies of tumor immunity have shown that the capacity to lyse tumor cells is not confined to lymphoid cells from tumor-bearing humans and experimental animals, but is found also in the circulation of normal subjects or experimental animals.

In particular, attention has been drawn to the existence in animals that have not been immunized of a population of lymphoid cells that has the capacity to kill a variety of syngeneic and allogeneic lymphomas (Kiessling *et al.*, 1975, 1976; Herberman *et al.*, 1975a,b). Peak activity is found in mice aged 1–3 months. Activity is greatest in the spleen, is found also in peripheral blood cells, and to a lesser extent in peritoneal exudate cells. Herberman *et al.* (1975a,b) found activity in lymph node cells, whereas Kiessling *et al.* were unable to demonstrate activity in lymph node cells. Thymus cells have low activity. Treatment with anti-θ serum plus complement, followed by removal of surface Ig-positive cells by filtration through anti-Ig columns, leaves between 1 and 5% of the original spleen cell population from normal mice. These have the appearance of small lymphocytes and contain all, or nearly all, of the natural cytotoxicity of the spleen cell population. Congenitally athymic (nude) mice have high activity in their spleens. The cytotoxic cells are not phagocytic or adherent. Originally shown to have activity against Moloney leukemia cells, the natural cytotoxic cells were later shown to have activity against a range of tumor cell types. Cytotoxicity does not appear to depend on Fc receptors, since it is not blocked by immune complexes and is trypsin sensitive. Indeed, incubation at 37°C markedly reduces the cytotoxic capacity of the cells, whereas antibody-dependent effector cell activity and cytotoxicity mediated by T lymphocytes is unaffected.

In view of the importance of Freund's complete adjuvant (containing tubercle bacilli) in the induction of experimental autoimmune disease, it is interesting that intraperitoneal inoculation of BCG into mice results in the appearance, in the peritoneal cavity, of nonspecific cytotoxic cells as defined above (Wolfe *et al.*, 1976). If natural cytotoxic cells are able to lyse normal cells *in vivo,* they could well contribute to autoimmune disease. Conceivably, Freund's complete adjuvant stimulates the formation of natural cytotoxic cells, and the specific immune response following concurrent administration of autoantigen favors the accumulation of these cells in the target organ. In human autoimmune disease, there may be the selective concentration of natural cytotoxic cells from the circulating blood in target organs. Unfortunately, two properties of natural cytotoxic cells, their sensitivity to proteolytic enzymes and lability in culture, make it more difficult to demonstrate natural cytotoxic cells in affected organs.

IV. AUTOIMMUNE DISEASES MEDIATED BY AUTOANTIBODIES

A. Inhibition of Intrinsic Factor Activity

Taylor (1959) and Schwartz (1960) showed that sera from some patients with pernicious anemia are able to block the absorption of vitamin B_{12} when fed to other patients with pernicious anemia. The inhibitory factor was shown to be a γ-globulin. It was subsequently established that there are two types of antibody to intrinsic factor: a blocking antibody (type 1) which combines with intrinsic factor at or near the site of vitamin B_{12} binding and blocks the formation of the vitamin B_{12}–intrinsic factor complexes, and a binding antibody which reacts with the intrinsic factor molecule at a site distant from the vitamin-binding site (Roitt *et al.*, 1969; Ashworth *et al.*, 1967). Type 2 binding antibodies may prevent the absorption of vitamin B_{12} in the distal ileum. Type 1 antibodies are detectable by radioimmunoassay (Ardeman and Chanarin, 1963) and type 2 antibodies by immunoelectrophoresis (Jeffries *et al.*, 1962). Some 40–60% of patients with pernicious anemia have type 1 intrinsic factor antibodies in the serum, and more have these antibodies if gastric juice as well as serum is examined (Chanarin and James, 1974). Intrinsic factor antibodies occur very rarely in the general population. Often intrinsic factor antibodies are associated with antibodies to gastric parietal cells (Irvine, 1975).

B. Autoimmunity to Sperm in Infertility

Animals immunized with autologous spermatozoa or testis homogenate in complete adjuvant form autoantibodies against spermatozoa, detectable in agglutination, immobilization, complement fixation, immunofluorescence, skin-sensitizing, cytotoxicity, and other tests. The immunized animals may develop autoimmune orchitis with aspermatogenesis. In 1954, Wilson and Rumke independently found agglutination in the ejaculated sperm of some infertile males and showed that this was due to the presence of antibodies in the serum. These antibodies could agglutinate normal spermatozoa from other persons, as well as those of the subjects, and could be absorbed out of the serum by spermatozoa but not by other cell types. Further properties were reviewed by Rumke and Hekman (1975). Microscopic examination of sperm incubated with serum that contained antibodies shows various patterns of agglutination. Head-to-head agglutination can be distinguished from tail-to-tail agglutination, which is more common. The sperm-agglutinating factor is usually antibody, as shown by fractionation and mixed antiglobulin reactions. Head agglutinins are often IgM, tail agglutinins IgG, and agglutinins in seminal plasma probably IgA. The relationship with sperm immobilization and cytolysis is discussed in the section on antibody and complement.

Rumke and Hekman (1975) found that the probability of men with normal sperm counts becoming fathers was inversely correlated with titers of sperm-agglutinating antibodies. Fifty or sixty per cent of vasectomized men form sperm antibodies, as well as weak antibodies to protamine, the sperm-specific nuclear protein. Although, in experimental animals, vasectomy can lead to autoimmune orchitis, the only clear implication of antibody responses after vasectomy in man is the possibility of immunologic infertility when reanastomosis has been performed.

C. Thyroid-Stimulating Antibodies

Graves' disease has many features suggestive of autoimmunity, including lymphoid infiltration of the thyroid and retroorbital tissues, the presence of thyroid-specific autoantibodies and deposition of immunoglobulins in the follicular basement membrane. However, the pathogenesis of the hyperthyroidism was not explained until the discovery of thyroid-stimulating antibodies. The long-acting thyroid stimulator (LATS) was found by Adams and Purves (1956) when serum from a thyrotoxic patient, injected into guinea pigs prepared for bioassay of TSH, was observed to cause unexpectedly prolonged stimulation of thyroid function. This was confirmed by McKenzie (1958) using mice instead of guinea pigs, providing a standard *in vivo* procedure for estimation of LATS. Mouse thyroid glands prelabeled with radioactive iodine can also be stimulated *in vitro* by LATS. Evidence has accumulated that LATS is an IgG antibody reacting with the TSH receptor of thyroid cells and stimulating the synthesis of cyclic AMP. This, in turn, leads to increased endocytosis of colloid which is degraded to liberate the thyroid hormones, T_3 and T_4, into the blood stream (see Kendall-Taylor, 1974). The capacity to stimulate lies in the Fab part of the molecule, although this stimulation with the univalent fragment is less prolonged than with the intact molecule. Thyroid stimulation by LATS does not require the participation of complement. This is seen from the stimulation produced by isolated Fab fragments, the detection of LATS in complement-depleted serum, and LATS responses in complement-deficient mice.

LATS can be absorbed by human thyroid preparations, and Adams and Kennedy (1967) observed that this *in vitro* reaction is blocked by the addition of sera from some thyrotoxic patients. The name LATS protector (LATS-P) was suggested because this factor, which proved to be a γ-globulin, protected the LATS from neutralization by the binding protein. LATS-P did not influence the response of the mouse thyroid to LATS, and LATS-P was not absorbed by mouse thyroid preparations. The possibility that LATS-P might be a human thyroid antibody, not reacting with mouse thyroid, was supported by the observations of Adams and his colleagues (1974) that sera containing LATS-P, but not LATS, stimulated thyroid function in human volunteers. Thus, LATS is a powerful mouse thyroid stimulator but does not stimulate the human thyroid, although it is bound by it. In contrast LATS-P is a human thyroid stimulator. Adams *et al.* (1975) propose in future to use the term thyroid-stimulating antibodies (TSAb) for both, human thyroid stimulator (HTS) for LATS-P, and mouse thyroid stimulator (MTS) for LATS. HTS is found in at least 90% of cases of diffuse toxic goiter, and there is now strong evidence that it is the direct cause of the thyroid hyperactivity in this condition (see Chapter 21). This is a common autoimmune disease, the pathogenesis of which is well understood.

V. COLLABORATION OF AUTOANTIBODIES AND COMPLEMENT

A. Autoimmune Hemolytic Anemias

Antibodies alone agglutinate but do not lyse cells, so that as a rule collaboration between antibodies and complement components or the appropriate effector cells is required for hemolysis. Some cells are more sensitive than others to lysis in the presence of antibodies and complement; e.g., erythrocytes from patients with paroxysmal nocturnal hemoglobinuria are more sensitive than normal human erythrocytes (Hinz *et al.*, 1961). For autoimmune disease to be produced by this mechanism, three components are necessary: antibodies of a complement-fixing subclass, sensitive cells, and complement. Complement is fixed efficiently by antibodies of the IgM class and IgG1 and IgG3 subclasses. Only a single molecule of IgM is required to activate complement by the classical pathway, whereas two closely apposed IgG molecules, which can be bridged by complement, are required. Erythrocytes of several species, including man, are relatively resistant to hemolysis by antibody and complement, so that many molecules of C1 have to be activated nearly simultaneously for lysis to occur (see Schreiber and Frank, 1972a).

The role of complement in autoimmune hemolysis is illustrated by the paroxysmal hemoglobinurias. In cold hemoglobinuria, there is a special kind of cold agglutinin, first studied by Donath and Landsteiner (1925), which combines with the alloantigen of human erythrocytes at lowered temperatures. When the complex is returned to body temperature, the bound antibody can activate complement and produce lysis. Binding of C1 in the cold phase stabilizes the complex at body temperature. The sequence of events in the classical pathway of complement activation is then set in motion (Hinz *et al.*, 1961).

Complement sensitization by high-affinity antibodies reacting with abundant antigenic sites on the surface of the erythrocyte can certainly result in intravascular lysis. Thus, most anti-A and anti-B antibodies are hemolytic *in vitro* and can produce rapid intravascular lysis *in vivo* (Mollison, 1972). This type of lysis may well occur in severe, acute autoimmune episodes. However, activation of the complement system by cell-bound autoantibodies does not always result in hemolysis.

Complement components bound to erythrocytes *in vivo* have been demonstrated in some patients with autoimmune hemolytic anemias using agglutination by antisera against C3 (see Fischer *et al.*, 1974). Complement components are found on the red cells of all patients with cold agglutinin disease (about 22% of autoimmune hemolytic anemias) and 44% of patients with warm antibody autoimmune hemolytic anemias. There are differences between results with anti-immunoglobulin and anti-complement Coombs' tests. Thus, cells from patients with cold agglutinin disease always give positive results with anti-C3 sera and negative results with anti-immunoglobulin sera. In contrast, cells from patients with autoimmune hemolytic anemias associated with administration of Aldomet (Worlledge *et al.*, 1966) or penicillin (Petz and Fudenberg, 1966) are strongly agglutinated by anti-immunoglobulin sera, but rarely by anti-C3. Immune hemolytic anemia in patients with systemic lupus erythematosus is regularly associated with the presence of complement on erythrocytes, usually accompanied by IgG. The demonstration of complement components bound to erythrocytes *in vivo* is an important contribution to the diagnosis of autoimmune hemolytic anemias in human patients. They may also have low levels of serum complement and increased fractional catabolic rates of C3.

Fischer and his colleagues used an immunochemical method to measure the number of C3 molecules bound to human erythrocytes *in vivo* and *in vitro*. The agglutination test, using antisera against C3, became positive with about 100 molecules of C3 per cell and was strongly positive with 1000 molecules per cell. Of 11 patients with more than 1100 molecules of C3 per cell, 61% had hemolytic anemia, whereas only 14% of 14 patients with less than 100 molecules of C3 per cell had hemolysis. Thus, the amount of C3 per cell is generally, but not always, related to the degree of hemolysis in human autoimmune hemolytic anemias.

The question arises how red cells coated with complement components survive in the circulation. In the next section, evidence will be presented that red cells coated with C3b are attached to specific receptors on mononuclear phagocytes but not endocytosed. In fact, C3b can be degraded to C3c and C3d and the attachment reversed. These *in vitro* experiments have counterparts in experimental animals and humans. Schreiber and Frank (1972a,b) found that about 60 IgM molecules, each a complement-fixing site, are required on a guinea pig erythrocyte for immune clearance. Most cells so sensitized were cleared by the liver in 5 minutes and were then slowly returned to the circulation where they survived normally. With continued exposure of the IgM:C site to fresh serum, the capacity to be cleared was lost. Likewise, there is evidence that, under certain circumstances, human erythrocytes coated with complement components may, after temporary sequestration in the liver, survive normally (Mollison, 1972). Collaboration of IgG antibodies and complement in the initiation of endocytosis is discussed in the next section.

The mechanism of resistance of erythrocytes to complement-mediated hemolysis in some patients with chronic cold agglutinin disease has been analyzed by Engelfriet *et al.* (1972). The authors conclude that, when red cells react with cold autoagglutinins *in vivo*, they are either hemolyzed immediately or, for unknown reasons, escape hemolysis. In the latter case, β_1E and β_1A disappear from the membrane. To the sites where these proteins have been attached, no further β_1E or β_1A molecules can be attached, so that generation of biologically active complement components is impossible. Specific antisera show that red cells from patients with autoimmune hemolytic anemia sensitized *in vivo* with C3 have only C3b in the surface (Engelfriet *et al.*, 1970).

B. Immobilization and Lysis of Spermatozoa

Microscopic tests allow the detection of antibodies immobilizing spermatozoa (Rumke and Hekman, 1975). Although some agglutinating sera may not show immobilizing activity, in general there is a close correlation between the presence of agglutinins and immobilizins. The immobilization requires more antibody as well as more complement, with rare exceptions. Cytotoxic antibodies to spermatozoa, detected by the trypan blue exclusion method, are also complement dependent.

VI. COLLABORATION OF AUTOANTIBODIES AND MONONUCLEAR PHAGOCYTES

Following the recommendations of the World Health Organization (van Furth *et al.*, 1972), it is now customary to use the term "mononuclear phagocyte system," rather than "reticuloendothelial system." Mononuclear phagocytes arise from stem cells in the bone marrow which can also differentiate into polymorphonuclear phagocytes (Metcalf and Moore, 1971). When suitably stimulated by colony-forming factors, the stem cells differentiate in the bone marrow into promonocytes, which adhere to glass and are phagocytic. These differentiate further into monocytes, which circulate in the peripheral blood and contribute to the population of mononuclear phagocytes in various tissues, e.g., the macrophages of the peritoneal and pleural cavities and pulmonary alveoli and the Kupffer cells which span the hepatic sinusoids.

Human monocytes and peritoneal macrophages have on their surfaces receptors for C3b and for the Fc regions of IgG1 and IgG3, but not for IgM, IgA, or the other subclasses of IgG. Erythrocytes to which IgG1 or IgG3 antibodies are bound are attached to monocytes, and this attachment is rapidly followed by phagocytosis (Huber and Weiner, 1974). In contrast, erythrocytes sensitized with IgM antibodies and C3 are attached to monocytes and form rosettes, but phagocytosis does not follow. Thus, the attachment to the Fc receptor of appropriate IgG subclasses triggers the contraction of the actomyosin system that moves the plasma membrane over the erythrocyte, whereas the attachment of C3b to the corresponding receptor on the plasma membrane does not.

A similar specificty is shown in the collaboration of antibodies and mononuclear phagocytes to lyse erythrocytes. For example, human erythrocytes of blood group A treated with IgG isoantibody to the A antigen are lysed by purified human peripheral blood monocytes or peritoneal macrophages in the absence of the complete complement sequence. Monocytes were able to lyse an excess of erythrocytes. In contrast, purified peripheral blood lymphocytes added to similarly sensitized erythrocytes at a lymphocyte: erythrocyte ratio of 25:1 have no effect under the same experimental conditions (Holm and Hammarström, 1973). Further studies of the class and subclass specificity of the lysis have been published by Holm *et al.*

(1974). IgM antibody (anti-A or cold agglutinin) was unable to collaborate in monocyte-mediated hemolysis. Lysis occurred with approximately equal efficiency when anti-D antibodies of subclasses IgG1 or IgG3 were used to sensitize the cells. The lytic reaction was inhibited by IgG1 or IgG3 myeloma proteins, native or heat-aggregated. IgG2 or IgG4 had only very weak inhibitory effects, possibly due to a low level of contamination with IgG1 or IgG3. Lysis of erythrocytes sensitized by IgG1 or IgG3 anti-D was equally well inhibited by IgG1 or IgG3 myeloma proteins, suggesting that the same receptor for Fc reacts with the CH_2 domain of IgG or requires interaction of the CH_2 and CH_3 domains.

Since the specificity of the monocyte receptors for Fc is the same as required for phagocytosis, it is not surprising that, during the incubation giving rise to lysis, there is some phagocytosis of erythrocytes. This is one factor in the lysis, but many erythrocytes are lysed by contact with monocytes in the absence of phagocytosis. Indeed, binding of erythrocytes sensitized with anti-D antibodies by human monocytes, with subsequent sphering of erythrocytes, is well known (Lo Buglio *et at.*, 1967). The mechanism of killing of erythrocytes by human mononuclear phagocytic cells apparently requires contact (Holm *et al.*, 1974). However, this was thought to be true in the case of mouse peritoneal mononuclear phagocytes, which when cultured for 8 hours acquire the ability to lyse syngeneic or allogeneic erythrocytes (Melsom *et al.*, 1974). Under ordinary culture conditions with serum in the medium, the lysis requires contact or close proximity of effector cells and target cells. However, by using a medium containing mercaptoethanol and lacking serum, it was possible to demonstrate a soluble lytic factor released from the mononuclear phagocytes. This factor is unstable and, therefore, not detected under ordinary conditions. It is a dialyzable substance which resists heating at 60°C for 30 minutes.

The effectiveness of IgG (but not IgM) antibodies in bringing about immune clearance of erythrocytes *in vivo* has been shown in C4-deficient guinea pigs, in which biologically active complement components are not generated (Atkinson and Frank, 1974). This complement-independent clearance was blocked by cortisone, which appears to inhibit the attachment of erythrocytes coated with IgG to splenic macrophages. The effectiveness of the cortisone block depended on the number of antibody molecules per cell; in the presence of many antibody molecules, the clearance could not be suppressed by cortisone. These observations may help to explain the effectiveness of corticosteroid therapy in some patients with autoimmune hemolytic anemias.

In the presence of small numbers of IgG molecules, especially with IgG antibodies of relatively low affinity, clearance is enhanced by complement (Schreiber and Frank, 1972a,b). About 2000 IgG molecules were required to form a complement-fixing site on the guinea pig erythrocyte surface, and about 1.4 complement-fixing sites were required for immune clearance of IgG-sensitized cells. Progressive trapping in the spleen was responsible for most of the clearance of IgG-sensitized cells. The contribution of the complement system to clearance was shown by its impairment in guinea pigs with C4 deficiency or depleted of late (C3–9) components with cobra venom factor. Splenic clearance of cells sensitized by IgG and complement was not readily reversed (unlike that of cells sensitized with IgM and complement; see previous section). Likewise IgG:complement attachment sites were more stable when incubated with fresh serum than the IgM:complement attachment sites. Possibly C3b molecules in the former are protected to some extent from degradation to C3d.

In general, it is likely that collaboration of autoantibodies with mononuclear phagocytes plays a major role in the pathogenesis of autoimmune hemolysis. The use of subclass-specific antisera shows that human erythrocytes can be coated by antibodies of all IgG subclasses. Erythrocytes coated with IgG1 and IgG3, with rare exceptions, become attached to monocytes, and the patients have signs of hemolytic anemia; erythrocytes coated only with IgG2 do not become attached to monocytes, and the patients do not show signs of hemolysis (C. P. Engelfriet, personal communication, 1976).

In some situations, especially with IgG antibodies, fixation of complement facilitates attachment of sensitized erythrocytes to mononuclear phagocytes, and this occurs in the spleen more readily than in other sites. Because the same subclasses of antibodies (IgG1 and IgG3) sensitize cells for attachment to mononuclear phagocytes and fix complement, these two processes tend to go together. It has long been known that sera containing complement-fixing autoantibodies promote phagocytosis of human erythrocytes, whereas sera containing other autoantibodies do not (Bonnin and Schwartz, 1954). However, the two processes may not always be correlated.

Presumably, contact of erythrocytes and mononuclear phagocytes results in phagocytosis in some cases, whereas, in other cases, the erythrocytes are lysed in an extracellular position. Some erythrocytes may be released as spherocytes before lysis is complete. Spherocytosis is prominent in many cases of autoimmune hemolytic anemia.

VII. PATHOGENESIS OF DISEASE BY AUTOANTIBODIES GENERATING IMMUNE COMPLEXES

A. Immune Complexes Containing DNA

The role of immune complexes in the pathogenesis of glomerulonephritis, vasculitis, and arthritis in SLE has been discussed by many investigators (see Feltkamp, 1975). Thus, Winfield *et al.* (1975) quote several lines of evidence suggesting that circulating complexes of DNA and anti-DNA antibodies are important in the pathogenesis of tissue injury in this disease. Increased titers of serum antibodies against native DNA (nDNA) and, to a lesser extent, single-stranded DNA (sDNA in general, are correlated with clinical activity and hypocomplementemia. Both nDNA and sDNA have been found to alternate with the presence of circulating antibody in the serum. Renal biopsies from cases of SLE with glomerulonephritis have shown the presence of immunoglobulins, complement components, and single-stranded DNA determinants in renal glomeruli. All patients examined had IgG and C3, while IgM, C1q, and sDNA determinants were present inconsistently but were usually associated with one another. Talal (1976) has recently reported correlation of serum IgG antibodies to nDNA and severity of disease.

Winfield and his colleagues isolated glomeruli from autopsy kidneys of patients with severe SLE glomerulonephritits and treated them with acid buffer or deoxyribonuclease. All eluates contained IgG, in most cases having antibodies against nDNA and sDNA in concentrations higher than those in serum. Antiribonucleoprotein was detected in 5 out of 10 eluates and was selectively concentrated in 3. These observations extend previously published reports that nDNA and sDNA and their complexes are present in the kidneys of patients with glomerulonephritis associated with SLE.

Recently, evidence has accumulated that serum cryoprecipitation may be a manifestation of immune complex formation (Brouet *et al.*, 1974). In SLE, cryoprecipitation is associated with hypocomplementemia and nephritis. Winfield *et al.* (1975) were able to show IgG antibodies against polynucleotides, as well as IgM rheumatoid factor and C1q in most cryoprecipitates. They suggest that complexes of DNA–anti DNA, IgM rheumatoid factor, and C1q may have the maximum potential for tissue damage.

This is now the conventional explanation of the pathogenesis of glomerulonephritis associated with SLE. However, the last word on the subject has not yet been said. Antibodies to highly purified DNA are probably not pathonomonic for SLE (Davis, 1975). There is no simple relationship between the presence of anti-DNA antibodies fixing complement and glomerulonephritis. Jokinen and Makitalo (1960) found complement-fixing antibodies to DNA in 5 out of 20 sera from cases of SLE. All five of the cases had LE cells and four of the five had arthritis and rash but only two of the patients had nephritis. although patients with persistent high levels of anti-DNA and hypocomplementemia more often show exacerbations of disease, including renal complications, this does not always occur (Lightfoot *et al.*, 1975). Hence, it is still not clear why the presence of autoantibodies against DNA sometimes gives rise to immunopathological manifestations and at other times does not. Perhaps antigen affinity and other properties of the antibodies will provide an explanation.

B. Immune Complexes in Exophthalmos

Two distinct lesions in endocrine exophthalmos are myositis of the extraocular muscles and increased bulk of retrobulbar connective tissue, especially fat. The latter is probably due to stimulating antibodies.

The extraocular myositis is characterized by edema and lymphoid infiltration, with necrosis of muscle fibers (Riley, 1972). Patients with exophthalmos have high concentrations of antibodies against thyroglobulin which leaves the thyroid via the lymphatics. Kriss (1970) demonstrated a connection between the lymphatic channels draining the thyroid gland with those draining the orbit. This suggested that soluble complexes of thyroglobulin and antibody might be involved in the lesions of exophthalmos. Konishi *et al.* (1974) found that complexes of thyroglobulin and antibody are more strongly bound to plasma membranes isolated from extraocular muscles than to membranes from other muscles or liver, and that the immune complexes are much more firmly bound than is thyroglobulin. Since T_3 and T_4 are present on the surface of the thyroglobulin molecules, the affinity for extraocular muscle membranes may be due to the large number of thyroid hormone-binding sites on these cells, reflecting a high level of physiological activity (Doniach and Florin-Christensen, 1975).

VIII. COLLABORATION OF AUTOANTIBODIES WITH NONSPECIFIC EFFECTOR CELLS (K CELLS)

Certain lymphoid cells with receptors for the Fc region of IgG can kill target cells coated with IgG antibody (see Perlmann and Holm, 1969). The capacity to kill target cells coated with antibody is exhibited by mononuclear phagocytes (especially when erythrocytes are used as targets, see Holm and Hammarström, 1973), but also by cells with the appearances of lymphocytes. The properties of these cells, which are termed K cells, have recently been described by Perlmann *et al.* (1975) and Cordier *et al.* (1976). In the human, they are found in peripheral blood, spleen, and bone marrow, but not thymus, lymph nodes, and tonsils. They have high-affinity receptors for Fc, belonging mostly to the small subset of peripheral blood lymphocytes with this property (about 1.5% of the total). Removal of most monocytes by adherence, or T or B lymphocytes by specific antisera, did not deplete the effector cell activity. Hence, the K cells lack conventional B or T lymphocyte markers. At least some of them bear receptors for C3, but C3 bound to target cells does not induce cytolysis (Perlmann *et al.*, 1975). Evidence is accumulating that, in both experimental autoimmune thyroiditis and Hashimoto's disease, there is collaboration of antibodies and K cells in the pathogenesis of lesions.

The mononuclear cell infiltrates in the thyroids of patients with Hashimoto's disease and animals with autoimmune thyroiditis were formerly interpreted as evidence that the damage was likely to be due to cytotoxic T lymphocytes. More recent observations have made that interpretation unlikely.

Electron microscopic observations of experimental autoimmune thyroiditis and Hashimoto's disease do not show appearances characteristic of T lymphocyte-mediated immunopathology. In fact, T lymphocyte infiltration is deficient, and cells of the B lymphocyte lineage are conspicuous (Wick and Graf, 1972; Söderström and Björklund, 1974). These include plasma cells closely applied to the follicular basement membranes, some penetrating into the follicles themselves (Kalderon *et al.*, 1973; Fig. 4).

The situation is shown diagramatically in Fig. 5. The plasma cells in the thyroid are secreting antibody against thyroglobulin (Tg) and other thyroid autoantigens. Tg released from the acini reacts with the antibodies. In experimental autoimmune thyroiditis, complexes of Tg and antibody along the basement membrane are readily demonstrable (Clagett and Weigle, 1974). Complexes of immunoglobulins and complement are seen on the acinar basement membrane in practically all thyrotoxic glands; these are similar to those found in the glomeruli in immune complex nephritis. They occur in small patches and are situated in the vicinity of areas of focal thyroiditis (Doniach, 1975). In Hashimoto's glands, they are less conspicuous because the lesions are more advanced, but electron-dense deposits are consistently observed in thickened follicular basement membranes, often associated with closely apposed plasma cells (Fig. 4).

Thus, the appearance of the glands are consistent with an antibody-mediated disease, and other evidence supports this view. In several animal species, experimental autoimmune thyroiditis has been transferred by immune serum (Nakamura and Weigle, 1969; Tomazic and Rose, 1975). When lymphoid cells from rabbits immunized with heterologous Tgs and developing thyroiditis are incubated with the heterologous proteins, macrophage migration-inhibition factor is liberated, whereas, when the cells are incubated with rabbit Tg, no such activity is released (Clinton and Weigle, 1972). This is evidence that T lymphocytes of the rabbit do not respond to autoantigenic Tg determinants. In rats, mice, and genetically predisposed obese chickens, thymectomy accelerates and accentuates autoimmune thyroiditis, whereas bursectomy in the chicken abolishes the disease (see above).

Thus, evidence from several sources suggest that autoimmune thyroiditis is an antibody-mediated, rather than a cell-mediated, immunopathological process. Since thyroiditis is as severe in animals depleted of C3 or congenitally lacking C5, as in intact animals, there is no indication that collaboration of antibodies and the complement system is required for pathogenesis. Hence, the question arises as to whether antibodies collaborate with K cells in damaging thyroid acinar cells, as shown diagramatically in Fig. 5. For

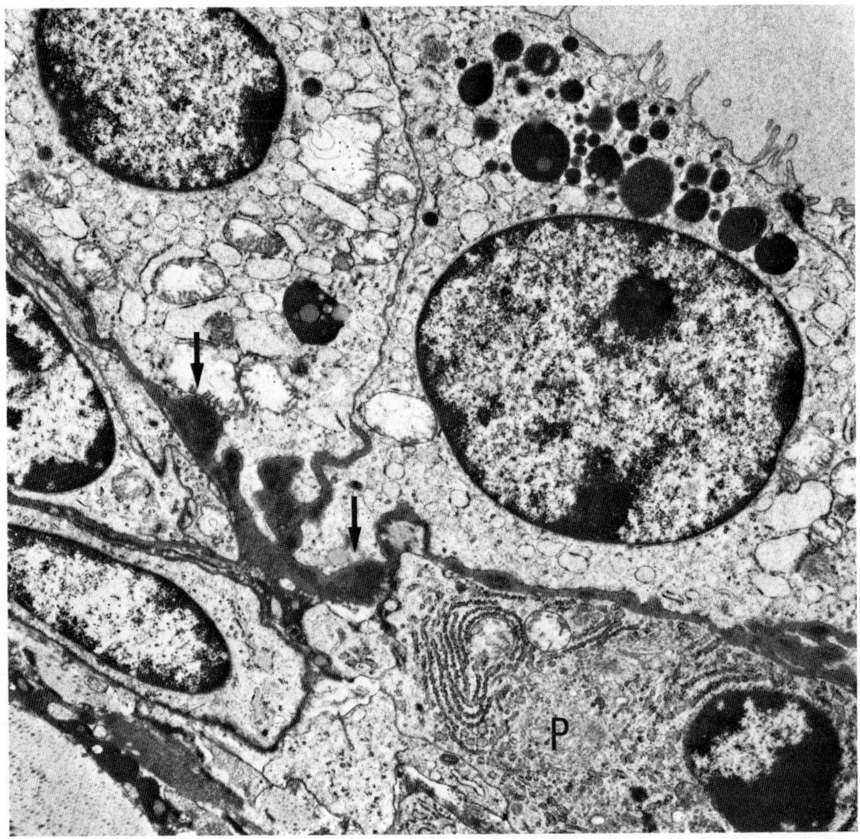

Fig. 4. The follicular basement membrane in Hashimoto's thyroiditis showing electron-dense deposits (arrows). Note penetration of the basement membrane containing deposits between two neighboring follicular cells (× 11,200). (From Kalderon *et al.* (1973), by kind permission of the author and publishers.)

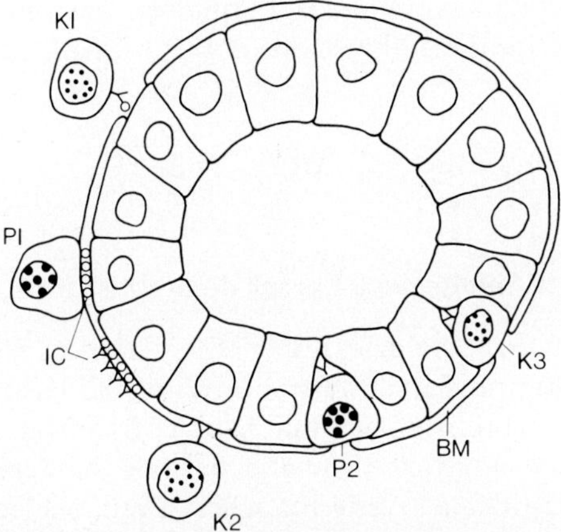

Fig. 5. Diagram showing the collaboration of plasma cells producing antibody against thyroid antigens and K cells in the pathogenesis of autoimmune thyroiditis. Plasma cells alongside the basement membrane (P1, compare Fig. 4) produce antibodies reacting against thyroid antigens. These form immune complexes (IC). At sites where the basement membrane is breached, antibodies can become attached to the base of follicular cells, and K cells (K2) can bind the antibodies. Alternatively, K cells can become specifically sensitized by immune complexes in antibody excess (K1). Plasma cells (P2) and K cells (K3) can penetrate through breaches in the basement membrane into the follicles, eventually destroying the follicular cells.

this interpretation to be tenable, it must be shown, first, that K cells can lyse target cells passively sensitized with thyroid antigens and antibodies and, second, that K cells accumulate in the gland during the course of the disease. Evidence has accumulated in support of both of these propositions.

Ringertz *et al.* (1971) induced thyroiditis by immunization of guinea pigs with homologous Tg in Freund's complete adjuvant. In the presence of sera from such animals, chicken erythrocytes coated with Tg were lysed by lymphoid cells from normal guinea pigs. Calder and Irvine (1975) have summarized observations that peripheral blood lymphocytes from normal persons are able to lyse Tg-coated target cells when serum from patients with autoimmune thyroid disease is added to the culture medium. Sera from control patients negative for Tg antibody do not cause target cell lysis. Within groups of patients with Hashimoto's thyroiditis, significant positive correlations have been found between cytotoxicity and Tg-hemagglutinating antibody titers. The cells released from surgical specimens of Hashimoto's thyroiditis include K cells able to lyse antibody-coated ^{51}Cr-labeled target cells (Allison, 1974). Thus, the antibodies and effector cells that form a lytic system are all present in the thyroids of patients, as well as experimental animals with autoimmune thyroiditis, and this provides the most likely mechanism for the pathogenesis of the disease.

IX. AUTOIMMUNE DISEASE MEDIATED BY T LYMPHOCYTES

A. Experimental Autoimmune Encephalomyelitis (EAE)

This is an immunopathological reaction induced in experimental animals by injection of central nervous tissue myelin, the basic protein of myelin (BP, MW 18,000 daltons), or certain peptide fragments derived from it, in Freund's complete adjuvant. The use of well-characterized antigens has made possible progress in several branches of immunology. EAE is the only autoimmune disease for which detailed information is available on the chemical composition of the antigen and the activity of various fragments. The experiments have been complicated by the fact that BPs from several species (bovine, human, guinea pig, and rat), which differ in composition, have been used. Several species of experimental animals have shown certain differences in response, and, within a species, strains differ in susceptibility to EAE. This has allowed the accumulation of information of genetic control of susceptibility to EAE and the underlying immunopathological mechanisms. Traditional approaches suggested that EAE is a cell-mediated immunopathological process, and recent experiments, in general, support this view, although with some reservations, which will be mentioned. Antibodies can certainly produce demyelination under appropriate circumstances, and their role in human disease must not be overlooked.

The evidence in support of cell-mediated immunity (CMI) can be summarized briefly. The disease is transferred by lymph node or thoracic duct cells, but not by sera, from animals with EAE (Paterson, 1967; Stone, 1961). Animals show delayed hypersensitivity to BP or central nervous tissue antigens (Shaw *et al.*, 1965). The *in vitro* migration of peritoneal cells from animals with EAE is specifically inhibited by nervous tissue antigens (Rauch *et al.*, 1969). Production of EAE in agammoglobulinemic chickens has been reported (Blaw *et al.*, 1967).

In rats, the major encephalitogenic determinant (ED) of BP is contained in a fragment containing 43 amino acids, residues 45–87. The capacity of rats to develop EAE is under the control of a gene, designated by Williams and Moore (1973) as the Ir–EAE gene, which is linked to the major histocompatibility locus. Lewis rats, which are highly susceptible, are homozygous for this gene, whereas resistant BN rats lack the susceptibility gene. McFarlin *et al.* (1975) have presented evidence that only Lewis rats have the capacity to mount a CMI against ED, but that both strains have the capacity to make antibodies against other parts of the BP molecule. Antibody production was greater in Lewis rats, suggesting that the encephalitogenic determinant recognized by T lymphocytes of the rat may function as a helper determinant in the production of antibody. Tests for CMI included delayed hypersensitivity skin tests, mitogenesis when lymphoid cells were cultured with antigen, and production of macrophage migration-inhibitory factor.

In guinea pigs, encephalitogenic activity is confined almost exclusively to

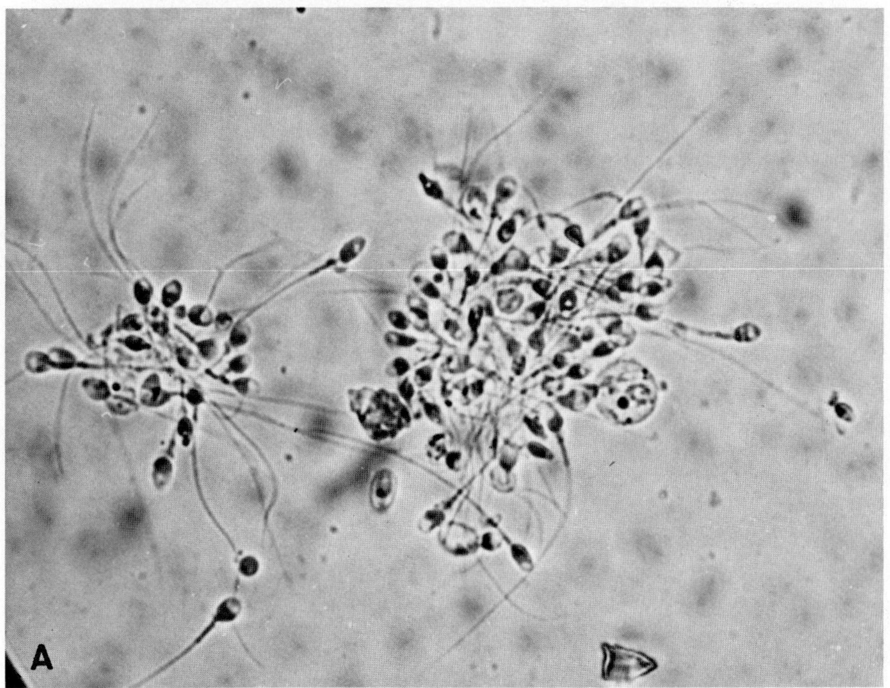

Fig. 6. Agglutination of human spermatozoa by different types of autoantibodies. (A) Mixed-type agglutination in an ejaculate of a patient with sperm agglutinins in his serum and seminal plasma. This is a common form of agglutination seen both in ejaculates and after incubation of normal semen with patient's serum. (B) Head-to-head agglutination of normal spermatozoa by serum of an infertile man (phase contrast). This form of agglutination is rare and is hardly ever seen in an ejaculate. (C) Tail tip-to-tail tip agglutination of normal spermatozoa by serum of an infertile man (phase contrast). This form of agglutination is rare and only clearly visible at the beginning of the agglutination. After prolonged incubation the whole tail seems to be involved. It has never been observed in an ejaculate.

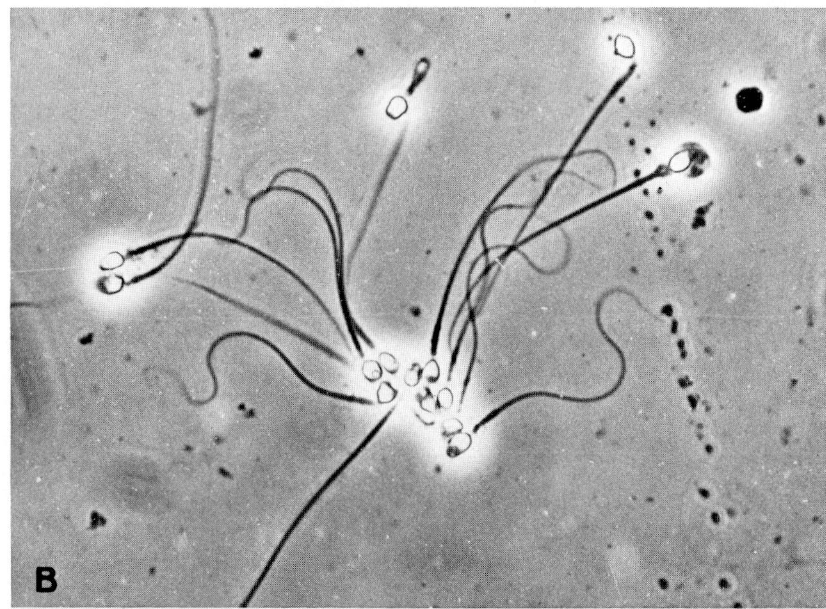

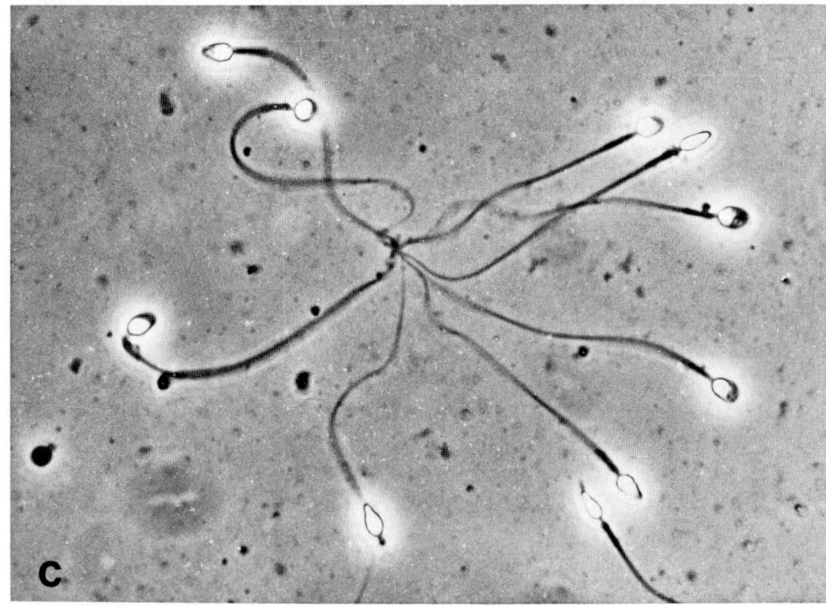

Fig. 6 (Continued)

a nonapeptide immediately surrounding the single tryptophan residue in the molecule, residues 114–122. Spitler *et al.* (1975) produced EAE in guinea pigs with human BP and the major encephalitogenic peptide (residues 114–122). Guinea pigs immunized with BP developed EAE but did not show CMI to the encephalitogenic peptide, as measured by skin-test reactivity, lymphocyte stimulation, or macrophage-migration inhibition. They did, however, show CMI to the intact BP. Animals immunized with the peptide regularly developed EAE and showed CMI to the peptide, but not to the BP. The authors conclude that, since CMI to the disease-producing determinant of the molecule could not be demonstrated, CMI, as measured by the three commonly used tests, may not necessarily be correlated with the production of EAE. They suggest that other possible mechanisms, including production of mediators or of antibodies, should be considered. An alternative explanation would be that EAE can be produced by T lymphocyte recognition of different determinants when the intact BP molecules and encephalitogenic peptide are used for immunization. For example, the folding of the polypeptide chain in the vicinity of the tryp-

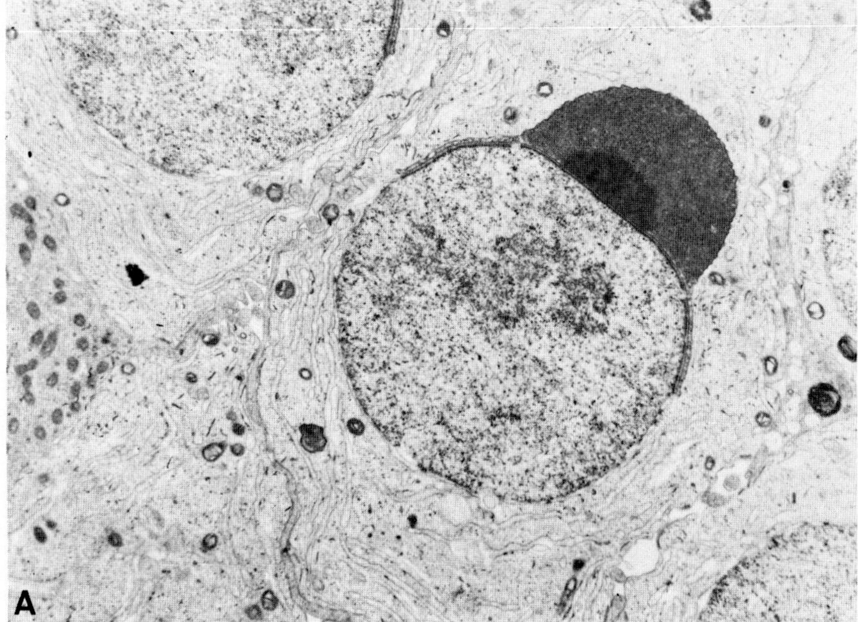

Fig. 7. Electron micrograph of a normal guinea pig spermatid, showing (A) the normal appearance of the electron-dense acrosome alongside the nucleus, and (B) the distorted acrosome in a guinea pig with experimental autoimmune orchitis (× 10,500). (From Brown *et al.* (1972) by kind permission of the author and publishers.)

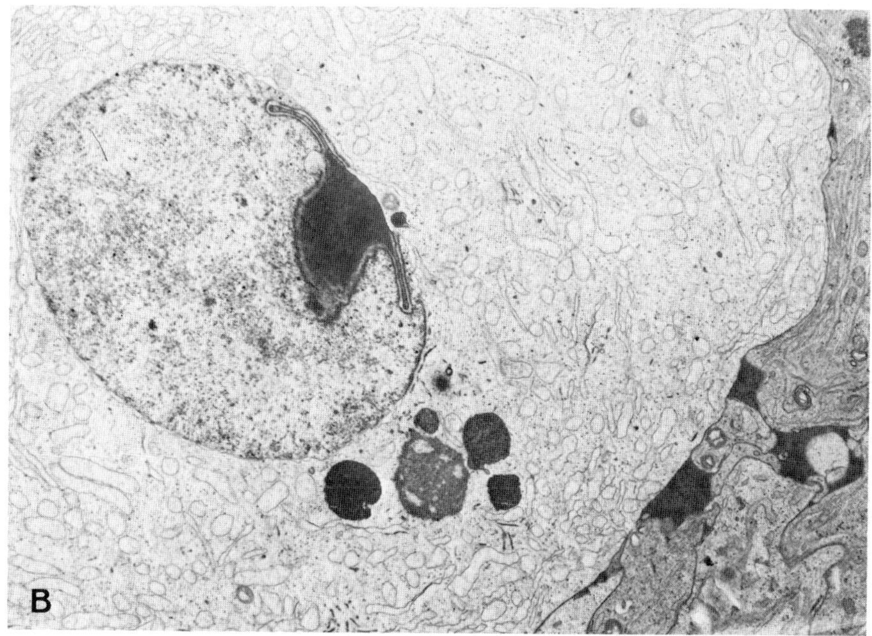

Fig. 7 (Continued)

tophan residue may be different. Further work with fragments should make it possible to decide whether EAE is mediated by T lymphocytes.

Another interesting development is the suppression of EAE by certain immunizing procedures. For example, the disease can be suppressed by administration of BP without Freund's complete adjuvant, even after the administration of BP in the complete adjuvant. Immunization with some nonencephalitogenic fragments of BP, and even synthetic peptides (such as a copolymer of alanine, glutamic acid, lysine, and tyrosine) can suppress the disease in monkeys as well as other experimental animals (Teitelbaum *et al.*, 1974). Whether these effects are mediated by suppressor T lymphocytes or other mechanisms is currently under investigation.

X. COLLABORATION OF AUTOANTIBODIES AND CELL-MEDIATED IMMUNITY

According to Brown *et al.* (1972; Brown and Glynn, 1969), experimental allergic orchitis in the guinea pig develops only when autoantibodies and sensitized lymphocytes giving delayed hypersensitivity are simultaneously present. The purified antigen used with Freund's complete adjuvant to induce this condition is acrosomal glycoprotein. In animals with the disease, immunofluorescence shows autoantibody bound to the acrosomes of the developing spermatids in the seminiferous tubules (Fig. 6). Ultrastructural studies show failure of accumulation of acrosomal material to form an acrosome, with consequent arrest of maturation of the cells (Fig. 7). The tubular basement membrane is not breached, and blood-borne cells are not seen within the tubules. Hence, the lesion is apparently antibody mediated. However, antibodies injected into the blood do not penetrate into the seminiferous tubules and produce disease. The first appearance of antibody bound to acrosomes in the tubules coincides with the development of delayed hypersensitivity in the caput epididymis, where traces of antigen meet sensitized lymphocytes. The permeability factors released apparently facilitate the penetration of antibody into the target organ.

REFERENCES

Adams, D. D., and Kennedy, T. H. (1967) *J. Clin. Endocrinol. Metab.* **27,** 173.

Adams, D. D., and Purves, H. D. (1956) *Proc. Univ. Otago Med. Sch.* **34,** 11.

Adams, D. D., Fastier, J. B., Howie, J. B., Kennedy, T. H., Kilpatrick, J. A., and Stewart, R. D. H. (1974) *J. Clin. Endocrinol. Metab.* **39,** 826.

Adams, D. D., Dirmikis, S., Dorniack, D., El Kabir, D. J., Hall, R., Ibbertson H. K., Irvine, W. J., Kendall-Taylor, P., Marley, S. W., Mehdi, S. Q., Munro, D. S., Purves, H. D., Smith, B. R., and Stewart, R. D. H. (1973). *Lancet* **1,** 1201.

Adelmann, B. C., Kirrane, J. A., and Glynn, L. E. (1972). *Immunology* **23,** 723.

Aho, K., and Wager, P. (1961). *Acta Med. Exp. Biol. Fenn.* **39,** 79.

Alarçon-Segovia, D., Wakim, K. G., Worthington, J. W., and Ward, C. G. (1967). *Medicine* (*Baltimore*) **46,** 1.

Albini, B., and Wick, G. (1973). *Immunology* **24,** 545.

Allison, A. C. (1971). *Lancet* **2,** 1401.

Allison, A. C. (1973). *Immunopotentiation, Ciba Found. Symp., 1973* p. 19.

Allison, A. C. (1974). *In* "Immunological Tolerance" D. H. Katz and B. Benacerraf, eds.), p. 25. Academic Press, New York.

Allison, A. C., Denman, A. M., and Barnes, R. D. (1971). *Lancet* **2,** 135.

Amos, H. E., Garner, B. W., Olds, R. J., and Coombs, R. R. A. (1967). *Int. Arch. Allergy Appl. Immunol.* **32,** 496.

Andersen, P., and Andersen, H. K. (1975). *Clin. Exp. Immunol.* **22,** 22.

Anderson, C. L., and Rose, N. R. (1971) *J. Immunol.* **107,** 1341.

Andersson, B., and Wigzell, H. (1971) *Eur. J. Immunol.* **1,** 384.

Ardeman, S., and Chanarin, I. (1963) *Lancet* **2,** 1350.

Aronson, M., Phillips, C. A., and Beeken, W. (1974). *Gastroenterology* **66,** 661.

Asherson, G. L. (1968). *Prog. Allergy* **12,** 192.

Asherson, G. L., and Mayhew, B. (1976). *Isr. J. Med. Sci.* **12,** 454.

Ashworth, L. A. E., England, J. M., Fisher, J. M., and Taylor, K. B. (1967). *Lancet* **2,** 1160.

Atkinson, J. P., and Frank, M. M. (1974). *Blood* **44,** 629.

Bach, J. F., Dardenne, M., and Salomon, J.-C. (1973). *Clin. Exp. Immunol.* **14,** 247.

Bankhurst, A. D., Torrigiani, G., and Allison, A. C. (1973). *Lancet* **1,** 226.

Barthold, D. R., Kysela, S., and Steinberg, A. D. (1973). *J. Immunol.* **2,** 133.

Baumgarten, A., and Geizy, A. F. (1970). *Immunology* **19,** 205.

Beeken, W. L., Mitchell, D. N., and Cave, D. R. (1976). *Clin. Gastroenterol.* **5,** 289.

Bell, E. B. (1973). *Eur. J. Immunol.* **3,** 267.

Bendixen, G., and Söborg, M. (1969). *Dan. Med. Bull.* **16,** 1.

Blaw, M. E., Cooper, M. D., and Good, R. A. (1967). *Science* **158,** 1198.

Blomgren, S. E., Condemi, J. J., and Vaughan, J. H. (1972). *Am. J. Med.* **52,** 338.

Bolten, P. M., Heatley, R. V., Owen, E., Heatley, R. V., Jones Williams, W., and Hughes, L. E. (1973). *Lancet* **2,** 1122.

Bonnin, J. A., and Schwartz, L. (1954). *Blood* **9,** 773.

Bonomo, L., Tursi, A., Trimisbiozzi, G., and Daniacco, F. (1965). *Br. Med. J.* **11,** 689.

Boyse, E. A., Bressler, E., Iritani, C. A., and Lardis, M. (1970). *Transplantation* **9,** 339.

Brostoff, J. (1974). *Proc. R. Soc. Med.* **67,** 514.

Brouet, J. C., Clauvel, J.-P., Danon, F., Klein, M., and Seligmann, M. (1974). *Am. J. Med.* **57,** 775.

Brown, P. C., and Glynn, L. E. (1969). *J. Pathol.* **98,** 277.

Brown, P. C., Dorling, J., and Glynn, L. E. (1972). *J. Pathol.* **176,** 229.

Burnet, F. M. (1949). "The Clonal Theory of Acquired Immunity." Cambridge Univ. Press, London and New York.

Burns, W. H., and Allison, A. C. (1975). *In* "The Antigens" (M. Sela, ed.), Vol. 3, p. 479. Academic Press, New York.

Burrell, R. G. (1963). *Am. Rev. Respir. Dis.* **87,** 389.

Busci, R. A., and Strausser, R. (1972). *Experientia* **82,** 194.

Calder, E., and Irvine, W. J. (1975). *Clin. Endocrinol. Metab.* **4,** 287.

Cannat, A., and Seligmann, M. (1968). *Clin. Exp. Immunol.* **3,** 99.

Cannat, A., and Varet, B. (1973). *Biomedicine* **19,** 108.

Cantor, H. (1972). *Cell. Immunol.* **3,** 461.

Cantor, H., Asofsky, R., and Talal, N. (1970). *J. Exp. Med.* **131,** 223.

Cave, D., Kane, S. P., and Mitchell, D. N. (1973). *Lancet* **2,** 1120.

Chanarin, I., and James, D. (1974). *Lancet* **1,** 1078.

Chiller, J. M., Habicht, G. S., and Weigle, W. O. (1970). *Science* **171,** 813.

Christian, C. L. (1963). *J. Exp. Med.* **118,** 827.

Chused, T. M., Steinberg, A. D., and Parker, L. M. (1973). *J. Immunol.* **111,** 52.

Clagett, J. A., and Weigle, W. O. (1974). *J. Exp. Med.* **139,** 643.

Clinton, B., and Weigle, W. O. (1972). *J. Exp. Med.* **136,** 1605.

Cochrane, A. M. G., Maussouros, A., Thompson, A. C., Eddleston, A. L. W. F., and Williams, R. (1975). *Lancet* **1,** 441.

Cock, A. G., and Simonsen, M. (1958). *Immunology* **1,** 103.

Cordier, G., Samarut, C., Brochier, J., and Revillard, J. P. (1976). *Scand. J. Immunol.* **5,** 233.

Cotes, P. M., Hobbs, K. E., and Bangham, D. R. (1966). *Immunology* **11,** 185.

Cracchiolo, A., III, Michaeli, D., Goldberg, L. S., and Fudenberg, H. H. (1975). *Clin. Immunol. Immunopathol.* **3,** 567.

Cunningham, A. J. (1976). *Transplant. Rev.* **31,** 23.

Dacie, J. V. (1963). "The Haemolytic Anaemias, Congenital and Acquired," Part II. Churchill, London.

Dauphinee, M. J., Talal, N., Goldstein, A. L., and White, A. (1974). *Proc. Natl. Acad. Sci. U.S.A.* **71,** 2637.

Davie, J. M., Paul, W. E., Katz, D. H., and Benacerraf, B. (1972). *J. Exp. Med.* **136,** 426.

Davis, J. S. (1975). *Scand. J. Rheumatol., Suppl.* **11,** 20.

De Heer, D. H., and Edgington, T. S. (1976). *Transplant. Rev.* **31,** 116.

De Horatius, R. J., and Messner, R. P. (1975). *J. Clin. Invest.* **55,** 1254.

Donath, J., and Landsteiner, K. (1925). *Muench. Med. Wochenschr.* **51,** 1590.

Doniach, D. (1975). *Clin. Endocrinol. Metab.* **4,** 267.

Doniach, D., and Florin-Christensen, A. (1975). *Clin. Endocrinol. Metab.* **4,** 341.

Dowden, S. V., and Sercarz, E. (1968) . *J. Immunol.* **101,** 1308.

Dresser, D. W., and Mitchison, N. A. (1968). *Adv. Immunol.* **8,** 129.

Dubois, E. L. (1969). *Medicine* (*Baltimore*) **48,** 217.

Eddleston, A. W. L. F., and Williams, R. (1974). *Lancet* **2,** 1543.

Eibl, M., and Sitko, C. (1972). *Z. Immunitaetsforsch., Exp. Klin. Immunol.* **144,** 352.

Eldredge, N. T., Robertson, W. van B., and Miller, J. J., III. (1974). *Clin. Immunol. Immunopathol.* **3,** 263.

Engelfriet, C. P., Ponsman, K. W., Walters, G., van dem Borne, A. E. G., Beckers, D., Misset-Groenfeld, G., and van Loghem, J. J. (1970). *Clin. Exp. Immunol.* **6,** 721.

Engelfriet, C. P., van dem Borne, A. E. G., Beckers, D., Reyniesse, E., and van Loghem, J. J. (1972). *Clin. Exp. Immunol.* **11,** 255.

Feizi, T., Taylor-Robinson, D., Shields, M. D., and Carter, R. A. (1969). *Nature* (*London*) **222,** 1253.

Feltkamp, T. G. W., (1975). *Scand. J. Rheumatol., Suppl.* **11.**

Fialkow, P. J., Gilchrist, C., and Allison, A. C. (1973). *Clin. Exp. Immunol.* **13,** 479.

Fischer, J. T., Petz, L. D., Garratty, G., and Cooper, N. R. (1974). *Blood* **44,** 359.

Frimmel, P. J. (1975). *J. Immunol.* **15,** 135.

Garrido, F., Schirrmacher, V., and Festenstein, H. (1976). *Nature* (*London*) **259,** 228.

Gershwin, M. E., and Steinberg, A. D. (1975). *Clin. Immunol. Immunopathol.* **4,** 38.

Gleichmann, E., and Gleichmann, H. (1976). *Z. Krebsforsch.* **85,** 91.

Gleichmann, E., Gleichmann, H., and Wilke, W. (1976). *Transplant. Rev.* **31,** 156.

Hämmarstrom, L., Smith, E., Prinii, D., and Möller, G. (1976). *Nature* (*London*) **263,** 60.

Harboe, A., and Haukenes, G. (1966). *Acta Pathol. Microbiol. Scand.* **68,** 98.
Herberman, R., Nunn, M., and Lavrin, D. (1975a). *Int. J. Cancer* **16,** 216.
Herberman, R., Nunn, M., Holden, H., and lavrin, P. (1975b). *Int. J. Cancer* **16,** 230.
Hinz, C. F., Picken, M. E., and Lepow, I. H. (1961). *J. Exp. Med.* **113,** 193.
Holborow, E. J., Hemsted, E. H., and Mead, S. V. (1973). *Br. Med. J.* **3,** 323.
Holm, G., and Hammarström, S. (1973). *Clin. Exp. Immunol.* **13,** 29.
Holm, G., Engwall, E., Hammarström, S., and Nativig, J. B. (1974). *Scand. J. Immunol.* **3,** 173.
Hopf, U., Meyer zum Buschenfelde, K. H., and Freudenberg, J. (1974). *Clin. Exp. Immunol.* **16,** 117.
Huber, H., and Weiner, M. (1974) *In* "Activation of Macrophages" (W. H. Wagner and H. Halum, eds.), p. 54. Excerpta Med. Found., Amsterdam.
Irvine, J. (1975). *Clin. Endocrinol. Metab.* **4,** 351.
Iverson, G. M. (1970). *Nature* (*London*) **227,** 273.
Iverson, G. M., and Lindenmann, J. (1972). *Eur. J. Immunol.* **2,** 195.
Jacobs, M, E., Gordon, J. K., and Talal, N. (1971). *J. Immunol.* **107,** 359.
Jeffries, G. H., Haskins, D. W., and Sleisinger, M. H. (1962). *J. Clin. Invest.* **41,** 1106.
Jokinen, E., and Makitalo, R. (1960). *Proc. Scand. Rheum. Congr., 8th, 19??* p. 103.
Kalderon, A. E., Bogaars, H. A., and Diamond, I. (1973). *Am. J. Med.* **55,** 485.
Kaplan, M. E., and Tan, E. M. (1968). *Lancet* **1,** 561.
Kapp, J. A., Pierce, C. W., Schlossman, S., and Benacerraf, B. (1974). *J. Exp. Med.* **137,** 967.
Katz, D. H. (1972). *Transplant. Rev.* **12,** 141.
Kendall-Taylor, P. (1975). *Clin. Endocrinol. Metab.* **4,** 319.
Kiessling, R., Klein, E., Pres, H., and Wigzell, H. (1975). *Eur. J. Immunol.* **5,** 117.
Kiessling, R., Petranyi, P., Kärre, K., Jondal, M., Tracey, D., and Wigzell, H. (1976). *J. Exp. Med.* **143,** 772.
Kölsch, E., Stumpf, R., and Weber, G. (1975). *Transplant. Rev.* **26,** 56.
Konishi, J., Herman, M. M., and Kriss, J. P. (1974). *Endocrinology* **95,** 434.
Korsmeyer, S., Strickland, R. G., Wilson, I. D., and Williams, R. C., Jr. (1974). *Gastroenterology* **67,** 578.
Korsmeyer, S. J., Williams, R. C., Jr., Wilson, I. D., and Strickland, R. D. (1976). *N. Engl. J. Med.* **293,** 1117.
Kotkes, P., and Pick, E. (1974). *Clin. Exp. Immunol.* **19,** 105.
Kreisler, M. J., Hirata, A. A., and Terasaki, P. I. (1970). *Transplantation* **10,** 411.
Kriss, J. P. (1970). *J. Clin. Endocrinol. Metab.* **31,** 315.
Kuzumaki, N., Kodama, T., Takeuchi, N., and Kobayashi, H. (1974). *Int. J. Cancer* **14,** 483.
Kysela, S., and Steinberg, A. D. (1973). *Clin. Immunol. Immunopathol.* **2,** 133.
Lerner, R. A., and Dixon, F. J. (1966). *J. Exp. Med.* **124,** 431.
Lightfoot, R. W., Redecha, P. B., and Levesanos, N. (1975). *Scand. J. Rheumatol., Suppl.* **11,** 52.
Lindenmann, J., and Klein, D. A. (1967). *J. Exp. Med.* **126,** 93.

Lindholm, L., Rydberg, L., and Strannegård, O. (1973). *Eur. J. Immunol.* **3,** 511.

Lo Buglio, A. F., Cotran, R. S., and Jandl, J. H. (1967). *Science* **158,** 1582.

McFarlin, D. E., Hsu, S. C.-L., Slemenda, S. B., Chou, F. C. H., and Kibler, R. F. (1975). *J. Exp. Med.* **141,** 72.

McKenzie, J. M. (1958). *Endocrinology* **63,** 372.

MacKinney, A. A., and Booker, H. E. (1972). *Arch. Intern. Med.* **129,** 988.

Mellors, R. C., and Mellors, J. W. (1976). *Proc. Natl. Acad. Sci. U.S.A.* **93,** 233.

Melsom, H., Kearny, G., Gruca, S., and Seljelid, R. (1974). *J. Exp. Med.* **140,** 1085.

Menninger, H., Fehr, K., Böni, A., and Otto, K. (1976) *Immunochemistry* **13,** 633.

Metcalf, D., and Moore, M. A. S. (1971). "Haemopoietic Cells." North-Holland Publ., Amsterdam.

Mitchell, D. N., Rees, R. J. W., and Goswami, K. K. A. (1976). *Lancet* (in press).

Mittal, K. K. K., Rossen, R. D., Sharp, J. T. *et al.* (1970). *Nature* (*London*) **225,** 1255.

Mollison, P. L. (1972). "Blood Transfusion in Clinical Medicine." Blackwell, Oxford.

Monier, J. C., and Septjian, M. (1975). *Ann. Immunol.* (*Paris*) **126c,** 63.

Morse, H. C., Steinberg, A. D., Schur, P. H., and Reed, N. D. (1974). *J. Immunol.* **113,** 688.

Nakamura, R. M., and Weigle, W. O. (1969). *J. Exp. Med.* **130,** 263.

Nilsson, L. A., and Rose, N. R. (1972). *Immunology* **22,** 13.

Nishizuka, Y., Tanaka, T., Sakakura, T., and Kojima, A. (1973). *Experientia* **29,** 1396.

Obata, Y., Stockert, E., Boyse, E. A., Tung, J.-S., and Litman, G. W. (1976). *J. Exp. Med.* **144,** 533.

Oliner, H., Schwartz, R., and Dameshek, W. (1961). *Blood* **17,** 20.

Packalen, T., and Wassermann, J. (1971). *Int. Arch. Allergy. Appl. Immunol.* **41,** 790.

Panijel, J., and Barbu, E. (1960). *C. R. Hebd. Seances Acad. Sci.* **250,** 232.

Paterson, P. Y. (1967). *Proc. Soc. Exp. Biol. Med.* **119,** 267.

Pearsall, H. R., Ewalt, J., Tsoi, M. S., Sumida, S., Packinos, D., Winterbauer, R. H., Webb, D., and Jones, H. (1974). *J. Lab. Clin. Med.* **83,** 728.

Penhale, W. J., Farmer, A., McKenna, R. P., and Irvine, W. J. (1973). *Clin. Exp. Immunol.* **15,** 225.

Penhale, W. J., Farmer, A., and Irvine, W. J. (1975). *Clin. Exp. Immunol.* **21,** 362.

Perlmann, P., and Holm, G. (1969). *Adv. Immunol.* **11,** 117.

Perlmann, P., Perlmann, H., and Müller-Eberhard, H. J. (1975). *J. Exp. Med.* **141,** 287.

Petz, L. D., and Fudenberg, H. H. (1966). *N. Engl. J. Med.* **274,** 171.

Rauch, H., Ferranesi, R. W., Raffel, S., and Einstein, R. R. (1969). *J. Immunol.* **102,** 1431.

Riley, F. C. (1972). *Mayo Clin. Proc.* **47,** 975.

Ringertz, B., Wasserman, J., Packalen, T. L., and Perlmann, P. (1971). *Int. Arch. Allergy Appl. Immunol.* **40,** 918.

Rocklin, R. E., McDermott, R. P., Chess, L., Schlossmann, S. F., and David, J. R. (1974). *J. Exp. Med.* **140,** 1303.

Roitt, I. M., Doniach, D., and Shapland, C. (1969). *Lancet* **2,** 469.
Rose, N. R. (1975). *Ann. N.Y. Acad. Sci.* **249,** 116.
Rumke, P. (1954). *Vox Sang.* **4,** 135.
Rumke, P., and Hekman, A. (1975). *Clin. Endocrinol. Metab.* **4,** 473.
Sayoc, A. S., and Howland, W. J. (1974). *Radiology* **111,** 579.
Schrader, J. W., Cunningham, B. A., and Edelman, G. M. (1975). *Proc. Natl. Acad. Sci. U.S.A.* **72,** 5066.
Schreiber, A. D., and Frank, M. M. (1972a). *J. Clin. Invest.* **51,** 575.
Schreiber, A. D., and Frank, M. M. (1972b). *J. Clin. Invest.* **51,** 583.
Schwartz, M. (1960). *Lancet* **2,** 1263.
Shaw, C. M., Albord, E. C., Keku, J., and Kies, M. W. (1965). *Ann. N.Y. Acad. Sci.* **122,** 318.
Shirai, T., Yoshiki, T., and Mellors, R. C. (1973). *J. Immunol.* **110,** 517.
Silverman, D. A., and Rose, N. R. (1974). *Science* **184,** 162.
Silverstein, A. M., Prendergast, R. A., and Kraner, K. L. (1964). *J. Exp. Med.* **119,** 955.
Singer, H. C., Anderson, J. G. D., Frischer, H., and Kirsner, J. B. (1971). *Gastroenterology* **61,** 423.
Siskind, G. (1974). *In* "Immunological Tolerance" (D. H. Katz and B. Benacerraf, eds.), p. 181. Academic Press, New York.
Söderström, N., and Björklund, A. (1974). *Scand. J. Immunol.* **3,** 295.
Spitler, L., Huber, H., and Fudenberg, H. H. (1969). *J. Immunol.* **102,** 404.
Spitler, L. E., von Muller, C. M., and Young, J. D. (1975). *Cell. Immunol.* **15,** 143.
Steffen, C. (1969). *Ann. Immunol.* **1,** 47.
Steward, M. W. (1976). *In* "Infection and Immunology in the Rheumatic Diseases" (D. C. Dumonde, ed.), Blackwell, Oxford.
Stites, D. P., and Leikola, J. (1971). *Semin. Hematol.* **8,** 243.
Stone, S. H. (1961). *Science* **134,** 619.
Strand, M., and August, J. T. (1974). *J. Virol.* **14,** 1584.
Streilein, J. W., Stone, M. J., and Duncan, W. R. (1975). *J. Immunol.* **114,** 255.
Szegedy, G., and Petranyi, G. (1972). *Ann. Immunol. Hung.* **16,** 433.
Talal, N. (1976). *Transplant. Rev.* **31,** 240.
Tan, E. M. (1968). *Arthritis Rheum.* **11,** 515.
Taub, R. N., Sachor, D. B., and Siltzbach, L. E. (1974). *Trans. Assoc. Am. Physicians* **87,** 219.
Taylor, K. B. (1959). *Lancet* **2,** 106.
Taylor, R. B. (1969). *Transplant. Rev.* **1,** 114.
Teitelbaum, D., Webb, C., Bree, M., Meshorer, A., Arnon, R., and Sela, M. (1974). *Clin. Immunol. Immunopathol.* **3,** 256.
Teppo, A.-M., Haltia, K., and Wager, O. (1976). *Scand. J. Immunol.* **5,** 249.
Terasaki, P. I., Motteroni, V. D., and Barnett, E. V. (1970). *N. Engl. J. Med.* **283,** 724.
Theis, G. A., and Siskind, G. W. (1968). *J. Immunol.* **100,** 138.
Thomas, D. B. (1972). *Lancet* **1,** 399.
Tomazic, V., and Rose, N. R. (1975). *Clin. Immunol. Immunopathol.* **4,** 511.

Torrigiani, G., Doniach, D., and Roitt, I. M. (1969). *J. Clin. Endocrinol. Metab.* **29,** 305.

Unanue, E. R., and Dixon, F. J. (1967). *Adv. Immunol.* **6,** 1.

van Furth, R., Cohn, Z. A., Hirsch, J. G., Humphrey, J. H., Spector, W. G., and Landevoort, H. L. (1972). *Bull. W. H. O.* **46,** 845.

Weigle, W. O. (1961). *J. Exp. Med.* **114,** 111.

Weigle, W. O. (1965). *J. Exp. Med.* **122,** 1049.

Weigle, W. O. (1971). *Clin. Exp. Immunol.* **9,** 437.

Weigle, W. O., High, G. J., and Nakamura, R. M. (1969). *J. Exp. Med.* **130,** 243.

Wick, G., and Graf, J. (1972). *Lab. Invest.* **27,** 400.

Wick, G., Kite, J. H., Jr., and Witebsky, E. (1970a). *J. Immunol.* **104,** 45.

Wick, G., Kite, J. H., Jr., and Witebsky, E. (1970b). *J. Immunol.* **104,** 54.

Wick, G., Kite, J. H., Jr., and Witebsky, E. (1970c). *J. Immunol.* **104,** 344.

Williams, R. C., and Kunkel, H. G. (1963). *Proc. Soc. Exp. Biol. Med.* **112,** 554.

Williams, R. M., and Moore, M. J. (1973). *J. Exp. Med.* **138,** 775.

Wilson, L. (1954). *Proc. Soc. Exp. Biol. Med.* **85,** 652.

Winfield, J. B., Winchester, R. J., Wernet, P., Fu, S. M., and Kunkel, H. G. (1975). *Arthritis Rheum.* **18,** 1.

Winfield, J. B., Koffler, D., and Kunkel, H. G. (1975). *Scand. J. Rheumatol., Suppl.* **11,** 59.

Witebsky, E., and Rose, N. R. (1956). *J. Immunol.* **74,** 408.

Wolfe, S. E., Tracey, D. E., and Henney, C. S. (1976). *Nature* (*London*) **262,** 584.

Worlledge, S. M., Carstairs, K. C., and Dacie, J. V. (1966). *Lancet* **2,** 135.

Yamashita, U., Takami, T., Hamaska, T., and Kitagaura, M. (1976). *Cell. Immunol.* **25,** 32.

Yoshiki, T., Mellors, R. C., Strand, M., and August, J. T. (1974). *J. Exp. Med.* **140,** 1011.

Zabriskie, J. B. (1976). *In* "Infection and Immunology in the Rheumatic Diseases" (D. C. Dumonde, ed.), p. 97. Blackwell, Oxford.

Zinkernagel, R. M., Dunlop, M. B. C., Blanden, R. V., Doherty, P. C., and Shreffler, D. C. (1976). *J. Exp. Med.* **144,** 519.

Chapter 5

Cellular Events in Experimental Autoimmune Thyroiditis, Allergic Encephalomyelitis and Tolerance to Self

WILLIAM O. WEIGLE

I. INTRODUCTION

Autoimmunity observed in both clinical and experimental circumstances can best be defined as an apparent termination of a natural unresponsive state to self. The available data suggests that the immune response is the result of a finely tuned network of regulatory mechanisms (Jerne, 1974) involving numerous cellular events that include the release of a number of mediators which enhance or suppress the response (Waksman and Namba, 1976), in addition to antibody itself (cited in Weigle, 1975). It is some malfunction or imbalance in this network that undoubtedly is responsible for the immunologic event that leads to the induction and perpetuation of immunity to self. Although the subcellular events that occur in such malfunctions are too complex to even attempt to dissect, the basic cellular events can be delineated into three general categories. Autoimmune states could possibly arise as the result of (1) a bypass of either T cell specificity or the need for T cells in the presence of competent B cells, (2) a stimulation of competent T cells and/or B cells in cases of self-antigens that are ordinarily sequestered from the lymphoid system, or (3) a loss of suppressor activity which ordinarily limits the ability of lymphoid cells to respond to self-antigens (Allison, 1974; Gerber *et al.*, 1974; Barthold *et al.*, 1974). Depending on the disease, any one or a combination of these possibilities may be at play involving a host of mediators that result secondarily to the cellular events. Furthermore, the autoimmune state may result from either a humoral response involving any one or a combination of immunoglobulin classes and subclasses, or cell-mediated hypersensitivity.

II. IMMUNOLOGIC TOLERANCE

Since autoimmunity appears to be a state in which a natural immunologic tolerance to self-constituents is nonoperative, a discussion of some of the cellular events involved in the induction, maintenance, and termination of acquired immunologic tolerance may give some insight into the basic mechanism involved in at least some autoimmune phenomena. It has become obvious that there is a diversity of tolerant states, in which unresponsiveness is the end result, but the mechanisms at play differ markedly. It has been suggested that there are two general mechanisms of immunologic tolerance (Weigle *et al.*, 1974a). One results in a central unresponsive state, which is characterized by an irreversible loss of competent lymphocytes, while the other is a peripheral inhibition where competent cells are present, but are suppressed. This review will be concerned mainly with central unresponsiveness, since it appears that it is the mechanism responsible in most part for the specific unresponsive state that the host enjoys to self-components. The experimental model that best represents unresponsiveness to self is that induced to heterologous serum proteins during neonatal life and to deaggregated preparations of heterologous γ-globulin in adults. An apparent central unresponsive state can be induced in adult A/J mice to human γ-globulin (HGG) by a single injection of deaggregated HGG (DHGG) during adult life (Habicht *et al.*, 1970). Not only do these mice not respond to the DHGG, but they fail to respond to a subsequent injection of aggregated HGG (AHGG) given as late as 4–5 months after the DHGG.

A. Kinetics of Induction

It is well established that a state of immunologic unresponsiveness can be induced in both the T and B cells (Chiller *et al.*, 1970). A single dose of 2.5 mg of DHGG induced an unresponsive state in thymus cells, bone marrow (BM), and in peripheral T and B cells, although the kinetics of induction and spontaneous termination may differ (Table I). The induction of unresponsiveness in the intact animal takes 4–5 days for completion, albeit the unresponsiveness is 75% complete within 12 hours after injection of the tolerogen (DHGG) (Chiller and Weigle, 1971). The induction of unresponsiveness in either the thymus cells or peripheral T cells is also rapid and parallels the kinetics of induction observed in the intact mouse. On the other hand, there is a latent period of 8–9 days after injection of the tolerogen before a noticeable unresponsive state appears in the BM cells, and the unresponsive state is not complete in these cells until day 21 (Chiller *et al.*, 1971). In comparison to BM cells, the induction in peripheral B cells is rapid, being only slightly longer than that observed in thymus and T cells. Of more importance for this review is the marked difference in the kinetics of the termination of the unresponsive state in peripheral T and B cells. Similar to the intact host, the unresponsive state remains in the peripheral T cells for 100–150 days, while B cells return to complete competency between 50 and 60 days after injection of tolerogen. Using a different

TABLE I

Temporal Pattern of Immunologic Unresponsiveness to HGG in A/J Mice[a]

Site	Days of Induction	Days of Maintenance
Thymus	<1	120–135
Bone marrow	8–15	40–50
Spleen		
T cells	<1	100–150
B cells	2–4	50–60
Whole animal	<1	130–150

[a] Injected with 2.5 mg DHGG on day 0.

model, Rajewsky and Brenig (1974) have also reported a similar difference in the kinetics of the spontaneous termination of acquired unresponsiveness in T and B cells. Thus, it appears that a period of time exists during the late unresponsive state to HGG when the T cells are tolerant and the B cells are competent. This immune status of T and B cells readily lends itself to investigation of the cellular events involved in both the termination of immunologic unresponsiveness and certain autoimmune phenomena.

B. Dose Response

T cells are also rendered unresponsive in the presence of competent B cells when small doses of tolerogen are used. It was demonstrated by Chiller *et al.* (1971) that the dose of DHGG required to induce unresponsiveness in BM cells was much greater than that required for thymus cells. A similar difference in the dose required for induction of tolerance to bovine serum albumin (BSA) in thymus and BM cells (Katsura *et al.*, 1972) and in peripheral T and B cells (Rajewsky and Brenig, 1974) has more recently been reported. Thus, when unresponsiveness is induced with small doses of antigen, B cells remain competent, while T cells become unresponsive. Similar events may occur with self-antigens, where those antigens present in low concentrations in the body fluid would be expected to induce unresponsiveness only in T cells, while those in high concentrations should induce unresponsiveness in both cell populations.

C. Macrophages

In addition to T and B cells, macrophages apparently also play a major role in the establishment of unresponsiveness. The role of macrophages is nonspecific and is under genetic control. In certain strains of mice, unresponsiveness to DHGG (Golub and Weigle, 1969) and deaggregated bovine γ-globulin (Das and Leskowitz, 1974) is readily induced, while in other strains it is difficult to induce with these antigens. It was suggested that this difference is the result of the variability in the different strains to nonspecifically handle the antigen (Golub and Weigle, 1969). More recently, it has been demonstrated that macrophages are responsible for the nonspecific handling (Lukić *et al.*, 1975a; Fujiwara and Cinader, 1974) and that their function in this capacity is under genetic control (Lukić *et al.*, 1975b).

D. Suppressor T Cells

Suppressor T cells and the products of such cells have been implicated in the maintenance of tolerance in certain experimental models, while in other models such suppressor activity could not be demonstrated (reviewed in Gershon, 1973; Weigle *et al.*, 1975). Similarly, in mice unresponsive to HGG, suppressor activity has been observed by some workers (Basten *et al.*, 1975; Benjamin, 1975; Doyle *et al.*, 1976) but not by others (Chiller *et al.*, 1974; Zolla and Naor, 1974). In any event, it does not appear that such suppressor activity is required in order that an unresponsive state is maintained *in vivo*. Recently, Doyle *et al.* (1976) observed suppressor activity to AHGG in spleens of mice unresponsive to HGG. The suppressor activity observed by these investigators was present in the spleen cells of mice injected 10 days previously, but such activity disappeared by day 40, a time at which complete tolerance was still maintained. Furthermore, complete suppression required large numbers of tolerant cells. Basten *et al.* (1975) also demonstrated a transient suppressor activity in spleen cells of mice tolerant to HGG when large numbers of cells from tolerant mice were transferred with normal cells to irradiated recipients. The degree of either suppression or central unresponsiveness which occurred markedly depended on the method of deaggregation, and these authors concluded, as did Doyle *et al.* (1976) that suppression was not obligatory for the maintenance of the unresponsive state to HGG.

E. Fate of Antigen-Binding Cells (ABC)

The fate of ABC during the induction of immunologic tolerance gives some additional insight into the induction and maintenance of the unresponsive state. ABC specific for a given antigen can be detected and enumerated with the use of radiolabeled antigen and autoradiography (Ada *et al.*, 1970; Humphrey and Keller, 1970). Depending on the experimental model, ABC have been observed to increase, decrease, or remain the same after induction of immunologic unresponsiveness (reviewed in Weigle *et al.*, 1972). The failure to demonstrate a reduction in antigen-binding cells with T cell-independent antigens (Ada *et al.*, 1970; Humphrey and Keller, 1970) suggests that competent B cells are present, albeit their immunocompetence is suppressed by the persisting antigen (Howard, 1972). On the other hand, the failure to show a decrease in ABC in animals tolerant to T-dependent antigens may be because functionally immunocompetent B cells are present, but immunologic unresponsiveness is the result of tolerance at the T cells, and, with the procedures used, ABC are detected only in the B cell population. This controversy has been resolved by studying the fate of ABC in the HGG-mouse model where the state of unresponsiveness in both the T and B cells can be monitored. In the case of unresponsiveness induced in mice to HGG, there were no significant ABC detected in the spleens at a time (5–20 days) when it was shown that both T and B cells are unresponsive. The kinetics of the loss of ABC after injection of the tolerogen parallels the loss in the function of B cells. The failure to find ABC after induction of unresponsiveness is not compatible with the suggestion that suppressor T cells are responsible for the unresponsiveness observed in B cells. Whether these cells have been eliminated or stripped of their receptors or the receptors have been covered by antigen cannot be answered at the present time. Recently, it has been suggested that the mechanism of B cell tolerance may be that of blockage of receptors by the tolerogen, since B cell tolerance is dependent on relatively large concentrations of tolerogen (Weigle and Skidmore, 1975). Others have presented experimental data which also indicate that antigen blockade may be a mechanism of B cell tolerance (Aldo-Benson and Borel, 1974; Gronowicz and Coutinho, 1975).

F. Termination of Immunologic Unresponsiveness

In the case of T cell-dependent antigens, the unresponsive state can be terminated by several maneuvers, providing that unresponsiveness exists in only the T cells and competent B cells are present. The manipulations have to be such that either the need for or the specificity of T cells is bypassed. Thus, the B cells may then be triggered, either by nonspecifically activated T cells or directly, in the absence of T cells. In either event, antibody specific for the tolerated antigen is produced in the presence of T cells tolerant to the same antigen.

1. Thymus (T) Cells

Normal thymus cells are capable of terminating the unresponsive state in spleen cells of mice unresponsive to HGG, and such termination is dependent on the immune status of the B cells. It has not been possible to terminate the unresponsive state in mice tolerant to HGG simply by injecting tolerant mice with normal thymus cells, even at a time when it is known that the B cells are competent. However, the unresponsive state of spleen cells tolerant to HGG can be overcome by injecting these cells along with normal thymus cells into irradiated recipients, provided the spleen cells are taken at a time (81 days after tolerogen) when unresponsiveness resides in the T but not the B cells. On the other hand, reconstition failed to occur when normal thymus cells were injected along with spleen cells obtained at a time (17 days after tolerogen) when unresponsiveness was present in both T and B cells. Miller and Mitchell (1970) have also been able to demonstrate that injection of normal spleen cells hastens the recovery from the tolerant state in mice. Similarly, it was shown by Benjamin (1974) that the unresponsive state to BSA induced in neonatal rabbits could be terminated by injecting normal sibling thymocytes prior to challenge with BSA, providing that the thymocytes were injected at a time when it could be assumed that the B cells were competent.

2. *Allogeneic Cells*

It is well established that the injection of allogeneic cells in the appropriate temporal relation to injection of antigen results in a marked enhancement of the immune response (Katz *et al.*, 1971), presumably because of nonspecific activation of T cells as a result of a graft versus host reaction. Such activation of T cells by allogeneic cells has been shown to result in the termination of tolerance in rats to SRBC (McCullagh, 1970). Similarly, the unresponsive state induced to HGG in adult B6A F_1 mice can be terminated with allogeneic (A/J) cells, but only if the allogeneic cells are injected at a time when B cells are competent (Weigle *et al.*, 1974b). No effect is observed if the allogeneic cells are injected at a time when both T and B cells are unresponsive. These results suggest that unresponsive T cell populations are nonspecifically activated by allogeneic cells, allowing stimulation of the competent B cells to differentiate and synthesize antibody to HGG.

3. *Lipopolysaccharide (LPS)*

LPS is capable of terminating the unresponsive state if injected with antigen at a time when tolerance is only in the T cells and competent B cells are present. Besides being a good adjuvant for antibody production (Landy and Baker, 1966; Rudbach, 1971), LPS is a mitogen for B cells (Gery *et al.*, 1972; Andersson *et al.*, 1972). It has been shown by several investigators that LPS can substitute for the T cell helper function in animals devoid of functional T cells (reviewed by Coutinho and Möller, 1975), suggesting that LPS may bypass the need for T cells by otherwise thymus-dependent antigens. Thus, it is not surprising that injection of LPS with immunogen causes the termination of the unresponsive state (Chiller and Weigle, 1973). The injection of LPS and AHGG into mice that are unresponsive to HGG results in the termination of the unresponsive state, providing that unresponsiveness is maintained only to T cells and the B cells are competent (143 days after tolerogen). When both the T and B cells are unresponsive (25 days after tolerogen), injection of LPS and AHGG does not result in the termination of the unresponsive state. With LPS, it appears that T cells play no specific role in the termination of unresponsiveness and that B cells are stimulated directly through a combination of a signal supplied by the immunogen and another by LPS. LPS could theoretically play a role in the circumvention of natural tolerance to self-antigens if the cellular basis for natural unresponsiveness to self-antigens present in low concentrations in the body fluids is that of unresponsive T cells and competent B cells. Thus, any means that renders the response independent of the specific T cells would be expected to permit antibody formation to these self-antigens. This is not to imply that the immunologic consequences of infection with gram-negative bacteria will always result in autoimmunity, but rather to suggest that under the appropriate temporal release of sufficient self-antigen and bacterial products, the homeostatic balance of self-tolerance could be altered.

4. Related Immunogens

The unresponsive state can be readily terminated with antigens or complexes that cross react with the tolerated antigen. Although the termination of immunologic unresponsiveness with related immunogens is well established and has been shown in a number of different models of tolerance (reviewed in Weigle, 1973), it is best documented in the unresponsive state induced to BSA in neonatal rabbits. Neonatal rabbits injected shortly after birth with 500 mg of BSA remain completely unresponsive to subsequent injections of BSA for at least 6 months. On the other hand, this unresponsive state can be readily terminated after immunization with either chemically altered preparations of BSA (Weigle, 1962) or heterologous albumins, which cross react with BSA (Weigle, 1961). Although the mechanism involved in both cases is probably the same, the data obtained with cross-reacting albumins is both more informative and easier to interpret. Rabbits immunized with aqueous preparations of heterologous albumins 3 months after the induction of tolerance to BSA lose their unresponsive state in that they produce circulating antibodies to the heterologous albumins (which also reacts with BSA). The antibody directed to BSA in the unresponsive rabbits is quantitatively and qualitatively the same as antibody produced in normal rabbits injected with these albumins (Benjamin and Weigle, 1970a). These observations can only be explained by the presence of a normal complement of precursors of antibody-forming cells in the unresponsive animal and imply that the unresponsiveness is present in the T cell but not the B cell. If the kinetics of the spontaneous termination of unresponsiveness induced in neonatal rabbits to BSA can be extrapolated from that observed in adult mice injected with DHGG, it appears likely that at the time of immunization (90 days of age) with cross-reacting antigens, the B cell population would have regained competence. Termination of the unresponsive state then could be explained by a bypass of the need for specific T cells. In this situation, the unrelated determinants on the cross-reacting albumins would activate T cells, permitting stimulation of B cells competent for both BSA and the unrelated determinants, and the B cells would produce a normal complement of antibodies reactive with BSA. The competence of the B cell population is further demonstrated by the ability of simultaneous injections of BSA with the cross-reacting albumins to inhibit the termination of the unresponsive state (Weigle, 1964; Benjamin and Weigle, 1970b). It appears most likely that the simultaneous injection of BSA reinduced an unresponsive state in the competent B cells before they could effectively be stimulated by either antigen or activated T cells. In support of this contention is the observation of Paul *et al.* (1969), who demonstrated that termination of unresponsiveness with chemically altered preparations depended on the temporal relationship between the last injection of tolerogen and the challenge with the altered BSA. Benjamin and Hershey (1974) also showed that tolerance introduced to a fragment of BSA obtained by cleavage with cyanogen bromide could be terminated by immunization with intact BSA. All of the above results can be readily explained by a bypass of the specificity of T cell unresponsiveness, resulting in stimulation of B cells to produce circulating antibody.

In order to further test the above suggestion, attempts were made to terminate the unresponsive state to BSA in rabbits by immunization with native BSA complexed with a heterologous carrier. Rabbits unresponsive to BSA were injected at 3 months of age with complexes formed between BSA and guinea pig anti-HSA (Habicht *et al.*, 1975). This combination permitted the unrelated antigen portion (guinea pig γ-globulin) of the complexes to activate T cells, while allowing the free BSA determinants (unrelated to HSA) to stimulate the BSA competent cells. As postulated by the above hypothesis, injection in the footpads with such complexes resulted in the appearance of PFC to BSA in the popliteal nodes (Table II).

III. AUTOIMMUNITY

The cellular mechanisms involved in the termination of acquired unresponsiveness to serum protein antigens by means of bypassing T cell tolerance may be similar to the cellular mechanisms involved in certain autoimmune diseases, a possibility that seems likely with self-components which are of limited concentration in the body fluids. As mentioned previously, with limited concentrations of self-components, an unresponsive state may be maintained in the T cells, but not in the B cells. A further limitation in the availability of self-antigens in the body fluid to the extent that they are sequestered from the lymphoid system would result in the presence of both competent T and B cells. The remainder of the present review will be devoted to a discussion of the cellular events in experimental autoimmune thyroiditis (EAT) and experimental allergic encephalomyelitis (EAE). Although the cellular basis for these two experimental autoimmune diseases is the immune status of T and B lymphocytes, the cellular events leading to the initiation and progression of these diseases appear to be quite different.

A. Experimental Autoimmune Thyroiditis (EAT)

EAT is an excellent example of an autoimmune phenomenon which is the result of termination of an unresponsive state to a self-antigen as the result

Termination of Immunologic Unresponsiveness to BSA Using Immune Complexes Made with Heterologous Antibody[a]

Group	Challenge	No. of animals	Indirect PFC/10^6 LN[b] cells	Percent Inhibition of PFC by:	
				BSA	HSA
A	GP anti-HSA[c] + BSA	8	296(71–609)[c]	100	14
B	BSA	8	6(0–31)	—	—
C	GPGG[d]	5	0	—	—

[a] Reprinted from Habicht *et al.* (1975).
[b] LN, lymph node.
[c] Numbers in parentheses indicate range of values.
[d] All groups challenged with GPGG made a PFC response to GPGG in the draining lymph node.

of bypass of unresponsive T cells. Experimental autoimmune thyroiditis was first produced in rabbits (Rose and Witebsky, 1956) but has since been produced in a number of different species (reviewed in Shulman, 1971). The classical procedure for production of experimental thyroiditis is injection of homologous thyroglobulin (Tg) incorporated into complete Freund's adjuvant (CFA) (Rose and Witebsky, 1956). The quantitative and qualitative aspects of the *in vivo* behavior of Tg suggests that tolerance to this thyroid protein is maintained by T cell tolerance, while the B cells are competent (Weigle, 1971).

Mammalian Tg is present in the circulation (Daniel *et al.*, 1967) and equilibrates between the intra- and extravascular fluid spaces persisting with a finite half-life (Nakamura *et al.*, 1968). The concentration observed in normal humans (Roitt and Torrigiani, 1967) is comparable with that required to maintain an unresponsive state in the T cells (Nakamura and Weigle, 1967), but not the B cells of rabbits. Furthermore, B cells capable of binding homologous Tg have been demonstrated in the human (Bankhurst *et al.*, 1973), and B cells capable of binding syngeneic Tg have been observed in the mouse (Clagett and Weigle, 1974) and in the rat (Penhale *et al.*, 1975). Because of the immune status of the T and B cells to autologous Tg, it is reasonable to suggest that experimental autoimmune thyroiditis may be induced as a result of the termination of self-tolerance to autologous thyroglobulin.

1. Induction with Cross-Reacting Tg

a. *Rabbits.* As is the case in the termination of the unresponsive state to BSA after immunization with cross-reacting albumins, the natural unresponsive state to autologous Tg in rabbits can be terminated by immunization with heterologous (cross-reacting) Tg. Normal adult rabbits immunized with aqueous preparations of heterologous Tg produce circulating antibody reactive with rabbit Tg and develop thyroid lesions characterized by infiltration of inflammatory cells (Weigle and Nakamura, 1967; Nakamura and Weigle, 1967) (Table III). As with the termination of unresponsiveness to BSA, simultaneous injections of native rabbit Tg with the heterologous Tg inhibits both the production of antibody to rabbit Tg and the development of lesions. As would be expected, antibody is still produced to the determinants on the cross-reacting Tg unrelated to rabbit Tg. Furthermore, although once the unresponsiveness is terminated the rabbits respond to a subsequent injection of rabbit Tg, multiple injections result in cessation of antibody production and regression of lesions. It appears that injection of rabbit Tg, either simultaneous with heterologous Tg or in multiple doses after termination of the unresponsive state to rabbit Tg,

TABLE III

The Production of Thyroiditis and Antibody to Rabbit Thyroglobulin (Tg) in Rabbits Injected with Heterologous Thyroglobulin

Tg injected	Antibody (μg/ml)	Lesions[a]			
		–	+	++	+++
Bovine	76.3	6	9	5	0
Human	56.3	3	4	3	0
Porcine	12.6	7	3	1	0
Mixture	120.0	2	8	8	4

[a] Number of rabbits showing lesions of different degrees.

results in a refractiveness possibly characterized by the induction of an unresponsive state in the previously competent and/or responsive B cells.

Additional information on the cellular events involved in the induction of thyroiditis after immunization with heterologous thyroglobulin was obtained by enumeration of the appearance of antibody-producing cells (Clinton and Weigle, 1972). Lymphocytes synthesizing antibody to Tg were detected as plaque-forming cells (PFC) by a modification of the hemolytic plaque assay. In these studies, rabbits received a series of five injections of an aqueous preparation of bovine Tg, and, after a 2-week rest period, the series of injections was repeated. At various times during and after the injections, the spleen and thyroid gland were assayed for PFC to both bovine and rabbit Tg (Fig. 1).

The peak of PFC to both bovine and rabbit Tg in the spleens occurred 34 days after initiation of the injections, and the ratio of PFC to bovine Tg was 20 times greater than that observed to rabbit Tg. The nature of the cellular events was revealed by the pattern of development to PFC to Tg in the thyroid gland. Although a small number of PFC to both bovine and rabbit Tg was observed at the same time as the peak of PFC in the spleen, the major peak of PFC appeared in the thyroid gland 7 days later, and the ratio of PFC to bovine and rabbit Tg was similar. It appeared that the thyroid gland was acting as an *in vivo* immunoabsorbant which specifically selected memory B lymphocytes to rabbit Tg which were initially stimulated in the spleen. After a latent period of 7 days, these lymphocytes were stimulated by the Tg in the gland and developed into antibody-producing cells. A similar latent period has been observed in rabbits undergoing cyclical production of PFC after a single injection of aggregated human IgG (Romball and Weigle, 1973). Of further importance is the direct correlation between the appearance of lesions and PFC to rabbit Tg in the glands (Fig. 2). Appreciable lesions did not appear with the appearance of PFC, and the severity of lesions was not optimal until 1 day after the peak of PFC was observed in the gland. It is likely that Tg released locally from the gland permitted absorption of memory cells and that the release of antibody from these stimulated cells within the gland causes more severe lesions. Serum levels of precipitating antibody to rabbit Tg correlated with the appearance of lesions (Fig. 3). Precipitating antibody appeared in the serum prior to the appearance of lesions, and once lesions began to appear, there was a precipitous drop in the level of antibody in the serum, apparently because of its removal by rabbit Tg either released into the body fluid or exposed in the thyroid gland. In contrast to the production of circulating autoantibody, cell-mediated hypersensitivity to rabbit Tg could not be detected in rabbits immunized with aqueous preparations of bovine thyroglobulin. Attempts to

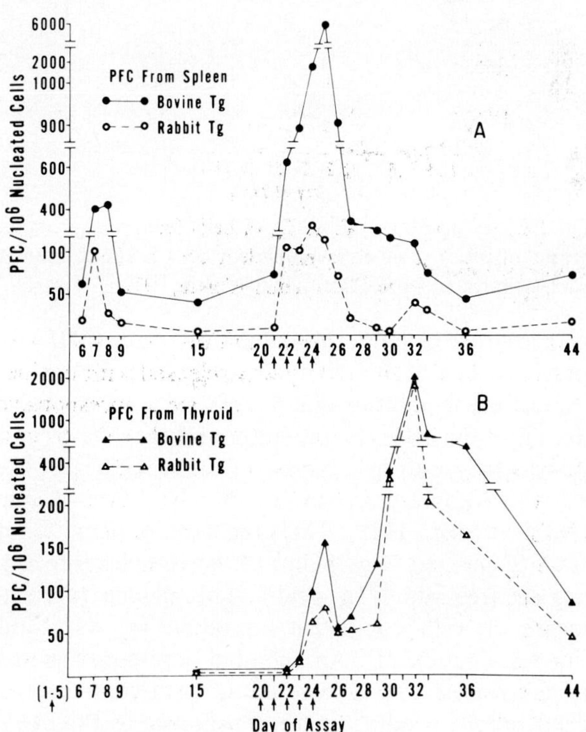

Fig. 1. The PFC response to bovine and rabbit Tg by the spleen (A) and thyroid gland (B). The arrows (↑) indicate injections performed on the various days. (Reprinted from Clinton and Weigle, 1972.)

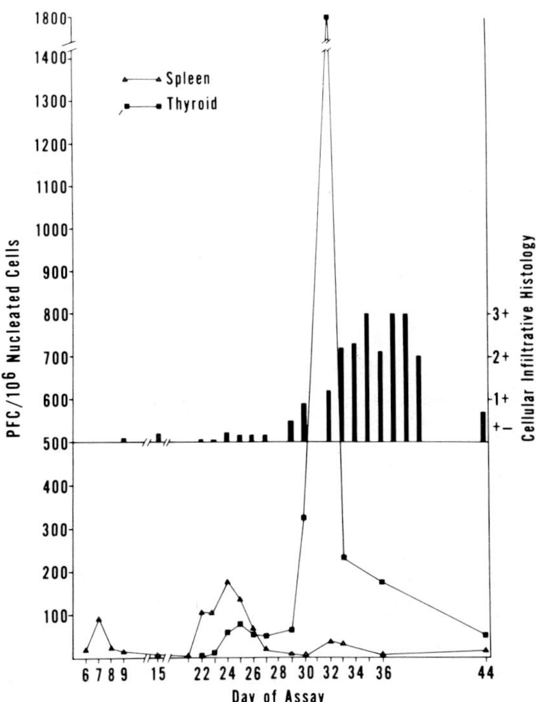

Fig. 2. The PFC response to rabbit Tg of cells from the spleen and the thyroid gland. The degree of infiltration of mononuclear cells in the thyroid gland is shown by the solid bars. (Reprinted from Clinton and Weigle, 1972.)

demonstrate the release of migration-inhibition factor (MIF) with rabbit Tg were unsuccessful, albeit MIF activity was released with bovine Tg.

In order to test the hypothesis that T cells were unresponsive and B cells competent to Tg in the self-tolerant state, and that the termination of the tolerant state was the result of a bypass of the specificity of T cells, rabbits were injected with complexes composed of rabbit Tg and guinea pig anti-bovine Tg (Habicht *et al.*, 1975). This combination permitted the unrelated antigen portion (guinea pig γ-globulin) of the complexes to activate T cells while allowing the free rabbit Tg-specific determinants (unrelated to bovine Tg) to stimulate the cells competent for rabbit Tg. As postulated by the hypothesis for termination of both acquired unresponsiveness to BSA and natural unresponsiveness to Tg, injection of such complexes into the footpads of normal rabbits resulted in the appearance of PFC to rabbit thyroglobulin and thyroiditis (Table IV).

b. *Mice.* EAT is also readily produced in mice immunized with aqueous preparations of a mixture of heterologous thyroglobulins (Nakamura

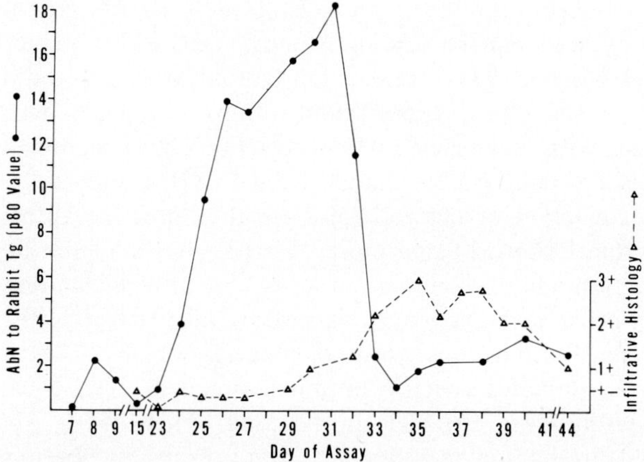

Fig. 3. A comparison of precipitating antibody in the circulation with appearance of thyroid lesions. (Reprinted from Clinton and Weigle, 1972.)

and Weigle, 1968; Clagett and Weigle, 1974). Such immunized mice produce autoantibody to mouse Tg and develop thyroid lesions consisting of infiltration of inflammatory cells. Studies at the cellular level in mice suggest that unresponsiveness to autologous Tg exists in the T cells, while the B cells are competent. It was shown that the spleen and BM contain ABC for both autologous and heterologous Tg, while thymus cells contain ABC to heterologous, but not to autologous Tg. Thus, it appears that competent B cells are present in the mouse, albeit they cannot be stimulated to produce antibody to autologous Tg in the absence of responsive T cells. That

TABLE IV

Termination of Natural Immunologic Unresponsiveness to RTg Using Immune Complexes Made with Heterologous Antibody[a, b]

Group	Challenge	No. of animals	Anti-RTg: Hemagglutination	Anti-RTg: ppt (Preer test)	Thyroid lesions
A	GP anti-BTg + RTg	10	9/10(16–5,120)[c]	6/10	6/10
B	RTg	11	2/11(16)	0/11	0/11
C	GPGG	6	0/6	0/6	0/6

[a] Reprinted from Habicht *et al.* (1975).

[b] These results represent data pooled from two different experiments. No differences were observed between the two experimental sets, although one set received three injections of RTg totaling 2400 μg RTg, while the other set received two injections of RTg totaling 1066 μg RTg.

[c] Numbers in parentheses indicate range of values.

thyroiditis induced in mice is the result of a B cell product has been established by studying the role of B and T cells in the induction of EAT (Clagett and Weigle, 1974). Neither autoantibody nor thyroiditis is induced in A/J mice that have been thymectomized, lethally irradiated, and reconstituted with syngeneic BM cells (TxXBM) before injection of heterologous Tg. On the other hand, if the TxXBM mice are given thymus cells before injection of heterologous Tg, they produce autoantibody and develop thyroid lesions. Furthermore, it is possible to inhibit both autoantibody production and development of lesions by prior incubation of BM, but not thymus cells, with syngeneic Tg heavily labeled with ^{125}I. It has been shown previously that incubation of heavily labeled (^{125}I) antigen with lymphocytes eliminates specific immunocompetent cells because of local irradiation (Ada *et al.*, 1970; Humphrey and Keller, 1970). The prevention of EAT and production of autoantibody to Tg by incubation of the BM cells with autologous ^{125}I-Tg demonstrates that the B cells or a B cell product (antibody) is involved in thyroiditis in the mouse. As has been suggested for the rabbit model, immunization of mice with heterologous Tg apparently bypasses the specificity of the T cells, and T cells activated by heterologous Tg supply a second signal needed for differentiation of competent B cells that have reacted with self-related determinants of the heterologous Tg.

Histological examination of thyroid lesions in A/J mice immunized with aqueous preparations of heterologous Tg further implicates humoral antibody as the causative agent in EAT (Clagett *et al.*, 1974). There was a direct correlation between the temporal appearance and quantity of serum autoantibody and the presumed *in situ* formation of complexes in the interstitium of the thyroid glands. After intense immune complex formation in which the complement-fixing antibody belongs exclusively to the IgG class, the glands were briefly invaded by an intense infiltration of neutrophils, which was replaced by chronic monocytic elements. By combination of fluorescent microscopy and autoradiography, Tg was demonstrated to be at least one of the antigens in the interstitial immune complexes. These complexes were granular to lumpy in appearance and formed at the basal area of the follicular cells in intimate association with the follicular basement membrane. Electron microscopy revealed electron-dense deposits, presumably immune complexes, between the follicular basement membrane and the plasma membrane. The presumed *in situ* formation of immune complexes in this model is similar to that which occurs in the Arthus reaction, and is a different mechanism of immune complex injury than that caused by tissue deposition of circulating immune complexes as occurs in serum sickness.

2. *Induction with Altered Tg*

EAT can also be readily induced by immunization of rabbits with chemically altered preparations of rabbit thyroglobulin (Weigle, 1965a). Rabbits given a series of injections of aqueous preparations of rabbit Tg conjugated to diazonium derivatives of arsanilic and sulfanilic acid (arsanil–sulfanil–Tg) produce antibody reactive to native rabbit Tg and develop thyroid lesions (Weigle, 1965b). The phenomenon is similar to that observed with EAT resulting from immunization with heterologous Tg in that (1) it spontaneously regresses in the absence of continued immunization, (2) simultaneous injections of native rabbit Tg inhibit the development of EAT, and (3) the rabbits respond to a subsequent injection of native rabbit Tg, but multiple injections result in the induction of unresponsiveness in the B cells (Weigle, 1967). It is apparent that termination of unresponsiveness to autologous Tg in rabbits by arsanil–sulfanil–Tg is also the result of a bypass of the specificity of T cells.

The induction of EAT following the immunization of rabbits with rabbit Tg incorporated into CFA is also apparently the result of altered Tg bypassing unresponsiveness at the T cell level (Weigle *et al.*, 1969). Although CFA probably plays a role in experimental autoimmune phenomena by enhancing the overall antigenicity, and in some species, by specifically enhancing cell-mediated hypersensitivity, with thyroiditis there has been speculation as to whether the components of the mycobacteria also cause alteration in Tg, since mycobacteria are an essential ingredient for the production of thyroiditis with homologous Tg. If such alteration takes place, it appears to be the result of the reaction of the host to the mycobacteria after injection, rather than to direct effects of the mycobacteria on the Tg (Weigle *et al.*, 1969). Mycobacteria incorporated into CFA with rabbit Tg causes no detectable changes in the biological, antigenic, or physical properties of the Tg. It seems most likely that alteration of Tg injected into CFA occurs *in vivo* and is initiated shortly after injection. Significant amounts of both BSA and rabbit Tg were released from CFA within the first 24–48 hours after injection; however, the BSA, but not the Tg, persisted in the circulation. Apparently, the Tg was sufficiently altered in the developing granuloma so that it either did not enter the circulation or was rapidly eliminated shortly after it did enter. Alteration of Tg *in vivo* is most likely the result of infiltration of neutrophils. It may be that cathepsins and other proteolytic enzymes released from the lysosomes of the neutrophils are responsible for the alteration. Since the cathepsins are active at only a relatively high hydrogen ion concentration, the pH at the site of degradation would have to be low. Such a low pH in the local environment of

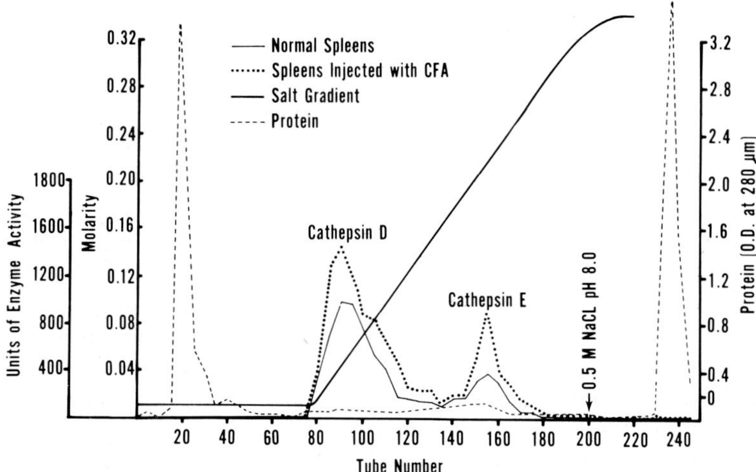

Fig. 4. Isolation of cathepsins D and E by DEAE-cellulose chromatography from extracts of spleens obtained from either normal rabbits or rabbits injected in the spleen with complete Freund's adjuvant (CFA). (Reprinted from Weigle *et al.*, 1969.)

neutrophils is well documented (Rous, 1925; Sbarra *et al.*, 1961; Cohn and Morse, 1960; Strauss and Stetson, 1960; McCarty *et al.*, 1966). A similar drop in the local pH may well occur in granuloma formed by CFA. Rabbit spleens injected with such adjuvant contained a marked infiltration of neutrophils around the adjuvant deposits, whereas infiltration of neutrophils in spleens injected with incomplete adjuvant (without mycobacteria) was insignificant. Likewise, rabbits injected with Tg incorporated into CFA develop both thyroid lesions and autoantibodies, whereas neither is produced in rabbits injected with Tg in incomplete adjuvant. Furthermore, significantly greater amounts of cathepsins D and E were isolated from extracts of rabbit spleens injected with CFA than with incomplete adjuvant (Fig. 4). Tg is much more susceptible to degradation by cathepsins at pH 2.5 than are proteins such as BSA, possibly because Tg, but not BSA, is denatured at this pH. In agreement with the preceding postulation is the induction of thyroid lesions and production of autoantibody in rabbits following injections of aqueous preparations of homologous Tg partially degraded by either pepsin (Weigle *et al.*, 1969) or papain (Anderson and Rose, 1971).

3. *Progressive Thyroiditis*

Although EAT produced in rabbits following a series of injections with aqueous preparations of either heterologous thyroglobulin or arsanil-sulfanil–rabbit Tg is a self-limiting experimental disease and recovery from lesions and disappearance of antibody occurs within 2 or 3 months after the last injection, the disease can be perpetuated. Thyroiditis produced by injections of aqueous preparations of either arsanil–sulfanil–rabbit Tg (Weigle and Nakamura, 1969) or heterologous Tg (Weigle and Romball, 1975) has been perpetuated by injections of aqueous preparations of the respective Tg over a prolonged period of time (6–12 months). In both cases, progressive lesions, which were present in all the rabbits and involved over 50% of the thyroid gland, developed. In addition, most of the rabbits developed relatively high levels of circulating antibody to rabbit Tg. Rabbits given 12 monthly injections of bovine thyroglobulin apparently lost the unresponsive state to rabbit Tg in the T cell population. Once the progressive thyroiditis was established, the rabbits responded readily to multiple monthly injections of native rabbit Tg, and no significant reductions in either the severity of lesions or level of circulating antibody resulted from the injections of native thyroglobulin. A continued response to homologous Tg indicates specific T cell helper activity. Furthermore, cell-mediated hypersensitivity to rabbit Tg, as evidenced by MIF activity, developed in rabbits after prolonged immunization with either the altered or heterologous Tg. The data suggest that the persistence of circulating antibody to autologous Tg sequesters the circulating Tg from lymphoid tissue and after a period of 12 months, the unresponsive state is lost in the T cell. Despite the apparent activation of T cells in progressive thyroiditis, this experimental disease is characterized by lesions and cellular infiltrations similar to that observed in Arthus reactions. It is suggested that similar events may be involved in the development of cell-mediated hypersensitivity in thyroiditis of humans (Brostoff, 1970; Calder *et al.*, 1972).

These studies suggest that if progressive immune diseases like Hashimoto's thyroiditis are the result of an immune response to altered self-antigens, it would be required that the altered antigen persist. Transient trauma or infection may be expected to result only in a transient disease that may be perpetuated by unaltered tissue antigens for only a limited period of time. Shortly after the insult that caused the alteration was corrected, however, the autoimmune state would cease. Such may be the case in acute transient forms of acquired hemolytic anemia and idiopathic thrombocytopenic purpura. If altered tissue components are responsible for autoimmunity, it appears that the alteration would have to be permanent in progressive autoimmune diseases.

4. Secondary Phenomena

In addition to the thyroid lesions induced in rabbits after immunization with aqueous preparations of either heterologous Tg or altered Tg, secondary tissue damage may result from complexes formed between Tg released from the gland and antibody synthesized by the animal (Weigle and High, 1967). Both antibody to autologous Tg and the lesions produced after immunization of rabbits with aqueous preparations of either arsanil–sulfanil–rabbit Tg or heterologous Tg disappear within 2 or 3 months. Such rabbits when injected with a large amount of Na-^{131}I (3–6 mCi), after being on an iodine-free diet, take up sufficient ^{131}I to cause destruction of the thyroid by internal irradiation. Autologous ^{131}I-Tg is released into the circulation, resulting in a stimulation of the immune system with production of circulating antibody to autologous Tg, which complexes with the ^{131}I-Tg in the circulation (Fig. 5). A number of rabbits develop proteinuria and at autopsy show mild glomerular changes in the kidney, accompanied by localization of rabbit immunoglobulin (antibody) and thyroglobulin along the glomerular basement membrane. The events leading to kidney injury appear to be similar to those involved in serum sickness. In both the present model and serum sickness, circulating complexes are formed between newly synthesized antibody and circulating antigen. The complexes are eliminated from the circulation, with deposits of both antigen and antibody along the glomerular basement membrane resulting in subsequent glomerular injury. Secondary glomerular injury is also observed in progressive thyroiditis. Rabbits that received periodic injections of altered homologous thyroglobulin over a 6-month period developed chronic glomerular lesions in additions to progressive EAT (Weigle and Nakamura, 1969). The lesions probably result from the localization of complexes formed in the circulation between circulating antibody and the injected arsanil–sulfanil–Tg, the native

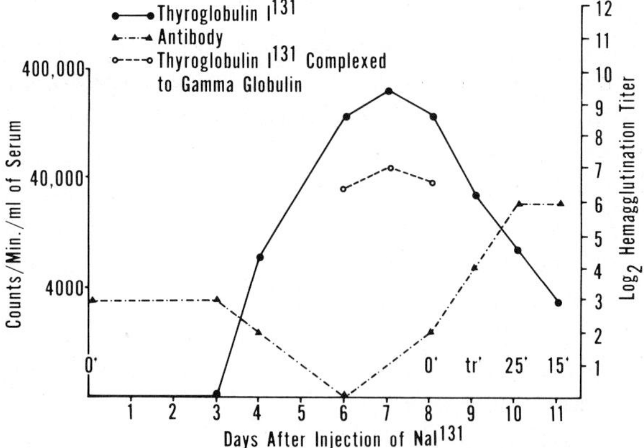

Fig. 5. Changes in the serum and urine of a rabbit immunized with arsanil–sulfanil–Tg (rabbit) and subsequently injected with Na-^{131}I. (Reprinted from Weigle and High, 1967.)

Tg released from the damaged glands, or both. Using fluorescent microscopy, IgG immunoglobulin, the C3 component of complement and Tg were found localized along the glomerular basement membrane.

Although secondary tissue injury resulting from circulating antigen–antibody complexes is a component of some autoimmune diseases in humans, little is known concerning the presence of such complexes or their biologic significance in thyroiditis of humans. R. S. Schwartz (personal communication, 1967) observed complete renal failure in a patient with thyroiditis which apparently resulted from deposition of autologous Tg and antibody along the glomerular basement membrane. D. Koffler (personal communication, 1968) also observed glomerular injury with deposition of Tg and immunoglobulin in the kidney of a patient with chronic thyroiditis. Similar phenomena have been more consistently observed in other diseases. Tan *et al.* (1965) and Krishman and Kaplan (1966) were first to implicate complexes formed between DNA and anti-DNA as a causative agent for renal injury in patients with systemic lupus erythematosus. Kunkel *et al.* (1961) observed the presence of immunoglobulin complexes in the sera of patients with rheumatoid arthritis. Since these early observations, similar complexes have been observed in other disease states.

5. *Mechanism*

The available data indicate that EAT is the result of the termination of a natural unresponsive state to thyroglobulin where the tolerant state is the result of unresponsive T cells in the presence of competent B cells. The competent B cells are capable of both binding autologous Tg and synthesizing antibody to self if appropriately stimulated as a result of bypassing the specificity of T lymphocytes. Evidence has also been presented which suggests that anti-Tg synthesized by B lymphocytes and specifically absorbed by the thyroid gland is responsible for the thyroid lesions. Cells containing and apparently forming antibody also have been observed in the mononuclear infiltrate in chronic thyroiditis in man (Mellors *et al.*, 1962). In any event, the above data overwhelmingly support the dominant role of antibody in EAT. A role for antibody is further supported by the passive transfer of thyroiditis with antibody in the rabbit (Nakamura and Weigle, 1969) and mouse (Anderson and Rose, 1971), and by spontaneous thyroiditis that naturally occurs in certain strains of chickens. This latter disease was first observed in less than 1% of the Cornell C-strain of white leghorn chickens (Van Tienhoven and Cole, 1962). By selective breeding of individual chickens with phenotypic symptoms of hypothyroidism, the incidence of the disease has been increased to 80–90%. Because of the obesity of these chickens, they have been referred to as the "obese strain" (OS). This disease has since been shown to be of an autoimmune nature and similar to

Hashimoto's thyroiditis. Both IgM and IgG antibodies, which react with autologous thyroglobulin, were present in the serum (Witebsky *et al.*, 1969). The interesting feature of the OS chickens is that bursectomy inhibits both the development of lesions and the production of antibody to Tg (Wick *et al.*, 1970a), while thymectomy causes an increase in the severity of lesions and levels of antibody (Wick *et al.*, 1970b). These results suggest (1) that the lesions are caused by circulating antibody and not by cell-mediated immunity and (2) that the thymus has some control function over the bursa's role in this disease. Neonatal thymectomy has also been shown to lead to earlier onset and increased severity of spontaneous thyroiditis in the OS chickens (Welch *et al.*, 1973). Similarly, the spontaneous occurrence of thyroiditis in rats (Penhale *et al.*, 1973) and mice (Miller and Mitchell, 1969) is favored by neonatal thymectomy. These latter results suggest that the T suppressor cell may act as a nonspecific "fail-safe" mechanism against the spontaneous occurrence of thyroiditis.

B. Experimental Allergic Encephalomyelitis (EAE)

Experimental allergic encephalomyelitis is an autoimmune disease of the central nervous system that was first observed following injection of experimental animals with brain tissue incorporated into CFA (Morgan, 1946; Kabat *et al.*, 1946; Wolf *et al.*, 1947). The disease is a neurological disorder involving the central nervous system and is characterized by demyelination of nerve fibers and infiltration of inflammatory cells in central nervous tissue (reviewed in Paterson, 1966; Rauch and Roboz Einstein, 1974). In addition, fibrin deposition occurs, which has been suggested to be a specific determinant in the clinical neurological signs of the disease (Paterson, 1976). EAE has been considered to be a prototype experimental disease for multiple sclerosis in humans because of the associated chemical and pathological changes observed in the central nervous system in this disease and EAE. Since the early experiments with brain tissue, EAE has been produced by immunization with CFA containing basic protein (encephalitogenic) of myelin (reviewed in Rauch and Roboz Einstein, 1974), encephalitogenic peptides isolated from myelin (Eylar *et al.*, 1970; Carnegie, 1971; Lamoreux *et al.*, 1972) and the corresponding peptides synthesized *in vitro* (Eylar, 1970). Since the immunologic aspect of EAE is characterized by a number of parameters of cell-mediated hypersensitivity and because it readily transferred with sensitized lymphocytes (Paterson, 1960; Waksman and Morrison, 1951; Paterson *et al.*, 1975) but not by serum antibody (reviewed in Paterson, 1966), it has been assumed that this experimental disease is the result of cell-mediated hypersensitivity. Thus, the mechanism involved in EAE may be quite different than that involved in EAT discussed above. It is, therefore, of considerable importance to understand the cellular events involved in EAE and compare these events with those described for EAT. Experiments were initiated recognizing the possibility that the encephalitogenic agents responsible for induction of EAE may be, at least in part, sequestered antigens, and both T and B cells may have some degree of competence to these self-antigens.

1. Role of T Lymphocytes as Effector Cells

It was previously reported that rats depleted of T cells by thoracic duct drainage were unresponsive to basic protein (BP) of myelin in that they failed to develop EAE when immunized with BP incorporated into CFA (Gonatas and Howard, 1974). Recently, the requirement of T cells in EAE in Lewis rats injected with syngeneic BP in CFA was studied in thymectomized, irradiated rats given passive transfer of a combination of normal spleen and lymph node cells (Ortiz-Ortiz *et al.,* 1976b). It was shown that pretreatment of the mixture of lymphoid cells with an antiserum specific for rat thymocytes (ATS) and complement prevented both the clinical symptoms and histological lesions in the recipient rats injected with BP–CFA, while recipients receiving untreated cells developed the classical lesions and clinical symptoms of EAE. The failure to develop EAE in the Tx, irradiated recipients that received ATS-treated spleen cells further emphasizes the necessity of T cells in the development of this autoimmune disease. However, neither the latter experiment, nor the experiment utilizing thoracic duct drainage, discriminates between a role for the T cells as an effector cell or as a helper cell in the antibody response.

In order to determine if T cells are the effector cells, attention was directed at studying the effect of ATS on the ability of sensitized lymphocytes to transfer competence to develop EAE to Tx irradiated recipients. When Tx irradiated recipients were injected with a mixture of spleen and lymph node cells obtained from syngeneic rats immunized 9 days previously with BP–CFA, they developed typical clinical symptoms of EAE with histological lesions in the cortex and cerebellum characterized by perivascular infiltrates accompanied by varying degrees of demyelination. On the other hand, when the sensitized lymphocytes were first treated with ATS and complement, no clinical symptoms of EAE or perivascular infiltrates of the brain were detected. It was of special interest that sera from both recipients receiving treated or untreated cells contained similar levels of antibody to BP. Thus, it appears that lymphocytes transferred 9 days after sensitization were already committed to the production of antibodies to BP and needed no further T cell help, since ATS treatment of these cells did not alter their capacity to produce antibody. Furthermore, in spite of the synthesis of antibody to BP, EAE did not develop, indicating that antibody to BP by itself was incapable of inducing EAE, which is in agreement with the failure to transfer EAE with passive antibody (Kabat *et al.*, 1948; Morgan, 1947; Waksman and Morrison, 1951). It is clear from these studies that induction of EAE is dependent on T effector cells and that cell-mediated immunity plays a major role in EAE. It is reasonable to assume that the myelin damage observed results from a direct effect of sensitized T lymphocytes or from mediators released from the activated cells.

2. *Cellular Events Involved in the Induction of EAE*

The immune status of the T cell to BP of myelin is quite different than that to autologous Tg. With the use of ^{125}I-labeled syngeneic BP and autoradiography, ABC to BP were detected in both the thymus and spleen cells of Lewis rats. Furthermore, the elimination of T cells from the spleen cell population by treatment with ATS and complement indicated that ABC in the spleen constituted both T and B cells. Thus, it appears that competent T and B cells to BP are present in the Lewis rat. Coates and Lennon (1973) were able to detect ABC to BP in guinea pigs; however, attempts to detect similar ABC in rats failed, probably as a result of the insensitivity of the assay used. In the above experiments, which show ABC to BP in Lewis rats, the receptors of the ABC in both the spleen and thymus appear to be an immunoglobulin related to the IgM class, since anti-μ and anti-light chain, but not anti-γ-chain antisera blocked binding of ^{125}I-BP. This finding of both T and B cells capable of binding BP further suggested that BP is sequestered from the lymphoid system in that even small amounts of BP capable of inducing and maintaining unresponsiveness in T lymphocytes is not available in the body fluids.

The role of T and B cells in the induction of EAE was further defined by antigen-suicide experiments where ABC for BP with either T or B cell functions were specifically eliminated by treatment with BP heavily labeled with ^{125}I (Ortiz-Ortiz and Weigle, 1976a). As mentioned above, Tx irradiated rats were readily reconstituted with normal thymus and BM cells in that such rats injected with BP–CFA developed clinical symptoms, typical histological lesions in the brain, and antibody to BP. On the other hand, clinical symptoms, lesions or antibody were not produced when the thymus cells were suicided with high specific ^{125}I-BP activity and transferred to Tx irradiated rats reconstituted with BM and challenged with BP–CFA, indicating pretreatment with the ^{125}I-BP eliminated specific T cells and, thus, abrogated cell-mediated immunity. Treatment of the thymus cells with the ^{125}I-BP also inhibited the formation of antibody to BP, but not to burro red blood cells (BRBC), suggesting that specific helper T cells were also eliminated. Supplementation of the ^{125}I-BP-inactivated thymus cells with normal thymus cells restored the appearance of clinical symptoms of EAE, histological lesions in the brain, and serum antibody to BP. More precise evidence for cell-mediated immunity in EAE was obtained by suiciding B cells. When the BM cells were treated with the heavily ^{125}I-labeled BP and injected into Tx irradiated recipients along with normal thymus cells, antibody formation to a subsequent challenge with BP–CFA was inhibited. In contrast, both clinical symptoms of EAE and histological lesions were similar to those observed in rats receiving both normal thymus cells and normal BM cells. The absence of antibody production in the presence of EAE again is in agreement with the failure to passively transfer EAE with sera from sensitized animals and with the ability to induce EAE in bursectomized (agammaglobulinemic) chickens (Blaw *et al.*, 1967). In fact, passive antibody has been shown to interfere with the development of EAE (Paterson and Harwin, 1963). In any event, the present results indicate that whether antibodies inhibit the induction of EAE or enhance the disease after it is initiated by cell-mediated immunity, they are not a requisite for the induction of EAE.

Additional insight into the diversity of the cellular events that may lead to autoimmunity are disclosed by studies in Brown Norway (BN) rats, which unlike Lewis rats, are resistant to the induction of EAE by sensitization with BP–CFA (Levine and Sowinski, 1975; Gasser *et al.*, 1973; Williams and Moore, 1973). Not only is this strain of rats resistant to induction of EAE with BP–CFA, but it lacks ABC in T cells (Ortiz-Ortiz and Weigle, 1976a). However, Pitts *et al.* (1975) were able to induce antibody production, but not EAE, after immunizing BN rats with BP–CFA and pertussis vaccine, an adjuvant known to stimulate B cell proliferation (Murgo and Athanassiades, 1975). This model may resemble that of EAT where the T cells are unresponsive, while the B cells are competent. Then, as in EAT, the T cells may be bypassed and the B cells stimulated directly, resulting in antibody production (but not EAE) to BP.

Since suppressor T cell activity has been implicated as a mechanism in the regulation of the immune response including autoimmune phenomena (Gershon, 1973), the possibility that suppressor T cells are involved in maintenance of tolerance to basic protein has to be considered. A role of suppressor T cells is intriguing in view of the presence of immunocompetence to BP in both the T and B cells. Suppressor T cell activity has been shown to be lost with age in New Zealand mice (Allison, 1974; Barthold *et al.*, 1974; Gerber *et al.*, 1974), and the loss was associated with the spontaneous induction of autoimmune disease. It was reported that thymocytes from rats immunized with bovine γ-globulin (BGG) could, upon transfer to normal rats, specifically suppress both cell-mediated and humoral antibody responses to BGG (Ha and Waksman, 1973). It is well established that the injection of BP without antigen, or incorporated into incomplete Freund's adjuvant (IFA), results in the suppression of the immune response to injections of BP–CFA (reviewed in Rauch and Roboz Einstein, 1974). Recently, a population of suppressor cells present in the lymph nodes and stimulated by injection of rats with BP in IFA, was suggested to be responsible for controlling the development of EAE in rats (Swierkosz and Swanborg, 1975). In other studies, adoptive transfer experiments provided no evidence for the presence of suppressor cells in either the spleens or lymph nodes of rats protected against EAE by injection of aqueous preparations of BP, or BP incorporated in IFA (Ortiz-Ortiz and Weigle, 1976a). The difference between the former and latter observations may result from the use of syngeneic BP in the latter studies, in contrast to the use of allogeneic BP in the former studies. Although the latter data suggest that suppressor T cell activity is not involved in the abrogation of EAE afforded by nonencephalitogenic BP, these observations cannot be interpreted to mean that suppressor T cells play no role in regulation of autoimmune phenomena similar to that observed in New Zealand mice.

IV. SUMMARY

The cellular events involved in the induction of immunologic tolerance to serum protein antigens were discussed and related to tolerance to self-components and autoimmunity. On the basis of the immune status of T and B cells, the cellular parameters of induction of experimental autoimmune thyroiditis (EAT) and experimental allergic encephalomyelitis (EAE) were described and compared. Although unresponsiveness to human γ-globulin (HGG) is induced in both T and B cells in mice injected with deaggregated HGG (DHGG), the unresponsive state in B cells was less stable in that it was spontaneously terminated in a relatively short period of time and required large amounts of DHGG to induce. Thus, conditions could be readily selected in which a state of unresponsive T cells and competent B cells prevailed. This unresponsive state was readily terminated by manipulations that resulted in a bypass of T cell specificity. Similarly, unresponsive T cells and competent B cells were shown to be the cellular parameters of self-unresponsiveness to Tg. This unresponsive state was terminated in rabbits and mice by bypassing the specificity of the T cells by immunization with cross-reacting Tg, resulting in thyroid lesions and circulating autoantibody. Analysis of the cellular events involving T and B cells during the induction of EAT established that this experimental disease was solely the result of antibodies of Tg and did not involve effector T cells. In contrast, similar analysis of EAE induction in Lewis rats revealed that effector T cells, rather than antibody, were responsible for the clinical symptoms and histological lesions resulting from immunization with CFA containing the basic protein (BP) of myelin. In contrast to the unresponsive state to Tg, neither T nor B cells appeared to be unresponsive to BP in that specific antigen-binding cells to BP were detected in both cell populations. By deleting either T or B cells that specifically bound BP from these populations, it was demonstrated that T cells, and not antibody, were responsible for induction of EAE. In addition, the protection against the induction of EAE by injections of nonencephalitogenic preparations of BP was shown not to be the result of suppressor cells.

ACKNOWLEDGMENTS

This is Publication No. 1070 from the Departments of Immunology, Scripps Clinic and Research Foundation, La Jolla, Calif. This work was supported by USPHS Grant AI-07007, Atomic Energy Administration Contract E (04-3)-410, NIH Grant AI-12449, and American Cancer Society Grant IM-42E.

Author is recipient of a USPHS Research Career Award 5-K6-GM-6936.

REFERENCES

Ada, G. L., Byrt, P., Mandel, T., and Warner, N. (1970). *In* "Developmental Aspects of Antibody Formation and Structure" (J. Sterzl and I. Riha, eds.), Vol. 1, p. 503. Academic Press, New York.

Aldo-Benson, M., and Borel, Y. (1974). *J. Immunol.* **112,** 1793.

Allison, A. C. (1974). *Contemp. Top. Immunobiol.* **3,** 227.

Anderson, C. L., and Rose, N. R. (1971). *J. Immunol.* **107,** 1341.

Anderson, J., Möller, G., and Sjöberg, O. (1972). *Cell. Immunol.* **4,** 381.

Bankhurst, A. D., Torrigiani, G., and Allison, A. C. (1973). *Lancet* **1,** 226.

Barthold, D. R., Kysela, S., and Steinberg, A. D. (1974). *J. Immunol.* **112,** 9.

Basten, A., Miller, J. F. A. P., and Johnson, P. (1975). *Transplant. Rev.* **26,** 130.

Benjamin, D. C. (1974). *J. Immunol.* **113,** 1589.

Benjamin, D. C. (1975). *J. Exp. Med.* **141,** 635.

Benjamin, D. C., and Hershey, C. W. (1974). *J. Immunol.* **113,** 1593.

Benjamin, D. C., and Weigle, W. O. (1970a). *J. Exp. Med.* **132,** 66.

Benjamin, D. C., and Weigle, W. O. (1970b). *J. Immunol.* **105,** 1231.

Blaw, M. E., Cooper, M. D., and Good, R. A. (1967). *Science* **158,** 1198.

Brostoff, J. (1970). *Proc. R. Soc. Med.* **63,** 905.

Calder, E. A., McLeman, D., Barnes, E. W., and Irvine, W. J. (1972). *Clin. Exp. Immunol.* **12,** 429.

Carnegie, P. R. (1971). *Biochem. J.* **123,** 57.

Chiller, J. M., and Weigle, W. O. (1971). *J. Immunol.* **106,** 1647.

Chiller, J. M., and Weigle, W. O. (1973). *J. Exp. Med.* **137,** 740.

Chiller, J. M., Habicht, G. S., and Weigle, W. O. (1970). *Proc. Natl. Acad. Sci. U.S.A.* **65,** 551.

Chiller, J. M., Habicht, G. S., and Weigle, W. O. (1971). *Science* **171,** 813.

Chiller, J. M., Louis, J. A., Skidmore, B. J., and Weigle, W. O. (1974). *In* "Immunological Tolerance" (D. H. Katz and B. Benacerraf, eds.), p. 373. Academic Press, New York.

Clagett, J. A., and Weigle, W. O. (1974). *J. Exp. Med.* **139,** 643.

Clagett, J. A., Wilson, C. B., and Weigle, W. O. (1974). *J. Exp. Med.* **140,** 1439.

Clinton, B. A., and Weigle, W. O. (1972). *J. Exp. Med.* **136,** 1605.

Coates, A. S., and Lennon, V. A. (1973). *Immunology* **24,** 425.

Cohn, Z. A., and Morse, S. I. (1960). *J. Exp. Med.* **111,** 667

Coutinho, A., and Möller, G., (1975). *Adv. Immunol.* **21,** 113.

Daniel, P. M., Pratt, O. E., Roitt, I. M., and Torrigiani, G. (1967). *Immunology* **12,** 489.

Das, S., and Leskowitz, S. (1974). *J. Immunol.* **112,** 107.

Doyle, M. V., Parks, D. E., and Weigle, W. O. (1976). *J. Immunol.* **117,** 1152.

Eylar, E. H. (1970). *Proc. Natl. Acad. Sci. U.S.A.* **67,** 1425.

Eylar, E. H., Caccam, J., Jackson, J. J., Westall, F. C., and Robinson, A. B. (1970). *Science* **168,** 1220.

Fujiwara, M., and Cinader, B. (1974). *Cell. Immunol.* **12,** 194.

Gasser, D. L., Newlin, C. M., Palm, J., and Gonatas, N. K. (1973). *Science* **181,** 872.

Gerber, N. L., Hardin, J. A., Chused, T. M., and Steinberg, A. D. (1974). *J. Immunol.* **113,** 1618.

Gershon, R. K. (1973). *Contemp. Top. Immunobiol.* **3,** 1.

Gery, I., Kruger, J., and Spiesel, S. Z. (1972). *J. Immunol.* **108,** 1088.

Golub, E. S., and Weigle, W. O. (1969). *J. Immunol.* **102,** 389.

Gonatas, N. K., and Howard, J. C. (1974). *Science* **186,** 839.

Gronowicz, E., and Coutinho, A. (1975). *Eur. J. Immunol.* **5,** 413.

Ha, T. Y., and Waksman, B. H. (1973). *J. Immunol.* **110,** 1290.

Habicht, G. S., Chiller, J. M., and Weigle, W. O. (1970). *In* "Developmental Aspects of Antibody Formation and Structure" (J. Sterzl and I. Riha, eds.), p. 893. Academic Press, New York.

Habicht, G. S., Chiller, J. M., and Weigle, W. O. (1975). *J. Exp. Med.* **142,** 312.

Howard, J. G. (1972). *Transplant. Rev.* **8,** 50.

Humphrey, J. H., and Keller, H. U. (1970). *In* "Developmental Aspects of Antibody Formation and Structure" (J. Sterzl and I. Riha, eds.), p. 485. Academic Press, New York.

Jerne, N. K. (1974). *Ann. Immunol.* (*Paris*) **125c,** 373.

Kabat, E. A., Wolf, A., and Bezer, A. E. (1946). *Science* **104,** 362.

Kabat, E. A., Wolf, A., and Bezer, A. E. (1948). *J. Exp. Med.* **88,** 417.

Katsura, Y., Kawaguchi, S., and Muramatsu, S. (1972). *Immunology* **23,** 537.

Katz, D. H., Paul, W. E., Goidl, E. A., and Benacerraf, B. (1971). *J. Exp. Med.* **133,** 169.

Krishman, C., and Kaplan, M. H. (1966). *Fed. Proc., Fed. Am. Soc. Exp. Biol.* **25,** 309.

Kunkel, H. G., Müller-Eberhard, H. J., Fudenberg, H. H., and Tomasi, T. B. (1961). *J. Clin. Invest.* **40,** 117.
Lamoreux, G., Thibault, G., Richer, G., and Bernard, C. (1972). *Union Med. Can.* **101,** 674.
Landy, M., and Baker, P. J. (1966). *J. Immunol.* **97,** 163.
Levine, S., and Sowinski, R. (1975). *J. Immunol.* **114,** 597.
Lukić, M. L., Cowing, C., and Leskowitz, S. (1975a). *J. Immunol.* **114,** 503.
Lukić, M. L., Wortis, H. H., and Leskowitz, S. (1975b). *Cell. Immunol.* **15,** 457.
McCarty, D. J., Jr., Phelps, P., and Pyenson, J. (1966). *J. Exp. Med.* **124,** 99.
McCullagh, P. J. (1970). *J. Exp. Med.* **132,** 916.
Mellors, R. C., Brzosko, W. J., and Sonkin, L. S. (1962). *Am. J. Pathol.* **41,** 425.
Miller, J. F. A. P., and Mitchell, G. F. (1969). *Transplant. Rev.* **1,** 3.
Miller, J. F. A. P., and Mitchell, G. F. (1970). *J. Exp. Med.* **131,** 675.
Morgan, I. M. (1946). *J. Bacteriol.* **51,** 614.
Morgan, I. M. (1947). *J. Exp. Med.* **85,** 131.
Murgo, A. J., and Athanassiades, T. J. (1975). *J. Immunol.* **115,** 928.
Nakamura, R. M., and Weigle, W. O. (1967). *J. Immunol.* **98,** 653.
Nakamura, R. M., and Weigle, W. O. (1968). *Proc. Soc. Exp. Biol. Med.* **129,** 412.
Nakamura, R. M., and Weigle, W. O. (1969). *J. Exp. Med.* **130,** 263.
Nakamura, R. M., Spiegelberg, H. L., Lee, S., and Weigle, W. O. (1968). *J. Immunol.* **100,** 376.
Ortiz-Ortiz, L., and Weigle, W. O. (1976a). *J. Exp. Med.* **144,** 604.
Ortiz-Ortiz, L., Nakamura, R. M., and Weigle, W. O. (1976b). *J. Immunol.* **117,** 567.
Paterson, P. Y. (1960). *J. Exp. Med.* **111,** 119.
Paterson, P. Y. (1966). *Adv. Immunol.* **5,** 131.
Paterson, P. Y. (1976). *Fed. Proc., Fed. Am. Soc. Exp. Biol.* **35,** 2428.
Paterson, P. Y., and Harwin, S. M. (1963). *J. Exp. Med.* **117,** 755.
Paterson, P. Y., Richardson, W. P., and Drobish, D. G. (1975). *Cell. Immunol.* **16,** 48.
Paul, W. E., Thorbecke, G. J., Siskind, G. W., and Benacerraf, B. (1969). *Immunology* **17,** 85.
Penhale, W. J., Farmer, A., McKenna, R. P., and Irvine, W. J. (1973). *Clin. Exp. Immunol.* **15,** 225.
Penhale, W. J., Farmer, A., Urbanick, S. J., and Irvine, W. J. (1975). *Clin. Exp. Immunol.* **19,** 179.
Pitts, O., Varitek, V. A., and Day, E. D. (1975). *J. Immunol.* **115,** 1114.
Rajewsky, K., and Brenig, C. (1974). *Eur. J. Immunol.* **4,** 120.
Rauch, H. C., and Roboz Einstein, E. (1974). *Rev. Neurosci.* **1,** 283.
Roitt, I. M., and Torrigiani, G. (1967). *Endocrinology* **81,** 421.
Romball, C. G., and Weigle, W. O. (1973). *J. Exp. Med.* **138,** 1426.
Rose, N. R., and Witebsky, E. (1956). *J. Immunol.* **76,** 417.
Rous, P. (1925). *J. Exp. Med.* **41,** 399.
Rudbach, J. A. (1971). *J. Immunol.* **106,** 993.
Sbarra, A. J., Bardawil, W. A., Shirley, W., and Gilfillan, R. F. (1961). *Exp. Cell Res.* **24,** 609.
Shulman, S. (1971). *Adv. Immunol.* **14,** 85.

Strauss, B. S., and Stetson, C. A. (1960). *J. Exp. Med.* **112,** 653.
Swierkosz, J. E., and Swanborg, R. H. (1975). *J. Immunol.* **115,** 631.
Tan, E. M., Schur, P. H., and Kunkel, H. G. (1965). *J. Clin. Invest.* **44,** 1104.
Van Tienhoven, A., and Cole, R. K. (1962). *Anat. Rev.* **142,** 111.
Waksman, B. H., and Morrison, L. R. (1951). *J. Immunol.* **66,** 421.
Waksman, B. H., and Namba, Y. (1976). *Cell. Immunol.* **21,** 161.
Weigle, W. O. (1961). *J. Exp. Med.* **114,** 111.
Weigle, W. O. (1962). *J. Exp. Med.* **116,** 913.
Weigle, W. O. (1964). *Immunology* **7,** 239.
Weigle, W. O. (1965a). *J. Exp. Med.* **121,** 289.
Weigle, W. O. (1965b). *J. Exp. Med.* **122,** 1049.
Weigle, W. O. (1967). *Immunology* **13,** 241.
Weigle, W. O. (1971). *Clin. Exp. Immunol.* **9,** 437.
Weigle, W. O. (1973). *Adv. Immunol.* **16,** 61.
Weigle, W. O. (1975). *Adv. Immunol.* **21,** 87.
Weigle, W. O., and High, G. J. (1967). *J. Immunol.* **98,** 1105.
Weigle, W. O., and Nakamura, R. M. (1967). *J. Immunol.* **99,** 223.
Weigle, W. O., and Nakamura, R. M. (1969). *Clin. Exp. Immunol.* **4,** 645.
Weigle, W. O., and Romball, C. G. (1975). *Clin. Exp. Immunol.* **21,** 351.
Weigle, W. O., and Skidmore, B. J. (1975). *Transplant. Rev.* **23,** 250.
Weigle, W. O., High, G. J., and Nakamura, R. M. (1969). *J. Exp. Med.* **130,** 243.
Weigle, W. O., Chiller, J. M., and Louis, J. A. (1972). *Transplant. Proc.* **4,** 373.
Weigle, W. O., Chiller, J. M., and Louis, J. A. (1974a). *Prog. Immunol., Int. Congr. Immunol., 2nd, 1974* Vol. 3, p. 187.
Weigle, W. O., Louis, J. A., Habicht, G. S., and Chiller, J. M. (1974b). *Adv. Biosci.* **12,** 93.
Weigle, W. O., Sieckmann, D. G., Doyle, M. V., and Chiller, J. M. (1975). *Transplant. Rev.* **26,** 186.
Welch, P., Rose, N. R., and Kite, J. H., Jr. (1973). *J. Immunol.* **110,** 575.
Wick, G., Kite, J. H., Jr., Cole, R. K., and Witebsky, E. (1970a). *J. Immunol.* **104,** 45.
Wick, G., Kite, J. H., Jr., and Witebsky, E. (1970b). *J. Immunol.* **104,** 54.
Williams, M. R., and Moore, M. J. (1973). *J. Exp. Med.* **138,** 775.
Witebsky, E., Kite, J. H., Jr., Wick, G., and Cole, R. K. (1969). *J. Immunol.* **103,** 708.
Wolf, A., Kabat, E. A., and Bezer, A. E. (1947). *J. Exp. Med.* **85,** 117.
Zolla, S., and Naor, D. (1974). *J. Exp. Med.* **140,** 1421.

Chapter 6

Suppressor T Cell Dysfunction as a Possible Cause for Autoimmunity

RICHARD K. GERSHON

I. INTRODUCTION

Although it has been known for a long time that T cells can act to diminish the immune response, as well as to augment it (see Gershon, 1974), it has been only recently that the "suppressor T cell" has passed from a concept to a distinct entity. Thus, it was not until the definition of distinct T cell subclasses with preprogrammed functions, by the use of anti-Ly antiserum, that the suppressor T cell has been shown to represent a unique subclass (for reviews, see Cantor and Boyse, 1976; Cantor, 1977). It can now be stated, with little reservation, that a separate subclass of T cells exists whose principal function is to suppress the response of other immunologically competent cells. What role the dysfunction of this particular subclass of T cells may play in the development of autoimmune diseases is essentially unknown, although much speculation abounds. There is considerable information in the literature describing situations where T cell dysfunction and certain types of autoimmune diseases are associated, as discussed elsewhere in this volume, although the cause and effect nature of the two associated phenomena have not been definitively demonstrated. Nonetheless, in recent years, there has been such a plethora of demonstration of T cell-mediated suppressor effects in all kinds of immunologic phenomena that it would seem reasonable to assume that at least some autoimmune diseases result from a malfunction of this particular T cell subclass. There have been many recent reviews and symposia on suppressor T cells (Singhal and St. C. Sinclair, 1975; Möller, 1976a; Kapp and Pierce, 1977; Dresser, 1976), and it is not the purpose of this article to catalogue the voluminous literature. Rather, I would like to distill what I consider to be the salient points presently known that might help the reader to interpret the more specific articles on autoimmunity contained herein and to help them to consider the possible role that suppressor T cell malfunction may play in some of these diseases.

Since the subclassification of T cells has been most extensively studied in the mouse, I will concentrate on murine phenomena but will assume that these may be representative of human conditions. Certainly, it is now known that suppressor T cell activity can be demonstrated in humans (Waldmann *et al.*, 1974; Shou *et al.*, 1976).

II. DEFINITION OF T CELL SUBCLASSES WITH ANTI-LY SERA

In 1968, Boyse and his colleagues defined a series of differentiation antigens in the mouse which they called Ly, because they were found exclusively on lymphocytes. It was found that all mice studied had one of two alleles at each genetic locus which codes for these antigens, i.e., the Ly antigens were similar to the θ antigen, which has subsequently come to be known as Thy-1. Thus, by cross-immunization of mice with different alleles at each Ly locus and by the subsequent backcrossing of the alternative alleles, making congenic mice, three Ly antigens were defined. Subsequent work has shown three of the Ly antigens are expressed exclusively on T cells. Since many more lymphocyte differentiation antigens are being uncovered, and, since not all of these are expressed exclusively on T cells (in fact, some are expressed exclusively on B cells), it is perhaps wise to subdivide the Ly differentiation antigens into Ly T and Ly B. In any case, the most extensively studied of the Ly antigens are Ly 1, 2, and 3, which are all T cell markers. Using antisera against these antigens and tested for specificity on backcrossed congenic mice, four distinct T cell subclasses have been defined (for detailed references, see Cantor and Boyse, 1976; Cantor, 1977).

One subclass expresses all three of the Ly antigens as well as the TL antigen [see Schreffler and David (1975) for discussion of the TL antigen system]. This subclass of T cells is found almost exclusively in the cortex of the thymus and not in the peripheral lymphoid tissue. Its immunologic function is basically unknown, and it is considered to be a very immature cell. Nonetheless, it has been clearly shown to express at least some immunologic reactivity so that it is not totally immunologically inert (Tigelaar *et al.*, 1975). It may be the precursor of all T cells.

A second subclass of T cells expresses all three of the Ly antigens, but not the TL antigen. Most, if not all, of the peripheral T cells of mice between birth and 2 weeks of age are composed of this T cell subclass. Around the age of 2 weeks, two other T cell subclasses start to appear.

One expresses the Ly 1 antigen exclusively, and another expresses the Ly 2 and the Ly 3 antigens. No Ly 2^+ 3^- or 3^+ 2^- T cells have thus far been described. At maturity, which is around 8 weeks of age in the mouse, the distribution of peripheral T cell subclasses is as follows: Ly 123 about 50%, Ly 1 about 30%, Ly 23 about 5–10%. Thus, not all θ-positive cells express the three Ly antigens thus far studied, and, therefore, more T cell subclasses are bound to be discovered in the future. There is no significant information available on the role of the Ly 123 negative, θ-positive T cells in the immune response. The functions of the Ly 1 and the Ly 23 cells have been extensively documented.

The following functions have been shown for the Ly 1 cell. It is the helper cell in T–B interactions; it is both necessary and sufficient for producing delayed type hypersensitivity reactions; it is the helper of the cell which mediates killer effects, although it itself has not been demonstrated to have any killing effect. The latter function is mediated by an Ly 1^- Ly 23^+ cell (all of the above studies are based on using antisera against the Ly 1.2 allele). There are studies with antisera against the Ly 1.1 allele which indicate that there may be some Ly 1 antigen on killer cells (Beverley, 1977). (It is not clear in my mind whether this is antibody directed against the Ly 1.1 antigen or a contaminant in the antibodies raised against Ly 1.1 cells). The suppressor cell is also Ly 1^-, 23^+. This has been shown to be true with antisera directed against the Ly 2.1 and 2.2 alleles, as well as the Ly 3.1 and 3.2 alleles. To my knowledge, no activity against suppressor cells has been shown with anti Ly 1.1 antisera. Thus, for the most part, both cytotoxic effector cells and suppressor cells are phenotypically Ly 1^- Ly 23^+. A number of workers have shown that the Ly 23 suppressor cells can also be inactivated by anti-Ia serum (Eichmann, 1975; Vadas *et al.*, 1976;

Feldmann, 1976; Okumura *et al.*, 1976; Murphy *et al.*, 1976; Schreffler and David, 1975, for information on Ia antigens and antisera). Anti-Ia serum has not yet been shown to inactivate killer cells, which at first glance might indicate that these two functions, i.e., killing and suppressing, are mediated by different subclasses of T cells. Further support for this contention can be found by demonstrations of histamine receptors on suppressor (Eichmann, 1975; Shearer *et al.*, 1974) but not killer cells. Further preliminary evidence with new antiserum also indicates that the phenotype of suppressor and killer cells may be different in terms of new Ly antigens as well (M. Feldmann, personal communication).

There is an important proviso one must put on interpreting these results at their present stage; i.e., in order to define a functionally distinct subclass of cells, one must demonstrate the stability of the phenotypic markers one is using to define the subclass. For example, there is some evidence that the amount of Ia antigen on T cells may be a function of the state of activity of the cell within the subclass (Wagner *et al.*, 1975). By this, I mean mitogen activated cells seem to express more Ia antigens on their surface than do resting cells. Thus, it is possible that the different results obtained in studies between killer cells and suppressor cells expressing I region antigens may only be because these cells are expressing different functions during different developmental states within the life cycle of the same subclass. On the other hand, the Ly 23 phenotype has been shown to be a stable marker. Thus, Cantor and his co-workers have shown that purified Ly 23 cells, when activated by mitogens, exhibit both killer and suppressor activity and are killed with anti-Ly 23 antiserum and complement both before and after activation (Cantor and Boyse, 1976; Cantor, 1977). Not only that, they have taken Ly 1^{-} 23^{+} cells and parked them in B mice for extensive periods of time. At intervals thereafter, they have retrieved the cells and have shown both the functions and the Ly phenotype that the cells express remained stable. They have also shown the same stability with the Ly 1 phenotype and the helper effects as well. The stability of the Ia markers and the histamine receptors have not been extensively examined.

Another feature common to both the killer cell (Möller, 1976b; Gershon and Cantor, 1977) and the suppressor cell (Gershon and Cantor, 1977) is their preference for reactivity with cell-surface products coded for by the peripheral (K/D) portions of the major histocompatibility complex. On the other hand, the Ly 1 helper cell binds to and reacts preferentially with the central region or I region of the major histocompatibility complex. These findings might suggest that the receptors on the two subclasses of T cells are somewhat different. Interestingly, both the Ly 1 cell and the Ly 23 cell have many of the overlapping characteristics with those cells that had been previously referred to T2, i.e., the more mature recirculating type of T cell.

III. POTENTIAL ROLE OF THE LY 123 CELL

We, thus, are left with finding a function for the major T cell component of mice, the Ly 123 cell. This cell has many of the overlapping characteristics with the cell that had previously been classified as the immature T1 cell (Raff and Cantor, 1971). It is probable that future work will show that the Ly 123 subclass of T cell is a heterogenous population of cells, but at present no markers are available which can subdivide this cell population. Since the present discussion is oriented towards suppressor T cells, I will concentrate the rest of this discussion on the role this subclass of cells might play in the generation of suppressive phenomena. In this matter, there is very little direct evidence. The main reason for this is the difficulty in obtaining purified Ly 123 populations. Purified Ly 1 populations are obtained by treating T cells with anti-Ly 2 or anti-Ly 3 antiserum plus complement, which removes all the Ly 23 cells as well as the Ly 123 cells. Similarly, preparation of purified of Ly 23 cell is obtained by treatment with Ly 1 antiserum and complement, which also removes all the Ly 123 cells as well as the Ly 1 cells. Therefore, negative selection experiments cannot obtain purified Ly 123 cells for study. Positive selection experiments, which are much harder to do, are required. This work has been hampered somewhat by an acute shortage of Ly antiserum because of the great difficulty there is in making it. Thus, most of the evidence on the function of Ly 123 cells comes from inferences on the functions of T1 cells or from experiments where Ly 1 and Ly 23 cells are recombined. When they fail to return the functions of normal population from which they are taken, the missing effects can be tentatively assigned to the Ly 123 cell. Doing these types of experiments, it is reasonably clear that the Ly 123 cells play a very important regulatory role in the immune response. Basically, there are two ways by which the Ly 123 cell could play its regulatory role. One is by acting as a distinct class of cells that controls the activity of the other two cells. Another way in which it could function is by acting as a precursor of the more mature effector helper suppressor and killer cells. By preferentially differentiating into an Ly 1 cell, it would regulate the response in an upward fashion; by differentiating into a 23 cell, it would regulate the response in a negative fashion. There is suggestive evidence that both forms of regulation may be operative.

Before discussing the mechanism by which the Ly 123 cell may suppress the immune response, it would be worth briefly considering the evidence as to whether the Ly 123 suppresses the immune response at all.

1. It has been noted in a number of instances that, after adult thymectomy, the immune response to certain antigens is augmented

(Mosier and Cantor, 1971; Kerbel and Eidinger, 1972). The Ly 123 cell is preferentially depleted by adult thymectomy (Cantor and Boyse, 1976; Cantor, 1977).

2. Several workers have noted that spleen-seeking T cells often act to suppress the immune response of lymph node-seeking cells (Wu and Lance, 1974; Rich and Rich, 1974; Folch and Waksman, 1974; Gershon *et al.*, 1974a). Although the precise distribution of the Ly phenotype of the T cells in the various lymphoid organs is not known, it has been shown that immature T cells (previously referred to as T1 cells) have a preference for splenic localization. It is most likely that these are predominantly Ly 123 cells. (Note: the association of T1 cells with Ly 123 cells comes not only from the preferential fall of Ly 123 cells after adult thymectomy, which has been a time-honored way of removing T1-type cells, but also from the ontogenic studies mentioned above where Ly 123 cells precede the development of either Ly 1 or Ly 23 cells).

3. Pretreatment of mice with drugs such as cyclophosphamide (Askenase *et al.*, 1975; Debré *et al.*, 1976b) or cortisone (Cohen and Gershon, 1975; Nachtigal and Zan-Bar, 1973) has been shown to abolish suppressor T cell activity; these drugs preferentially effect T1-type cells.

4. With time, after adult thymectomy, it becomes increasingly difficult to demonstrate suppressor T cells in several different tolerance models (Nachtigal and Zan-Bar, 1973; Basten *et al.*, 1975). Thus, there is ample evidence that T1 cells are important contributors to suppressor T cell activity, and, as mentioned above, there is suggestive evidence that the Ly 123 subclass is the predominant constituent of the cells previously referred to as T1.

It should also be pointed out that there are many instances where T1 cells have been shown to exhibit amplifier, instead of suppressor, activity in a number of different immunologic assays. Thus, it seems that T1 and/or Ly 123 cells have a bidirectional regulatory capacity. Thus, it has been suggested that this subclass of cells could be thought of as hermaphrocytes (Gershon *et al.*, 1976). Since cell interactions between T cells are as important in generating suppressor cells as they are in generating helper cells, and since T1 cells are very important in cell interactions, it is very probable that they do play an important role in generating suppressor cells. Up to this moment, however, all suppressor systems examined with the use of Ly antiserum have failed to find a direct role in suppression for a cell with the Ly 1 antigen on it.

One general rule we have found is that, when T1-type cells are added to an immune response which is going very well or is at a high level, the T1 cells tend to act as suppressor cells. On the other hand, when they are added to immune responses that are going rather weakly they tend to act as helper cells. Thus, it seems that they are cells which are capable of recognizing the level or intensity of an immune response and, by recognition of the signals emitted during the immune response, feedback and regulate the response. As noted above, how they do so is a matter of conjecture. If they acted as a distinct subclass of their own, they could produce factors which could differentially affect preprogrammed Ly 1 helpers or Ly 23 suppressors. On the other hand, one of the factors determining their differentiation pathway could be the factors emitted from the more mature helper and suppressor cells, and this, in turn, could effect the differentiation of the Ly 123 into a reciprocal class, i.e., excess Ly 1 activity is recognized by Ly 123 cells which then differentiate into Ly 23 suppressor cells. On the other hand, a low level of signal from Ly 1 or high signaling activity from Ly 23 cells could cause a differentiation of the Ly 123 cell into an Ly 1 helper.

IV. POTENTIAL CAUSES OF BREAKDOWN IN T CELL REGULATION WHICH COULD LEAD TO AUTOIMMUNITY

All these interactions I have discussed would tend to modulate the immune response and allow it to set a reasonable level. Aberrant responses could be caused by two principal factors: (1) problems with differentiation, which set abnormal levels or ratios of the three subclasses, causing a breakdown of their regulatory interactions; (2) aberrant behavior due to genetic, hormonal, antigenic, viral, or other factors induced in any one of the subclasses. One point which must be considered is that, not only is the amount of suppressor T cell activity a factor in determining whether the immune response will take place, but there also must be a receptivity of the target cell for the suppressor effect. Thus, target cells could be affected in such a way that they lose receptors or develop resistance to signals from suppressor cells, and, thus, immune regulation could break down in the face of normal suppressor cell activity. Examples where different types of T cells display different levels of susceptibility to suppressor factors have been shown (Gershon *et al.*, 1974b). It seems that the more mature a T cell is, the harder it is to suppress. In a review I once wrote, when the concept of suppressor T cells was just getting off the ground, to illustrate the problems and complexities of theorizing when one has multiple subclasses of cells on which to build theories, I quoted an old saying: "With two variables one could build an elephant—with three the universe" (Gershon, 1974). Thus, one would think, with the definition by the use of the Ly antiserum of T cells into distinct subclasses with preprogrammed functions, one would have a clearer understanding of how suppressor T cells work. Paradoxically, the reverse is true because of the new potential and demonstrated interactions between the subclasses, including feedback interactions between the regulatees and the regulators. The added variable of sensitivity to regulatory signals also makes extremely difficult any coherent logical formulation to account for all the known phenomenology. At a minimum, it can be said that there is a distinct subclass of T cells which play an important role in regulating the level of the immune response. The activity of this subclass of cells is clearly affected by the activity of other subclasses, and the ability of this suppressor subclass to regulate the other subclasses is also dependent, to some degree, upon the maturational state on the regulatee. Thus, there are numerous places within this cascade of interactions where breakdowns could occur, leading either to the production of cells or antibodies reactive with self. It would seem probable at this stage of our understanding that suppressor dysfunction is a cause of at least some autoimmune diseases, and that, at least in some of those cases, the aberrant activity of the suppressor T cells is not due to inherent dysfunction of that cell but due to defects in other cells that regulate it or are regulated by it.

V. RELATION OF SUPPRESSOR ACTIVITY TO HISTOCOMPATIBILITY ANTIGENS

There are two other recent important developments in the understanding of how suppressor T cells function, which should be commented on in a general overview. One is their relation to Ir gene control. It has been clearly demonstrated that a number of diseases of suspected autoimmune etiology have highly skewed histocompatibility phenotypes (see Chapter 1). It is also known that the ability to respond to certain antigens is also related to histocompatibility phenotype and that, at least in some of these cases, nonresponsiveness is due to a predominance of suppressor T cell activity (Benacerraf *et al.*, 1975). The histocompatibility genes which determine immunologic responsiveness or unresponsiveness are called Ir genes, and, thus, one might suspect that certain people who lack Ir genes might be more susceptible to autoimmune disease. One problem with this hypothesis is that a lack of an Ir gene should lead to unresponsiveness and, thus, should not be a direct cause of excess anti-self responsiveness. However, a new finding could overcome this apparent paradox (Debré *et al.*, 1976a). There are certain antigens to which no inbred strains of mice make an immune response, although some outbreds strains do respond. One antigen under study, however, can be made immunogenic when it is complexed to methylated bovine serum albumin. The most interesting finding is that pretreatment of some strains of mice with the nonimmunogenic form of antigen raises suppressor cells that prevent the mice from responding to a subsequent challenge with the immunogenic form of antigen. This trait has also been linked to the histocompatibility locus. The genes responsible for this suppressive effect have been called Is genes (immune suppressor genes). Thus, if this phenomenon can be made general, the linkage of autoimmune phenomena to the histocompatibility locus in some cases could be due to malfunction of Is genes controlling responses against self antigens, which leads to malfunction of suppressor T cells and autoimmunity.

Another question to be considered is whether suppressor T cells act by direct contact with their target cell or whether they produce soluble mediators. Unfortunately, the answer to this question is unknown. A number of workers have demonstrated soluble factors which act to suppress immune responses. Basically, there are two classes of factors; one seems to lack antigen specificity and has no demonstrable histocompatibility antigenic determinants on it. The prototype for this factor is the one released from Ly 23 cells after stimulation with Con A and has been called SIRS (Cantor and Boyse, 1976; Cantor, 1977; Rich and Pierce, 1974). This factor is released into culture supernatants.

Another factor has antigen specificity and contains histocompatibility antigenic determinants—particular antigens coded for by the I region (Tada *et al.,* 1975) and, moreover, by a special class of I region antigen which is not represented on B cells or on helper T cells. This antigen is coded for by a special I subregion (I–J) and appears to be uniquely represented on the suppressor factor and the cells which bear it (Murphy *et al.,* 1976; T. Tada, M. Taniguchi, and C. S. David, unpublished observations). This factor has not been shown to be released into the supernatants of cultures, but must be extracted from the cells which bear it. This does not mean that it is released under some circumstances and can act as a soluble factor, but, up to now, this release has not been demonstrated. It has also been shown that there are special acceptor sites on other T cells for this factor which are coded for, at least in part, by genes mapping to the major histocompatibility locus (Taniguchi *et al.,* 1976). However, it is unknown whether the factor itself is a suppressive agent or whether the receptor cell acts as the suppressor cell. Interestingly, thymocytes have a large number of acceptor sites for this factor, and it could very well be that this factor is one of the substances which causes uncommited cells to differentiate into Ly 23 suppressor cells.

Thus, it can be seen that some very important new discoveries have been made in understanding the mechanism of T cell-mediated suppression, but that these new discoveries have raised at least as many questions as they have provided answers. A pessimist would throw up his hands and say with all these lymphocyte subclasses and interactions that a clear-cut understanding of today's phenomenology is unattainable with present-day technology. A more optimistic view would be that the development of antisera against differentiation antigens and factors augurs well for the future, in that many laboratories are busy trying to produce more and different antisera, which may produce more illumination (on the other hand, they could produce more confusion). I personally would adopt a middle position. I would not be as optimistic as the late President Johnson and his colleagues and say "Ah yes we can now see the light at the end of the tunnel," but at least I would go so far as to say that the light at the beginning of the tunnel is starting to dim. The question which remains is "How long is the tunnel?"

ACKNOWLEDGMENTS

I am grateful to Patricia Byfield for helpful suggestions in preparing this manuscript. My own research was supported by NIH Grants of CA-08593, CA-14216, and AI-10497.

REFERENCES

Askenase, P. W., Hayden, B. J., and Gershon, R. K. (1975). *J. Exp. Med.* **141,** 697.

Basten, A., Miller, J. F. A. P., and Johnson, P. (1975). *Transplant. Rev.* **26,** 130.

Benacerraf, B., Kapp, J. A., Debré, P., Pierce, C. W., and de la Croix, F. (1975). *Transplant. Rev.* **26,** 21.

Beverley, P. C. L. (1977). *In* "T and B Lymphocytes in Immune Recognition" (G. Roelants and F. Loor, eds.). Wiley, New York (in press).

Boyse, E. A., Miyazawa, A., Aoki, T., and Old, L. J. (1968). *Proc. R. Soc. London, B Ser.* **170,** 175.

Cantor, H. (1977). *Contemp. Top. Immunobiol.* **7** (in press).

Cantor, H., and Boyse, E. A. (1976). *Cold Spring Harbor Symp. Quant. Biol.* **41,** 23.

Cohen, P., and Gershon, R. K. (1975). *Ann. N.Y. Acad. Sci.* **249,** 451.

Debré, P., Waltenbaugh, C., Dorf, M., and Benacerraf, B. (1976a). *J. Exp. Med.* **144,** 272.

Debré, P., Waltenbaugh, C., Dorf, M. E., and Benacerraf, B. (1976b). *J. Exp. Med.* **144,** 277.

Dresser, D. W., ed. (1976). *Br. Med. Bull.* **32,** No. 2.

Eichmann, K. (1975). *Eur. J. Immunol.* **5,** 511.

Feldmann, M. (1976). *Cold Spring Harbor Symp. Quant. Biol.* **41,** 113.

Folch, H., and Waksman, B. H. (1974). *J. Immunol.* **113,** 127.

Gershon, R. K. (1974). *Contemp. Top. Immunbiol.* **3,** 1.

Gershon, R. K., and Cantor, H. (1977). *In* "Development of Host Defenses" (D. Dayton and M. Cooper, eds.). Rowen Press, New York (in press).

Gershon, R. K., Lance, E. M., and Kondo, K. (1974a). *J. Immunol.* **112,** 546.

Gershon, R. K., Orbach-Arbouys, S., and Calkins, C. (1974b). *Prog. Immunol., Int. Congr. Immunol., 2nd, 1974* Vol. 2, p. 123.

Gershon, R. K., Eardley, D. D., Naidorf, K. F., and Ptak, W. (1976). *Cold Spring Harbor Symp. Quant. Biol.* **41,** 85.

Kapp, J., and Pierce, C. W. (1976). *Contemp. Top. Immunol.* **5,** 91.

Kerbel, R. S., and Eidinger, D. (1972). *Eur. J. Immunol.* **2,** 114.

Möller, G., ed. (1976a). *Transplant. Rev.* **26,** 1.

Möller, G., ed. (1976b). *Transplant. Rev.* **29,** 1.

Mosier, D., and Cantor, H. (1971). *Eur. J. Immunol.* **1,** 459.

Murphy, D. B., Herzenberg, L. A., Okumura, K., Herzenberg, L. A., and McDevitt, H. O. (1976). *J. Exp. Med.* **144,** 699.

Nachtigal, D., and Zan-Bar, I. (1973). *Eur. J. Immunol.* **3,** 315.

Okumura, K., Herzenberg, L. A., Murphy, D. B., McDevitt, H. O., and Herzenberg, L. A. (1976). *J. Exp. Med.* **144,** 685.

Raff, M. C., and Cantor, H. (1971). *Progr. Immunol., Int. Congr. Immunol., 1st, 1971* p. 83.

Rich, R. R., and Pierce, C. W. (1974). *J. Immunol.* **112,** 1360.

Rich, S. S., and Rich, R. R. (1974). *J. Exp. Med.* **140,** 1588.

Schreffler, D. C., and David, C. S. (1975). *Adv. Immunol.* **20,** 125.

Shearer, G. M., Weinstein, Y., and Melmon, K. L. (1974). *J. Immunol.* **113,** 597.

Shou, L., Schwartz, S. A., and Good, R. A. (1976). *J. Exp. Med.* **143,** 1100.

Singhal, S. K., and St. C. Sinclair, N. K., eds. (1975). "Suppressor Cells in Immunity." Univ. Western Ontario Press, Ontario.

Tada, T., Taniguchi, M., and Takemori, T. (1975). *Transplant. Rev.* **26,** 106.

Taniguchi, M., Tada, T., and Tokuhisa, T. (1976). *J. Exp. Med.* **144,** 20.

Tigelaar, R. E., Gershon, R. K., and Asofsky, R. (1975). *Cell. Immunol.* **19,** 58.

Vadas, M. A., Miller, J. F. A. P., McKenzie, I. F. C., Chism, S. E., Shen, F.-W., Boyse, E. A., Gamble, J. R., and Whitelaw, A. M. (1976). *J. Exp. Med.* **144,** 10.

Wagner, H., Götze, D., Ptschelinzew, L., and Röllinghoff, M. (1975). *J. Exp. Med.* **142,** 1477.

Waldmann, T. A., Durm, M., Broder, S., Blackman, M., Blaese, R. M., and Strober, W. (1974). *Lancet* **2,** 609.

Wu, C.-Y., and Lance, E. M. (1974). *Cell. Immunol.* **13,** 1.

Chapter 7

Autoimmunity and Lymphoid Malignancy: Manifestations of Immunoregulatory Disequilibrium

NORMAN TALAL

I. INTRODUCTION

The physiological regulation of the various manifestations of immune reactivity involves a complex interaction of genetic, cellular, and probably viral components. When the immune system is functioning efficiently and its diverse components are well integrated, the normal events of antibody formation, delayed hypersensitivity, and self/nonself discrimination present a harmonious appearance. Control is manifest in the appropriate initiation and termination of immune responses involving T and B lymphocytes, in the regulated differentiation of B lymphocytes into plasma cells, in the switch from IgM to IgG production, and in the general utility of these responses to the host, who is protected from infectious agents and possibly from neoplasia. However, when this system is functioning abnormally, there is an appearance of immunologic chaos in which the clinical consequences may take the form of autoimmune diseases and/or malignant lymphoproliferation.

There is now extensive human and animal evidence to suggest that autoimmunity, monoclonal immunoglobulin production, and malignant lymphocytic or plasma cell proliferation may be related events. Many monoclonal immunoglobulins in humans and mice have antibody activity, frequently for autoantigens, suggesting that autoimmune mechanisms may contribute to the pathogenesis of monoclonal antibody production. The occurrence of lymphoid neoplasms in patients with autoimmune diseases, and the frequent appearance of autoantibodies in patients with lymphoma or chronic lymphocytic leukemia, is further evidence for a relationship between autoimmunity and malignant lymphoproliferation. The development of lymphomas in immunodeficiency diseases, following immunosuppression and following renal transplantation, suggests that disordered immunologic regulation may be an underlying pathogenetic factor in lymphoid neoplasia.

Abnormal regulation of the immune system is a feature of many autoimmune disorders, and is best demonstrated in NZB and NZB/NZW F_1 (B/W) mice which spontaneously develop diverse autoantibodies, immune complex glomerulonephritis, defective T cell function, monoclonal macroglobulinemia, and malignant lymphomas (Talal, 1974). The role of genetic factors and C-type viruses in the pathogenesis of this murine disorder is discussed, respectively, in the chapters by Warner and Levy. This chapter will focus on immunologic control of immune reactivity and autoantibody formation in these mice, particularly on the role of T lymphocytes. A major defect in T cell regulation may be an important mechanism promoting autoimmunity and lymphoid neoplasia, not only in experimental animals, but also in human diseases.

II. AUTOIMMUNITY AND LYMPHOID MALIGNANCY IN NZB AND NZB/NZW F_1 (B/W) MICE

A. Natural History

An outline of the course of spontaneous disease and associated immunologic deficits is presented schematically in Table I. The mice appear clinically normal at birth, although some aspects of immunologic hyperactivity are present even this early in life. They are capable of making adult levels of plaque-forming cells to sheep erythrocytes (SRBC) in their first week of life (Evans *et al.*, 1968). They have very active cellular immunity at this age and are highly efficient regressors of malignant tumors (Gazdar *et al.*, 1971).

This immune competence appears prematurely, compared to normal strains, and may reflect an abnormality of immunologic regulation that first develops *in utero*. Certainly, by 2 months of age, these mice are highly resistant to immunologic tolerance induced by disaggregated bovine or human γ-globulin (Staples and Talal, 1969). If the tolerogen is injected at 3 weeks of age, NZB and B/W mice escape from tolerance within weeks, whereas control strains develop long-lasting tolerance. The kinetics of escape suggests the behavior of B cells returning from tolerance to immune competence (see Chapter 5 by Weigle). This defect is not unique to the NZB,

TABLE I

Temporal Changes in Immunologic Status and Clinical Course in NZB and NZB/NZW F_1 Mice

Age of mice	Immunologic status	Clinical condition
Birth	Hyperactive (humoral and cellular)	Normal
2 months	Resistant to tolerance; escape from tolerance; decreased suppressor T function; decreased thymic humoral factor	Autoantibodies appear (to nucleic acids, RBC, thymocytes, and viral antigens)
5 months	Humoral hyperactivity to many antigens; IgM to IgG switching begins (first for anti-DNA in females)	Immune complex nephritis (worse in females); Coombs'-positive hemolytic anemia; lymphocytic tissue infiltrates
12 months	Hypoactive (humoral and cellular)	Malignant lymphoma; monoclonal IgM

is under genetic control (see Chapter 2), and may be related to a deficiency of suppressor T cells (Benjamin, 1975).

Suppressor T cell activity declines between 1–2 months of age in NZB mice, as shown in graft versus host (GVH) assays (Dauphinee and Talal, 1973; Hardin *et al.*, 1973), in the response to polyvinylpyrrolidone (see Chapter 1), and in the response to pneumococcal polysaccharide (Barthold *et al.*, 1974). The importance of suppressor T cells for the maintenance of immunologic tolerance and prevention of autoimmunity is discussed elsewhere (see Chapters 5 and 6).

The thymus gland produces humoral factors that normally play a role in the differentiation of T cells (see Chapter 8). These factors decline prematurely in NZB and B/W mice at the time when suppressor T cell activity decreases and the mice become resistant to tolerance induction. The administration of thymosin fraction 5 at this age can restore suppressor activity (Dauphinee *et al.*, 1974; Talal *et al.*, 1975). However, the injection of thymosin therapeutically is without benefit thus far on the course of disease.

The first clinical appearance of autoantibodies occurs at about 2–3 months of age, although they can be detected much earlier by more sensitive methods. Antibodies to erythrocytes and to lymphocyte surface antigens appear in almost every NZB mouse, whereas antibodies to nucleic acids are found in B/W mice. Antibodies cytotoxic to T lymphocytes occur commonly in young NZB mice (Shirai and Mellors, 1971), are characteristically IgM, and do not distinguish NZB T cells from other T lymphocytes. This antibody occurs less often in B/W mice, a strain in which individual animals may develop antibodies to nucleic acids without detectable serum levels of antibodies to T cells (Goldblum *et al.*, 1975).

There is a marked sex difference in B/W mice; females develop severe immune complex glomerulonephritis and die approximately 4 months earlier than males. The renal deposits contain complement, antibodies to DNA (Lambert and Dixon, 1968), and antibodies to the major glycoprotein (gp 69/71) or murine C-type viruses (Yoshiki *et al.*, 1974). The more accelerated disease of female B/W mice is associated with earlier appearance and greater amounts of IgG antibodies to DNA (Papoian *et al.*, 1976). The switch from IgM to IgG antibodies to both DNA and RNA, and the influence of sex hormones upon this switch, is discussed below.

The titers of autoantibodies rise progressively, associated with a general augmentation of humoral immunity. Adult NZB and B/W mice make excessive antibody responses to several experimental antigens, including foreign proteins, SRBC, and synthetic nucleic acids (Talal, 1970). However, responses to pig and chicken erythrocytes are within the range of normal strains (Playfair, 1968), indicating some selectivity in their humoral hyperactivity.

Normal antibody responses undergo maturational events characterized by an increasing affinity and decreased heterogeneity, indicative of clonal restriction. Maturation of the SRBC response is abnormal in NZB mice, which make predominantly low affinity antibody, both to SRBC and to erythrocyte autoantigens (DeHeer and Edgington, 1976).

The major disease manifestations become clinically apparent after 5 months of age (Howie and Helyer, 1968). NZB mice develop Coombs'-positive hemolytic anemia; B/W mice develop proteinuria and uremia. Both strains develop marked lymphocytic and plasmacytic infiltrates in many different organs. This extensive lymphoproliferation may suggest malignancy (Mellors, 1966).

Mice that survive the autoimmune disorder are susceptible to the development of malignant lymphomas, at times associated with the production of monoclonal IgM (Sugai *et al.*, 1973). The development of lymphoma is enhanced by the administration of immunosuppressive drugs, such as azathioprine and cyclophosphamide. These older mice often have marked deficiencies of cell-mediated immunity, as shown by impaired proliferative responses to phytomitogens, reduced capacity to induce graft versus host disease or to reject malignant tumors and skin grafts (reviewed in Talal, 1974). The number of T cells in their peripheral lymphoid organs are decreased, and their ability to mount antibody responses to SRBC and other experimental antigens may decline to levels below those of normal strains.

B. T Cell Regulation

Although there are differences of opinion as to the importance of suppressor T cells in the various forms of immunologic tolerance, there is general agreement that T cells exert a major role in immunologic regulation. The resistance to immunologic tolerance, the early loss of suppressor T cell function, and the rather generalized immunologic hyperactivity of NZB and B/W mice suggest a state of immunologic imbalance in which B cell hyperactivity arises as a consequence of impaired T cell regulation (Talal, 1970, 1976). The premature immune competence present in the first week of life suggests that the foundations of this imbalance may become established immediately after birth or even *in utero*.

NZB and B/W mice behave as if they are hyperstimulated or under the influence of an adjuvant. Indeed, they fail to demonstrate an augmented response to SRBC when the latter is given with a synthetic polynucleotide adjuvant (Jacobs *et al.*, 1972). Other experiments suggest that some T cell functions may be increased at certain periods. The proliferative response of spleen cells to a common alloantigenic stimulus is greater in NZB mice, as compared to other H-2^d strains (Palmer *et al.*, 1976). Increased helper T cell activity may contribute to the increased *in vivo* response to SRBC. Maturation of bone marrow precursors into alloantigen- and mitogen-responsive thymocytes occurs more rapidly in NZB than in another H-2^d control strain (Dauphinee *et al.*, 1975).

Thus, the experimental evidence suggests that B cell and helper T cell functions are increased, whereas suppressor T cell activity is decreased. The simplest explanation would be a defect in suppressor T cells which then fail to regulate helper T cells and B cells, or to control helper T cells alone. A hyperactivity of the latter could indirectly lead to B cell activation and autoantibody formation.

Helper T cells and suppressor T cells are stable populations that can be distinguished because they have different Ly alloantigens on their surface membranes (Cantor and Boyse, 1975). Helper T cells have Ly 1, whereas suppressor T cells have Ly 2,3. The latter cells also express cytotoxic activity. Both populations may arise from a pool of Ly 1,2,3 precursor cells which differentiate into the two more mature populations. Cantor found a decrease in Ly 1,2,3 cells in adult NZB mice compared to normal strains, suggesting some defect in T cell maturation (personal communication).

Based on a presumed deficiency of suppressor function, Krakauer *et al.* (1976) have presented evidence for a loss of a suppressor factor in adult B/W mice. They found that spleen T cells from normal strains and 1-month-old B/W mice produce a soluble factor in response to concanavalin A which can markedly decrease immunoglobulin synthesis by mouse lymphoid cells. This factor is not produced by old B/W mice, although spleen cells from old B/W mice can respond to suppressor factor derived from normal mice. They have treated B/W mice starting at 1 month of age with suppressor factor from Balb/c mice and observed marked suppression of autoimmunity and glomerulonephritis accompanied by prolongation of survival (T. Waldmann, personal communication).

C. Regulation of Spontaneous Antibodies to Nucleic Acids

Antibodies to DNA and RNA can be detected as early as 4 weeks of age in B/W mice, using a sensitive filter radioimmunoassay and sucrose density gradient ultracentrifugation to fractionate serum (Papoian *et al.*, 1976). Antibodies to DNA are both IgM and IgG, whereas antibodies to RNA [polyadenylic acid, poly(A)] are exclusively IgM in these young mice. There is a striking difference between female and male animals in the Ig distribu-

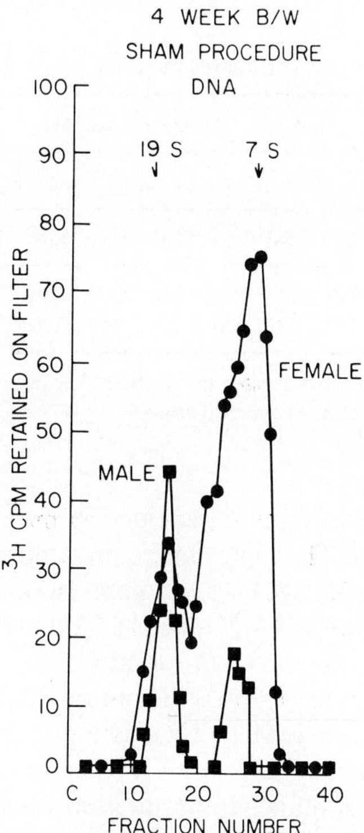

Fig. 1. The distribution of antibodies binding ^{3}H-DNA (from KB cells) after separation of serum from male and female B/W mice by sucrose density gradient ultracentrifugation. The bottom of the gradient is on the left. Binding of radioactive antigen is directly proportional to antibody concentration. The peak in the 19 S region contains IgM; DNA binding is inhibited by anti-μ chain antiserum. The peak in the 7 S region contains IgG; DNA binding is inhibited by anti-γ chain antiserum. The major difference is the greater IgG activity in the female.

tion of antibodies to DNA (Fig. 1). Females have much more IgG anti-DNA than do males.

Antibodies to DNA increase slowly from 1 to 4 months, as shown by progressively greater serum binding activity. The Ig distribution of anti-DNA antibodies remains relatively unchanged until 5–6 months when, in females, there is a sudden and marked increase in DNA binding by IgG antibodies. The radioactivity in the IgG region increases fourfold between 4 and 6 months (Table II). This does not occur in age-matched male mice. Furthermore, at 6–7 months in females, antibodies to poly(A) undergo a dramatic switch to IgG (Table III).

TABLE II

DNA Binding by IgM and IgG Antibodies in NZB/NZW F_1 Mice

	Age in months													
	1		2		4		6		9		11		13	
Sex	IgM	IgG	IgM	IgG	IgM	IgG	IgM	IgG	IgM	IgG	IgM	IgG	IgM	IgG
Female	210[a]	555[a]	440	720	1215	655	1690	2370	935	3590	—[b]			
Male	110	50	290	310	540	170	355	145	770	2165	595	2120	470	4050

[a] Total corrected cpm (^{3}H-DNA) under the 19 S or 7 S peaks respectively after fractionation by sucrose density gradient ultracentrifugation.

[b] No surviving mice.

This same sequence of events is repeated in males, but offset in time by approximately 4 months. The males make predominantly IgM antibodies to DNA until 9 months of age, when there is an approximately 15-fold increase in IgG binding of DNA (Table II). The switch of IgG antibodies to RNA [poly(A)] occurs in males at 11 months of age (Table III).

This ordered appearance of antibodies to nucleic acids, with an age and sex-dependent switch from IgM to IgG, is highly reproducible in different series of experiments. It suggests the presence of a regulatory mechanism acting to control the spontaneous production of antibodies to DNA and RNA. The timing of the switch from IgM to greatly increased IgG antibodies to DNA correlates, in each sex, with the onset of severe glomerulonephritis leading rapidly to death. This switch appears to herald the onset of a severe exacerbation of disease, which occurs first in females and later

TABLE III

RNA [Poly(A)] Binding by IgM and IgG Antibodies in NZB/NZW F_1 Mice

	Age in months													
	1		2		4		6		9		11		13	
Sex	IgM	IgG	IgM	IgG	IgM	IgG	IgM	IgG	IgM	IgG	IgM	IgG	IgM	IgG
Female	145[a]	0	340	0	340	260	370	3040	535	2130	—[b]			
Male	125	0	205	0	230	0	295	0	185	0	340	1645	990	3175

[a] Total corrected cpm [^{3}H-poly(A)] under the 19 S or 7 S peaks, respectively, after fractionation by sucrose density gradient ultracentrifugation.

[b] No surviving mice.

in males. The Ig switch may represent the conversion from a partial to a more complete regulatory defect with further impaired ability to control disease expression.

The IgM to IgG switch in antibody synthesis is a major event in B cell differentiation. The two factors that promote this event are antigen and T cells, probably acting together. Very little is known about the nature or origin of the immunogenic nucleic acids in B/W mice. We do not know whether the antigenic stimulus is mammalian or viral in origin, nor whether the antigenic load varies quantitatively throughout the life span of the animal. T cell control is mediated by factors which contain antigen binding sites as well as Ia determinants (Mozes, 1976). Exactly how and where these factors act is uncertain. The considerable information concerning T cell abnormalities in NZB and B/W mice suggests that the Ig switch might reflect disordered T cell control of immune reactivity.

In normal mouse strains, the switch from IgM to IgG is highly T cell dependent (although there are exceptions). T cells or T cell factors can convert strains that are genetically low responder to high responder status, an event accompanied by an IgM to IgG switch (Ordal and Grumet, 1972). Nude mice or thymectomized mice react to thymic-dependent antigens by producing predominantly IgM rather than the expected IgG antibodies (Davie and Paul, 1974). For these additional reasons, we presume that the IgM to IgG switch for nucleic acid antibodies reflects the activity of regulatory T cells, and may be an indirect but highly relevant way to study helper and suppressor T cell function.

D. Evidence for T Cell Regulation of Spontaneous Antibodies to DNA and RNA

A series of surgical ablation experiments were performed to test this concept. Neonatal thymectomy (performed on 2 or 3-day old B/W mice) had an opposite effect on survival of female and male animals (Table IV). Thymectomy significantly prolonged survival of the females, but increased mortality in the males (Roubinian *et al.*, 1977a). The thymectomized males had an immediate and persistent increase in antibodies to DNA, associated with an accelerated switch to IgG, which occurred at 4 rather than at 9 months (Fig. 2).

These results are consistent with the elimination of thymic suppressor influence in the males, resulting in an essentially female pattern of disease expression. By contrast, neonatal thymectomy of females had relatively little effect on antibodies to DNA, suggesting that this antibody response is already independent of a thymic suppressor mechanism at the time of sur-

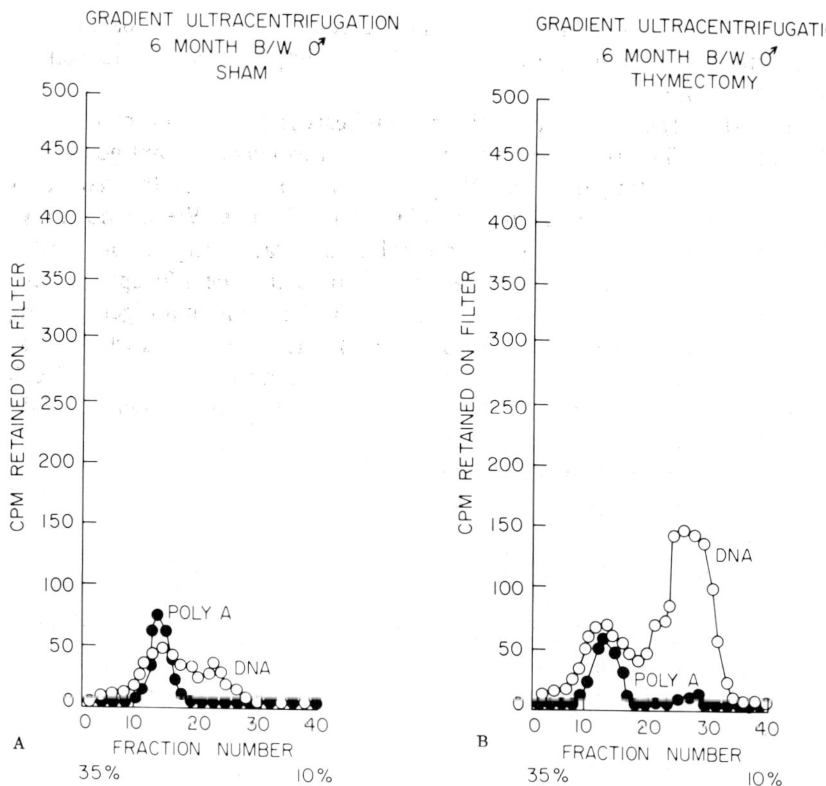

Fig. 2. The distribution of antibodies binding ^{3}H-DNA and ^{3}H-poly(A) in serum from (A) sham operated or (B) neonatally thymectomized male B/W mice. The major difference is the increase in IgG antibodies to DNA after thymectomy.

gery. Helper T cells for anti-DNA may be relatively more peripheralized in newborn female compared to male B/W mice; this would be consistent with the larger amount of IgG antibodies present in 4-week females (Fig. 1).

In contrast to the anti-DNA response, the RNA response is influenced by thymectomy in both sexes. Neonatal thymectomy almost completely prevented the switch to IgG anti-poly(A), suggesting a requirement for thymus-derived helper cells (Fig. 3). This result is particularly interesting because an early effect of neonatal thymectomy was an augmentation of IgM antibodies to poly(A), suggesting suppressor cell control. Thus, the poly(A) response may be controlled by both thymic suppressor and thymic helper cells. This result suggests that an antibody response may appear "thymic-independent" early in life (i.e., independent of helper T cells), but may become highly "thymic-dependent" later in life.

The spleen of male B/W mice also exerts a suppressor influence. Neonatal splenectomy significantly shortened the life span of males, but had no effect on females (Table IV). It also resulted in a premature switch to IgG anti-poly(A) antibodies (2 months earlier than in sham-operated controls). This switch might reflect the activity of helper T cells in lymph nodes, perhaps released from splenic suppression. Moreover, this switch to IgG anti-poly(A) occurred even in thymectomized mice, provided that splenectomy was also performed. Thus, the thymic-dependence of the poly(A) response is not absolute and can be circumvented if splenic suppressor influences are also eliminated.

These results suggest an important role for helper and suppressor T cells in regulating the amount and Ig class of antibodies to nucleic acids. Addi-

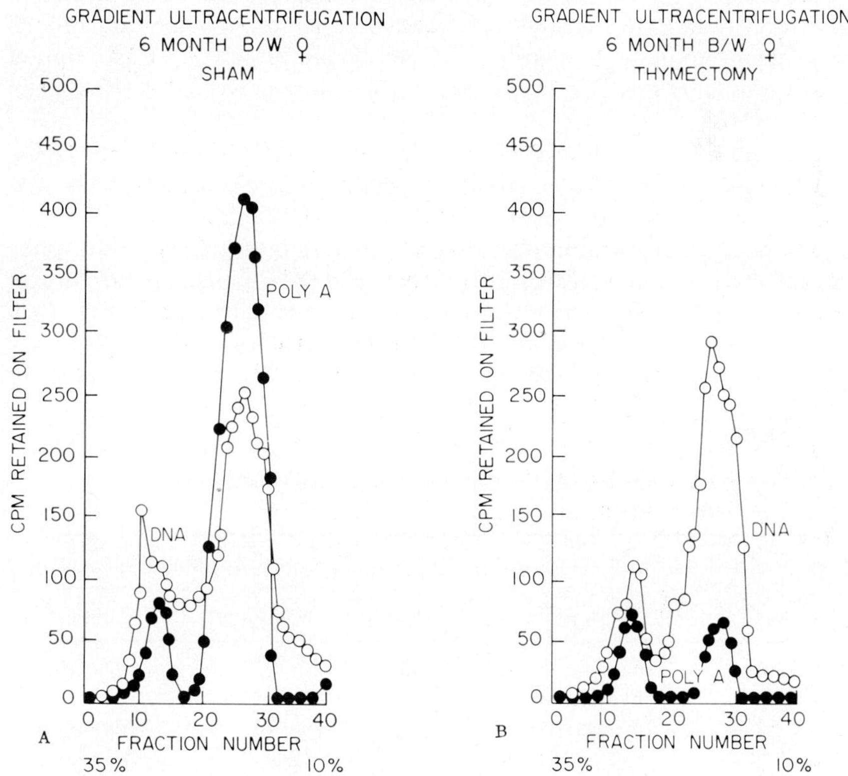

Fig. 3. The distribution of antibodies binding ³H-DNA and ³H-poly(A) in serum from (A) sham operated or (B) neonatally thymectomized female B/W mice. The major difference is the blunted IgG antibody response to poly(A) in the operated mice.

tional control experiments currently in progress attempt to confirm this interpretation by adoptive transfer of putative thymic or splenic suppressor populations into syngeneic test animals.

E. Modulation of T Cell Regulation by Sex Hormones

The milder disease of male B/W mice is associated with a later conversion to IgG antibodies to nucleic acids and more evidence of suppressor regulation. Prepubertal castration of males (performed at 2 weeks) resulted in significantly shortened survival, whereas castration had no effect in females (Table V). Castrated males had greater amounts of antibodies to DNA and poly(A) and showed a premature switch to IgG (Fig. 4). In these respects, they resembled thymectomized males and female B/W mice. Thus, castration of males, like thymectomy, caused a worsening of disease and accelerated appearance of IgG antibodies. However, castration differed from thymectomy with regard to IgG antibodies to poly(A). Castration of males promoted this switch, whereas thymectomy prevented it (Roubinian *et al.*, 1977b).

Castrated females showed only a slight decrease in antibodies to DNA, but failed to develop IgG antibodies to poly(A) (Fig. 5). In all respects, castration and thymectomy were similar in female B/W mice.

The effects of castration indicate that sex hormones greatly influence the spontaneous antibody response to DNA and RNA, and the severity of disease, in B/W mice. The major influence appears to be a protective effect of male hormone. Experiments currently underway will explore the potential therapeutic benefit of this observation. The protective effect of

TABLE IV

Effect of Neonatal Thymectomy or Splenectomy on Mortality in NZB/NZW F_1 Mice

		Mortality (%)		
Sex	Procedure	6 Months	9 Months	12 Months
Female	Sham	33	73	93
	Thymectomy	11	44[a]	61[a]
	Splenectomy	21	72	100
Male	Sham	0	10	50
	Thymectomy	35[a]	47[a]	70
	Splenectomy	0	55[a]	100[a]

[a] $p < 0.05$.

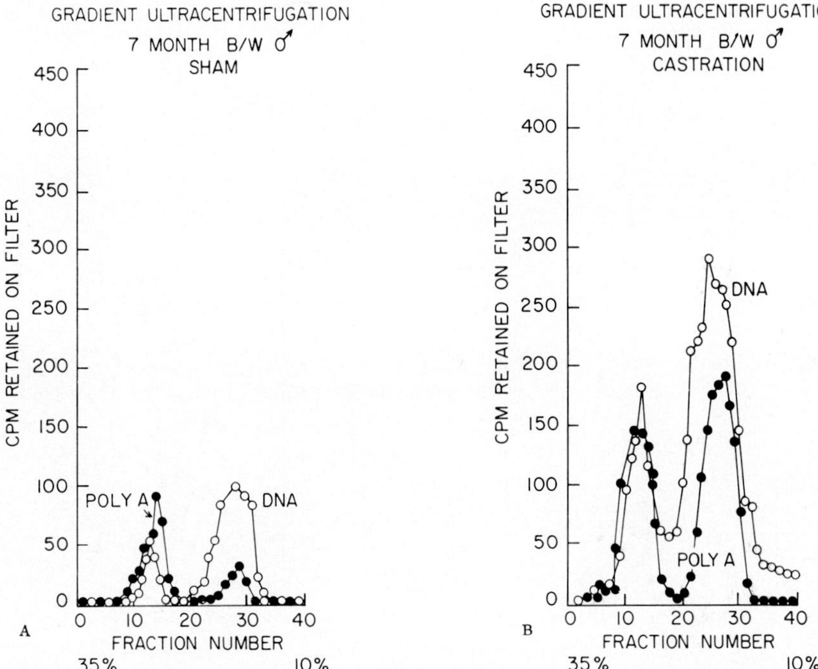

Fig. 4. The distribution of antibodies binding ^{3}H-DNA and ^{3}H-poly(A) in serum from (A) sham operated or (B) castrated male B/W mice. Castration resulted in greater binding activity and premature switch to IgG.

androgen probably explains why autoimmunity, in general, is more common in females.

Our results indicate similarities between castration and thymectomy, and help pinpoint the mechanism by which sex hormones influence these immune responses. The elimination of androgen was similar to removing a thymic suppressor mechanism, allowing an IgG switch for both antibodies to DNA and poly(A). The latter response is interesting because thymectomy had the opposite effect, i.e., prevented the development of IgG antibodies to poly(A).

In females, castration also resembled thymectomy in that it had little effect on anti-DNA antibodies or on the disease. This may relate to the premature peripheralization of the anti-DNA response in this sex. However, IgG antibodies to poly(A) in the female are not present early in life and require the thymus for their development (e.g., they fail to appear in neonatally thymectomized animals). These antibodies did not develop in castrated females, which is further evidence that sex hormones act at the level

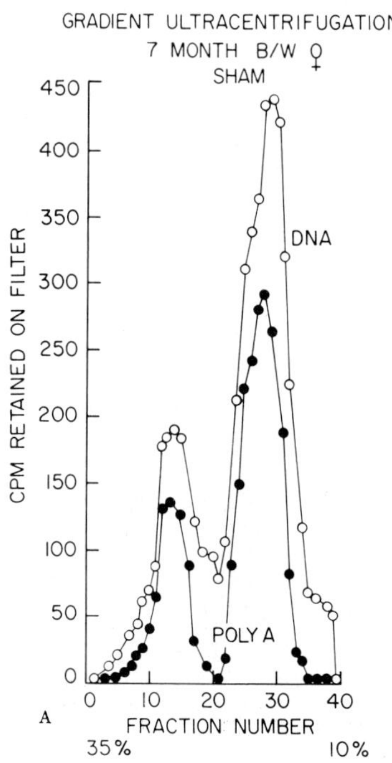

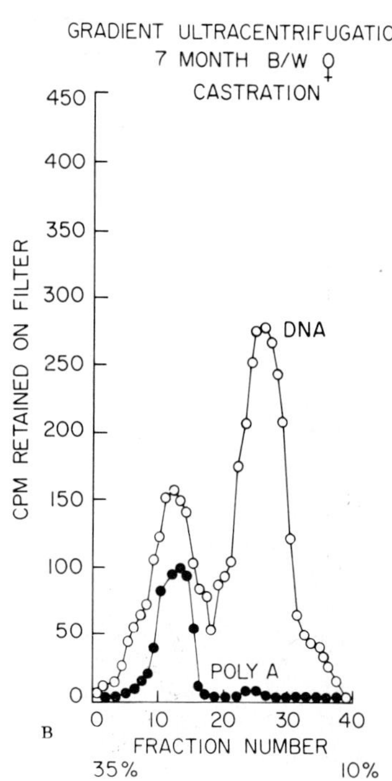

Fig. 5. The distribution of antibodies binding ^{3}H-DNA and ^{3}H-poly(A) in serum from (A) sham operated or (B) castrated female B/W mice. Castration prevented the development of IgG antibodies to poly(A).

of the thymus to modulate the immune response to nucleic acids. Furthermore, this result suggests that, even in the female, regulatory events that still depend upon the thymus are susceptible to modulating influences. The treatment of B/W mice with nucleoside conjugated to mouse γ-globulin to induce carrier-determined tolerance may be an example of such modulation (Borel, 1976).

These effects on autoantibodies are consistent with the known regulatory effects of sex hormones on normal immune responses. For example, female mice are less susceptible to immunologic tolerance than males. Female lymphocytes are more active in mixed lymphocyte responses. Female mice of various normal strains have higher antibody responses to several different antigens when compared with males (Eidinger and Garrett, 1972). Castrated male mice give an augmented "female" response to these antigens. After orchiectomy at 6 weeks of age, the thymus weight of operated mice increased greatly. Thymectomy abolished the enhanced antibody response seen after orchiectomy. These results in normal strains, like the results in

TABLE V

Effect of Prepubertal Castration on Mortality in NZB/NZW F_1 Mice

Sex	Procedure	Mortality at 8 months (%)
Female	Sham	78 (11/14)[a]
	Castration	87 (14/16)
Male	Sham	8 (1/12)
	Castration	60 (9/15)[b]

[a] Number of mice dead/total number.
[b] $p < 0.05$.

B/W mice, suggest that sex hormones act at the level of the thymus. Thus, sex differences in autoimmunity are probably aberrant expressions of the normal physiological effects that sex hormones exert on immune reactivity.

Our results, taken together, indicate that autoantibody responses are regulated by T cells, probably in a manner not very different from normal antibody responses. The equilibrium between helper and suppressor T cells may be modulated by sex hormones, with androgens favoring suppression. The pattern of earlier onset and more severe disease in female B/W mice seems predetermined from birth. How hormones act to modulate T cell regulation is, at the moment, a subject for speculation.

F. Malignant Lymphoproliferation and Monoclonal Immunoglobulins

Malignant and pseudomalignant lymphoproliferation and dysproteinemia are recognized features of disease in elderly NZB and B/W mice (Mellors, 1966; East, 1970). The extensive lymphocytic and plasmacytic infiltrations, and the hyperplasia of lymphatic organs, may give a false impression of neoplasia (pseudolymphoma).

The malignant lymphomas vary in degree of cellular differentiation, but appear to belong to the B cell line (Greenspan *et al.*, 1974). The serum often contains monoclonal immunoglobulins of the IgM class, frequently in small amounts, and not necessarily associated with an obvious tumor (Sugai *et al.*, 1973). Thus far, no antibody activity has been found for these monoclonal proteins. They are not antibodies to nucleic acids or rheumatoid factors. Idiotypic antisera prepared against one such monoclonal IgM (141) reacts specifically with determinants on the cell surface of the lymphoma producing that protein. These idiotypic membrane determinants behave as tumor-associated transplantation antigens (Sugai *et al.*, 1974).

The occurrence of monoclonal IgM and B cell neoplasms in old B/W mice suggests that malignant lymphoproliferation, like autoimmunity, may occur as a result of disordered immune regulation. Both the synthesis of autoantibodies by B cells and the malignant proliferation of B cells may arise as manifestations of disturbed T cell control of B cell function. It is interesting that NZB and Balb/c mice are the only strains susceptible to the induction of plasmacytomas and myeloma proteins by the injection of mineral oil (Potter, 1972; Warner, 1975). Genetic and viral factors (possibly C-type viruses) are involved in this unique susceptibility. Warner (1975) has suggested that the genetic resistance of NZB and Balb/c mice to tolerance induction is related to the development of plasmacytomas. He proposes that the mineral oil irritant leads to granuloma formation, with associated tissue destruction and release of autoantigens. The tolerance abnormality, possibly through a failure of T cell suppression, then results in autoimmunization, hypergammaglobulinemia, and B cell activation. The transformation of an activated B cell or plasma cell, possibly by a C-type virus, may be the final step in plasmacytoma formation.

III. MONOCLONAL IMMUNOGLOBULINS AND AUTOIMMUNITY

Monoclonal immunoglobulins having antibody activity occur in 5–10% of mineral oil-induced plasmacytomas in Balb/c mice (Potter, 1972), and in patients with lymphoproliferative malignancies, particularly Waldenström's macroglobulinemia and multiple myeloma (Seligmann and Brouet, 1973). Although several such proteins with low binding affinities probably lack true functional sites, others appear to be monoclonal antibodies. The specificity of these functional monoclonal proteins is often directed against autoantigens, suggesting that they arise through mechanisms involving autoimmunization.

In humans, these specificities include IgG ("monoclonal rheumatoid factor"), red blood cell antigens, lipoproteins, fibrin, transferrin, and albumin. Anti-IgG activity is found in 5% of random monoclonal IgM proteins (Seligmann and Brouet, 1973). In mice, these monoclonal immunoglobulins bind such antigenic determinants as phosphorylcholine, nitrophenyl ligands, 5-acetyl uracil, and carbohydrate antigens (including 1–6 linked galactans, and 1–3 linked dextrans). Some myeloma proteins with specificity for DNP protein conjugates cross-react with nucleic acid derivatives or with DNA

(Schubert *et al.*, 1968). An interesting IgA myeloma protein with antibody activity for DNA is the product of a lymphoid tumor that arose in a Balb/c × A/Jax F_1 mouse injected intraperitoneally with a spleen filtrate from a dog with lupus (Lewis *et al.*, 1973). The specificity of this monoclonal anti-DNA antibody is very similar to anti-DNA antibodies seen in lupus patients and in B/W mice (Dixon *et al.*, 1975).

The greatest number of oil-induced myeloma proteins are IgA. This high incidence of IgA synthesis, as well as the unusual specificities, suggest a nonrandom process of selection involved in plasmacytoma induction. The frequent occurrence of IgA is probably explained by the intestinal origin of the malignant plasma cells arising after intraperitoneal injection of the oil irritant. Microbial flora in the intestine may act as antigens and explain some aspects of the specificity. For example, phosphorylcholine is the major antigenic determinant in pneumococcal C polysaccharide.

Although autoimmunity and monoclonal Ig formation are related in the spontaneous diseases of NZB and B/W mice, in patients, and in the autoantibody activity of some myeloma proteins, many aspects of this relationship are unclear. Cells already producing autoantibodies may be more susceptible to neoplastic transformation, although the lack of autoimmunity in the Balb/c strain, the disappearance of autoantibodies in B/W mice developing monoclonal IgM (Sugai *et al.*, 1973), and the absence of antibody activity in the B/W monoclonal IgM's, argue against this simple explanation.

IV. OTHER EXPERIMENTAL MODELS OF AUTOIMMUNITY AND MALIGNANT LYMPHOPROLIFERATION

A. Aleutian Mink Disease

This disease in genetically susceptible mink homozygous for the Aleutian gene a is characterized by marked hypergammaglobulinemia, plasmacytosis, diffuse vasculitis, generalized lymphadenopathy, and glomerulonephritis. A viral etiology is suspect (Ingram and Cho, 1974). Autoantibodies and homogeneous γ-globulins have been reported (Porter *et al.*, 1965).

B. Murine Diseases

Several strains of mice develop autoantibodies and generalized lymphoproliferation in association with aging.

The SJL strain develops marked dysproteinemia, myelomalike immunoglobulins and reticulum cell lymphoid tumors (thought to resemble Hodgkin's disease). Anti-nuclear antibodies are present in 53% of mice at 11–12 months. As in B/W mice, anti-nuclear antibodies are less common in tumor-bearing animals (Haran-Ghera *et al.*, 1973).

A recently introduced strain, developed by Dr. E. D. Murphy at Bar Harbor and called MRL/1, is characterized by massive lymphoproliferation and immune complex glomerulonephritis. A single autosomal recessive gene determines the lymphoproliferation which has the characteristics of a pleomorphic lymphoma. This strain develops hypergammaglobulinemia, LE cells, and antibodies to DNA. Female mice die before males (at 120 days compared to 150 days for males).

The induction of a chronic graft versus host disease by the injection of parent cells into F_1 hybrid recipients leads to autoantibody formation and lymphoid tumors (Datta and Schwartz, 1976; Gleichmann *et al.*, 1976). Autoimmune hemolytic anemia and immune complex glomerulonephritis develop as a consequence of a persistent allogeneic effect. Parent T cells and a K-end difference in the H-2 region are required. F_1 B cells produce most of the autoantibodies, indicating involvement of host cells in the response. Many of the lymphomas, which have been called reticulum cell sarcomas, are probably also derived from host B cells and require an I region difference for induction.

V. CLINICAL EXPERIENCES WITH THE ASSOCIATION OF AUTOIMMUNITY AND LYMPHOMA

A. Sjögren's Syndrome

The clearest association between autoimmunity and lymphoma in the group of autoimmune diseases occurs in Sjögren's syndrome (SS), where the clinical experience parallels the example of NZB and B/W mice. This syndrome represents a lymphocytic attack on the salivary and lacrimal glands, and is accompanied by rheumatoid arthritis in half the cases. The disease is benign in over 90% of patients, and leads progressively to oral and ocular dryness. Some patients exhibit a more aggressive course in which lymphocytic infiltrates may involve parenchymal organs such as liver, lungs, and kidneys, and lymphadenopathy may be extreme (Talal, 1974). The histological picture in the lymph nodes is one of atypical and highly pleomorphic involvement, with erosion through the capsule and loss of nodal architecture. The term "pseudolymphoma" has been applied to this condition, which appears benign and generally responsive to corticosteroid or immunosuppressive therapy. However, some patients with SS develop malignant lymphomas, without necessarily passing through a pseudolymphoma stage. The lymphomas are often highly undifferentiated and may be associated with hypogammaglobulinemia and loss of autoantibodies. Serum β_2-microglobulin is increased in such patients (Michalski *et al.*, 1975). Monoclonal macroglobulinemia may be associated with pseudolymphoma or with a more malignant course like Waldenström's macroglobulinemia.

The similarity to NZB and B/W mice lies in the sequence of autoimmunity proceeding to lymphoma, in the existence of an intermediate stage of lymphocytic reactivity (pseudolymphoma), in the association with monoclonal IgM, and in the tendency to lose autoantibodies as the malignant disorder emerges.

B. Immunoblastic Lymphadenopathy

A pseudoneoplastic lymphocytic reaction to intense antigenic stimulation is not unique to autoimmune diseases. A recently described pathological entity, termed immunoblastic lymphadenopathy, suggests that this lymph node response may be a more general occurrence (Frizzera *et al.*, 1974; Lukes and Tindle, 1975; Dorfman and Warnke, 1974). Patients with this entity may be confused with those having Hodgkin's disease. They present with constitutional symptoms, generalized lymphadenopathy, and hepatosplenomegaly. Hyperglobulinemia, autoantibodies, mixed cryoglobulinemia, monoclonal gammapathy, and hemolytic anemia may be present. The lymph nodes show immunoblastic proliferation in the B lymphocyte–plasma cell series, proliferation of small vessels, and deposits of amorphous interstitial material. The prognosis is poor (median survival of 15 months in 18 fatal cases) even though the cellular proliferation appears benign. A hypersensitivity reaction to drugs may be involved in some patients, supporting the concept that this disorder represents an uncontrolled proliferation to an antigenic stimulus. A true neoplasm (immunoblastic sarcoma) may develop.

C. Diseases Associated with Epstein-Barr (EB) Virus

The DNA-containing EB virus is associated with both a benign self-limited form of lymphoproliferation (infectious mononucleosis, IM) and with the malignant proliferation seen in Burkitt's lymphoma (BL). In IM, EB virus preferentially infects B cells which then express viral antigens. These antigenically modified B cells stimulate T cells, which become specifically cytotoxic to EB virus-infected cells (Carter, 1975). The atypical lymphocytes seen in this disease are such stimulated T cells. The heterophile antibody and other autoantibodies appear, most often in the IgM class. There is no documented progression from IM to BL.

The IgM antibodies to EB virus in IM suggest a primary infection, whereas in BL the antibodies tend to be more IgG and suggest a chronic infection. In one African study, children with the highest antibody titers seemed most predisposed to the development of BL. IM is a polyclonal disease, possibly related to the ability of EB virus to act as a polyclonal activator of B cells. EB virus-positive B cell tissue culture lines established from IM patients are always diploid. However, cell lines from BL patients are not diploid and consistently contain an anomaly of chromosome number 14. The BL lines will grow when transplanted into nude mice, but the IM lines will not. Thus, the IM lines, although immortal in culture, are preneoplastic and lack the chromosomal change associated with the true neoplasia of BL (G. Klein, personal communication). This suggests a final chromosomal step superimposed upon a viral–autoimmune background as a necessary component in the conversion from a benign to a malignant lymphoproliferation.

VI. THEORETICAL CONSIDERATIONS

Immunoregulation depends upon the proper interaction and function of genetic and immunologic factors. Considerable evidence suggests that H_2 molecules on surface membranes act as adapters (Edelman, 1976) or receptors for viral antigens, tumor antigens, and chemical modifiers. This has led to the "altered-self" hypothesis in which H_2 + viral determinants create new antigenic sites which are specifically recognized by syngeneic lymphocytes (see Chapter 12). Syngeneic recognition may be a fundamental element in the integrated function of the immune system analogous to the self-recognition of parenchymal cells which permits the development of organ systems. Viewed from this perspective, autorecognition is a physiological event and far removed from the immunopathology of autoimmune diseases.

How then to explain the existence of these diseases? At this point, one must consider the extensive evidence that autoimmunity and immunopathology arise out of the interaction of viruses with the immune system. For the NZB disorder, the pertinent virus is the C-type particle whose antigens may play important roles in normal cellular differentiation events (see Chapter 14). We have recently studied the presence of C-type viral antigens on the surface membranes of a B/W B cell lymphoma (141) and on T and B spleen cells from normal and B/W mice. We can detect the major envelope glycoprotein (gp 69/71) and major core protein (p30) of leukemia virus using specific antisera and an antibody-dependent cellular cytotoxicity assay. Is there a cellular function for these surface viral antigens, apart from their incorporation into the virus particle? The molecular association of H_2 and gp 69/71 on tumor cell membranes has been shown by co-capping experiments (Schrader *et al.*, 1975). Possibly other surface antigens (e.g., Ia or even idiotype of Ig) can also associate with viral antigens at certain times in the life cycle of normal lymphocytes and, thereby, create new antigenic units whose recognition may initiate physiological or pathological immune reactivity.

The surface of a lymphocyte is shown schematically in Fig. 6. Antigenic determinants representing H_2, Ia, and idiotype of Ig are indicated, each in potential association with a viral antigen (gp 69/71). The recognition of an altered-self antigen (H_2 + gp 69/71) by a T cell is illustrated. Other theoretical altered self antigens are suggested in the figure.

Hypothetically, a T cell response to virally altered self-antigens might result in the generation of suppressor or helper factors. Suppressor factors might limit B cell proliferation and antibody synthesis, possibly leading to IgM antibody. Helper factors would stimulate B cell differentiation and result in IgG antibody. The factors determining whether the response is suppressor or helper are not known, but depend in part on the chemical structure of the antigen, presence of adjuvants, prior antibody response, activity of macrophages, etc. Autoimmunity might arise through the inappropriate insertion and expression of viral antigens on the lymphocyte membrane in association with self-determinants. This could act to modify the expression of self-antigens, alter membrane events, and generate a deficiency of suppressor or excess of helper T cells, resulting in autoantibody formation. Such a mechanism would conveniently explain the anti-lymphocyte antibodies that occur in NZB mice and in lupus patients.

A theoretical scheme for relating C-type virus expression to immunoregulation is illustrated in Fig. 7. Helper and suppressor T cells are shown as two populations with their characteristic Ly surface-cell antigens. These cells scan each other's MHC surface antigens and respond to new antigenic

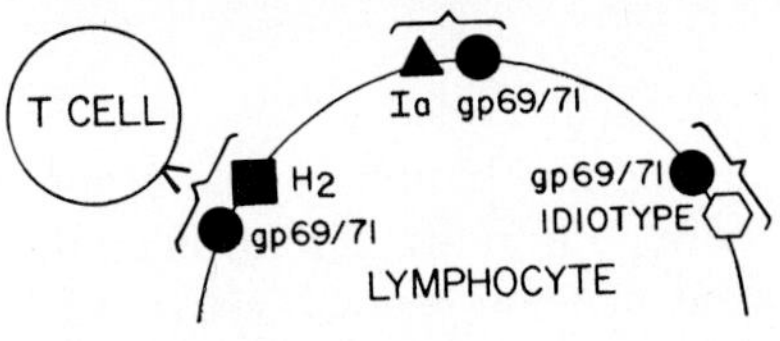

Fig. 6. The theoretical association of C-type viral antigen (gp 69/71) and self antigens on the lymphocyte surface. Recognition of "altered-self" antigens by T cells may lead to immunopathology.

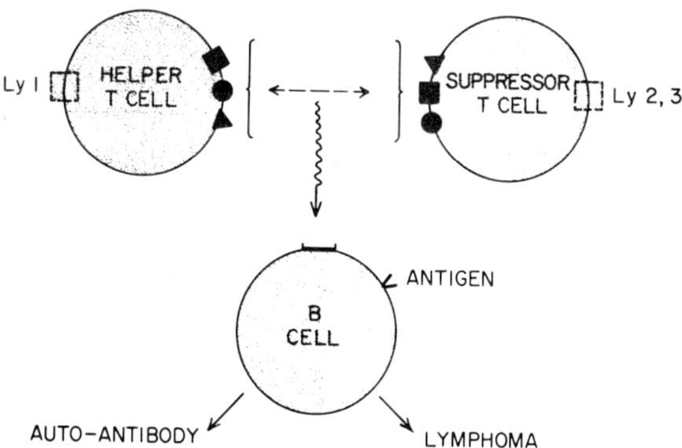

Fig. 7. A hypothetical scheme by which disordered immunologic regulation may lead to autoantibody formation and malignant lymphoma.

variations introduced by viral or other foreign antigens. The response can result in the generation of T cell signals, which are transmitted to B cells. These signals may be the T cell factors which contain antigen-combining sites plus Ia determinants (Mozes, 1976). The nature of these factors and the regulatory equilibrium so created, determines whether B cell proliferation and antibody synthesis is favored or suppressed. The inappropriate expression of viral antigens on the surface of one or another regulatory T cell population might perturb the normal helper/suppressor equilibrium, leading to autoantibody production and ultimately to malignant lymphoproliferation.

This theoretical scheme fits nicely with the following features of the antibody response to nucleic acids in B/W mice: (1) the existence of suppressor T cell control; (2) the switch from IgM to IgG representing the activation of helper T cells; (3) the suppression of helper T cells as well as B cells; and (4) the sex hormone modulation of regulation, with androgens favoring suppression.

VII. CONCLUSIONS

Experimental and clinical evidence suggests that autoimmunity and malignant and pseudomalignant lymphoproliferation may be manifestations of immunoregulatory disequilibrium. The balance between helper and suppressor T cells is dependent upon genetic, viral, and hormonal factors. The expression of viral antigens in association with MHC gene products on the lymphocyte surface may influence this regulatory equilibrium and may function normally to limit B cell proliferation and prevent autoantibody formation. The inappropriate insertion of viral or other foreign antigens on the lymphocyte surface may subvert normal regulatory mechanisms and lead to autoimmunity and lymphoma. This hypothesis may be generally applicable to a wide range of situations discussed in this chapter in which autoimmunity, monoclonal gammopathy, and malignant lymphoproliferation can be related.

REFERENCES

Barthold, D. R., Kysela, S., and Steinberg, A. D. (1974). *J. Immunol.* **112,** 9.

Benjamin, D. C. (1975). *J. Exp. Med.* **141,** 635.

Borel, Y. (1976). *Transplant. Rev.* **31,** 1.

Cantor, H., and Boyse, E. A. (1975). *J. Exp. Med.* **141,** 1376.

Carter, R. L. (1975). *Lancet* **1,** 846.

Datta, S. K., and Schwartz, R. S. (1976). *Transplant. Rev.* **31,** 44.

Dauphinee, M. J., and Talal, N. (1973). *Proc. Natl. Acad. Sci. U.S.A.* **70,** Part II, 37.

Dauphinee, M. J., Talal, N., Goldstein, A. L., and White, A. (1974). *Proc. Natl. Acad. Sci. U.S.A.* **71,** 2637.

Dauphinee, M. J., Palmer, D. W., and Talal, N. (1975). *J. Immunol.* **115,** 1054.

Davie, J. M., and Paul, W. E. (1974). *J. Immunol.* **113,** 1438.

DeHeer, D. H., and Edgington, T. S. (1976). *Transplant. Rev.* **31,** 116.

Dixon, J. A., Sugai, S., and Talal, N. (1975). *Clin. Exp. Immunol.* **19,** 347.

Dorfman, R. F., and Warnke, R. (1974). *Hum. Pathol.* **5,** 519.

East, J. (1970). *Prog. Exp. Res.,* **13,** 84–134.

Edelman, G. M. (1976). *Science* **192,** 218–226.

Eidinger, D., and Garrett, T. J. (1972). *J. Exp. Med.* **136,** 1098.

Evans, M. N., Williamson, W. G., and Irvine, W. J. (1968). *Clin. Exp. Immunol.* **3,** 375.

Frizzera, G., Moran, E. M., and Rappaport, H. (1974). *Lancet* **1,** 1070.

Gazdar, A. F., Beitzel, W., and Talal, N. (1971). *Clin. Exp. Immunol.* **8,** 501.

Gleichmann, E., Gleichmann, H., and Wilke, W. (1976). *Transplant. Rev.* **31,** 156.

Goldblum, R., Pillarisetty, R., and Talal, N. (1975). *Immunology* **28,** 621.

Greenspan, J. S., Gutman, G. A., Talal, N., Weissman, I. L., and Sugai, S. (1974). *Clin. Immunol. Immunopathol.* **3,** 32.

Haran-Ghera, N., Ben-Yaakov, M., Peled, A., and Bentwich, Z. (1973). *J. Natl. Cancer Inst.* **50,** 1227.

Hardin, J. A., Chused, T. M., and Steinberg, A. D. (1973). *J. Immunol.* **111,** 650.

Howie, J. B., and Helyer, B. J. (1968). *Adv. Immunol.* **9,** 215.

Ingram, D. G., and Cho, H. J. (1974). *J. Rheumatol.* **1,** 1.

Jacobs, M. E., Steinberg, A. D., Gordon, J. K., and Talal, N. (1972). *Arthritis and Rheum.* **15,** 201.

Krakauer, R. S., Waldmann, T. A., and Strober, W. (1976). *J. Exp. Med.* **144,** 662.

Lambert, P. H., and Dixon, F. S. (1968). *J. Exp. Med.* **127,** 507.

Lewis, R. M., Andre-Schwartz, J., Harris, G. S., Hirsch, M. S., and Black, P. M. (1973). *J. Clin. Invest.* **52,** 1893.
Lukes, R. J., and Tindle, B. M. (1975). *N. Engl. J. Med.* **292,** 1.
Mellors, R. C. (1966). *Int. Rev. Exp. Pathol.* **5,** 217.
Michalski, J. P., Daniels, T. E., Talal, N., and Grey, H. (1975). *N. Engl. J. Med.* **293,** 1228.
Mozes, E. (1976). *In* "The Role of Products of the Histocompatibility Gene Complex in Immune Responses," (D. H. Katz and B. Benacerraf, ed.). Academic Press, New York.
Ordal, J. C., and Grumet, F. C. (1972). *J. Exp. Med.* **136,** 1195.
Palmer, D. W., Dauphinee, M. J., Murphy, E., and Talal, N. (1976). *Clin. Exp. Immunol.* **23,** 578.
Papoian, R., Pillarisetty, R., and Talal, N. (1976). *Immunology* **32,** 75.
Playfair, J. H. L. (1968). *Immunology* **15,** 35.
Porter, D. D., Dixon, F. J., and Larsen, A. E. (1965). *Blood* **25,** 736.
Potter, M. (1972). *Physiol. Rev.* **52,** 631.
Roubinian, J. R., Papoian, R., and Talal, N. (1977a). *J. Immunol.* **118,** 1524.
Roubinian, J. R., Papoian, R., and Talal, N. (1977b). *J. Clin. Invest.* (in press).
Schrader, J. W., Cunningham, B. A., and Edelman, G. M. (1975). *Proc. Natl. Acad. Sci. U.S.A.* **72,** 5066.
Schubert, D., Jobe, A., and Cohn, M. (1968). *Nature* (*London*) **220,** 882.
Seligmann, M., and Brouet, J. C. (1973). *Semin. Hematol.* **10,** 163.
Shearer, G. M., Rehn, T. G., and Garbarius, C. A. (1975). *J. Exp. Med.* **141,** 1348.
Shirai, T., and Mellors, R. C. (1971). *Proc. Natl. Acad. Sci. U.S.A.* **68,** 1412.
Staples, P. J., and Talal, N. (1969). *J. Exp. Med.* **129,** 123.
Sugai, S., Pillarisetty, R. J., and Talal, N. (1973). *J. Exp. Med.* **138,** 989.
Sugai, S., Palmer, D. W., Talal, N., and Witz, I. P. (1974). *J. Exp. Med.* **140,** 1547.
Talal, N. (1970). *Arthritis Rheum.* **13,** 887.
Talal, N. (1974). *Prog. Clin. Immunol.* **2,** 101.
Talal, N. (1976). *Transplant. Rev.* **31,** 240.
Talal, N., Dauphinee, M. J., Pillarisetty, R., and Goldblum, R. (1975). *Ann. N.Y. Acad. Sci.* **249,** 438.
Warner, N. L. (1975). *Immunogenetics* **2,** 1.
Yoshiki, T., Mellors, R. C., Strand, M., and August, J. T. (1974). *J. Exp. Med.* **140,** 1011.

Chapter 8

Thymic Hormones and Autoimmunity

J. F. BACH, M. A. BACH, C. CARNAUD,
M. DARDENNE, AND J. C. MONIER

There is now compelling evidence that the thymus gland produces humoral factors. Recent data obtained in several laboratories indicate that these factors are probably involved, at some stage, in T cell differentiation. Their relevance to autoimmunity, which is the reason for this chapter, has arisen from several lines of evidence, including the demonstration of thymus hormone (TH) deficiency in autoimmune mice and the demonstration of a direct effect of thymus hormones on self-recognition. Before discussing in detail the implication of TH in the mechanism of autoimmunity, we shall review briefly the present status of the subject, since it is both rapidly moving and controversial.

I. THYMUS HORMONES: PRESENT STATUS

A. The Humoral Function of the Thymus

Not long after the role of the thymus in immunity had been discovered by J. Miller, the hypothesis was put forward that the thymus might act by producing soluble mediators or hormones. This hypothesis was supported by the fact that a thymus gland placed in a cell-impermeable Millipore chamber and introduced into neonatally thymectomized mice restored their immunocompetence (Osoba and Miller, 1963). The appearance of immunocompetence in neonatally thymectomized mice after pregnancy, probably associated with fetal thymus secretion, was in the same line (Osoba, 1965). These experiments were criticized for the imperfect cell impermeability of the Millipore chamber and the difficulty in reproducing the pregnancy experiments (Stutman *et al.*, 1970). In fact, all these experiments have been reproduced with satisfactory controls (Stutman and Good, 1973). In particular, it has been shown that one could restore the immunocompetence of neonatally thymectomized mice by injecting them with dissociated pure epithelial cells derived from a carcinogen-induced thymoma, whether or not enclosed within a Millipore chamber. Thymus grafts in man (which are always done in allogeneic combinations and do not allow a satisfactory lymphocyte survival), like grafts enclosed in Millipore chambers, probably also operate through the secretion of a humoral factor. The rapidity of T cell functional reconstitution in thymus-grafted patients with Di George syndrome (August *et al.*, 1970) is very much in favor of this interpretation.

The controversy raised by the Millipore chamber and the pregnancy experiments, as well as the presence of numerous lymphocytes in the thymus itself (it is indeed unusual to find the target cells of a hormone in the hormone-producing gland itself) led to a purely cellular theory of thymus action; T cell precursors enter the thymus where they differentiate after direct contact with the thymic epithelial microenvironment. Davies' experiments (1969) showing that a thymus graft (with a recognizable chromosomal marker) seeds PHA-responsive lymphocytes to the periphery supported this hypothesis, although the possibility of a local secretion of soluble mediators only active at high concentrations could not be excluded.

B. Direct Evidence for Thymic Hormone

More direct evidence for the existence of TH was obtained when it was shown that one could reconstitute immunocompetence by injecting cell-free thymus extracts. A. L. Goldstein and A. White (then in New York) and N. Trainin (in Israel) and their co-workers played a major role in that effort. Positive results were obtained *in vivo* (skin allograft rejection and graft versus host reaction) (Goldstein *et al.*, 1972) and especially *in vitro,* mitogen responsiveness (Thurman and Goldstein, 1975; Rotter and Trainin, 1975), mixed lymphocyte reaction (Umiel and Trainin, 1975), and graft versus host reaction (Trainin *et al.*, 1969). These results, however, led to several criticisms: (1) the doses of thymic extracts utilized were fairly high, at least in the first experiments, and might have represented a nonspecific immunologic stimulus, since they came from heterologous species; (2) the control experiments with extracts of other organs were not always completely negative; (3) contamination of the extracts with endotoxins (Kruger *et al.*, 1970) or other pharmacologically active products could be responsible for the demonstrated effects, the more so since neonatally thymectomized mice recover immune competence after treatment with polyribonucleotides such as poly(A:U) (Johnson, 1973). The fact is that all of these experiments supported a possible humoral function of the thymus, even if they could not be accepted as being definitive. It remained necessary to demonstrate the activity of pure materials with better controls than extracts of nonthymic organs and more refined reconstitution experiments in well-controlled T cell deficiency states. Data are now available on each of these three points.

1. In Vitro Induction of T Cell Markers by Thymic Factors

We reported in 1971 that thymic extracts induced the appearance of T cell markers (θ-antigen, azathioprine sensitivity) in bone marrow cells lacking these markers (Bach *et al.*, 1971). Initially, a criticism similar to that of earlier data could be made, since the extract used was relatively crude. However, the demonstration that normal serum contained a factor with the same activity as thymic extracts and the rapid disappearance of this activity following thymectomy (Bach and Dardenne, 1972, 1973) established proof of the exclusively thymic origin of the factor(s) detected by the θ-conversion assay. These data were further confirmed by the reestablishment of a normal serum thymic factor level after grafting a thymus or a thymic functional epithelium (Bach and Dardenne, 1972, 1973).

θ Induction does not involve all θ-negative cells and, in fact, the assay initially described had been performed, using the rosette test to detect relevant target cells of the hormone. Another way of showing θ-induction by thymic extracts was reported by Komuro and Boyse 2 years later (1973). In brief, normal spleen cells were separated in four layers on a BSA density gradient. The less dense cells proved to be essentially θ-negative and to include a large percentage of null cells, also Ig negative. When such cells were incubated with thymic extracts, it could be shown that 10–20% of them became θ-positive.

The neosynthesis of antigenic material, i.e., gene activation, is the most attractive hypothesis to explain these findings, although membrane rearrangements making the θ-antigen already present on the precursor cell more accessible to the antibody is also possible. One cannot exclude cell fragility, especially in the BSA gradient system where cells are manipulated for a long time before being typed; such fragility might make the cells more susceptible to the effects of small amounts of antibody and complement. On another level, one may discuss whether the changes are indeed associated with a true "differentiation." The reversibility of the θ-induction, observed *in vivo* in the rosette assay (Dardenne and Bach, 1973), indicates that θ-conversion is not a sufficient criterion for differentiation. The main consequence of these remarks is that any factor isolated or tested on the basis of conversion assays must be shown to be active by functional tests before being considered a thymopoietic hormone. This is not an easy matter, since complete T cell maturation takes several weeks in the normal animal.

2. *Biochemistry and Biologic Activities of Thymic Hormones*

Several of the polypeptide factors responsible for some of the biologic activities listed above have been isolated. A. L. Goldstein's thymosin is a 12,500 MW acidic polypeptide. It has been primarily isolated on the basis of its capacity to induce DNA synthesis *in vivo* and has been recently shown to be active in the rosette θ-conversion assay (Goldstein *et al.*, 1972). Thymosin has been reported to possess several biologic activities in man and in the mouse (in particular, rejection of skin allografts, graft versus host reaction, mitogen responsiveness, and mixed lymphocyte reaction), but it should be stressed that these activities have been mostly demonstrated with crude extracts (fraction V). N. Trainin's thymic humoral factor (THF) has been isolated from calf thymus on the basis of an *in vitro* graft versus host assay (Trainin *et al.*, 1969). It is a peptide of known amino acid composition, with an MW close to 3000 daltons. It is active in the rosette assay and in various functional assays (in particular, mixed lymphocyte reaction and PHA responsiveness). G. Goldstein's thymopoietin (formerly thymine) has been isolated on the basis of its unexpected depressive effect on neuromuscular conduction (Goldstein, 1975). Its sequence has been published recently (Schlesinger and Goldstein, 1975). Thymopoietin is active in the Komuro and Boyse assay, but has not yet been shown to possess any capacity to render T cell precursors functionally immunocompetent. One should await such demonstration before accepting it as a true thymopoietic hormone, since it is known that ubiquitin, a thymus protein found in other organs, can be positive in the Komuro and Boyse assay at low molarities. Our circulating thymic factor (TF) has been evenly sequenced (Bach *et al.*, 1977). It is a neutral peptide with an MW close to 1000 daltons. Its amino acid sequence allows us to ascertain that it is not a split product of thymopoietin. Such an association between thymosin and TF is possible, since release of low molecular weight products from thymosin has been demonstrated *in vivo* and *in vitro*. Biologic significance of TF is assessed by its capacity to induce mitogen responsiveness, to restore suppressor T cells in NZB mice (Bach and Niaudet, 1976) and in adult thymectomized rats (Bash *et al.*, 1976), to allow the rejection of MSV-induced sarcomas in thymectomized irradiated bone marrow reconstituted mice (J. F. Bach *et al.*, 1975), to reduce anti-μ-2 cytotoxic T-cell (M. A. Bach, 1977) and to correct the abnormally high level of autologous rosettes in adult thymectomized mice (Charreire and Bach, 1975).

Biochemical data are now also available on the mode of action of thymic hormones at the cellular level. It has been shown that cyclic AMP and products increasing intralymphocyte cAMP level, such as prostaglandins, mimic the effects of thymic hormones in various systems, such as the rosette θ-conversion assay (Bach and Bach, 1973; M. A. Bach *et al.*, 1975), the Komuro and Boyse assay (Scheid *et al.*, 1975) and the *in vitro* GVH assay (Kook and Trainin, 1974). A synergy has been demonstrated between thymic hormones and cAMP in the rosette assay, and preliminary data suggest that thymic hormones may increase cAMP level. This action on the adenyl cyclase system does not necessarily define the mode of action of thymic hormones. However, it is reminiscent of other data in other systems showing the involvement of cAMP in cellular differentiation. It could well be that the T lymphocyte precursors must raise their cAMP level before differentiation can occur.

3. *The Significance of Thymic Hormones (Relevance to T Cell Differentiation)*

The TH target cell is not definitively determined. One is struck by the relative facility with which T cell functions altered by adult thymectomy can be restored (θ-antigen, autologous rosettes, cytotoxin (T cells), contrasting with the difficulty of obtaining significant effects in nude mice. These data might indicate that TF acts at a relatively late stage of T cell differentiation, which would be compatible with the fact that thymus grafts in Millipore chambers work only in neonatally thymectomized mice (which have had a thymus gland during their fetal life) and not in nude mice (Stutman, 1975). More generally, Stutman's work indicates that thymic humoral function is mainly operating (at least in the small concentrations found in the periphery) on relatively differentiated T cells (such as those found at birth) and not on more primitive precursors (such as those found on the fourteenth day of gestation).

There is another difficulty in showing reconstitution of full T cell competence with thymic extracts, related to the long duration of some aspects of T cell maturation. Indeed, it takes several weeks to obtain the immunologic reconstitution of neonatally thymectomized mice with a fully

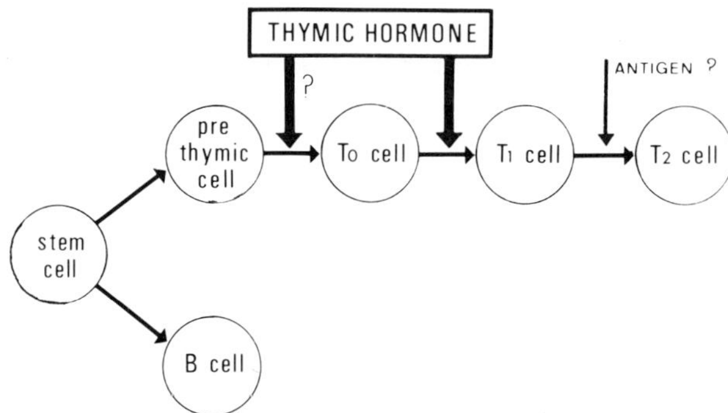

Fig. 1. Scheme of T cell differentiation.

functional thymus graft, which means that it will probably be necessary to give chronic long-term TH treatment for several weeks to obtain complete reconstitution. This still raises practical problems linked to the short life span or to the immunogenicity of the preparations used so far.

Finally, one may tentatively distinguish four steps in T cell maturation (Fig. 1): (1) from the primitive stem cell to the pre-T cell (also called prothymocyte). This stage might be largely thymus-independent, since one finds such cells (slightly θ-positive) in nude mice (Roelants *et al.*, 1976), (2) from the pre T cell to the T0 cell (also called postthymic). This step probably needs a direct contact with the thymic epithelial microenvironment, even if local secretion of humoral factor may play a role, (3) from the T0 cell to a T1 cell, the major step of TH action, which develops both in the thymus and in the periphery. The T1 cell already expresses most T cell markers and is probably endowed with suppressor T cell function, (4) from the T1 cell to the T2 cell, which is a lengthy step, taking place essentially outside the thymus and probably independently of thymic influence.

In this scheme, T0 and T1 cells are short-lived. Thus, a premature cessation of thymus function, as will be discussed in NZB mice, may lead to a selective deficiency of these cells, without major T2 cell defect (either helper cells or cytotoxic cells). T2 cell exacerbation may occur, due to a deficiency of (presumably T1) suppressor T cells.

II. THYMUS HORMONES AND THE CONTROL OF AUTOIMMUNITY

Increasing evidence, reviewed elsewhere in this volume, indicates that a T cell deficiency could be a major etiologic factor in the development of several autoimmune conditions. The question of the origin of such T cell deficiency may be raised. We shall present arguments indicative of an intrathymic defect, possibly bearing on thymic hormone secretion.

A. Thymus Dysfunction in Autoimmunity

1. Thymus Pathology

The thymus shows a number of pathological abnormalities in autoimmune states. The presence of germinal centers has impressed immunopathologists for a long time. The specificity is doubtful, however, since they are encountered in many experimental and clinical situations and appear only at relatively late stages of the diseases. The same comments apply to the finding of viruslike particles.

Perhaps more specific is the thymic atrophy noted early in the life of NZB and B/W mice (De Vries and Hijmans, 1967). This atrophy bears selectively on epithelial cells, which are probably the TH-secreting cells. Interestingly, this atrophy may be associated in NZB and Swan mice with the presence of crystalline inclusions of undetermined significance (Schmitt, 1974).

2. Depression of T Cell Function

Several abnormalities in T cell function have been described over the last few years in NZB, B/W, and Swan mice, as well as in various human diseases. These abnormalities, reviewed in more detail elsewhere in this volume, include the precocious failure of thymus cells to be rendered tolerant to heterologous red cells and proteins (Staples and Talal, 1969), the abnormality in the *in vivo* proliferative response of thymocytes to alloantigens (Dauphinee *et al.*, 1974), and the depression of *in vitro* mitogen and MLR responses (Rodey *et al.*, 1971). It is only later that one observes the decline in GVH reactivity in skin graft rejection and in the number of peripheral T cells (Stutman *et al.*, 1968).

Several types of deficiency have been put forward in human systemic lupus: decrease in cutaneous delayed hypersensitivity reactions (Block *et al.*, 1968), depression of *in vitro* proliferative response to phytohemagglutinin (Malave *et al.*, 1975), diminution of mixed lymphocyte reaction (Suciu-Foca *et al.*, 1974), and depression of the number of rosettes formed by T lymphocytes with sheep red blood cells, a specific T cell marker (Scheinberg and Cathcart, 1973). We have shown that E rosettes are diminished in 25–35% of SLE patients and in an even higher percentage when only active cases are considered.

The mechanism of the depression of these various T cell functions is obscure. A true decrease in T cell number is a possibility, although one should note that NZB mice retain a normal T cell number (as assessed by cytotoxic assays with anti-θ-serum) until the age of 1 year, well after they have shown anti-nuclear factors and glomerulonephritis. The recovery of normal E rosette values under the influence of steroid treatment, as we have noted in a few examples, as well as the *in vitro* increase in E rosette values after treatment with thymic hormone, argue against this interpretation. The action of lymphocytotoxic antibodies should be discussed, since these antibodies are found in a high percentage of NZB mice and lupus patients (Shirai and Mellors, 1972). However, we have not found a good correlation between the presence of these antibodies, shown by a lymphocytotoxicity test performed at 15°C, and low E rosette values. Moreover, the recovery of normal E rosette values under *in vitro* TH treatment contradicts this hypothesis. A last hypothesis to explain the abnormality of T cell functions seen in SLE involves the loss of thymic hormone peripheral action that we shall discuss later.

3. *Effects of Thymectomy and Thymus Grafting*

Neonatal thymectomy of normally nonautoimmune mouse strains is associated with an abnormal occurrence of autoantibodies; in particular, antinuclear antibodies after the age of 4–8 weeks (Thivolet *et al.*, 1967). The onset of autoantibodies is still more precocious in nude mice (Monier *et al.*, 1974) and is then associated with pathological signs of presumably immune complex glomerulonephritis (Pelletier *et al.*, 1975). The question has been raised as to the role of frequent infections in the development of autoimmunity in T cell deprived mice (Morel-Maroger and Salomon, 1974). It is indeed true that germfree, neonatally thymectomized, and nude mice show fewer autoimmune manifestations than conventionally reared mice, but germfree breeding does not suppress autoimmunity (Monier *et al.*, 1969). Adult thymectomy at the age of 1 month also favors the onset of autoimmunity (antinuclear antibodies) (Monier *et al.*, 1970) and glomerular Ig deposits (Markham *et al.*, 1973). Neonatal thymectomy aggravates the natural course of several spontaneous animal autoimmune diseases, such as the immune complex disease of female NZB and B/W mice (East *et al.*, 1967) and the autoimmune thyroiditis of the obese strain of chicken, a disease prevented by neonatal bursectomy (Wick *et al.*, 1970). Conversely, neonatal thymectomy prevents the development of experimentally induced autoimmune diseases such as experimental allergic thyroiditis (which probably involves helper T cells at some stages).

On the other hand, thymus grafting has been reported to correct several of the immunologic abnormalities of NZB mice, at least when one uses still-functional, newborn thymuses. Thus, thymus grafting restores PHA and Con A responsiveness (even when placed in a Millipore chamber) in NZB mice (Niaudet and Bach, 1976) and prevents the appearance of autoimmune hemolytic anemia in B/W mice (Kysela and Steinberg, 1973; Gershwin and Steinberg, 1975). Interestingly, this latter effect could only be obtained when thymus grafts were less frequent or started later in life. This comment is reminiscent of the finding that grafting nude mice with an irradiated NZB mouse thymus provides only a transient immunologic reconstitution, whereas restoration is long lasting when the grafted thymus is taken from a nonautoimmune strain (Blankwater and Lina, 1974).

B. Thymus Hormone in Autoimmune States

The serum level of the circulating thymus factor (assessed by the rosette assay mentioned above) has been tested in several experimental autoimmune conditions (Bach *et al.*, 1973; Dardenne *et al.*, 1974). NZB and B/W mice have a normal TH level at birth, but it decreases prematurely between the third and sixth week of life (Figs. 2 and 3). At 2 months, NZB and B/W mice have no significant TH, whereas TH is still at birth levels in control mouse strains and remains at this level until the fourth to sixth month. Six weeks after the decline of serum TH, NZB mice show disappearance of θ-positive lymph node RFC, and 2 weeks later, progressive decrease in spleen RFC sensitivity to anti-θ serum and azathioprine, as in neonatally thymectomized mice. Normal azathioprine and anti-θ-serum RFC sensitivity is reconstituted by *in vitro* or *in vivo* treatment with thymic extracts. Similarly, grafting a newborn NZB thymus to 6-month-old NZB mice leads to rapid normalization of the initially low level of circulating thymic factor. However, this restoration is transient (1 month). Injection of purified circulating TF also normalizes serum level, with the same kinetics as in normal mouse strains (Bach and Niaudet, 1977).

The mechanisms leading to low serum TH levels in NZB mice probably implicate a premature cessation of TH secretion, whatever its mechanism

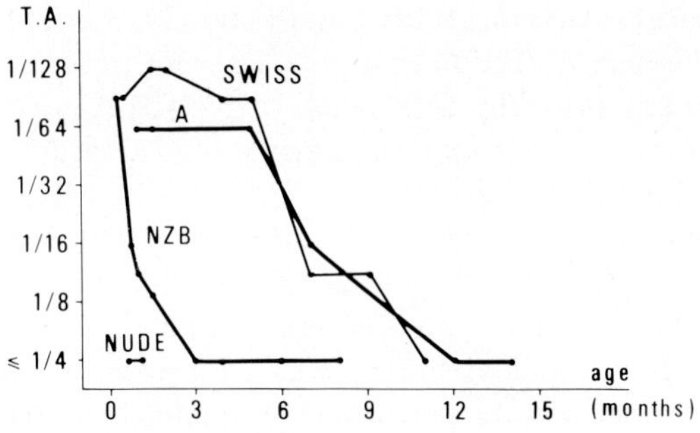

Fig. 2. Age dependence of serum TH level in Swiss, A, NZB, and nude mice.

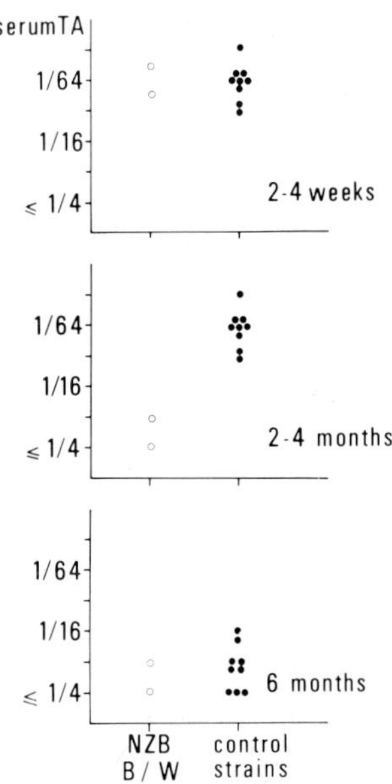

Fig. 3. Circulating TH level in NZB, B/W, and nine control strains at 2–4 weeks, 2–4 months, and 6 months.

may be. A peripheral destruction could theoretically be envisaged. Anti-thymus antibodies have indeed been described in NZB and B/W mice (Shirai and Mellors, 1972). Although these antibodies are not as often consistently found as the decrease in TH level (Goldblum *et al.*, 1975), one may argue that they induce a peripheral TH destruction. Using our rosette assay, Gershwin *et al.* (1975) have confirmed our data concerning the premature decrease in TH level in NZB and B/W mice.

In spite of such confirmatory data, Gershwin *et al.* reached the different conclusion that this apparent decrease in thymic hormone level was due to the action of natural thymocytotoxic antibody (NTA). This interpretation was based on the demonstration that a serum pool from 6-month-old NZB mice, having an exceptionally high NTA titer (1/512), was capable of suppressing the TH-like activity found in normal mouse serum. In our opinion, this is an oversimplified interpretation. One cannot extrapolate from the data obtained with a high-titered NTA serum from 6-month-old mice to the physiological condition of 1-month-old NZB mice, which show a disappearance of thymic hormone from the serum at an age when NTA is not yet found regularly (Shirai and Mellors, 1972). Moreover, one should note that Gershwin's experiments were performed by simple mixing of crude sera. This differs significantly from our own experimental procedures: before assaying mouse sera, we always remove molecules larger than 50,000 daltons with a CF-50 Amicon filter, and sometimes use PM-10 filters, which pass only molecules smaller than 10,000 daltons (Bach and Dardenne, 1973). These ultrafiltration steps remove the high molecular weight serum inhibitors as well as all immunoglobulins and, in particular, the IgM to which NTA belongs (Shirai and Mellors, 1972). One should also note that, under the same experimental conditions, using various NZB sera (1, 2, 4, and 8 months old) not selected for their NTA titers, we have not been able to reproduce Gershwin's data. The argument that NTA could be produced in young NZB mice but is not detected in the serum because it is bound to cells would not explain the peripheral destruction of the serum thymic hormones.

Other arguments prompt us to exclude the role of NTA in the premature decrease in thymic hormone level in NZB miçe: (1) grafting a neonatal NZB thymus into 6- to 8-month-old NZB mice, presumably presenting high NTA titers, provides a full reconstitution of thymic hormone level which lasts more than 3 weeks, which is not compatible with the concept of peripheral destruction (Niaudet and Bach, 1976); (2) injection of purified thymic hormone into 6- to 8-month-old NZB mice induces the appearance of serum levels comparable with those found under identical conditions in thymectomized C57BL/6 mice, with the same pharmacologic kinetics (Bach and Niaudet, 1976); (3) injection of purified thymic factor at nanogram levels reconstitutes the capacity of NZB mice to respond to PHA and Con A and to produce normal amounts of anti-PVP antibodies (Table 1), probably under the control of thymic hormone-induced suppressor T

TABLE I

Normalization of Suppressor T Cell Function in NZB Mice by Thymic Factor (Assessed by Antibody Production against Polyvinyl Pyrrolidone (PVP)[a]

	Day 5	Day 10
TF + CMC	0.277 ± 0.020	0.121 ± 0.008
CMC alone	0.364 ± 0.038	0.366 ± 0.037

[a] Serum antigen-binding capacity (micrograms PVP per milliliter of serum) in NZB mice treated from the age of 3 weeks for 5 weeks with a purified thymic factor J. F. Bach *et al.*, 1975) bound to carboxymethyl cellulose (to increase its half-life). Sera were collected 5 and 10 days after immunization with PVP (0.1 μg i.v.) at the age of 7 weeks (mean ± SE) (Bach and Niaudet, 1976).

cells (Bach and Niaudet, 1976). The same premature cessation of TH secretion has been found in Swan mice, genetically selected on the basis of spontaneous antibody production (Dardenne *et al.*, 1974).

Studies performed on human systemic lupus patients have also shown low TH serum levels. The variation among normal individuals makes a precise determination of the incidence of these low TH levels difficult, even in younger patients (before age-matched controls show declining serum TH) (J. F. Bach *et al.*, 1975). This low TH level is in keeping with the low E rosette values and their correction after *in vitro* TH treatment (our unpublished results). Other studies have unexpectedly shown increased TH level in rheumatoid arthritis (J. F. Bach *et al.*, 1975), which might indicate an increased level in T cell function in this disease. However, the nature of the factor detected merits further studies, since intense inflammatory reactions might release mediators active in the rosette assay. Results obtained in myasthenia gravis also indicate a tendency to higher levels than in normal subjects, irrespective of thymoma existence (Bach *et al.*, 1972). This augmentation, however, is moderate, much less than could be expected from the hypothesis giving a central role to TH in the pathogenesis of the disease.

The causal relationship of alteration in thymic hormone secretion and T cell deficiency is suggested by the correction of several T cell deficiencies by TH injections. Thus, administered twice or three times weekly, TH normalizes several of the T cell abnormalities mentioned above. These include spleen (Niaudet and Bach, 1976) and lymph node (Thurman *et al.*, 1975; Gershwin *et al.*, 1974) *in vitro* responses to PHA and Con A, abnormal pattern of thymus cell proliferation in irradiated allogeneic hosts (Dauphinee *et al.*, 1974), depression of antigen-induced DNA synthesis (Dauphinee and Talal, 1975), and, lastly, the augmentation of anti-PVP antibody responses probably associated with a loss of suppressor T cells (Bach and Niaudet, 1977). Interestingly, in all these models, the therapeutic effect was obtained only when the treatment was started early (before the age of 8–10 weeks) and continued for a sufficiently long time (2–4 weeks). In older animals, no effect was observed; in the PVP system, an increase in antibody production was even noted, perhaps linked to a stimulation of the amplifier T cells described by Baker (1975).

These difficulties, added to the possible immunogenicity of TH and to the need of using daily preparations made necessary by the rapid metabolism of the small peptides used, probably explain the lack of data concerning the prevention of autoimmunity. The only promising results are those reported by Dauphinee and Talal (Dauphinee *et al.*, 1974) showing a transient delay in appearance of RNA and DNA antibodies, as well as those of Monier (Monier and Robert, 1974) showing prevention of anti-nuclear antibody formation by thymosin treatment in Swan mice.

C. Possible Mechanisms of Action

1. TH Dependence of Experimental Model of Self-Recognition

The influence of thymic factors upon autoreactivity has been tested in three experimental models which we shall briefly describe.

a. *In Vitro* autosensitization. Cohen and Wekerle have shown that normal lymphoid cells cultured for 5 days on syngeneic fibroblast monolayers differentiate into specifically sensitized T cells able to mediate specific cytotoxicity against syngeneic (Cohen and Wekerle, 1973) or H-2-compatible target cells (Ilfeld *et al.,* 1975), and to induce a GVH-like reaction of splenomegaly or of lymph node enlargment after *in vivo* transfer into a syngeneic host (Cohen *et al.,* 1971; Cohen, 1975). Adsorption experiments on syngeneic fibroblasts, followed by transfer onto syngeneic or allogeneic sensitizing monolayers, have demonstrated that T cells endowed with specific recognition structures for self-antigens preexist in the spleen prior to *in vitro* sensitization. This raises the question of the control mechanism which normally prevents lymphocytes from being triggered by self-antigens *in vivo.* Cohen and Wekerle have suggested that serum blocking factors, such as soluble antigens or antigen–antibody complexes specifically inhibit potentially self-reactive lymphocytes (see Chapter 9). This hypothesis is supported by the fact that syngeneic serum prevents adherence of self-reactive lymphocytes on syngeneic monolayers, whereas allogeneic serum does not (Cohen and Wekerle, 1973).

The same experimental system has also been used by Trainin's group to investigate the effects of a calf thymus extract on autoreactivity (Trainin *et al.,* 1973). It has been found that addition of such an extract to the culture medium during the sensitization phase inhibited the generation of effector cells, as measured by cell-mediated cytotoxicity or by an *in vitro* GVH-like assay on syngeneic spleen fragments (Small and Trainin, 1975). Normal syngeneic serum also blocked the reaction. However, syngeneic serum from newborn thymectomized donors did not show any blocking activity. It was, therefore, assumed that the blocking factor present in normal serum was a humoral substance secreted by the thymus and disappearing from the blood stream after thymectomy.

b. *Autologous rosettes.* Further evidence for the role of the thymus in the control of autoreactivity is derived from the study of autologous rosettes (ARFC) formed between lymphocytes and autologous or syngeneic erythrocytes. Their dependence on the presence of the thymus was suggested by the observation that ARFC are found in higher numbers in thymus than in spleen or lymph nodes. Adult thymectomy increases more than 10 times the incidence of ARFC in the spleen (Charreire and Bach, 1975a). A high number of rosette-forming cells is also found in the spleen of athymic nude mice and aging mice, as well as among cortisone-sensitive thymocytes. The question of the nature and of the specificity of ARFC may be raised since, for example, human T lymphocytes bind sheep or human erythrocytes nonspecifically (Bach, 1973; Gluckman and Montambault, 1975). Such specificity is, however, suggested by the fact that the adsorption of ARFC on fibroblasts is restricted to monolayers bearing H-2 identical antigens. Moreover, ARFC depletion by centrifugation on a Ficoll gradient leads to a specific loss in autoreactive lymphocytes tested in a GVH-like reaction (our unpublished results). It is, thus, likely that ARFC formation expresses a true recognition event of self-antigenic determinants. The high number of rosettes found in the spleen of adult thymectomized animals is reduced to normal values after a single injection of purified circulating thymic factor 24 hours before the test, adding further support to the concept of a control exerted by the thymus upon ARFC, which are probably immature T cells.

c. *Autoreactivity in Thymectomized Animals.* Spleen cells from neo-

TABLE II

Biologic Activities of Thymic Hormones[a]

Biologic activity	Reference
Induction of alloantigenic T cell marker (rosette assay, cytotoxic assay)	(Bach and Dardenne, 1973; Komuro and Boyse, 1973; Touraine *et al.*, 1975).
Induction of E rosette formation in man	(Wara *et al.*, 1975; Goldstein *et al.*, 1975)
Mitogen responsiveness (PHA, Con A; *in vitro, in vivo*)	(Thurman and Goldstein 1975; Rotter and Trainin, 1975; Hooper *et al.*, 1975; Bach *et al.*, 1975)
Mixed lymphocyte reaction (*in vivo, in vitro*)	(Umiel and Trainin, 1975; Hooper *et al.*, 1975)
Antibody production	(Hooper *et al.*, 1975; Stobel, 1974; Ikehara *et al.*, 1975; Miller *et al.*, 1973)
Rejection of MSV-induced sarcoma	(Bach *et al.*, 1975; Hardy *et al.*, 1971)
Inhibition of autoreactivity (autologous rosettes, GVH)	(Charreire and Bach, 1975a; Carnaud *et al.*, 1975; Trainin *et al.*, 1973).
Restoration of suppressor T cells (PVP, antibody response, thymocyte proliferation in allogeneic recipients)	(Bach and Niaudet, 1977; Dauphinee *et al.*, 1974; Dauphinee and Talal, 1975).
Induction of anti-μ-2 cytotoxic cells	(M. A. Bach, 1977)

[a] A nonexhaustive list of successful trials of immunologic reconstitution of thymectomized mice. It should be realized that the quality of the restoration and the validity of controls are very variable according to experiments.

natally thymectomized mice are capable of inducing a GVH-like reaction measured either *in vitro* by enlargement of a cultured spleen explant or *in vivo* by evaluation of splenomegaly or popliteal lymph node swelling (Small and Trainin, 1975, our unpublished data). Interestingly, this capacity is lost after *in vitro* or *in vivo* contact with a thymic extract (Small and Trainin, 1975). The cell responsible for this effect has not yet been determined. However, our recent finding that adult thymectomy enhances manifestations of autoreactivity, as will now be outlined, suggests that this cell might be an immature T cell. Millipore chambers filled with mixtures of syngeneic spleen cells and fibroblasts were introduced into the peritoneal cavity of adult thymectomized and intact mice. Five days later, the lymphocytes were recovered from the chambers and tested for cytotoxicity against syngeneic target cells. Autoreactive cells were exclusively found in chambers that had been implanted into thymectomized mice (Carnaud *et al.*, 1975). Autosensitization could be prevented in those chambers by the intraperitoneal administration of a thymic extract (thymosin fraction V). Similarly, spleen cells appear, shortly after adult thymectomy, which can elicit a GVH-like reaction in syngeneic recipients (our unpublished results), as described above for spleen cells from neonatally thymectomized mice (Small and Trainin, 1975).

These experimental models give information on the mechanisms involved in the control of autoreactivity. One-hour incubation of the lymphocytes with thymic factors, prior to or at the beginning of the education process, prevents further differentiation into effector cells, suggesting that the thymic factors affect the early stages of autosensitization (Trainin *et al.*, 1973; Small and Trainin, 1975). Moreover, the results obtained with autologous rosettes support the view that TH may directly suppress the expression of membrane self-recognition receptors (Charreire and Bach, 1975a,b). One may wonder whether thymic factors will continue to prevent further stages of differentiation once recognition has occurred. Triggered lymphocytes obtained either after *in vitro* contact with syngeneic fibroblasts (Cohen, 1975) or from a thymectomized animal (Small and Trainin, 1975, our unpublished results) induce a GVH-like reaction *in vivo.* Recipient animals have a functional thymus and the transferred cells are, therefore, in contact with thymic humoral products. Yet the GVH reaction is not prevented. On the other hand, Trainin and Small have shown that lymphocytes from thymectomized donors lose their capacity to induce an *in vitro* GVH reaction after 1-hour incubation with a thymic extract (Small and Trainin, 1975). One cannot draw final conclusions about this important question until further investigation has been made.

Another open question is whether thymus factors involved in the preceding models and those shown to increase T lymphocyte immune competence are the same (Table II). The involvement of at least two different substances cannot be excluded, since the extracts used in these types of experiments are, in general, unpurified. An alternative explanation is to assume that the cells responsible for autoreactivity are different from those involved in allogeneic responses. Indeed, ARFC characterization, as well as the kinetics of ARFC appearance following thymectomy, suggests that they are very immature T cells, a hypothesis in keeping with the finding that cortical thymocytes can become autosensitized *in vitro*. This is in contrast with the fact that mostly medullary thymocytes are responsive in MLC. Thymic factors might, therefore, block the potential reactivity of immature T cells, while increasing the competence of more mature T1 or T2 cells. Small and Trainin have suggested that thymic factors deplete the pool of autoreactive T cells by pushing them toward a more mature stage of differentiation. Alternatively, thymic factors could promote the differentiation of two T-cell subsets, one ending as suppressor cells controlling autoreactivity and the other being responsible for helper and effector T cell functions.

2. *Conclusions*

Finally, TF control of autoimmunity assessed on the effect of thymectomy, thymus grafting, and TH injections, could have two main explanations.

A loss of suppressor T cells is the most current hypothesis. Suppressor T cells are short-lived and probably immature, and we have seen that their selective loss may well be explained by a premature thymus failure. TH treatment would restore suppressor T cell function or prevent their decline, as shown in the PVP system (Bach and Niaudet, 1977). Suppressor T cells, whether antigen-specific or not, normally exert a negative regulatory function on B cells and probably also other T cells. Their premature loss might explain autoantibody formation and, perhaps, the increase in self-reactivity, expressed by the number of autologous rosette-forming cells following adult thymectomy (Charreire and Bach, 1975a). A direct TH action on self-recognition cannot be excluded. It is possible that the loss of circulating TH enhances the degree of self-reactivity, in particular among immature T cells.

D. Potential Clinical Applications

All the preceeding data argue in favor of TH indications in SLE and related diseases. A few preliminary TH clinical trials have been made recently in various centers, mainly in immunodeficiency syndromes, using A. L. Goldstein's thymosin (Wara *et al.*, 1975; Goldstein *et al.*, 1975). It is too early to interpret the preliminary clinical results. The most clear-cut effects bear on the *in vivo* correction of low E rosette values, similar to what has been shown in *in vitro* experiments, in particular, in one trial in systemic lupus (Scheinberg *et al.,* 1975). It will probably take some time, however, before conclusive results are obtained with randomized trials using standardized preparations with well-defined half-lives (delay preparations will be necessary as for most peptidic hormones). In addition, it will perhaps be necessary to select those patients who do not have too advanced a disease, since in the NZB model, old mice do not appear to be TH sensitive.

III. SWAN MICE*

Several models exist of spontaneous autoimmune mice, including NZB, B/W, A/J, and nude mice. Studies in NZB mice have shown that genetic factors play a central role in the control of autoimmunity in these mice as in human lupus (Block *et al.,* 1975), resulting in the idea of producing autoimmune mice by genetic selection based on spontaneous antinuclear antibody production.

A. Swan Mice Production

Swiss/Gif mice often show low titers of anti-nuclear antibodies (ANA) as detected by immunofluorescence after 6 months of age (7.5% in a series of 120 mice). Two mice, one male and one female, were found with high ANA titers (respectively, 512 and 1024). These mice were mated and the six mice thus obtained all showed positive ANA test between the third and fifth months of life. F_2 generations provided mice showing ANA development consistently at the age of 3 months. Breeding difficulties did not allow continuation of the selection. All F_1 and F_2 survivors were randomly mated. The mouse colony that consistently developed ANA has now been maintained for 7 years.

B. Description of Autoimmune Manifestations

1. Autoantibodies

ANA are found at increasing frequency and titer with aging: 16% of mice already show ANA at 3 months; 100% of mice present ANA at 8 months, with titers of 512 or higher in more than 60% (with more than 20% presenting ANA titer higher than 1024). Females show ANA more precociously and at higher titers than males. The fluorescence is generally homogeneous.

* This Section was authored by J. C. Monier and J. F. Bach.

Anti-DNA antibodies (detected by immunofluorescence using trypanosome preparations) are positive in the majority of mice at 10 months of age (Monier and Sepetjian, 1975). Positive Coombs' tests are rarely found and only after the age of 10 months. Cryoglobulins are sometimes found after the sixth month.

2. *Renal Lesions*

Swan mice regularly develop a glomerulonephritis (GN) after the age of 9 months. Light and electron microscopy show a thickening of the glomerular basement membrane due to subendothelial deposits, and a proliferation and a hypertrophy of mesangial and endothelial cells (Schmitt *et al.*, 1972). Immunofluorescence reveals the presence of intense immunoglobulin and complement granular deposits (Monier *et al.*, 1969 ; Monier and Sepetjian, 1975) in the mesangium and in the subendothelial region. These deposits are also found in nonautoimmune mice (Markham *et al.*, 1973; Pelletier *et al.*, 1975), but Swan mice show much more intense deposits than age-matched controls. All these elements are very similar to the abnormalities described in the glomeruli of NZB mice and lupus patients.

3. *Skin Lesions*

After the 8 months of age, Swan mice present localized skin lesions, which become diffuse at 10 months, consisting of alopecia, erythema, and skin atrophy. Histological examination mainly shows a thickening of the basement membrane (Monier *et al.*, 1971). Immunofluorescence shows immunoglobulins and C3 deposits at the dermal–epidermal junction.

C. Thymus and T Cell Abnormalities

1. *Thymus Pathology*

In addition to autoimmune manifestations, Swan mice show early abnormalities in thymus function. The thymus itself is prematurely atrophic with rare Hassal's corpuscles. Epithelial cells show ultrastructural alterations with necrosis and vacuolization (Schmitt and Monier, 1974; Schmitt, 1974). Incorporation of radioactive sulfur is diminished (Monier *et al.*, 1975a). One does not find germinal centers like in NZB mice but, like in NZB mice (Schmitt *et al.*, 1975) the epithelial cells of 14- to 20-week-old Swan mice show crystalline inclusions in their cytoplasm (Schmitt and Monier, 1974; Schmitt, 1974). About 80% of the cells contain inclusions in mice with high antinuclear autoantibody titers (Fig. 4). The significance of these inclusions, which have never been found in age- and sex-matched Swiss mice, is still unknown.

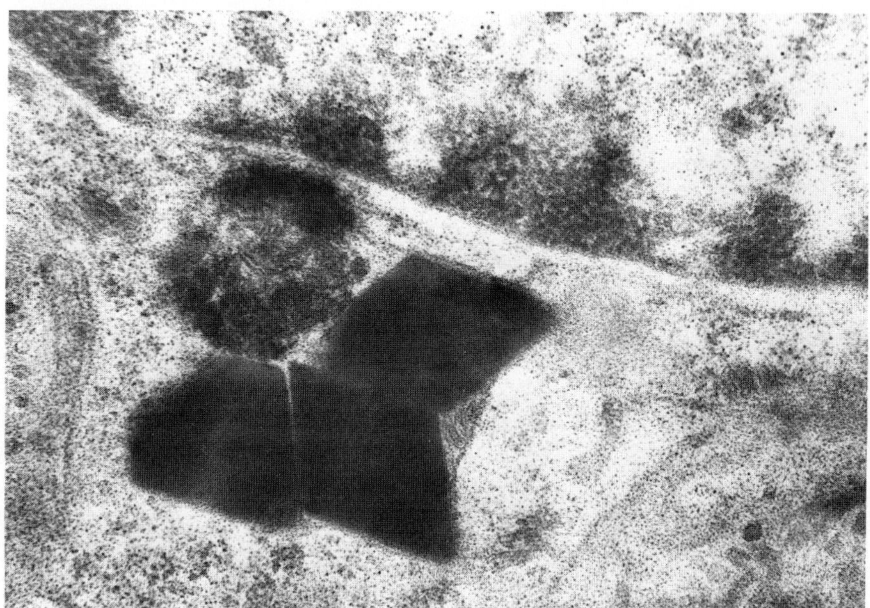

Fig. 4. Crystalline inclusion in a Swan mouse thymus.

2. Thymic Hormone Secretion

Parallel to these thymic abnormalities, one notes a premature cessation of thymic hormone secretion (Dardenne *et al.*, 1974). The serum level of the circulating factor detected by the rosette assay begins to decline prematurely at the age of 3 months, whereas nonautoimmune mouse strains do not show such decline until the sixth month (Fig. 5). Interestingly, Biozzi's mice, selected on the basis of their high antibody response to a variety of antigens, do not show the same early decline in thymus hormone production.

3. T Cell Functions

Last, one notes a low responsiveness of spleen cells to PHA at 6 months of age (Monier and Robert, 1974) suggesting the existence of a peripheral T cell functional deficiency. Other abnormalities, such as low antibody responsiveness to sheep erythrocytes and diminution in antigenic competition between heterologous erythrocytes (Monier *et al.*, 1975a), could also be related to a thymus dysfunction, since these two functions are both thymus dependent.

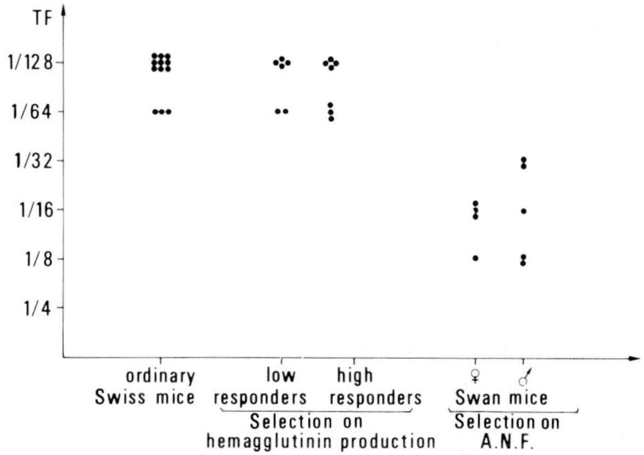

Fig. 5. TF serum level in genetically selected mice (at 4 months of age).

4. *Thymectomy and Thymic Hormone Treatment*

Neonatal thymectomy accelerates ANA appearance in Swan mice, since ANA are then found in 20% (3/15) of mice at 7 weeks and 100% at 16 weeks (10/10) (versus 45% in control Swan mice) (Monier *et al.*, 1971). Conversely, treatment of young Swan mice for 8 weeks with thymosin fraction V (Goldstein *et al.*, 1972) decreases ANA production very significantly, especially when the treatment is initiated early, at 8 weeks of age. Control mice injected with BSA do not show any alteration in ANA production (Monier *et al.*, 1975b).

D. Conclusions

Swan mice, genetically selected for spontaneous ANA production, show a clinical and immunologic picture very close to that of NZB and B/W mice. Autoimmune manifestations and thymus dysfunction are similar, although they appear slightly later and are less intense. A major role should probably be given to thymus dysfunction, and more precisely to suppressor T cell failure, perhaps associated with premature cessation of thymic hormone secretion. The determination of the nature of the thymic crystals and their possible relationship to thymic secretion, might be helpful in this respect. The role of viral factors should also be considered, since viruslike particles have been found in the thymus of Swan mice (Monier *et al.*, 1975b). In any case, the manner by which Swan mice have been obtained give a major role to genetic factors in the onset of their autoimmunity.

REFERENCES

August, C. S., Levey, R. H., Berkel, A. I., Rosen, F. S., and Kay, H. E. M. (1970). *Lancet* **1,** 1080.
Bach, J. F. (1973). *Transplant. Rev.* **16,** 196.
Bach, J. F., and Dardenne, M. (1972). *Transplant. Proc.* **4,** 345.
Bach, J. F., and Dardenne, M. (1973). *Immunology* **25,** 353.
Bach, J. F., Dardenne, M., Goldstein, A., Guha, A., and White, A. (1971). *Proc. Natl. Acad. Sci. U.S.A.* **68,** 2734.
Bach, J. F., Dardenne, M., Papiernik, M., Barois, A., Levasseur, P., and Le Brigand, H. (1972). *Lancet* **2,** 1056.
Bach, J. F., Dardenne, M., and Salomon, J. C. (1973). *Clin. Exp. Immunol.* **14,** 247.
Bach, J. F., Dardenne, M., and Clot, J. (1975). *Rheumatology* **6,** 242.
Bach, J. F., Dardenne, M., Plean, J. M., and Rosa, J. (1977). *Nature* (*London*) **266,** 55.
Bach, M. A. (1977). *Immunol.* (in press).
Bach, M. A., and Bach, J. F. (1973). *Eur. J. Immunol.* **3,** 778.
Bach, M. A., Fournier, C., and Bach, J. F. (1975). *Ann. N.Y. Acad. Sci.* **249,** 3.
Bach, M. A., and Niaudet, P. (1976). *J. Immunol.* **117,** 76.
Baker, P. J. (1975). *Transpl. Rev.* **26,** 3.
Basch, R. S., and Goldstein, G. (1975). *Cell. Immunol.* **20,** 218.
Bash, J. S., Dardenne, M., Bach, J. F., and Waksman, B. H. (1976). *Cell. Immunol.* **26,** 308.
Blankwater, M. J., and Lina, P. H. C. (1974). *In* "Proceedings of the First International Workshop on Nude Mice" (J. Rygaard and C. E. Povsen, eds.), p. 167. Fischer, Stuttgart.
Block, J. R., Gibbs, C. B., Stevens, M. B., and Shulman, L. B. (1968). *Ann. Rheum. Dis.* **27,** 311.
Block, S. R., Winfield, J. B., Lockshin, M. D., D'Angelo, W. A., and Christian, C. L. (1975). *Am. J. Med.* **59,** 533.
Carnaud, C., Ilfeld, D., Petranyi, G., and Klein, E. (1975). *Eur. J. Immunol.* **5,** 575.
Charreire, J., and Bach, J. F. (1975a). *Proc. Natl. Acad. Sci. U.S.A.* **72,** 3201.
Charreire, J., and Bach, J. F. (1975b). *In* "Biological Activity of Thymic Hormones" (D. W. Van Bekkum, ed.), p. 245. Kooyker Sci. Publ., Rotterdam.
Cohen, I. R. (1975). *Eur. J. Immunol.* **5,** 389.
Cohen, I. R., and Wekerle, H. (1973). *J. Exp. Med.* **137,** 224.
Cohen, I. R., Globerson, A., and Feldman, M. (1971). *J. Exp. Med.* **133,** 834.
Dardenne, M., and Bach, J. F. (1973). *Immunology* **25,** 343.
Dardenne, M., Monier, J. C., Biozzi, G., and Bach, J. F. (1974). *Clin. Exp. Immunol.* **17,** 339.
Dauphinee, M. J., and Talal, N. (1975). *Proc. Natl. Acad. Sci. U.S.A.* **114,** 1713.
Dauphinee, M. J., Talal, N., Goldstein, A. L., and White, A. (1974). *Proc. Natl. Acad. Sci. U.S.A.* **71,** 2637.
Davies, A. J. S. (1969). *Transplant. Rev.* **1,** 43.
De Vries, M. J., and Hijmans, W. (1967). *Immunology* **12,** 179.
East, J., De Sousa, M. A. B., Parrott, M. V., and Jaquet, H. (1967). *Clin. Exp. Immunol.* **2,** 203.

Gershwin, E. M., Ahmed, A., Steinberg, A. D., Thurman, G. B., and Goldstein, A. L. (1974). *J. Immunol.* **113,** 1068.

Gershwin, E. M., Steinberg, A. D., Woody, J. N., and Ahmed, A. (1975). *J. Immunol.* **115,** 1444.

Gershwin, M. E., and Steinberg, A. D. (1975). *Clin. Immunol. Immunopathol.* **4,** 38.

Gluckman, J. C., and Montambault, P. (1975). *Clin. Exp. Immunol.* **22,** 302.

Goldblum, R., Pillarisetty, R., and Talal, N. (1975). *Immunology* **28,** 621.

Goldstein, A. L., Guha, A., Zatz, M., Hardy, M. A., and White, A. (1972). *Proc. Natl. Acad. Sci. U.S.A.* **69,** 1800.

Goldstein, A. L., Thurman, G. B., Cohen, G. H., and Hooper, J. A. (1975). *In* "Biological Activity of Thymic Hormones" (D. W. Van Bekkum, ed.), p. 173. Kooyker Sci. Publ., Rotterdam.

Goldstein, G. (1975). *Ann. N.Y. Acad. Sci.* **249,** 177.

Goldstein, G., and Schlesinger, D. H. (1975). *Lancet* **2,** 256.

Hardy, M. A., Zisblatt, M., Levine, N., Goldstein, A. L., Lilly, F., and White, A. (1971). *Transplant. Proc.* **3,** 926.

Hooper, J. A., McDaniel, M. C., Thurman, B. G., Cohen, G. H., Schulof, R. S., and Goldstein, A. L. (1975). *Ann. N.Y. Acad. Sci.* **28,** 125.

Ikehara, S., Hamashima, Y., and Masuda, T. (1975). *Nature* (*London*) **258,** 336.

Ilfeld, D., Carnaud, C., and Klein, E. (1975). *Immunogenetics* **2,** 231.

Johnson, A. G. (1973). *J. Reticuloendothel. Soc.* **14,** 441.

Komuro, K., and Boyse, E. A. (1973). *Lancet* **1,** 740.

Kook, A., and Trainin, N. (1974). *J. Exp. Med.* **129,** 193.

Kruger, J., Goldstein, A. L., and Waksman, B. (1970). *Cell. Immunol.* **1,** 51.

Kysela, S., and Steinberg, A. D. (1973). *Clin. Immunol. Immunopathol.* **2,** 133.

Leung-Tack, J., Monier, J. C., Leung-Tack, K., and Thivolet, J. (1970). *Pathol. Eur.* **5,** 58.

Malave, I., Layrisse, Z., and Layrisse, M. (1975). *Cell. Immunol.* **15,** 231.

Markham, R. V., Sutherland, J. C., and Mardiney, M. R. (1973). *Lab. Invest.* **29,** 111.

Miller, H. C., Schmieze, S. K., and Rule, A. (1973). *J. Immunol.* **111,** 1005.

Monier, J. C., and Robert, M. (1974). *Ann. Immunol.* (*Paris*) **125c,** 405.

Monier, J. C., and Sepetjian, M. (1975). *Ann. Immunol.* (*Paris*) **126,** 63.

Monier, J. C., Thivolet, J., and Sepetjian, M. (1969a). *Rev. Fr. Etud. Clin. Biol.* **14,** 185.

Monier, J. C., Thivolet, J., and Sepetjian, M. (1969b). *Ann. Inst. Pasteur, Paris* **11,** 646.

Monier, J. C., Thivolet, J., and Sepetjian, M. (1970). *Experientia* **26,** 535.

Monier, J. C., Thivolet, J., Beyvin, A. J., Czyba, J. C., Schmitt, D., and Salussola, D. (1971). *Pathol. Eur.* **6,** 357.

Monier, J. C., Sepetjian, M., Czyba, J. C., Ortonne, J. P., and Thivolet, J. (1974). *In* "Proceedings of the First International Workshop on Nude Mice". (J. Rygaard and C. O. Polvsen, eds.), p. 243. Fischer, Stuttgart.

Monier, J. C., Quincy, C., Salussola, D., and Sepetjian, M. (1975a). *Experientia* **31,** 859.
Monier, J. C., Deschaux, P., and Fontanges, R. (1975b). *Nouv. Presse Med.* **4,** 507.
Morel-Maroger, L., and Salomon, J. C. (1974). *In* "Proceedings of the First International Workshop on Nude Mice" (J. Rygaard and C. O. Polvsen, eds.), p. 251. Fischer, Stuttgart.
Niaudet, P., and Bach, M. A. (1976). *Clin. Exp. Immunol.* **23,** 328.
Osoba, D. (1965). *Science* **147,** 298.
Osoba, D., and Miller, J. F. A. P. (1963). *Nature* (*London*) **199,** 633.
Pelletier, M., Hinglais, N., and Bach, J. F. (1975). *Lab. Invest.* **32,** 388.
Rodey, G. E., Yunis, E. J., and Good, R. A. (1971). *Clin. Exp. Immunol.* **9,** 305.
Roelants, G. E., Mayor, K. S., Hagg, L. B., and Loor, F. (1976). *Eur. J. Immunol.* **6,** 75.
Rotter, V., Globerson, A., Nakamura, I., and Trainin, N. (1973). *J. Exp. Med.* **138,** 130.
Scheid, M. P., Goldstein, G., Hammerling, U., and Boyse, E. A. (1975). *Ann. N.Y. Acad. Sci.* **249,** 531.
Scheinberg, M. A., and Cathcart, E. S. (1973). *Arthritis Rheum.* **16,** 566.
Scheinberg, M. A., Cathcart, E. S., and Goldstein, A. L. (1975). *Lancet* **1,** 424.
Schlesinger, D. H., and Goldstein, G. (1975). *Cell* **5,** 361.
Schmitt, D. (1974). *C.R. Hebd. Seances Acad. Sci.* **278,** 1649.
Schmitt, D., and Monier, J. C. (1974). *Experientia* **30,** 1349.
Schmitt, D., Monier, J. C., Perrot, H., and Thivolet, J. (1972). *C.R. Hebd. Seances Acad. Sci.* **275,** 623.
Schmitt, D., Monier, J. C., Viac, J., and Thivolet, J. (1975). *Ann. Immunol.* (*Paris*) **126c,** 399.
Shirai, T., and Mellors, R. C. (1972). *Cell. Immunol.* **15,** 231.
Small, M., and Trainin, N. (1975). *Cell. Immunol.* **20,** 1.
Staples, P. J., and Talal, N. (1969). *J. Exp. Med.* **129,** 123.
Stobel, C. (1974). *Eur. J. Immunol.* **4,** 621.
Stutman, O. (1975). *In* "Biological Activities of Thymic Hormones" (D. W. Van Bekkum, ed.), p. 87. Kooyker Sci. Publ. Rotterdam.
Stutman, O., and Good, R. A. (1973). *Contemp. Top. Immunobiol.* **2,** 299.
Stutman, O., Yunis, E. J., and Good, R. A. (1968). *Proc. Soc. Exp. Biol. Med.* **127,** 1204.
Stutman, O., Yunis, E., and Good, R. A. (1970). *J. Exp. Med.* **132,** 183.
Suciu-Foca, N., Buda, J., Theim, T., and Reemstma, K. (1974). *Clin. Exp. Immunol.* **18,** 296.
Thivolet, J., Monier, J. C., Ruel, J. P., and Richard, M. H. (1967). *Nature* (*London*) **214,** 1134.
Thurman, G. B., and Goldstein, A. L. (1975). *In* "Biological Activities of Thymic Hormones" (D. W. van Bekkum, ed.), p. 000. Kooyker Sci. Publ., Rotterdam.
Thurman, G. B., Ahmed, A., Strong, D. M., Gershwin, M. E., Steinberg, A. D., and Goldstein, A. L. (1975). *Transplant. Proc.* **7,** 299.

Touraine, J. L., Touraine, F., Incefy, G. S., and Good, R. A. (1975). *Ann. N.Y. Acad. Sci.* **249,** 335.

Trainin, N., Small, M., and Globerson, A. (1969). *J. Exp. Med.* **130,** 765.

Trainin, N., Carnaud, C., and Ilfeld, D. (1973). *Nature* (*London*), *New Biol.* **245,** 253.

Umiel, T., and Trainin, N. (1975). *Eur. J. Immunol.* **5,** 85.

Wara, D. W., Goldstein, A. L., Doyle, W., and Amman, A. J. (1975). *N. Engl. J. Med.* **292,** 70.

Wick, G., Kite, J. H., Jr., and Witebsky, E. (1970). *J. Immunol.* **104,** 54.

Chapter 9

Autoimmunity, Self-Recognition, and Blocking Factors

IRUN R. COHEN AND HARTMUT WEKERLE

I. INTRODUCTION

The immune system of an individual identifies and reacts against foreign substances. It does not normally react against components of the body itself. The term natural self-tolerance refers to this characteristic of the immune system.

Autoimmune diseases occur when the immune system of an individual loses self-tolerance and attacks the apparently normal constituents of its own body. The actual or potential targets of such an autoimmune process can be called self-antigens. A large number of clinical and experimental autoimmune diseases can be distinguished by the particular self-antigens involved and the nature of the autoimmune reaction (Samter, 1971). For example, autoantibodies produced by B cells against circulating red blood cells can produce hemolytic anemia (Weens and Schwartz, 1974). In contrast, the autoimmune lesions in experimental allergic encephalomyelitis (EAE) are caused by effector T lymphocytes (Paterson, 1966; Gonatas and Howard, 1974), and autoantibodies against the relevant self-antigen appear to protect against the disease. Thus, each autoimmune disease has its own pathological physiology. Nevertheless, a common feature of all autoimmune states is the recognition of self-antigens by activated effector lymphocytes or their products. Lymphocytes capable of reacting specifically against any antigen, foreign or self, must have receptors that can recognize complementary antigens. Therefore, a fundamental aspect of autoimmunity is the existence of effector lymphocytes with receptors for self.

The origin of self-recognizing lymphocytes is an important question in understanding the processes that lead to loss of self-tolerance and autoimmunity. Until recently, it was generally thought that the immune system was self-tolerant because there were no functional lymphocytes in immunologically competent animals with receptors for self-antigens. This notion, described most clearly by Burnet (1959), was based on the concept of clonal selection as the primary process activating the immune system. Specific antigen selected and activated those lymphocytes with complementary receptors. The immune response was determined by contact between lymphocyte receptors and their antigens. Burnet proposed that natural self-tolerance, the absence of reactivity to self-antigens, logically required either the absence of lymphocytes with receptors for self, or the inaccessibility of self-antigens to contact with lymphocytes. Autoimmunity was thought to result either from the development by somatic mutations of self-recognizing lymphocytes or from the contact of lymphocytes with normally inaccessible self-antigens (Burnet, 1959). These ideas were based on the principle that the major factors controlling the immune response were the available concentrations of lymphocyte receptors and antigens.

However, the original concepts of clonal selection have been modified by the impact of studies whose essential message is that the immune system is regulated and controlled by many and diverse factors. The outcome of an interaction between an antigen and receptor-bearing lymphocytes may be a response of variable intensity, a persistent state of tolerance to further contact with the antigen or no detectable response. Indeed, major efforts are being made at present to analyze the genetic, cellular, and molecular factors that regulate the expression of the immune system. In short, as with all organized biologic, behavioral, or physical systems, an understanding of the immune system requires knowledge of the regulation of its components.

Understanding regulation of the immune system is of particular importance to autoimmunity, since it now appears that lymphocytes with receptors for some accessible self-antigens do exist in healthy animals (Cohen and Wekerle, 1973; Bankhurst, *et al.*, 1973), and self-tolerance can no longer be explained in all instances as the mere absence of such lymphocytes. Of course, this does not deny the possibility that certain classes of potentially self-reactive lymphocytes are totally deleted. For example, no lymphocytes have been found with receptors for self-antigens, such as albumen, which circulates freely in high concentration (Bankhurst *et al.*, 1973). Thus, elimination of particular clones of lymphocytes (Nossal and Pike, 1974) may have a place together with other processes that produce self-tolerance.

The chapters of this book describe a number of mechanisms that appear to regulate self-tolerance and autoimmunity, such as the balance between suppressor and helper cells, hormones, genetic background, or viruses. In this chapter, we shall discuss the possible functions of blocking factors as regulators of self-tolerance. Since blocking factors, by definition, inhibit the reactivity of potentially reactive lymphocytes, we shall first briefly review some of the evidence supporting the conclusion that self-recognizing lymphocytes are normally present and threaten healthy individuals. This will be followed by a discussion of the role of blocking factors themselves. Finally, we shall consider possible functions for self-recognition in the physiology of the immune response. Much important work that bears upon these subjects will not be reviewed; rather, we shall concentrate upon a few experimental systems that conveniently illustrate selected points. The term tolerance will be used to describe any form of specific unresponsiveness caused by immunologic processes.

II. THE DETECTION OF LYMPHOCYTES THAT RECOGNIZE SELF-ANTIGENS

Direct evidence of self-recognition is based on observation of the binding of self-antigens to specific receptors of autologous or syngeneic lymphocytes.

The antigen-sensitive receptors of B lymphocytes are, without doubt, membrane-bound antibodies with the molecular features of immunoglobulins (Wigzell, 1973). The antigen-sensitive receptors of T lymphocytes, in all probability, may not be immunoglobulins (Crone *et al.,* 1972), although there exists some controversy on this point (Marchalonis *et al.,* 1972). Nevertheless, the results of recent studies indicate that the receptors of both T and B lymphocytes directed against the same antigens share common idiotypes; i.e., they bear common structures in the region of their combining site (Ramsier and Lindenmann, 1971; Binz and Wigzell, 1975). This suggests that the receptors of T and B lymphocytes have similar if not identical kinds of antigen-binding sites, even though the constant regions of the T and B receptor molecules may be unrelated, and the biologic effects that are produced, subsequent to recognition, may be vastly different. Since recognition itself is a functional property of similar subregions of both types of receptors, we shall discuss self-recognition and potential self-reactivity as an operation common to both T and B lymphocytes.

A. Self-Recognizing B Lymphocytes

Thyroglobulin is an iodine-containing protein produced by thyroid epithelial cells and stored in the thyroid gland. This material is broken down to form the active thyroid hormones, which are released into the blood. Autoantibodies to thyroglobulin are found in spontaneous autoimmune thyroiditis in humans, and thyroiditis can be produced in experimental animals by injecting them with homologous thyroglobulin in complete Freund's adjuvant (Ringertz *et al.,* 1971). The development of thyroiditis seems to be dependent on autoantibodies secreted by B lymphocytes, since the disease can be passively transferred by using serum from sick donors (Nakamura and Weigle, 1969; Vladutiu and Rose, 1971). Therefore, the recognition of homologous thyroglobulin by B lymphocytes is a factor in autoimmune thyroiditis. This example of a clinically significant disease has provided a model for studying the question of self-recognizing B lymphocytes.

Thyroglobulin should be accessible to lymphocytes, since it can be detected in the serum of normal humans (Torrigiani *et al.,* 1969). Are there lymphocytes, which can recognize thyroglobulin, in the circulation of normal individuals? The answer to this question appears to be yes. B lymphocytes from the peripheral blood of humans were found to specifically bind radioactively labeled human thyroglobulin (Bankhurst *et al.,* 1973). Similar findings have also been reported in inbred mice (Clagett and Weigle, 1974) and rats (Ada and Cooper, 1971).

Is thyroiditis caused by those lymphocytes which bind thyroglobulin? Allison (1974) and Clagett and Weigle (1974) studied this question by "suicide experiments" in which the specific receptor-bearing cells in suspensions of lymphocytes were killed *in vitro* by their selective binding of strongly radioactive thyroglobulin. The remaining viable lymphocytes were then injected into syngeneic mice that had been heavily irradiated. The immune system of these recipient mice was restored by the donor lymphocytes, and they were able to make immune responses to other antigens. However, the mice were unable to make antibodies to thyroglobulin or to develop autoimmune thyroiditis subsequent to injection of thyroglobulin. These findings indicate that the lymphocytes, which had been observed to bind thyroglobulin, were the cells responsible for the autoimmune disease. Therefore, it seems that healthy individuals possess competent B lymphocytes with receptors for a circulating self-antigen, and activation of these lymphocytes leads to autoimmunity.

Despite the fact that these self-recognizing B lymphocytes circulate together with their specific self-antigens, the vast majority of individuals never develop autoimmune thyroiditis. As convincingly argued by Allison (1971, 1974) and Weigle (1971), autologous thyroglobulin is immunogenic but will trigger the induction of antibody production by B lymphocytes only if help is provided by T lymphocytes. Thus, self-tolerance to thyroglobulin depends upon the control of B lymphocyte responsiveness by T lymphocytes. The mechanism that ensures the tolerance of T lymphocytes to thyroglobulin remains to be investigated. It has been shown, however, that relatively low concentrations of antigen render T lymphocytes unresponsive (Taylor, 1969; Chiller *et al.,* 1971). Thus, as proposed by Allison (1971) and by Weigle (1971), the low concentrations of circulating thyroglobulin produce tolerance by making T lymphocytes unresponsive, and, thereby, depriving B lymphocytes of their help.

However, autoantibodies to thyroglobulin are detectable in many persons without thyroid disease (Hill, 1961). Therefore, autoantibodies alone are not sufficient to produce thyroiditis. Hence, the absence of autoimmunity against the thyroid cannot be attributed entirely to lack of helper T cells for induction of such antibodies.

B. Self-Recognizing T Lymphocytes

We have studied the recognition by T lymphocytes of self-antigens, using an approach based on the induction of sensitization of T lymphocytes *in vitro* (Feldman *et al.,* 1972). This system was first developed by Ginsburg (1968) for the sensitization of rat lymphocytes against xenogeneic mouse fibroblasts. Later modifications made it possible to study sensitization of rat or mouse T lymphocytes against allogeneic or syngeneic fibroblasts (Cohen *et al.*, 1971a,b; Cohen and Wekerle, 1972, 1973, 1974; Wekerle *et al.*, 1973).

We used these methods to test whether healthy inbred rats or mice possessed lymphocytes with receptors for self-antigens, and if such lymphocytes could be activated to produce damage to self-target cells immunospecifically. We incubated spleen, thymus, or lymph node lymphocytes with monolayers of syngeneic fibroblasts obtained from embryos or with reticulum cells obtained from adult animals and found that autosensitization was induced *in vitro.* The developing effector lymphocytes lysed syngeneic target cells more effectively than they did foreign target cells. Injection of the autosensitized lymphocytes into syngeneic rats or mice produced enlargement of lymphoid organs, and, in some cases, caused runting of newborn animals (Cohen *et al.*, 1971b). In further studies, it was possible to demonstrate that lymphocytes from rat thymus glands could undergo sensitization *in vitro* against thymus reticulum cells isolated from the same thymuses. These autosensitized lymphocytes produced enlargement of draining popliteal lymph nodes when they were injected into the hind footpads of syngeneic rats. Suspensions of lymphocytes from these enlarged lymph nodes lysed syngeneic target cells to a greater degree than they did allogeneic target cells (Cohen and Wekerle, 1973).

To test whether this form of autosensitization is based on the preexistence of specific self-recognizing lymphocytes, we used immunoadsorption techniques developed to analyze recognition by T lymphocytes (Wekerle *et al.*, 1972). Syngeneic fibroblasts or thymus reticulum cells were used as absorbants for rat lymphocytes. We found that lymphocytes that adhered to syngeneic monolayer cells could be autosensitized. The nonadherent lymphocytes were depleted of their capacity to undergo autosensitization but could be sensitized against allogeneic cells. This indicates that autosensitization is the property of a fraction of self-recognizing T lymphocytes. Hence, normal rats have unsensitized lymphocytes with preformed receptors that specifically bind to self-antigens.

The identity of the self-antigens recognized on syngeneic fibroblasts *in vitro* is unknown. However, genetic analyses of this reaction suggest that products of genes of the major histocompatibility complex (MHC), H-2 in mice (Ilfeld *et al.*, 1975) and H-1 in rats (H. Wekerle, unpublished) may be the targets of this form of self-recognition. Lymphocytes autosensitized against syngeneic fibroblasts were found to kill best target fibroblasts that shared identical regions of the MHC. Thus, contact with syngeneic fibroblasts *in vitro* appears to trigger the immune differentiation of those effector T lymphocytes which recognize MHC markers of the individual himself.

It is noteworthy that these same MHC markers serve to trigger allogeneic lymphocytes in transplantation reactions against foreign cells (Anonymous, 1972). Thus, the survival of cells grafted into an allogeneic individual is markedly influenced by the MHC identity of the graft and the host. This suggests that the immune system is particularly responsive to products of genes of the MHC region.

A unique function for MHC markers has recently been observed in the immune response against syngeneic cells infected with certain viruses. Lymphocytes from mice infected with lymphocytic choriomeningitis (LCM) virus were found to kill LCM infected target cells only if the target cells shared identical subregions of the MHC with the attacking lymphocytes (Zinkernagel and Doherty, 1974). Modification of syngeneic lymphocytes with a chemical hapten such as TNP was shown to elicit an immune response *in vitro* against TNP modified target cells (Shearer, 1974). However, similar to autosensitization against normal, apparently unmodified syngeneic fibroblasts, the response against TNP-treated target cells involved recognition of self-MHC antigens. The significance of these forms of self-reactivity directed against MHC is unknown and will be discussed below (Section VI,B). Nevertheless, we can conclude that this immune system has a particular readiness to react against MHC markers, self as well as foreign. The potential reactivity against self-MHC must be controlled well *in vivo* to insure self-tolerance.

Despite the presence of MHC markers on most of the individual's cells, many clinical autoimmune diseases appear to be directed against self-antigens limited to only certain cells or organs. These diseases are organ specific. Can normal T lymphocytes also recognize organ-specific self-antigens? To approach this question, we have recently developed systems to study the induction of organ-specific autoimmunity *in vitro*. We have found that rat thymus lymphocytes can be sensitized *in vitro* against extracts of syngeneic rat brains. Intravenous injection of syngeneic recipient rats with these autosensitized lymphocytes led to the development of lesions in their brains similar to those found in EAE (Orgad and Cohen, 1974). This work is being extended to study sensitization *in vitro* against purified basic protein of myelin (see Section IV,A,3). The findings are compatible with the observation (Yung *et al.*, 1973) that a fraction of normal human lymphocytes specifically binds human encephalitogenic protein.

A second model of organ-specific autoimmunity involves sensitization *in vitro* of rat lymphocytes against cultures of syngeneic testicular cells (Wekerle and Begemann, 1976). The lymphocytes are found to damage testicular cells *in vitro* and produce lesions of orchitis after injection *in vivo*.

It, therefore, seems that autosensitization of T lymphocytes can be induced *in vitro* against both MHC products and organ-specific self-antigens. Normal human T lymphocytes have been found to bind human red blood cells (Baxley *et al.*, 1973).

III. BLOCKING FACTORS

The above findings (Section II,A and B) demonstrate that healthy individuals possess B and T lymphocytes capable of recognizing and of being triggered by accessible self-antigens. Among the diversity of competent lymphocytes are a fraction with receptors for self. Regulatory mechanisms, such as blocking factors, therefore, have a reason to exist: to prevent the immune differentiation and/or effects of such self-recognizing lymphocytes. The first question to be considered is: What is a blocking factor? In other words: How can blocking factors be distinguished experimentally from other processes that might regulate immune reactivity, such as active tolerogens or suppressor cells?

Blocking factors should be distinguishable from active tolerogens. The latter induce nonresponsiveness as a form of differentiation of the target lymphocytes. Active tolerogens render lymphocytes intrinsically tolerant so that they remain unreactive to specific immunogenic signals, whether or not the tolerogen continues to be present. The lymphocyte as a receiver of signals is itself modified or irreversibly inactivated. This tolerance can be broken only by a change in the state of differentiation of the tolerant lymphocytes or by entry into the system of new, nontolerant lymphocytes.

In contrast to active tolerogens, blocking factors exert inhibitory effects without actively modifying the state of the lymphocytes. They merely block transmission of specific immunogenic signals at some point in the immune response arc. Their effect is dependent on their continued presence and is reversible on a cellular level, once the blocking factors are removed. Active tolerogens can be said to produce changes within the lymphocyte, while the activity of blocking factors is limited to the membrane receptors.

Unresponsiveness caused by blocking factors must also be distinguished from that caused by suppressor cells. Tolerance in certain conditions has been found to be associated with the presence of T lymphocytes which function to inhibit the reactivity of other normal, nontolerant lymphocytes (Gershon, 1974). The mechanism by which suppressor T lymphocytes work is not clear. Furthermore, some evidence suggests that other types of cells such as macrophages (Kirchner *et al.*, 1974) or B lymphocytes (Kilburn *et al.*, 1974) may function as suppressors. Although much remains to be learned about suppressor cells, they would appear at first glance to be distinguishable from blocking factors which are not cells. However, as will be discussed in a later section, forms of tolerance believed to be associated with some kinds of blocking factors may, in fact, be related to tolerance involving certain active tolerogens or suppressor cells.

There appear to be four classes of materials that could fulfill the definition of blocking factors as immunospecific extracellular substances which reversibly block the immune activity of lymphocytes bearing specific receptors: antigens, antibodies, antigen–antibody complexes, and anti-idiotypes (Fig. 1).

1. Antigens

Molecules with a geometric configuration that allows them to bind to the receptors of lymphocytes are antigens (Wigzell, 1973). Antigens also interact with the combining sites of antibodies secreted by B lymphocytes, or with specific factors secreted by T lymphocytes (Munroe *et al.*, 1974). Antigens with properties sufficient to trigger the immune differentiation of

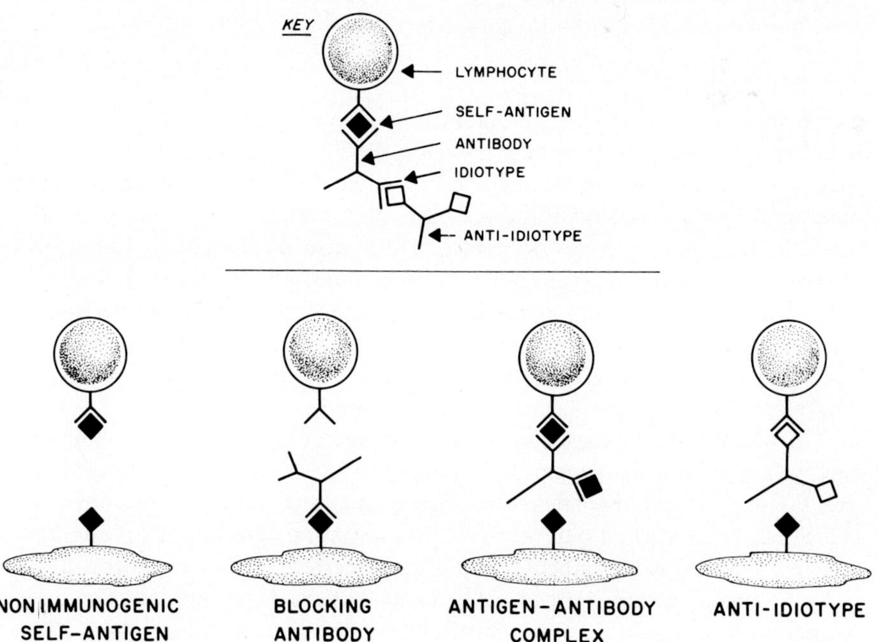

Fig. 1. Blocking factors. Immunogenic self-antigen is shown schematically by the diamond-shaped structure presented on a cell surface. The lymphocyte with a specific receptor is prevented from recognizing this immunogenic form of self-antigen by four blocking factors: soluble nonimmunogenic self-antigen, blocking antibody, antigen–antibody complex, and anti-idiotype. These interactions are discussed in the text (see Section IV).

lymphocytes are called immunogens. Antigens may also bind to receptors without triggering lymphocytes. Such nonimmunogenic antigens can be blocking factors by occupying specific lymphocyte receptors and so preventing contact between lymphocytes and immunogens.

2. *Antibodies*

The binding of preformed antibody molecules to an immunogen can hide the immunogen from lymphocyte receptors. In this way, antibodies can prevent the transmission of an effective signal to lymphocytes and, thus, function as blockers.

3. *Antigen–Antibody Complexes*

Blocking antibodies work by binding to the immunogen, while blocking antigens act by binding to the lymphocyte receptors. It has been suggested that antigen–antibody complexes combine both kinds of blocking activity. However, in addition to blocking, they may have a function in inducing active tolerance (Howard and Mitchison, 1975).

4. *Anti-Idiotypes*

An idiotype is a unique configuration of the variable portion (Fv) of a lymphocyte's receptor (Capra and Kehoe, 1975). Therefore, the idiotype is a structure that is close to, or includes, the actual site on the receptor which combines with antigen. Idiotypes can be immunogenic and stimulate specific antibodies against themselves (McKearn *et al.*, 1974). These antibodies, called anti-idiotypes, function as antibodies to receptors of lymphocytes. As such, they can bind to the receptors and block recognition of immunogens. It is likely that T lymphocytes can also recognize idiotypes (Janeway *et al.*, 1975) and, perhaps, even secrete anti-idiotype T cell factors (Ramsier, 1974).

These blocking factors can be defined operationally by the manner in which they inhibit the triggering of potentially reactive lymphocytes. Blocking factors can act theoretically at any point in the immune response arc. They can prevent the afferent phase, the initial recognition of an immunogen by a specific lymphocyte. They can interfere with the generation of effector cells, which is defined as the central phase of the immune response. In addition, blocking factors can prevent expression of the immune effect itself mediated by antibodies or cytotoxic lymphocytes.

Finally, blocking may be observed as a reversible first stage in the induction of a more active form of tolerance or suppression. In the next section, we shall review experimental examples of the various blocking factors and their modes of action.

IV. EXAMPLES OF BLOCKING FACTORS

A. Blocking Antigens

1. Foreign Antigens

Studies of experimental induction of tolerance to foreign antigens have provided the clearest evidence that antigens in certain forms can function as blocking factors. Free haptens, small, nonimmunogenic antigens, have been found to prevent the antibody response to the same haptens bound to an immunogenic carrier (Brownstone *et al.*, 1966; Feldmann, 1972). The mechanism of this tolerance appears to be competition for binding at the lymphocyte receptor between immunogenic and nonimmunogenic molecules of an antigen. This type of blocking by competition is readily demonstrable *in vitro,* using relatively high concentrations of free hapten. Hapten, in the form of an affinity label that combines covalently with receptors, blocks at much lower concentrations.

The blocking effects of haptens have been more difficult to demonstrate *in vivo,* probably because of the difficulty in achieving high enough concentrations of free hapten to compete with the binding of immunogenic hapten–carrier molecules (Howard and Mitchison, 1975). Intravenous injection of haptens has been found to prevent the induction of delayed hypersensitivity to an immunogenic form of the antigen (Asherson and Ptak, 1968). However, this type of unresponsiveness may be mediated by suppressor cells rather than by blocking (Zembala and Asherson, 1973).

Bacterial antigens, such as pneumococcal capsular polysaccharide type III (Howard and Mitchison, 1975) or lipopolysaccharide from *Escherichia coli* (Sjöberg, 1972), provide examples of blocking *in vivo.* Injection of these materials into mice in an appropriate dosage schedule leads to specific unresponsiveness that may last a year or more. This tolerance is accompanied by the persistence of increased numbers of antigen-binding B lymphocytes, and it can be reversed within a few hours to a few days by incubation of the lymphocytes *in vitro* or by their transfer to normal recipients. These bacterial polysaccharides are relatively poorly degradable, and it is conceivable that they persist in the body for long periods of time in blocking form. The blocked lymphocytes become unblocked by incubating them *in vitro* and/or transferring them into new animals, maneuvers which presumably lower the effective concentration of blocking antigens.

Undegradable synthetic antigens made with amino acids in the D configuration also induce unresponsiveness (Nossal *et al.,* 1973). This may be another example of the ability of nonmetabolized persisting antigens to block lymphocyte receptors.

2. *Tumor Antigens*

The actions of blocking antigens described above involved unphysiological experimental manipulations of the immune system. A role for antigens as blocking factors in a clinical situation has been found in advanced cancer (Currie and Basham, 1972). Some human patients with widespread tumors appear to have tumor-associated antigens freely circulating uncombined with antibodies. Such antigens seem to block the patient's lymphocyte receptors and inhibit a cytotoxic reaction against the tumor cells. These blocking antigens can be removed by repeated washing to the patient's lymphocytes, and their cytotoxic activity against tumor target cells can be restored *in vitro*.

These findings indicate that blocking by antigen can be produced experimentally and that it may even occur spontaneously in cancer patients. The experimental studies suggest that antigen blockade can prevent the afferent sensitization phase of the antibody immune response, while the tumor studies indicate that the effector function of sensitized potentially cytotoxic T lymphocytes may be blocked by free antigen.

3. *Self-Antigens*

There is much logic to the notion that nonimmunogenic self-antigens act to block potentially self-recognizing lymphocytes. The constant turnover and shedding (Doljanski, 1973) of normal cell membrane components would seem to provide an inexhaustable source of soluble fragments of self-antigens to compete with immunogenic membrane-bound forms of these antigens. The concentration of blocking self-antigens would be highest near the very cells which bear the respective immunogenic self-antigens. Thus, negative-feedback blocking would be guaranteed to be most efficient at the most critical point when a potentially self-recognizing lymphocyte approaches the cell. In both persistence and effective concentration, soluble self-antigens should be superior to either bacterial polysaccharides (Sjöberg, 1972) or synthetic haptens (Howard and Mitchison, 1975) as blocking factors.

Blocking self-antigens would appear to have a further advantage for the individual, compared to the other kinds of potential blocking factors. To be produced, blocking antibodies, antigen–antibody complexes, and anti-idiotypes, as well as suppressor T cells—in contrast to blocking antigens—all require an immune response of the individual against his own self-components. Therefore, blocking self-antigens would seem to recommend themselves as a first line of defense against potentially self-recognizing lymphocytes.

Is there indeed any evidence that blocking self-antigens have a role in maintaining self-tolerance?

We first approached this question by using the system described in Section II,B which had demonstrated the existence of T lymphocytes with receptors for self-antigens on fibroblasts or thymus reticulum cells (Wekerle *et al.*, 1973; Cohen and Wekerle, 1973). If such lymphocytes could bind to and be triggered by these self-antigens *in vitro,* there had to be a mechanism to prevent similar autosensitization *in vivo.* Furthermore, this putative inhibitory mechanism had to be lost during incubation *in vitro.*

To investigate the control of self-recognition, we studied the kinetics of lymphocyte binding to self-immunoadsorbent monolayer cells, compared to the kinetics of their binding to foreign cells. We found that receptor-bearing lymphocytes bound to allogeneic or xenogeneic fibroblasts in about ½ to 1 hour (Wekerle *et al.*, 1972). In contrast, it required from 3 to 5 hours for lymphocytes to bind specifically to syngeneic monolayers (Cohen and Wekerle, 1973). Therefore, it appeared that self-recognizing lymphocytes, upon removal from the rat, were relatively inhibited in their ability to recognize membrane-bound self-antigens. Further delay in self-recognition could be produced by incubating the lymphocytes with fresh autologous serum before assaying their specific adherence to syngeneic monolayer cells. Incubation with allogeneic rat serum did not inhibit recognition of self, and autologous serum did not inhibit recognition of foreign monolayer cells. Treatment of the immunoadsorbent monolayers with serum did not prevent their recognition by lymphocytes. Therefore, autologous serum appeared to contain factors that acted in a reversible manner on those lymphocytes with specific receptors capable of recognizing self-antigens. The blocking factors did not bind to the self-antigens themselves. Hence, we concluded that the blocking factors were probably serum-soluble self-antigens and not antibodies or complexes. This conclusion was strengthened by our finding that the blocking activity was mediated by material with a molecular weight (MW) of less than 50,000 daltons as determined by fractionation of autologous serum through a graded membrane (Cohen and Wekerle, 1974). A similar fraction of allogeneic serum did not block self-recognition. The serum-blocking activity was found to be lost after incubation for several hours at 37°C, or after freezing and thawing (unpublished). This has made it difficult to characterize satisfactorily the blocking factors, and the evidence that the factors are self-antigens remains circumstantial.

Besides blocking self-antigen, the only other substance with the properties needed to account for these results are anti-idiotypes, antibodies to receptors for self-antigens (see below, Section IV,D). However, to be smaller than 50,000 daltons, the anti-idiotypes would have to be fragments of antibody molecules, or T cell factors with anti-anti-self specificity. Such entities have not yet been demonstrated to exist naturally.

In addition to blocking recognition of syngeneic fibroblasts or thymus reticulum cells, fresh autologous serum has been found to inhibit autosensitization *in vitro* against cultures of testicular cells (Wekerle and Begemann, 1976). The presence of as little as 1% of a rat's own serum in the culture medium completely prevented his spleen or lymph node lymphocytes from developing into cytotoxic effector cells during 3 days of culture with autologous testis cells. Serum from female rats appeared to inhibit primarily that part of the reaction which was directed against MHC (H-1) antigens present on syngeneic testis cells. The component of the reaction that seemed to be directed against testis-specific self-antigens was inhibited to a much greater degree by male serum. The lower inhibitory capacity of female rat serum reasonably can be attributed to a lower concentration of antigens cross-reactive with testis in the circulation of female rats. The experimental finding is, therefore, compatible with concept of blocking antigen.

These studies showing inhibition of self-reactivity by factors in serum suggested, but could not prove a role for blocking self-antigens. In the systems used, the self-antigens involved either as immunogens or as blocking factors were undefined. The fundamental question remained as to whether soluble nonimmunogenic self-antigens can, and do compete for lymphocyte receptors with immunogenic forms of the same self-antigens.

We have attempted to approach this question directly by developing a system of autosensitization *in vitro* directed against a defined self-antigen. Experimental allergic encephalomylitis (EAE) is an autoimmune disease of the central nervous system in which T lymphocytes appear to be involved (Paterson, 1966). EAE has been produced classically by injecting susceptible guinea pigs, rats, mice, or monkeys with heterologous or isologous brain tissue emulsified in complete Freund's adjuvant (CFA). Similar pathological lesions were caused in rats by the intravenous injection of rat thymus lymphocytes, which had been autosensitized *in vitro* for 18 hours against a crude extract of syngeneic brain tissue, in the absence of adjuvants (Orgad and Cohen, 1974). These findings led to the conclusion that T lymphocytes with receptors for brain antigens exist in normal rats (Section II,B).

A useful feature of the EAE model is that the encephalitogenic self-antigen has been identified as myelin basic protein (Einstein *et al.*, 1962). The molecular composition of encephalitogenic determinants of basic protein has been characterized (Bergstrand and Källén, 1972). Therefore, investigation of the recognition of basic protein by lymphocytes *in vitro* might provide a system to analyze the suggested role of a blocking self-antigen.

We have been able to induce autosensitization *in vitro* of lymphocytes (probably T cells) from susceptible strain 13 guinea pigs against purified basic protein (Steinman *et al.*, 1977). The results relating to the problem of blocking self-antigen as yet are incomplete but contribute to elucidation of the question. Basic protein was found to be immunogenic for lymphocytes after uptake by syngeneic macrophages. Triggering of the lymphocytes by these macrophages, however, could be specifically inhibited by the presence of soluble basic protein in the culture medium.

These results illustrate several points. A self-antigen can be rendered immunogenic by syngeneic macrophages. The cultures were done in the absence of serum or other foreign macromolecules that could function as potentially immunogenic "carriers" (Habicht *et al.*, 1975) for basic protein. Therefore, a reasonably pure syngeneic system can produce autosensitization *in vitro* against a defined self-antigen. Furthermore, the soluble nonimmunogenic form of the self-antigen could prevent triggering by the immunogenic self-antigen. The mechanism of inhibition has to be investigated; however, the finding certainly argues for the possibility that soluble self-antigens can compete with immunogenic self-antigens for lymphocyte receptors. Studies of *in vitro* systems might provide an insight into the molecular bases of immunogenicity and of blocking. How does the association of a self-antigen with syngeneic macrophages lead to activation of lymphocytes, while the self-antigen in soluble form inhibits activation?

Another important question is whether this process does, in fact, occur physiologically. The results of the studies of serum blocking in the anti-fibroblast and anti-testis autosensitization systems would predict that soluble basic protein or its fragments be present in body fluids, and that such materials would serve as blocking factors. Nevertheless, even if blocking self-antigens could be assigned a physiological function in maintaining self-tolerance, it is very likely that additional mechanisms operate to ensure nonreactivity against self.

B. Blocking Antibodies

The paradigm of antibodies as blocking factors regulating the immune response is the so-called enhancement phenomenon. The growth of transplanted allogeneic tumor cells was found to be enhanced by the presence of preformed antibodies directed against the particular allogeneic antigens (Kaliss, 1966). Evidence suggested that the antibodies bound to the foreign transplantation antigens and blocked the ability of host lymphocytes to recognize them. Antibodies were found to block the primary sensitization of lymphocytes against foreign fibroblasts *in vitro* (Cohen and Feldman,

1971a), as well as to inhibit mediation of the cytotoxic effects of already sensitized lymphocytes (Cohen and Feldman, 1971b). Thus, blocking antibodies could act on both the afferent and efferent phases of the cell-mediated response.

The concept of blocking antibodies was extended greatly by the work of Voisin (1971) and of the Hellströms (1974) and their colleagues. It was found that newborn or transplanted animals made tolerant to allogeneic cells developed serum blocking factors with the characteristics of antibodies to the allogeneic antigens (Hellström *et al.,* 1971). Similar blocking antibodies could be detected in the sera of animals bearing tumors. As expected, the antibodies in such animals were directed against tumor-associated antigens (Hellström and Hellström, 1969). Much work was also done in characterizing the molecular nature of blocking antibodies both in tumor systems (Ran and Witz, 1972) and in tolerance to allogeneic cells (Voisin *et al.,* 1972). However, the question of interest in this discussion is whether or not blocking antibodies have a function in maintaining self-tolerance.

An attempt to study this question was made using tetraparental mice. These mice are created by fusing early embryos of two allogeneic strains and transplanting the mixture of cells back into the uterus for completion of fetal development. The mice that are born are found to be chimeras containing cells of two different allogeneic origins. It was felt that these mice were examples of the induction of allograft tolerance at an extremely early point in development and could be models for studying the mechanisms of self-tolerance. The results of one set of studies by Wegmann, Hellström, and Hellström (1971) indicated that the lymphocytes of tetraparental mice were cytotoxic *in vitro* against target cells of either parental strain. This cytotoxicity was inhibited by the serum of the tetraparental mice, but not by normal serum of either parent or of F_1 hybrid mice. This suggested that blocking factors, probably antibodies, were involved in the allogeneic tolerance of tetraparental mice. However, further studies of the tetraparental model failed to produce consistent results. Phillips and Wegmann (1973) found that active suppression might have a role in tetraparental tolerance, while Meo, Matsunaga, and Rijnbeek (1973) could find no evidence of lymphocyte reactivity *in vitro* against the allogeneic parental strains. They concluded that elimination of potentially reactive clones of lymphocytes had probably occurred. Barnes (1976) has stressed the dynamic relationship between chimeric cell populations in tetraparental mice. The proportions of the two different allogeneic cells, e.g., in the skin, can vary markedly in the course of the history of a single mouse. Furthermore, the mice tend to be populated with lymphoid cells of only one parental strain. Barnes could find no evidence of either blocking factors or suppressor cells in these mice. In short, the tetraparental system seems to be an unsuitable model for studying stable, natural self-tolerance to syngeneic cells.

There have not been many extensive studies which conclude unequivocally that blocking antibodies alone protect against autoimmunity. The Hellströms (1972) have reported that normal mouse lymphocytes may injure syngeneic brain cells *in vitro* and that a blocking factor inhibits this damage. Since the blocking factor could be absorbed by brain tissues, it seemed possible that blocking antibodies might be involved. However, antigen–antibody complexes could have produced the same result. Indeed, a number of investigators (Sjögren *et al.*, 1971; Baldwin *et al.*, 1972) have concluded that blocking activity, demonstrable in tumor systems, is mediated by antigen–antibody complexes, rather than by antibodies alone.

C. Antigen–Antibody Complexes

Studies of a number of different experimental systems show that antigen–antibody complexes are involved in certain types of reversible tolerance. As mentioned above (Section IV,B), blocking factors which develop spontaneously during the natural history of some tumors have been shown to be antigen–antibody complexes. In a totally different system, Diener and Feldmann (1972) investigated induction of B lymphocyte tolerance *in vitro* to a foreign protein, monomeric or polymerized flagellin. They found that an otherwise immunogenic concentration of antigen could induce tolerance in the presence of a suitable concentration of specific antibodies to the antigen. This tolerance was reversible up to 2 days after induction by trypsinization of the lymphocytes *in vitro* or by their transfer to irradiated recipient mice. Therefore, antigen–antibody complexes seemed to be important in blocking receptor-bearing B lymphocytes. However, continued incubation *in vitro* led to irreversible tolerance. This suggests that blockade by antigen–antibody complexes may be only the first step in the induction of a more active form of tolerance.

Studies reported by Gorczynski and colleagues (1974) indicate that T lymphocytes, too, can carry complexes of antigen and antibody on their surfaces and that these blockaded lymphocytes have a role in reversible tolerance. The evidence for this assertion is not strong, being based on investigations of retention and release by T lymphocytes of protein antigens *in vitro*. Nevertheless, it is compatible with the conclusions derived from studies of the tumor systems.

What is the relationship of these models of tolerance to the question of natural tolerance to self-antigens? At present, there are no studies that associate antigen–antibody complexes with tolerance to normal body components. Nevertheless, understanding the mechanism by which complexes block may be important to this inquiry for at least two reasons. This type of blocking appears spontaneously in tolerance to some tumor-associated antigens, and its function in maintaining self-tolerance is, therefore, theoretically conceivable. In addition, even if complexes cannot be implicated in self-tolerance, the mechanism of their action might teach us about tolerance mediated by other factors, such as blocking antigen or anti-idiotypes.

Diener and Feldmann (1972) have proposed that the critical factor in induction of tolerance is immobilization of lymphocyte receptors in the fluid cell membrane brought about by cross-linking of the receptors and formation of a lattice. Antigen molecules with the necessary density and configuation of epitopes (receptor-binding regions) readily induce tolerance by themselves. Antigens that do not have the configuration for proper cross-linking of receptors can be aided by complexing with bivalent antibodies. The antibodies, thus, serve to arrange the antigens so that the complex can cross-link and freeze the lymphocyte receptors to produce tolerance. These concepts emphasize the primary importance of the nature of the interaction between receptors and antigens in tolerance.

However, does the antibody moiety of the complex serve merely to focus antigen on the membrane, or does the antibody itself actively help shut off the lymphocytes?

The importance of antibody as a carrier in the blockade of lymphocyte receptors has been highlighted by studies carried out by Borel and his colleagues (Borel, 1971; Golan and Borel, 1971) and others (Moorhead *et al.,* 1973). A hapten, such as dinitrophenyl (DNP), was bound covalently to autologous mouse IgG, and the conjugate was injected into mice. The recipient mice were then observed to be unresponsive to injection with DNP, coupled to a carrier such as keyhole limpet hemocyanin (KLH), an otherwise strong immunogen. The nature of the tolerance produced by the hapten–IgG conjugate appears to be of interest to this discussion for a number of reasons. (1) DNP coupled to other autologous serum proteins, such as albumen, did not produce tolerance. (2) The whole IgG molecule had to be present. Tolerance could not be produced *in vivo* when the Fc region was cleaved from the DNP–IgG conjugate (Borel *et al.,* 1976). (3) There appeared to be specificity with regard to the place on the IgG molecule to which the hapten was bound. DNP coupled to the ϵ-amino groups of lysine was tolerogenic. In contrast, DNP bound to histidine or tyrosine by azo linkage, or to free carboyxyl groups by a mustard reagent created an immunogenic molecule that produced no tolerance at all (Paley *et al.,* 1975). The mode of hapten binding was found to be much more important than the density of hapten on the IgG carrier. (4) Both T and B lymphocytes were rendered tolerant by the DNP–IgG conjugate (Borel *et al.*, 1975). (5) The tolerance was reversible by incubation of the lymphocytes *in vitro* and appeared to be related to blockade of receptors (Aldo-Benson and Borel, 1974). The state of nonreactivity was associated with the presence of lymphocytes binding the DNP–IgG, and loss of tolerance *in vitro* was correlated with loss of DNP–IgG from the surface of the lymphocytes (Aldo-Benson and Borel, 1976). In short, autologous IgG appears to serve as a specific tolerogenic carrier for haptens bound to it in a particular way. The tolerance seems to be produced by a reversible surface interaction between the conjugate and specific receptor-bearing T and B lymphocytes.

Of particular importance to autoimmunity was the finding that the spontaneous lupuslike nephritis of (NZB $\times$ NZW)F_1 mice could be prevented by injecting the mice with NZB mouse IgG coupled to the nucleosides of DNA (Borel *et al.*, 1973). Thus, clinically effective tolerance to denatured DNA was produced by a conjugate of the "self-antigen" with "self-IgG." In this way, the nephritis resulting from the accumulation of antigen–antibody complexes was avoided. More recent results (Y. Borel, personal communication) suggest that appropriate treatment with the IgG–carrier conjugate can reverse nephritis as well as prevent it prophylactically.

These findings suggest that immunoglobulins have a unique function among plasma proteins in blocking lymphocytes. The characteristics of immunoglobulins responsible for this function are presently unclear. It is conceivable that a common mode of action might underlie the tolerance produced by hapten–IgG conjugates and that produced by antigen–antibody complexes. The concept developed by Diener and Feldmann (1972) from their studies of antigen–antibody complexes *in vitro* pictures the antibody as a passive scaffold for focusing antigen on the lymphocyte membrane. However, a more intrinsic role for the IgG molecule is indicated by studies of the hapten–IgG conjugate *in vivo*. For example, a combination of hapten and immunoglobulin might interact at the same time with diverse receptors on the lymphocyte membrane. The antigen could bind to the antigen-sensitive receptor, while the immunoglobulin could bind to the Fc receptors of either B (Dickler and Kunkel, 1972) or T lymphocytes (Stout and Herzenberg, 1975). This double binding might produce a stable form of peripheral blockade, and it could also trigger, in time, a form of central tolerance involving differentiation of the lymphocyte. This could be expressed as irreversible nonreactivity, or development of the lymphocyte into an active suppressor cell. It has been suggested that suppressor T lymphocytes operate via complexes (Gorczynski *et al.*, 1974). Indeed, recent findings hint that lymphocytes blocked with hapten–IgG have an active function in mediating tolerance (Y. Borel, personal communication).

The proposed function for the Fc portion of the immunoglobulin may be more important *in vivo* than *in vitro* where much higher concentration of antigen–immunoglobulin can be maintained. The $F(ab')_2$ fragments of antibody were effective in the *in vitro* system of Diener and Feldmann (1972), and blocking with DNP-$F(ab')_2$ conjugates has been achieved in the Borel system *in vitro,* although not *in vivo* (Borel *et al.*, 1976). The Fc portion of the immunoglobulin may be critical *in vivo* to stabilize the binding of the complex or conjugate to the lymphocyte.

D. Anti-Idiotypes

Tolerance involving immunoglobulin binding to lymphocytes can also be produced by antibodies to lymphocyte receptors, anti-idiotypes (Nisonoff and Bangasser, 1975). Anti-idiotypes can be produced experimentally by isolating homogeneous specific antibodies from one or a group of animals and immunizing another animal of the same or of a different species against the antibodies. Absorption of the resulting antiserum can be used to obtain antibodies reactive against specific idiotypes present on the immunizing antibodies. Anti-idiotypes can also be produced against receptors on T lymphocytes (Ramsier and Lindenmann, 1971; Binz and Wigzell, 1975).

Spontaneous synthesis of anti-idiotype antibody has been detected during sensitization of an animal to a particular antigen (Kluskens and Köhler, 1974; Köhler, 1975). In such a case, the anti-idiotype is a true autoantibody produced by an individual against one or several of its own receptors.

Anti-idiotypes may be related to this discussion, both by the mechanism by which they produce tolerance and by their potential function as autoantibodies.

Information regarding the first question has been derived mostly from experimentally induced anti-idiotypes. Injection of animals with anti-idiotypic antibodies led to suppression of the particular T or B lymphocytes which had receptors bearing the idiotype (Nisonoff and Bangasser, 1975). The nature of the inhibition appeared to depend upon the stage of development of the recipient animal. Mice suppressed as adults showed reversible inhibition of idiotypes suggestive of blocking. In contrast, injection of newborn mice with anti-idiotypes appeared to produce permanent inactivation of those clones of lymphocytes bearing the idiotype (Strayer *et al.*, 1974; Köhler *et al.*, 1974).

Blocking of adult lymphocytes by anti-idiotypes showed certain characteristics similar to blocking produced *in vivo* by hapten–IgG conjugates, and possibly to that produced by antigen–antibody complexes. The blocking was reversible, lasting for a number of weeks (Pawlak *et al.*, 1973). Continued presence of the anti-idiotype was needed to maintain suppression. Intact antibody was required, and Fab or $F(ab')_2$ fragments of anti-idiotypes did not inhibit the idiotypes. The effect of the anti-idiotype was reversed by incubation *in vitro*. Finally, evidence suggested that inhibition of the idiotype-bearing lymphocytes was mediated by suppressor cells (Eichmann, 1975). Suppression could be adoptively transferred into mildly irradiated (200 rads) recipients but was abolished by treating the transferred cells with anti-θ serum plus complement. This implicated suppressor T cells. However, Bangasser and colleagues (1975) found that successful adoptive transfer of suppression depended on priming the donors with antigen before transfer of their lymphocytes and raised the possibility that transferred B cells might be involved. Suppressor T cells have been shown to mediate suppression of immunoglobulin allotypes (Herzenberg *et al.*, 1973).

The irreversible tolerance produced in newborn mice was considered by Strayer *et al.* (1974) to result from elimination of idiotype-bearing lymphocytes, possible by way of antibody-dependent cell-mediated cytotoxicity.

Raff and his colleagues (1975) have found that immature mouse B lymphocytes respond differently than mature cells to suppression induced *in vitro* by anti-immunoglobulin antibodies. Anti-immunoglobulin antibodies may be related conceptually to anti-idiotypes. The latter are antibodies to hypervariable regions of the Fv portions of antibodies or receptors. Anti-immunoglobulins represent, for the most part, antibodies to constant portions of antibodies or B cell receptors. IgM-bearing B cells in fetal liver or adult bone marrow were irreversibly suppressed by exposure to anti-immunoglobulin antibodies. In contrast, such cells in adult spleen or lymph nodes were only reversibly suppressed by the same treatment. It is conceivable, therefore, that intrinsic properties in the lymphocytes themselves determine the outcome of the binding of specific antibodies to lymphocyte receptors.

A speculative but heuristically useful generalization might be made regarding the essential role of immunoglobulins in the various modes of suppression described above. Antigen–antibody complexes, hapten–IgG conjugates, anti-idiotype antibodies, and antibodies to constant regions of immunoglobulins can all be seen as immunoglobulins, products of the immune system, which, by way of various ligands, are bound to lymphocyte receptors. Antigen–antibody complexes and hapten–IgG conjugates bind to those lymphocytes with receptors for the antigen or hapten. Anti-idiotypes bind to lymphocytes whose receptors bear the specific idiotypes. Anti-immunoglobulins bind to all B lymphocytes that express the particular immunoglobulin class marker on their surface. One common result of this binding is to block the immune reactivity of the lymphocytes. The blocking can be transient and reversible, so that the agents fulfill the operational definition of blocking factors. However, a second more active phase may be generated; irreversible inactivation of susceptible lymphocytes caused by antibody-dependent cell-mediated cytotoxicity (Köhler *et al.*, 1974), or intrinsic changes in the lymphocyte (Raff *et al.*, 1975) can occur. Blocked lymphocytes also might be induced to become suppressor cells (Gorczynski *et al.*, 1974).

Another result of the binding of these agents may be activation of lymphocytes. Anti-idiotypes (Trenkner and Riblet, 1975), hapten–IgG conjugates (Yamashita and Kitagawa, 1974), and anti-immunoglobulin antibodies (Parker, 1975) have been shown to trigger lymphocytes under special circumstances.

Hapten–IgG conjugates are experimental artifacts that are instructive, and could be extremely useful as therapeutic agents to induce tolerance (Borel *et al.*, 1973; Stollar and Borel, 1975). Antigen–antibody complexes and spontaneous anti-idiotypes are physiological products of the immune system and, therefore, might be agents of negative feedback, which function to regulate the immune response.

Some evidence hints at such a role for anti-idiotypes. McKearn, Stuart, and Fitch (1974) found that Lewis rats which had been repeatedly injected with BN rat tumor cells developed, at first, idiotypic anti-BN antibodies, but, after continued injections, the Lewis rats also produced antibodies to their own idiotype. Thus, Lewis anti- (Lewis anti-BN) was spontaneously formed. Kluskens and Köhler (1974) gave multiple injections of pneumococcal vaccine to BALB/c mice and detected two kinds of antibody responses: one directed against antigen and the other directed against self-antibody to the antigen.

These findings are compatible with the stimulating ideas of a regulatory network of idiotypes and anti-idiotypes put forth by Jerne (1973, 1974a,b). However, Nisonoff and Bangasser (1975) have urged caution in interpreting the physiology of anti-idiotypes. They point out that detectable anti-idiotypes are induced with difficulty, that idiotypes can persist for months or years upon prolonged immunization, and that circulating idiotypes might be expected to tolerize the individual and render him unable to make anti-idiotypes. Nevertheless, whether or not a network (see Section VI,A) of idiotypes and anti-idiotypes exists, it is clear that spontaneous anti-idiotypes are true autoantibodies and can function as blocking factors.

V. DO BLOCKING FACTORS REGULATE SELF-TOLERANCE?

The above review (Section IV) shows in essence that several kinds of blocking factors do exist and can be demonstrated to influence the behavior of the immune response in certain systems. It also seems very likely that healthy individuals are populated with lymphocytes that can recognize at least certain unhidden self-antigens (Section II). However, at present, there is no direct evidence that proves that the immune reactivity of such lymphocytes is indeed regulated by blocking factors. Blocking factors do appear to inhibit recognition of immunogenic self-antigens (Cohen and Wekerle, 1973) and development of effector lymphocytes *in vitro* (Wekerle and Begemann, 1976). But we lack the critical link to connect this observation with the physiology of the intact animal. No autoimmune disease, spontaneous or experimental, has been demonstrated to be caused by, or even to involve a dysfunction of blocking factors. The failure to detect such a dysfunction, however, may be related either to the unsuitability of the experimental systems used, or to the pathophysiology of autoimmunity. Nevertheless, an interim appreciation of the potential role of blocking factors may be made.

Blocking antigens seem to constitute a first line of defense against self-recognizing T lymphocytes. We have demonstrated *in vitro* that autologous serum can inhibit the initial recognition of self-antigens, most probably products of the MHC, on fibroblasts or thymus reticulum cells. Testis self-antigens in serum or soluble myelin basic protein in culture medium were shown to inhibit triggering of T lymphocytes by the respective self-antigens in cell-bound immunogenic forms (See Section IV,A,3).

In addition to natural antigens, synthetic antigens might be used therapeutically to suppress autoimmunity. For example, Teitelbaum and her colleagues (1971, 1972) have reversed EAE by injecting animals with a copolymer of basic amino acids cross-reactive with myelin basic protein (Webb *et al.*, 1973).

The blocking effects of soluble self-antigens on self-recognizing B lymphocytes has not been studied. Wiegle (1971) and Allison, Denman, and Barnes (1971) have proposed that self-recognizing B lymphocytes are prevented from producing autoantibodies by want of help from self-tolerant T lymphocytes. It is conceivable that these T lymphocytes are rendered tolerant by blocking self-antigens. Thus, soluble self-antigens could block T lymphocytes directly and indirectly deprive B lymphocyts of the help they need to make autoantibodies.

Impairment of blocking might explain the induction of organ specific autoimmune diseases following injection of self-antigens in adjuvants. For example, the subcutaneous injection of brain tissue in CFA causes EAE (Paterson, 1966). This procedure might expose potentially reactive lymphocytes to immunogenic brain antigens in the absence of the fragments of shed soluble brain antigens that block self-recognition in the intact brain (Orgad and Cohen, 1974). In addition, CFA might stimulate macrophages to take up and process brain antigen and so tilt the local balance of self-antigen in the direction of the immunogenic form (see above, Sections II,B and IV,A,3). In this way, self-recognizing lymphocytes could be triggered and recruit other effector T lymphocytes (Cohen, 1973a,b) to mediate encephalitis. We have observed that differentiated effector T lymphocytes are much less susceptible to blocking by antigen than are resting, unsensitized lymphocytes (unpublished results). Therefore, once they are triggered, effector lymphocytes might injure target cells, despite the presence of shed soluble antigens.

In contrast to blocking antigens, it is difficult to make a case for blocking antibodies alone as agents of self-tolerance (See Section IV,B).

Although the most definitive studies of blocking by antigen–antibody complexes have been done in tumor systems (Sjögren *et al.,* 1971; Baldwin *et al.,* 1972), complexes seem to be excellent candidates for a second line of defense against autoimmunity after failure of blocking self-antigens. First, complexes would be expected to form as soon as autoantibodies were secreted. Such complexes would most likely be soluble because of the relative excess of self-antigens present in the individual. Second, the complexes would have a number of beneficial effects. Similar to conjugates, they could block production of autoantibody by B lymphocytes (Borel *et al.,* 1973). In addition, they would block potentially cytotoxic autosensitized T lymphocytes, just as they can block cytotoxicity against tumor cells (Baldwin *et al.,* 1972). Complexes probably block differentiated T lymphocytes much better than blocking antigen alone. Finally, as we discussed above (Section IV,C), antigen–antibody complexes might induce the differentiation of suppressor T cells (Gorczynski *et al.,* 1974). This would add an active element to the peripheral blocking of autoreactivity. However, there is a paucity of work which actually relates complexes to autoimmunity. Russell, Liburd, and Diener (1974) have reported that non-θ-bearing lymphocytes from young mice of NZB or other strains can inhibit the cytotoxic effects against fibroblasts *in vitro* of T lymphocytes from old autoimmune NZB mice. The authors speculated that this inhibition could be due to autoantibody released from B cells complexing with self-antigens from the target fibroblasts.

Anti-idiotypes are theoretically attractive as regulators of self-reactivity. The great volume of work presently devoted to anti-idiotypes may yet uncover evidence to support this notion. At the present time, however, evidence of functional blocking rests mostly on soluble antigen and antigen–antibody complexes.

The blocking effects of soluble antigens and of antigen–antibody complexes, and the inhibition mediated by suppressor cells seem to have evolved to protect the individual in a more dynamic and resiliant series of checks to autoimmunity than could be provided by elimination of "forbidden clones"

(Burnet, 1959) alone. However, these physiological processes may be subverted by tumor cells bearing otherwise foreign antigens and allow them to evade surveillance by the immune system (Cohen *et al.*, 1974; Alexander, 1974). Tumor antigens (Currie and Basham, 1972), antigen–antibody complexes (Baldwin *et al.*, 1972), and suppressor T lymphocytes (Treves *et al.*, 1974) have all been implicated in the pathophysiology of the tumor–host relationship.

VI. DOES SELF-RECOGNITION HAVE A NORMAL FUNCTION IN THE IMMUNE SYSTEM?

We have assumed that recognition of self-antigens by the receptors of lymphocytes can lead to harmful autoimmunity and, thus, is guarded against by various controls, including blocking factors. This is undoubtedly true regarding most self-antigens, particularly the organ specific antigens associated with autoimmune diseases. However, there is reason to believe that recognition of some self-antigens may be an integral feature of the immune system itself. Two such classes of self-antigens are the receptors of lymphocytes and, possibly, certain products of the MHC genes.

A. Self-Recognition of Idiotypes

Antibodies or T cell factors directed against the individual's own receptors are the essential ingredients in the network theories of immune regulation proposed by Jerne (1973, 1974a,b) and extended by others, including Köhler (1975), Richter (1975), and Hoffmann (1975). These investigators attempt to explain the behavior of the immune system by the interactions of antigens, idiotypes, and anti-idiotypes. The configuration of every antigen-sensitive receptor or idiotype allows interaction with either of two structurally complementary substances: one is the specific antigen (or family of cross-reactive antigens), and the other is the receptors of another clone of lymphocytes, the anti-idiotype. The idiotypes and anti-idiotypes may be either B or T cells and their antigen reactive products, antibodies, or T factors. Logically, the anti-idiotypes themselves can also recognize structurally complementary antigens and be recognized in turn by other receptors, anti-anti-idiotypes. Interactions between various components can facilitate or suppress their biosynthesis or immune reactivity. Therefore, this web of mutually interacting components forms a dynamic network that regulates itself. The details of the system differ according to the different theories. Since idiotypes are self-antigens, the motivating forces of the network, in general, are self-recognition and autoreactivity.

B. Self-Recognition in Interactions between Initiator and Recruited T Lymphocytes

A second example of self-recognition in the immune system can be found in the interactions between subsets of T lymphocytes. The laboratory of one of us (I.R.C.) has been investigating the nature of the cellular events that take place during the development of effector T lymphocytes in an allograft reaction (Cohen, 1973b,c; Treves and Cohen, 1973; Livnat and Cohen, 1975a,b). The strategy was to separate the induction of sensitization by antigen, the afferent phase, from the differentiation of effector lymphocytes, the central phase of the cell-mediated immune response arc. The results of these studies are published elsewhere (Cohen and Livnat, 1976a). Pertinent to this discussion was the finding that the generation of effector T lymphocytes involved the sequential interaction of two distinct subclasses of T lymphocytes that differ in their organs of residence, migration patterns, surface properties, and function within the immune response arc.

A conceptual outline of the sequence of events is that the afferent phase of the response is mediated by initiator T lymphocytes (ITL). The ITL are capable of recognizing and being sensitized by antigens presented on allogeneic fibroblasts *in vitro*. The central phase involves recruitment of the precursors of effector and memory lymphocytes by the sensitized ITL. These recruited T lymphocytes (RTL) appear to recognize and be triggered by a double signal that includes the sensitized syngeneic ITL or its products, plus a piece of the antigen, an epitope. The RTL cannot be activated by allogeneic fibroblasts alone either *in vitro* or *in vivo*. Thus, a chain reaction is produced when a second T lymphocyte (RTL) recognizes the state of immune differentiation of a preceding T lymphocyte (ITL).

What is the nature of the ITL substance that is recognized by syngeneic RTL in addition to the epitope? Preliminary evidence (S. D. Waksal, S. Livnat, and I. R. Cohen, unpublished) indicates that, for successful recruitment, ITL and RTL must be congenic at subregions of the MHC, particularly at the K end of H-2 in the mouse. This suggests that RTL recognize a combination of epitope plus a product of the MHC genes (Fig. 2).

In support of this concept is the finding that antigen-specific T cell factors (Munroe *et al.*, 1974; Armerding *et al.*, 1974) involved in interactions with B cells bear antigens coded for in the I region of the H-2 complex termed I-associated or Ia antigens (Shreffler and David, 1975). Part of the ITL signal recognized by syngeneic RTL may therefore be Ia structures. This would explain the need in recruitment for syngeny at the K end of the H-2 region, which could contain I subregions.

The particular sensitivity of T lymphocytes to syngeneic MHC products has been demonstrated in two additional systems. Shearer (1974) found that

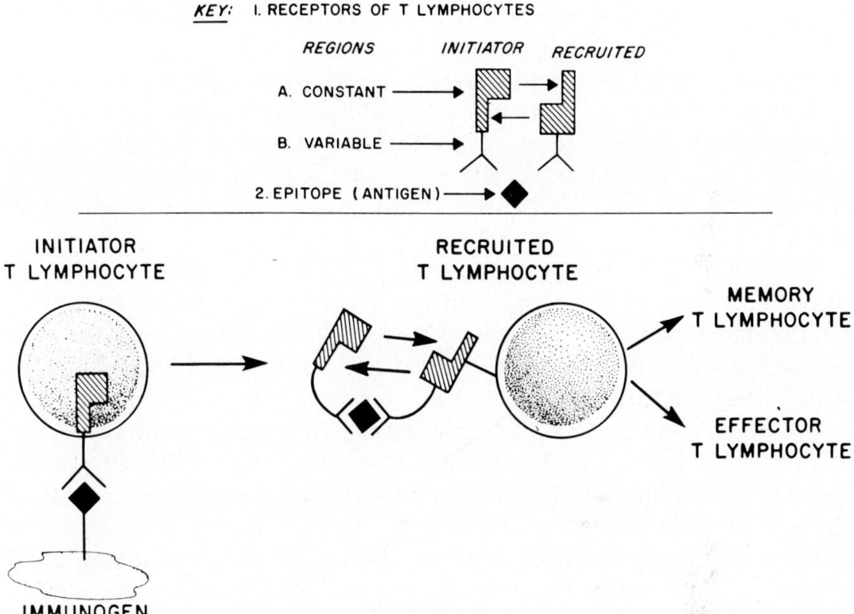

Fig. 2. Recruited T lymphocyte-activated by-product of sensitized syngeneic initiator T lymphocyte. The receptors of the initiator and recruited T lymphocytes are shown as complexes of constant and variable regions. The variable regions include the receptors that recognize the complementary epitope or antigen. The variable regions, therefore, comprise the specific idiotype which the two lymphocytes have in common. The constant regions of their receptors are presumed to interact in a form of self-recognition (after Cohen and Livnat, 1976a). These constant regions could differ in a way characteristic for initiator or recruited T lymphocytes, consonant with their different immune functions. The constant regions might be the products of immune response (I) genes of the major histocompatibility complex. The initiator T lymphocyte is activated by epitope presented on the surface of a cell (e.g., an allogeneic fibroblast or antigen-bearing syngeneic macrophage). The recruited T lymphocyte is activated by the double signal of the sensitized syngeneic initiator T lymphocyte (or its product) plus the epitope. Memory and effector T lymphocytes are then generated.

modification of lymphocytes with trinitrophenyl (TNP) endowed them with the ability to stimulate normal unmodified syngeneic lymphocytes to differentiate into effector cells. These effector lymphocytes were active only against TNP-modified target cells that were identical with the stimulating cells at certain H-2 complex subregions. Forman (1975) studied the effects of F_1 hybrid lymphocytes against TNP-modified target cells of the parental strains. Since the F_1 expresses the H-2 haplotypes of both parental strains, it was possible to test whether H-2 identity served merely to allow cell contact or whether the particular H-2 product was recognized as a component of the TNP-modified target. He found that only parental target cells syngeneic with the particular parental stimulator cells were lysed; the other parental target cells were not killed even though they were H-2 compatible. Thus, recognition of H-2 subregions was involved in the killing reaction, and the requirement for H-2 identity was not merely to allow cell contact.

Zinkernagel and Doherty (1974) have found that syngeneic lymphocytes infected with lymphocytic choriomengitis (LCM) virus stimulated a cytolytic response against LCM-infected target cells. The target cells were not recognized unless they shared parts of the H-2 complex with the attacking lymphocytes (see Chapter 12).

The observation by Opelz and colleagues (1975) that human T cells are stimulated by autologous B cells suggests that recognition of self may be involved in T–B interactions as well as in T–T interactions. Further study of this system might clarify this possibility.

In short, findings derived from a number of different experimental systems indicate that recognition of syngeneic MHC products, possibly Ia structures (Katz and Benacerraf, 1972; Benacerraf and McDevitt, 1972) is necessary for interactions between T lymphocytes, as well as between T and B lymphocytes. The ITL–RTL recruitment system suggests that this type of recognition of self has a physiological function in the sequential chain reaction of T lymphocytes (Cohen and Livnat, 1976a). The ready induction of autosensitization against MHC products on fibroblasts or thymus reticulum cells discussed above (Section II,B) is another example of this predisposition. It is conceivable, therefore, that the blocking factors (self-MHC antigens?), which we detected in autologous serum (Cohen and Wekerle, 1973), have a physiological role in regulating cellular interactions as well as autosensitization.

A corollary of the concept that recognition of self can activate the immune response is that the strength of some immunogenic stimuli may be related more to their resemblance to "self" than to their degree of "foreignness." The GVH reaction may provide a working example. This reaction develops when competent T lymphocytes are grafted into a host that is antigenically foreign to the lymphocytes (Simonsen, 1962). A susceptible host is one that is unable to reject the grafted lymphocytes and, so, is either immature, immunosuppressed, or the F_1 hybrid of the strain of the grafted lymphocytes with another parental strain. The grafted lymphocytes are stimulated and attack the host to produce a GVH reaction.

The strongest GVH reactions are stimulated when the host is allogeneic for MHC genes. Paradoxically, a xenogeneic host, with a relatively greater antigenic disparity stimulates, as a rule, a much weaker GVH response than an allogeneic host (Lafferty *et al.*, 1972). This anomaly may result from a greater cross-reactivity of allogeneic lymphocytes with sensitized self-ITL. We have found that RTL activated by sensitized syngeneic ITL include the precursors of specific GVH reactive lymphocytes (Cohen and Livnat, 1976a,b). This means that the same RTL that recognize allosensitized syngeneic ITL also recognize allogeneic stimulator lymphocytes in the GVH. RTL recognize the double signal of sensitized ITL (an Ia product?) plus an epitope. Hence, allogeneic lymphocytes probably provide both components of this double signal. Since they are foreign, their MHC products present epitopes. In addition to the degree to which their MHC products cross-react with activated syngeneic ITL, allogeneic lymphocytes provide the required second part of the signal. Allogeneic lymphocytes, thus, bypass syngeneic ITL and directly activate RTL-, GVH-reactive lymphocytes. Xenogeneic or "weak" allogeneic histoincompatible lymphocytes are less cross-reactive with self-ITL. Hence, their epitopes activate the immune response arc by way of ITL as do conventional foreign antigens. Thus, the unique strength of the allogeneic GVH reaction may be due to cross-reactivity between allogeneic and self-Ia products (Cohen and Livnat, 1976b).

Lafferty and Cunningham (1975) have proposed that strong allogeneic stimulator cells bear a species-specific proliferation signal in addition to antigen. They also suggest that this signal has a physiological function in interactions between syngeneic lymphocytes.

What kind of RTL receptor molecules recognize the double signal of ITL structure (Ia?) plus an epitope, and how is this signal prepared and presented by the ITL to the RTL? These questions should be answered as we develop sensitive *in vitro* systems capable of analyzing the ITL–RTL interaction.

C. An Immune System

At least two generalizations may be derived from the material reviewed in this chapter. The first is that the immune system is a true system, and, as such, obeys the fundamental principle that its components are regulated by the products of the system itself, in addition to responding to inputs from outside of the system, the antigens (Fig. 3). Antibodies, one of the outputs of the immune system, function as regulatory inputs when combined with antigen as complexes or when recognized, in turn, as antigens to stimulate anti-idiotypes, or even rheumatoid factors (Pope *et al.*, 1974). Products of the MHC, possibly parts of the receptors or extracellular factors of certain T cells, are recognized by other lymphocytes, which may be helped, sup-

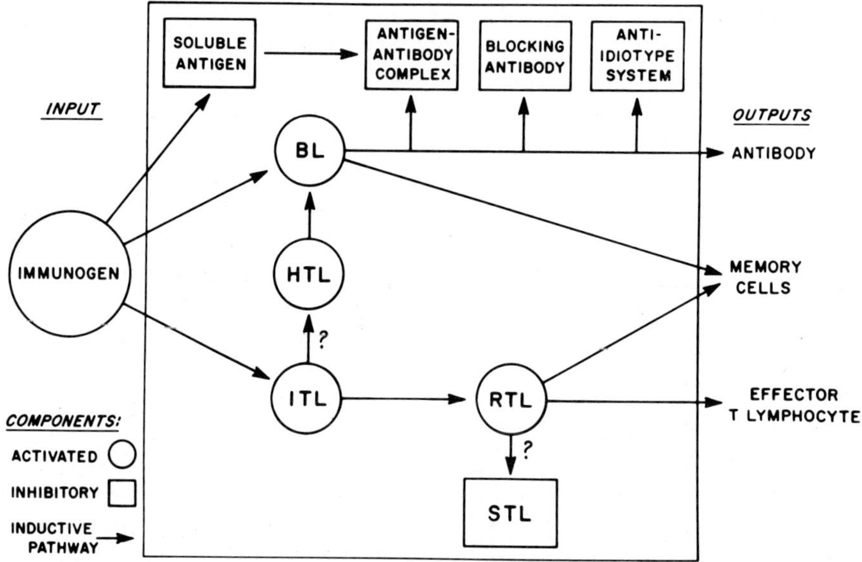

Fig. 3. An immune system. A block diagram illustrates points discussed in the text. Immunogen is the input into the immune system. The outputs are antibody, the product of B lymphocytes (BL); effector T lymphocytes (ETL); and memory cells, comprising both B and T lymphocytes. Activated components of the system, which facilitate development of the outputs, are written in circles. The squares signify inhibitory components which are agents of negative feedback. The arrows indicate inductive pathways between input, components, and outputs. Immunogen activates BL and initiator T lymphocytes (ITL). BL produce antibody and memory B cells. ITL activate recruited T lymphocytes (RTL) and possibly helper T lymphocytes (HTL). The latter facilitate the induction of antibody production by BL. RTL give rise to ETL and memory T cells. Suppressor T lymphocytes (STL) are shown as hypothetically resulting from the activation of RTL. Other negative feedback components include soluble blocking antigen that is a product of the immunogen itself; antigen–antibody complex; and blocking antibody. The anti-idiotype system represents a regulatory subsystem in which the idiotype of the antibody (or the receptors of the activated lymphocytes) function as inputs to activate an anti-idiotype response by other B or T lymphocytes.

pressed, or recruited. Receptors may be stimulated or blocked by antigen, or by-products of the immune system alone, or by combinations of the two.

The second generalization is that knowledge of the details of these regulatory interactions is woefully incomplete. Each method we use to analyze the immune system probably activates above the threshold of detection only a different selected small number of the system's components. The call to consider the immune system as a network analogous to the nervous system is timely and should stimulate the development of new experimental methods (Jerne, 1974a,b). The biologic functions of blocking factors discussed in this chapter might then be tested.

ACKNOWLEDGMENTS

We thank Drs. B. David Stollar, Yves Borel, Chaim Shustik, and Syamal Datta for editorial comments and discussions. Dr. Robert S. Schwartz was particularly helpful in providing the intellectual and physical environment that made possible the writing of this chapter. Finally, we thank our Chiefs, Professors, Herbert Fischer, and Michael Feldman for their continued support and guidance.

REFERENCES

Ada, G. L., and Cooper, M. G. (1971). *Ann. N.Y. Acad. Sci.* **181,** 96–107.

Aldo-Benson, M., and Borel, Y. (1974). *J. Immunol.* **112,** 1793–1803.

Aldo-Benson, M., and Borel, Y. (1976). *J. Immunol.* **116,** 223–226.

Alexander, P. (1974). *Cancer Res.* **34,** 2077–2082.

Allison, A. C. (1971). *Lancet* **2,** 1401–1403.

Allison, A. C. (1974). *In* "Immunological Tolerance" (D. H. Katz and B. Benacerraf, eds.), pp. 25–49. Academic Press, New York.

Allison, A. C., Denman, A. M., and Barnes, R. D. (1971). *Lancet* **2,** 135–140.

Anonymous. (1972). *Transplant. Rev.* **12,** 3–228.

Amerding, D., Sachs, D. H., and Katz, D. H. (1974). *J. Exp. Med.* **140,** 1717–1722.

Asherson, G. L., and Ptak, W. (1968). *Immunology* **15,** 405–416.

Baldwin, R. W., Price, M. R., and Robins, R. A. (1972). *Nature* (*London*), *New Biol.* **238,** 185–187.

Bangasser, S. A., Kapsalis, A. A., Fraker, P. J., and Nisonoff, A. (1975). *J. Immunol.* **114,** 610–614.

Bankhurst, A. D., Torrigiani, G., and Allison, A. C. (1973). *Lancet* **1,** 226–230.

Barnes, R. D. (1976). *Transplant. Proc.* **8,** 359–362.

Baxley, G., Bishop, G. B., Cooper, A. G., and Wortis, H. H. (1973). *Clin. Exp. Immunol.* **15,** 385–392.

Benacerraf, B., and McDevitt, H. O. (1972). *Science* **175,** 273–279.

Bergstrand, H., and Källén, B. (1972). *Cell. Immunol.* **3,** 660–671.

Binz, H., and Wigzell, H. (1975). *J. Exp. Med.* **142,** 197–211, 1218–1230, and 1231–1240.

Borel, Y. (1971). *Nature* (*London*), *New Biol.* **230,** 180–182.

Borel, Y., Lewis, R. M., and Stollar, B. D. (1973). *Science* **182,** 76–78.

Borel, Y., Reinisch, C. L., and Schlossman, S. F. (1975). *J. Exp. Med.* **142,** 1254–1262.

Borel, Y., Golan, D. T., Kilham, L., and Borel, H. (1976). *J. Immunol.* (in press).

Brownstone, A., Mitchison, N. A., and Pitt-Rivers, R. (1966). *Immunology* **10,** 481–492.

Burnet, F. M. (1959). "The Clonal Selection Theory of Acquired Immunity." Vanderbilt Univ. Press, Nashville, Tennessee.

Capra, H. D., and Kehoe, J. M. (1975). *Adv. Immunol.* **20,** 1–40.

Chiller, H. M., Habicht, G. S., and Weigle, W. O. (1971). *Science* **171,** 813–815.

Clagget, J. A., and Weigle, W. O. (1974). *J. Exp. Med.* **139,** 643–660.

Cohen, I. R. (1937a). *Nature* (*London*), *New Biol.* **242,** 60–61.

Cohen, I. R. (1973b). *Cell. Immunol.* **8,** 209–220.

Cohen, I. R. (1973c). *Eur. J. Immunol.* **3,** 829–833.

Cohen, I. R., and Feldman, M. (1971a). *In* "Morphological and Fundamental Aspects of Immunity" (K. Lindahl-Kiessling, M. G. Hanna, Jr., and G. V. Alm, eds.), pp. 371–377. Plenum, New York.

Cohen, I. R., and Feldman, M. (1971b). *Cell. Immunol.* **1,** 521–535.

Cohen, I. R., and Livnat, S. (1976a). *Transplant. Rev.* **29,** 24–58.

Cohen, I. R., and Livnat, S. (1976b). *Transplant. Proc.* **8,** 393–397.

Cohen, I. R., and Wekerle, H. (1972). *Science* **176,** 1324–1325.

Cohen, I. R., and Wekerle, H. (1973). *J. Exp. Med.* **137,** 224–238.

Cohen, I. R., and Wekerle, H. (1974). *Prog. Immunol., Int. Congr. Immunol., 2nd, 1974,* Vol. 5, pp. 5–14.

Cohen, I. R., Globerson, A., and Feldman, M. (1971a). *J. Exp. Med.* **133,** 821–833.

Cohen, I. R., Globerson, A., and Feldman, M. (1971b). *J. Exp. Med.* **133,** 834–845.

Cohen, I. R., Wekerle, H., and Feldman, M. (1974). *Isr. J. Med. Sci.* **10,** 1024–1032.

Crone, M., Koch, C., and Simonsen, M. (1972). *Transplant. Rev.* **10,** 36–56.

Currie, G. A., and Basham, C. (1972). *Br. J. Cancer* **26,** 427–438.

Dickler, H. B., and Kunkel, H. C. (1972). *J. Exp. Med.* **136,** 191–196.

Diener, E., and Feldmann, M. (1972). *Transplant. Rev.* **8,** 76–103.

Doljanski, F. (1973). *Isr. J. Med. Sci.* **9,** 251–257.

Eichmann, K. (1975). *Eur. J. Immunol.* **5,** 511–517.

Einstein, E. R., Robertson, D. M., DiCapro, J. M., and Moore, W. (1962). *J. Neurochem.* **9,** 353–361.

Feldman, M., Cohen, I. R., and Wekerle, H. (1972). *Transplant. Rev.* **12,** 57–90.

Feldmann, M. (1972). *J. Exp. Med.* **136,** 532–545.

Forman, S. (1975). *J. Exp. Med.* **142,** 403–417.

Gershon, R. K. (1974). *Contemp. Top. Immunobiol.* **3,** 1–40.

Ginsburg, H. (1968). *Immunology* **14,** 621–635.

Golan, D. T., and Borel, Y. (1971). *J. Exp. Med.* **134,** 1046–1061.

Gonatas, N. K., and Howard, J. C. (1974). *Science* **186,** 839–841.

Gorczynski, R., Kontiainen, S., Mitchison, N. A., and Tigelaar, R. E. (1974). *In* "Cellular Selection and Regulation in the Immune Response" (G. M. Edelman, ed.), pp. 143–154. Raven, New York.

Habicht, G. S., Chiller, J. M., and Weigle, W. O. (1975). *J. Exp. Med.* **142,** 312–320.

Hellström, I., and Hellström, K. E. (1969). *Int. J. Cancer* **5,** 195–201.

Hellström, I., and Hellström, K. E. (1972). *Nature* (*London*) **240,** 471–473.

Hellström, I., Hellström, K. E., and Allison, A. C. (1971). *Nature* (*London*) **230,** 49–50.

Hellström, K. E., and Hellström, I. (1974). *Adv. Immunol.* **18,** 209–277.

Herzenberg, L. A., Chan, E. L., Ravitch, M. M., Riblet, R. J., and Herzenberg, L. A. (1973). *J. Exp. Med.* **137,** 1311–1324.

Hill, O. W. (1961). *Br. Med. J.* **1,** 1793–1796.

Hoffmann, G. W. (1975). *Eur. J. Immunol.* **5,** 638–647.

Howard, J. G., and Mitchison, N. A. (1975). *Prog. Allergy* **18,** 43–96.

Ilfeld, D., Carnaud, C., and Kiein, E. (1975). *Immunogenetics* **2,** 231–240.

Janeway, C. A., Jr., Sakato, N., and Eisen, H. N. (1975). *Proc. Natl. Acad. Sci. U.S.A.* **72,** 2357–2360.

Jerne, N. K. (1973). *Sci. Am.* **229,** 52–60.

Jerne, N. K. (1974a). *In* "Cellular Selection and Regulation in the Immune Response" (G. M. Edelman, ed.), pp. 39–48. Raven, New York.

Jerne, N. K. (1974b). *Ann. Immunol.* (*Paris*) **125,** 373–389.

Kaliss, N. (1966). *Ann. N.Y. Acad. Sci.* **129,** 155–163.

Katz, D. H., and Benacerraf, B. (1972). *Adv. Immunol.* **15,** 1–94.

Kilburn, D. G., Smith, J., and Gorczynski, R. (1974). *Eur. J. Immunol.* **4,** 784–788.

Kirchner, H., Chused, T. M., Herberman, R. B., Holden, H. T., and Larvin, D. H. (1974). *J. Exp. Med.* **139,** 1473–1487.

Kluskens, L., and Köhler, H. (1974). *Proc. Natl. Acad. Sci. U.S.A.* **71,** 5083–5087.

Köhler, H. (1975). *Transplant. Rev.* **27,** 24–56.

Köhler, H., Kaplan, D. R., and Strayer, D. S. (1974). *Science* **186,** 643–644.

Lafferty, K. J., and Cunningham, A. J. (1975). *Aust. J. Exp. Biol. Med. Sci.* **53,** 27–42.

Lafferty, K. J., Walder, K. Z., Scollay, R. G., and Killby, V. A. A. (1972). *Transplant. Rev.* **12,** 198–228.

Livnat, S., and Cohen, I. R. (1975a). *Eur. J. Immunol.* **5,** 357–360.

Livnat, S., and Cohen, I. R. (1975b). *Eur. J. Immunol.* **5,** 389–394.

McKearn, T. J., Stuart, F. P., and Fitch, F. W. (1974). *J. Immunol.* **113,** 1876–1882.

Marchalonis, J. J., Cone, R. E., and Artwell, J. L. (1972). *J. Exp. Med.* **135,** 956–971.

Meo, T., Matsunaga, T., and Rijnbeek, A. M. (1973). *Transplant. Proc.* **5,** 1607–1610.

Moorhead, J. W., Walters, C. S., and Claman, H. N. (1973). *J. Exp. Med.* **137,** 411–423.

Munroe, A. J., Taussig, M. J., Campbell, R., Williams, H., and Lawson, Y. (1974). *J. Exp. Med.* **140,** 1579–1587.

Nakamura, R. M., and Weigle, W. O. (1969). *J. Exp. Med.* **130,** 263–283.

Nisonoff, A., and Bangasser, S. A. (1975). *Transplant. Rev.* **27,** 100–134.

Nossal, G. J. V., and Pike, B. L. (1974). *In* "Immunological Tolerance" (D. H. Katz and B. Benacerraf, eds.), pp. 351–364. Academic Press, New York.

Nossal, G. J. V., Pike, B. L., and Katz, O. H. (1973). *J. Exp. Med.* **138,** 312–317.

Opelz, G., Kiuchi, M., Takasugi, M., and Terasaki, P. I. (1975). *J. Exp. Med.* **142,** 1327–1333.

Orgad, S., and Cohen, I. R. (1974). *Science* **183,** 1083–1085.

Paley, R. S., Leskowitz, S., and Borel, Y. (1975). *J. Immunol.* **115,** 1409–1413.

Parker, D. C. (1975). *Nature* (*London*) **258,** 361–363.

Paterson, P. Y. (1966). *Adv. Immunol.* **5,** 131–208.

Paterson, P. Y., and Harwin, S. M. (1963). *J. Exp. Med.* **117,** 755–774.

Pawlak, I. L., Hart, D. A., and Nisonoff, A. (1973). *J. Exp. Med.* **137,** 1442–1458.

Phillips, S. M., and Wegmann, T. G. (1973). *J. Exp. Med.* **137,** 291–300.

Pope, R. M., Teller, D. C., and Mannik, M. (1974). *Proc. Natl. Acad. Sci. U.S.A.* **71,** 517–521.

Raff, M. C., Owen, J. J. T., Cooper, M. D., Lawton, A. R., III, Megson, M., and Gathings, W. E. (1975). *J. Exp. Med.* **142,** 1052–1064.

Ramsier, H. (1974). *J. Exp. Med.* **140,** 603–618.

Ramsier, H., and Lindenmann, J. (1971). *J. Exp. Med.* **134,** 1083–1094.

Ran, M., and Witz, I. P. (1972). *Int. J. Cancer* **9,** 242–247.

Richter, P. H. (1975). *Eur. J. Immunol.* **5,** 350–354.

Ringertz, B., Wasserman, J., Packalou, T. L., and Perlmann, P. (1971). *Int. Arch. Allergy Appl. Immunol.* **40,** 918–927.

Russell, A. S., Liburd, E. M., and Diener, E. (1974). *Nature* (*London*) **249,** 43–45.

Samter, M. (1971). "Immunological Diseases," 2nd ed. Little, Brown, Boston, Massachusetts.

Shearer, G. M. (1974). *Eur. J. Immunol.* **4,** 527–533.

Shreffler, D. C., and David, C. S. (1975). *Adv. Immunol.* **20,** 125–195.

Simonsen, M. (1962). *Prog. Allergy* **6,** 349–467.

Sjöberg, O. (1972). *J. Exp. Med.* **135,** 850–859.

Sjögren, H. O., Hellström, I., Bansal, S. C., and Hellström, K. E. (1971). *Proc. Natl. Acad. Sci. U.S.A.* **68,** 1372–1375.

Steinman, L., Cohen, I. R., Teitelbaum, D., and Arnon, R. (1977). *Nature* (*London*) **265,** 173–175.

Stoller, B. D., and Borel, Y. (1975). *J. Immunol.* **115,** 1095–1100.

Stout, R. D., and Herzenberg, L. A. (1975). *J. Exp. Med.* **142,** 611–621.

Strayer, D. S., Cosenza, H., Lee, W. M. F., Rowley, D. A., and Köhler, H. (1974). *Science* **186,** 640–643.

Taylor, R. B. (1969). *Transplant. Rev.* **1,** 114–149.

Teitelbaum, D., Meshorer, A., Hirshfield, T., Arnon, R., and Sela, M. (1971). *Eur. J. Immunol.* **1,** 242–248.

Teitelbaum, D., Webb, C., Meshorer, A., Arnon, R., and Sela, M. (1972). *Nature* (*London*) **240,** 564–566.

Torrigiani, G., Doniach, D., and Roitt, I. M. (1969). *J. Clin. Endocrinol. Metab.* **29,** 305–314.

Trenkner, E., and Riblet, R. (1975). *J. Exp. Med.* **142,** 1121–1132.

Treves, A. J., and Cohen, I. R. (1973). *J. Natl. Cancer Inst.* **51,** 1919–1925.

Treves, A. J., Carnaud, C., Trainin, N., Feldman, M., and Cohen, I. R. (1974). *Eur. J. Immunol.* **4,** 722–727.

Vladutiu, R. O., and Rose, N. R. (1971). *J. Immunol.* **106,** 1139–1142.
Voisin, G. A. (1971). *Prog. Allergy* **15,** 328–485.
Voisin, G. A., Kinsky, R. G., and Duc, H. T. (1972). *J. Exp. Med.* **135,** 1185–1203.
Webb, C., Teitelbaum, D., Arnon, R., and Sela, M. (1973). *Eur. J. Immunol.* **3,** 279–286.
Weens, J. H., and Schwartz, R. S. (1974). *Ser. Haematol.* **7,** 303–327.
Wegmann, T. G., Hellström, I., and Hellström, K. E. (1971). *Proc. Natl. Acad. Sci. U.S.A.* **68,** 1644–1647.
Weigle, W. O. (1971). *Clin. Exp. Immunol.* **9,** 437–477.
Wekerle, H., and Begemann, M. (1976). *J. Immunol.* **116,** 159–177.
Wekerle, H., Lonai, P., and Feldman, M. (1972). *Proc. Natl. Acad. Sci. U.S.A.* **69,** 1620–1624.
Wekerle, H., Cohen, I. R., and Feldman, M. (1973). *Nature* (*London*), *New Biol.* **241,** 25–26.
Wigzell, H. (1973). *Contemp. Top. Immunobiol.* **3,** 77–96.
Yamashita, U., and Kitagawa, M. (1974). *Cell. Immunol.* **14,** 182–192.
Yung, L. L. L., Diener, E., McPherson, A., Barton, M. A., and Hyde, H. A. (1973). *J. Immunol.* **110,** 1383–1387.
Zembala, M., and Asherson, G. L. (1973). *Nature* (*London*) **244,** 227–228.
Zinkernagel, R., and Doherty, P. (1974). *Nature* (*London*) **248,** 701–702.

Chapter 10

Self-Recognition: The Basic Principle in the Immune System

HEINZ KÖHLER AND DONALD A. ROWLEY

I. INTRODUCTION

Plato's imperative of self-recognition (γνῶτον σεαυτόν) has had its impact on western philosophy and formed our humanistic view on life and matter. Freud followed this call for self-recognition, attempting to penetrate into the area of subconsciousness. The school of Lorenz and his followers, studying inherited instinctive behavior, enlightened us further on the mechanics of animal and human behavior and motivation.

In more recent times, other examples of self-recognition have been recognized, and models have been designed to account for phenomena, such as cell–cell recognition during differentiation and ontogeny, or the construction of circuits and cell networks in the central nervous system through cell–cell contacts. While the molecular basis of self-recognition in these systems is still largely unresolved, we may learn more about the molecular and cellular basis of a self-recognizing system by considering self-recognition in the immune system. This system consists of specialized cells carrying receptor molecules, some of them producing immunoglobulin molecules that are copies of the receptors. The chemical and three-dimensional structure of the immunoglobulins is known in great detail (Poljak, 1975), and the specification of cells in the immune system that produce immunoglobulins or are required for their production can also be defined with precision. Thus, the immune system, being one of the best understood "cellular organs" at the molecular level, could serve as an excellent model for studying the phenomenon of self-recognition. While we believe the knowledge of this system will be essential for understanding the pathology of autoimmunity, we suspect that autoimmune diseases are only aberrations of a system whose primary function may be as much concerned with self-recognition as with defense against agents that are not self.

The concept of self-recognition in the immune system was first discussed by Jerne (1955) and Burnet (1959). Both authors concluded that certain clones of immunocompetent cells can distinguish between self-antigens and non-self-antigens, and that this discrimination served as the operational basis for selecting and favoring clones recognizing nonself over clones which recognize self. The first demonstration that antibodies can be the target for recognition by immune cells was made (Oudin and Michell, 1963; Kunkel *et al.*, 1963) by showing that antigen-specific structures of antibodies can be antigenic in the same or different species. Recent work by several investigators (Sirisinha and Eisen, 1971; Yakulis *et al.*, 1972; Rodkey, 1974) shows that an animal can recognize its own immunoglobulins and mount an immune response against them, which is specific for the antigen-specific portion of the molecule (V region). Thus, the potential of self-recognition has been clearly demonstrated in the immune system. The following discussion will deal with this phenomenon and will attempt to indicate the biologic and evolutionary significance of autoimmunity in the function and evolution of the immune system.

II. SELF-RECOGNITION IN THE IMMUNE SYSTEM

The immune system can be described in most general terms as an ensemble of lymphoid cells and immunoglobulin molecules, both of which collectively are endowed with the capacity to recognize a great diversity of different structures, the antigens. During an immune response, several different cell types of the system interact. For example, B and T cells have to collaborate for the production of antibodies. Since both cell types have receptors for different portions of the antigen, it has been reasoned that antigen provides the link between T and B cells. However, recent evidence shows that B and T cells also can interact with each other in the absence of exogenous antigen. The target in this latter kind of interaction are the receptors on the cell surface. B cell receptors are immunoglobulins that are close copies of the antibodies secreted by the cells.

The existence of unique structures of the antigen receptors was demonstrated by using antisera directed against the antigen-specific portion of antibody molecule (V region); such anti-antibodies are referred to as "anti-idiotypic antibody." These studies suggest that B and T cells can have identical antigen-specific idiotypic structures (Ramseier and Lindemann, 1972; McKearn, 1974; Binz and Wigzell, 1975). B and T cells can be stimulated or suppressed by anti-idiotypic antibody (Cosenza and Köhler, 1972; Hart *et al.*, 1972; Eichmann, 1975), and T or B cells primed by the anti-idiotype or the idiotype can suppress or stimulate each other (Eichmann and Rajewski, 1975; Eichmann, 1975).

Though the interactions of different cells of an organism, based on the recognition of cell surface determinants, are common events during differentiation, the mutual recognition by different immune cells deserves special consideration, since these interactions are interrelated with the discrimination of self and nonself by the immune system.

To exemplify the phenomenon of autorecognition during the immune response, we will discuss the response of mice to the small epitope, phosphorylcholine (PC) (Köhler, 1975). Mice have antibodies against phosphorylcholine, which occur in two forms: one is a family of myeloma proteins which binds PC; the other, antibodies induced in normal mice by immunization with PC-containing antigens. Some of the PC–myeloma proteins share specific determinants with the induced anti-PC antibodies. These shared determinants are collectively referred to as the TEPC-15 (T15) idiotype. Normal Balb/c mice, the mouse strain from which the transplantable myeloma tumor TEPC-15 originated, can be immunized with the T15 idiotype to produce antibodies against the T15 idiotype (Beatty *et al.*, 1976). If Balb/c mice are immunized with PC antigen, they produce first antibodies to PC and, subsequently, antibodies against the T15 idiotypes (Kluskens and Köhler, 1974, Cosenza, 1976). Furthermore, small amounts of idiotype and anti-idiotype can be detected in serum of normal Balb/c mice (H. Köhler, unpublished). Thus, Balb/c mice have the potential to produce the idiotype and the anti-idiotype, and both can be produced by the same animal at the same time. Since idiotype and anti-idiotype are defined as unique structures of an individual or inbred strain, the finding of an idiotype–anti-idiotype response represents a case of autorecognition in the immune response. Similar observations on the simultaneous production of idiotype and anti-idiotype have been made in rats (McKearn *et al.*, 1974).

III. THE EFFECTS OF AUTOIMMUNE RESPONSES: CONTROL OF THE EXPRESSION OF RECEPTORS

To study the influence an anti-idiotypic antibody might have on the expression of the idiotype in Balb/c, we first used a "reagent" anti-idiotypic serum prepared in a different strain of mice, the A strain. Giving reagent anti-idiotypic antibody to Balb/c mice passively, or adding the antibody to spleen cells from Balb/c before or at the time of immunization with PC antigen, suppresses the response to PC completely (Cosenza and Köhler, 1972). In the animal, the suppression lasts as long as the passively given antibody persists; however, a long-lasting unresponsiveness to PC is induced by giving anti-idiotype sera to neonatal Balb/c mice (Strayer *et al.*, 1975). Those treated animals, as adults, seem to lack the T15 clone and are unable to respond to PC (Köhler *et al.*, 1974), though cells from these unresponsive animals can suppress the response in culture to PC by normal cells. The suppressing cells may include B cells, as well as T cells (DuClos *et al.*, 1976). Most investigators would interpret this to indicate active suppression, which maintains a state of apparent clonal depletion. But it is equally possible that the anti-idiotypic serum given neonatally may, in fact, decrease the clone of cells responding to PC, while leaving the "complementary" or regulating clone unchanged or amplified in number. The preservation of this regulating clone is then demonstrable by adding cells of the unresponsive mice to normal cells.

These experiments using "reagent" anti-idiotypic sera as anti-receptor antibody (ARA) suggested that ARA might be involved in the autoregulation of the immune response (Köhler, 1975). The following observations demonstrate that this phenomenon occurs: repeated immunization with PC induced T15-specific ARA and a concomitant suppression of the response to PC (Lee and Köhler, 1974; Kluskens and Köhler, 1974). If mice were immunized with the idiotype T15 and produced ARA, they could not respond to PC (Rowley *et al.*, 1976). Alternatively, if mice are first immunized with PC to produce the T15 idiotype, they were suppressed to subsequent immunization with T15. These results show that the first induced antibody response may function as an anti-receptor antibody for a subsequently induced response when both responses have an idiotype–anti-idiotype relationship. But it was also observed that, when both responses were induced at about the same time, both responses could be detected in the same animal at the same time (Rowley *et al.*, 1976). It might be possible to correlate ARA-induced suppression with observations of modulation of membrane receptors. Microaggregation of receptor molecules can be induced by the ligand or by specific antibody against the receptor. This modulation of receptors may be an *in vitro* correlate of suppression by auto-ARA in the same way as antigen is believed to trigger the cell by inducing receptor modulation (Edelman, 1976).

Using specific antisera against the receptor idiotype, we have observed receptor movement with indirect fluorescence staining of idiotype-bearing cells. The antisera used suppressed specifically the response to PC and, thus, could function as anti-receptor antibody (ARA). The demonstration of auto-ARA during the immune response or even in the nonstimulated animal suggests that, depending on the amount of idiotype and anti-idiotype in the circulation at a given time, the receptor molecules might be modulated to different degrees. Thus, varying the net activities of auto-ARA during the immune response might control the expression of receptors by keeping the cell-surface receptor in different states of modulation. If the arrangement of receptors on the surface is important for the stimulation of the cell, then this proposed mechanism of modulation by auto-ARA would be an effective way to control the response.

IV. THE CONCEPT OF THE INTERACTION OF COMPLEMENTARY CLONES

The identity of an antibody can be described in two ways: by its epitope having a K_a value of 10^{-5} or higher and by the presence of unique determinants, which are recognized by specific antibody (anti-idiotypes). Very close association between the epitope specificity and the idiotype determinants has been observed (Hopper and Nisonoff, 1971). Idiotypic determinants very near the binding site are described as ligand modifiable. But even for idiotypic determinants more removed from the binding site, a stringent linkage to the epitope specificity seems to be the rule. Thus, it is reasonable to assume that the binding of an anti-idiotypic antibody to an idiotypic receptor determinant that is not the binding site produces blocking or stimulation. These effects would be the same as those produced by an anti-idiotype binding exactly to the binding site of the receptor. Therefore, in a functional sense, only the linkage of epitope and idiotype is of importance. With the same reasoning, no difference may occur in the effects generated by the interaction of idiotype and anti-idiotype, whether or not the epitope–idiotype linkage is found on the receptor or the anti-receptor. In both cases, similar effects of suppression or stimulation of the receptor-bearing cells may be expected. Thus, the fact that cells have receptors and can produce antibodies, which bind to receptors specifically, enables certain cell clones to interact with each other in a specific way. The specificity of this clonal interaction is based on the complementarity of receptor and anti-receptor, which resides for both in the variable sequence portion of the immunoglobulin molecule. In the traditional view, and for practical reasons, one antibody is described as "idiotype," and the specific anti-antibody for it as the "anti-idiotype," but, within the concept of a functional relationship between clones of the immune system, this distinction may be nonexistent. An idiotype can be antigen or anti-receptor antibody (ARA), depending entirely on the difference in the activity of complementary clones. The concept of clonal interactions based on complementary idiotype of receptor and anti-receptor is derived from functional interactions and should not be taken to indicate a structural complementarity of the entirety of two binding sites. Complementarity of clones is the minimum requirement for effective interaction of cells but may not be sufficient to achieve regulation of the immune response. In addition, the class of anti-receptor antibody, the amount and duration of activity of the antibody, and the sequence of occurrence of complementary responses may be important in determining whether suppression or stimulation results.

The model of interaction of complementary clones is based on observations in two different species in the response to two different antigens (Köhler, 1975; McKearn *et al.*, 1974). Together, the data support the concept that a clone of cells which carries immunoglobulin receptors may interact with antigen or ARA to induce either suppression or stimulation of the cell. If the ARA is produced by another clone (complementary clone) present in the same organism, both clones may engage in an active "spiel" of stimulation and suppression. In this circumstance, "external" antigen is not required for interaction of the clones; however, exogenous antigen may disturb the equilibrium of complementary clones to initiate events that are observed as response or tolerance.

V. COMPLEMENTARY CLONAL INTERACTION DURING EVOLUTION

Observations in other immune responses are indicative or compatible with the concept of a dual complementary response for each antigen (Bankert and Pressman, 1976; Strosberg, 1976). Clonal interaction may regulate, not only the state of immunity of an individual, but may also have constituted an important force in the evolution of the immune system. The existence of mutual cross-stimulating clones should provide a potent factor in evolution that would select for complementarity. Selection for antigen fit would not necessarily reinforce selection for fit for receptor complementarity; rather, it might counteract selection for strict clonal complementarity and prevent the evolutionary convergence of complementary clones to one set of perfectly complementing clones.

We can attempt to reconstruct the evolutionary development of the immune system by assuming that histocompatibility antigens and immunoglobulins have a common evolutionary origin (Gally and Edelman, 1972). Recent data on the structural homology between immunoglobulins and histocompatibility antigens support the hypothesis that both proteins have evolved from a primordial cell-surface protein, which had the function of a cell recognition marker (Peterson *et al.,* 1975). Mutual cell recognition by surface receptor complementarity should favor development of polymorphism in this locus. Such polymorphism would allow binding to structures not controlled by the receptor locus, i.e., by antigens in a conventional sense. In this way, interaction with external antigen may be a force in the evolution of this locus, which provides protection against exogenous antigens. This evolutionary force would be in addition to the forces that select for external and internal complementarity. Since mutations in one clone not only affects antigen binding, but also the clonal complementarity, the linked selection for external and internal complementation would presumably mount strong selective pressures for a balance between external and internal complementarity. This development, in turn, would lead to the establishment of clusters of clones and anti-clones, which are functionally interconnected by stimulatory and suppressive stimuli (Köhler *et al.,* 1976).

The delineation of complementary idiotype clusters of clones through an evolutionary process permits two statements about the basic function and development of the immune system: (1) stimulation with antigen induces a dual response, one complementary to the antigen and the other complementary to the antigen-specific response; (2) the entire potential for response of a mature organism has developed by evolution and not by ad hoc adaptation during ontogeny. The essential point of this theory leads to the deduction that clonal diversity could evolve and be maintained without external antigenic stimulation. An interesting aspect of this reasoning is that the immune system may be preadapted to new antigens as a consequence of the selection for clonal complementarity. However, the preadaption to external antigen is only apparent and not real, since there is a fundamental structural difference between self-antigens (idiotope) and non-self-antigens (epitope). Because of this, exogenous antigen may increase the diversity of responses by mechanisms discussed above. Still, the question can be asked whether the combination of autoimmunelike interactions of complementary clones and exogenous antigenic stimulation is sufficient to explain antibody diversity. The hypothesis made by Lewontin (1974) that arranging genetic loci into linkage groups favors genetic polymorphism appears to be an argument in support of the germ-line theory of antibody diversity. The proposed dichotomy of clones and anticlones in the immune system lends itself easily to a model in which the genes of complementary clones are arranged in a certain order, allowing Lewontin's principle to become active.

VI. CONCLUSION

The role of autorecognition in the immune system has been discussed in light of recent experimental data. These findings indicate that the recognition of self-determinants on antigen receptors and antibodies is normal, and that self-recognition plays an essential role in the homeostasis of immunity and the control of the immune response. It is proposed that self-recognition played an important role in the evolution of the immune system, permitting the development of clonal diversity by the balance of two selective processes: selection for antigen fit and clonal complementarity. Since autorecognition is normal in a functioning immune system, autoimmune disease may result from an imbalance or other aberration of complementary responses.

REFERENCES

Bankert, R. B., and Pressman, D. J. (1976). *Immunol.* **117,** 457.

Beatty, P. G., Kim, B. S., Rowley, D. A., and Coppleson, L. W. (1976). *J. Immunol.* **116,** 1391.

Binz, H., and Wigzell, H. (1975). *J. Exp. Med.* **142,** 197.

Burnet, F. M. (1959). "The Clonal Selection Theory of Acquired Immunity." Cambridge Univ. Press, London and New York.

Cosenza, H. (1976). *Eur. J. Immunol.* **6,** 114.

Cosenza, H., and Köhler, H. (1972). *Proc. Natl. Acad. Sci. U.S.A.* **69,** 2701.

DuClos, T., Kim, B. S., and Rowley, D. A. (1976). *Fed. Proc., Fed. Am. Soc. Exp. Biol.* **35,** 789.

Edelman, G. M. (1976). *Science* **192,** 218.

Eichmann, K. (1975). *Eur. J. Immunol.* **5,** 511.

Eichmann, K., and Rajewski, K. (1975). *Eur. J. Immunol.* **5,** 661.

Gally, J. A., and Edelman, G. M. (1972). *Annu. Rev. Genet.* **6,** 1.

Hart, D. A., Wang, A. L., Pawlak, L. L., and Nisonoff, A. (1972). *J. Exp. Med.* **135,** 1293.

Hopper, J. E., and Nisonoff, A. (1971). *Adv. Immunol.* **13,** 57.

Janeway, C. A., Sakato, N., and Eisen, H. (1975). *Proc. Natl. Acad. Sci. U.S.A.* **72,** 2357.

Jerne, N. K. (1955). *Proc. Natl. Acad. Sci. U.S.A.* **41,** 849.

Köhler, H. (1975). *Transplant. Rev.* **27,** 26.

Köhler, H., Strayer, D. S., and Kaplan, D. R. (1974). *Science* **186,** 643.

Köhler, H., Rowley, D. A., DuClos, T., and Richardson, B. (1976). *Fed. Proc., Fed. Am. Soc. Exp. Biol.* **36,** 221.
Kluskens, L., and Köhler, H. (1974). *Proc. Natl. Acad. Sci. U.S.A.* **71,** 5083.
Kunkel, H. G., Mannik, M., and Williams, R. C. (1963). *Science* **140,** 1218.
Lee, W., and Köhler, H. (1974). *J. Immunol.* **113,** 1644.
Lewontin, R. C. (1974). "The Genetic Basis of Evolutionary Change." Columbia Univ. Press, New York.
McKearn, T. J. (1974). *Science* **183,** 94.
McKearn, T. J., Stuart, F. P., and Fitch, F. W. (1974). *J. Immunol.* **113,** 1876.
Oudin, J., and Michel, M. (1963). *C. R. Seances Acad. Agric. Fr.* **257,** 805.
Peterson, P. A., Rask, L., Sege, K., Klareskog, L., Anundi, H., and Östberg, L. (1975). *Proc. Natl. Acad. Sci. U.S.A.* **72,** 1612.
Poljak, R. J. (1975). *Adv. Immunol.* **21,** 1.
Ramseier, H., and Lindemann, J. (1972). *Eur. J. Immunol.* **2,** 109.
Rodkey, L. S. (1974). *J. Exp. Med.* **139,** 712.
Rowley, D. A., Köhler, H., Schreiber, H., and Lorbach, I. (1976). *J. Exp. Med.* **144,** 946.
Sirisinha, S., and Eisen, H. N. (1971). *Proc. Natl. Acad. Sci. U.S.A.* **68,** 3130.
Strayer, D. S., Lee, W., Rowley, D. A., and Köhler, H. (1975). *J. Immunol.* **114,** 728.
Strosberg, A. D. (1976). *Biochem. Soc. Trans.* **4,** 41.
Yakulis, V., Bhoopalam, N., and Heller, P. (1972). *J. Immunol.* **108,** 1119.

Chapter 11

The Biology of Immune Complexes

ALAN O. HAAKENSTAD AND MART MANNIK

I. INTRODUCTION

Immune complexes or antigen–antibody complexes are formed by the interaction of antigenic substances and antibodies with specificity to the antigenic substance. The production of antibodies is an important host defense mechanism for neutralizing and removing infectious microorganisms and other foreign materials that enter the internal milieu of the host. It is clear, however, that the formation of antigen–antibody complexes in circulation or in tissues may lead to tissue injury.

The principles underlying the pathogenic mechanism of immune complexes were first suggested by von Pirquet in 1911 in his classical description of "serum disease" in both humans and experimental animals. The experimentally induced serum sickness in rabbits has been the most important model for understanding the pathogenesis of immune complex disease. With the use of these models, Dixon *et al.* (1958) proved that antigen–antibody complexes existed in the circulation at the time the animals developed glomerulonephritis, vasculitis, synovitis, and heart lesions. Furthermore, the development of these lesions was associated with the deposition of antigen and antibodies in the glomeruli and in other vascular sites, where they were detected by immunofluorescence microscopy (Dixon *et al.,* 1958). On the basis of these observations, a number of human diseases of varied etiology have been proven to be caused by immune complexes.

In this chapter, the factors involved in the formation of antigen–antibody complexes as well as the biologic properties of immune complexes will be considered. The experimental models of immune complex disease will be reviewed, and the evidence that induction of disease requires the persistence of circulating complexes with a large-lattice structure will be emphasized. Finally, the available methods for detecting immune complexes will be reviewed.

II. FORMATION OF ANTIGEN–ANTIBODY COMPLEXES

A. Characteristics of Antigens

Antigens were commonly defined (1) as substances that elicit an immune response when administered to a suitable host, and (2) as substances that interact specifically with available antibodies or sensitized lymphocytes. Since the characteristics of substances that can elicit an immune response differ from the characteristics of materials that interact with already available antibodies, the terms immunogen and antigen have been employed.

Immunogens are defined as substances that upon administration to a suitable host will elicit an immune response. The characteristics of substances that can behave as immunogens are considered elsewhere in this text. Antigens are defined as substances that will react specifically with available antibodies or with sensitized lymphocytes. For the discussion of antigen–antibody complexes, the nature and reactivity of antigens with antibodies is of concern.

The early investigations on antigenicity utilized complex protein or polysaccharide molecules or microorganisms. A number of studies have searched for the smallest molecule that can effectively and specifically react with an antibody molecule (see Kabat, 1968, for further details). Among carbohydrates, hexa- or heptasaccharides react optimally with antibodies. Smaller saccharides of similar composition are not as effective as saccharides composed of six or seven units. On the other hand, increasing the size of polysaccharides above heptasaccharides does not increase the efficacy of the reaction. Similar studies of natural or synthetic polypeptides indicate that five or six amino acids form the optimal antigenic molecule. A further increase in the size of the peptide will not increase the antigen–antibody reactivity, but a smaller peptide will be less effective in the interaction. These observations define the size of the antigenic determinant, defined as that portion of the antigenic substance which interacts with the binding site of an antibody or with a receptor of a sensitized lymphocyte. Therefore, large protein, polysaccharide, polynucleotide, or other molecules may have different antigenic determinants or many repeating, identical antigenic determinants. Thus, an antigenic substance has a valence in respect to each immunochemically distinct antigenic determinant.

Antigenic determinants on antigenic substances may be generated by the primary sequence of amino acids, saccharides, or nucleic acids. For example, a single amino acid difference between human hemoglobin A and S generates different antigenic determinants. Alterations of secondary and tertiary structure may lead to loss of antigenic determinants. These conclusions have been illustrated by loss of antigenicity by unfolding synthetic polypeptides and by cleaving disulfide bonds in ribonuclease, hemoglobins, etc. Finally, antigenic determinants may be constituted by the close proximity of polypeptide chains in complex protein molecules. Such antigenic determinants are not recognized in the separated polypeptide chains.

Turning from molecules to microorganisms, cells, and tissues, it is apparent that the potential for antigenic determinants increases with the complexity of the structures. The union of antibody and antigen can lead to immune complexes with varying degree of complexity, depending on the complexity of the antigen. The size and valence of the antigenic substance can alter the physical size of immune complexes, ranging from soluble complexes to fixed tissue structure covered by antibody molecules. The pathogenic role of such complexes varies considerably. Soluble complexes, as will be discussed below, can deposit in various organs, whereas complexes formed by fixed tissue structures will lead to inflammation in the location of such structures.

B. Characteristics of Antibodies

Upon exposure to an immunogen, an individual responds by synthesizing specific antibodies and by developing delayed hypersensitivity. The current concepts of the chemical basis of antibody specificity and the basic principles of immunoglobulin structure and function are beyond the scope of this chapter. The features of antibody molecules that are important to formation and function of antigen–antibody complexes are the valence of various classes of immunoglobulins for a specific antigen, the association constant for the union of specific antibody and antigen, and the biologic properties that are generated as a result of this union.

On structural basis, the antigen-binding site on antibody molecules is formed by the appropriate conformation and association of one light and one heavy polypeptide chain. Amino acids in the hypervariable regions of the variable domains of the light and heavy chain constitute the antigen-binding sites of antibody molecules. Thus, the basic four-chain unit of immunoglobulins has a valence of two for combining with an antigen. Accordingly, the valence of IgG, monomeric IgA, IgD, and IgE is two. The valence of IgM is ten, and the valence of dimeric secretory IgA is four (Table I).

The valence of two for the IgG class of antibodies has been documented experimentally in many ways, including the binding with two small antigenic molecules (haptens) and the binding of each Fab fragment (consisting of the light chain and the amino-terminal half of the heavy chain) to the specific antigen. With polyvalent antigens, however, the bivalent antibody molecule may behave as monovalent molecule because both binding sites may interact with a repeating antigenic determinant on the same antigenic molecule. Such functional valence of one was termed "monogamous bivalence" by Klinman and Karush (1967). At high degrees of antigen excess, some immune complexes with IgG class of antibodies are composed of one antigen and one antibody molecule, using human serum albumin as an antigen and rabbit antibodies to human serum albumin (Arend *et al.*, 1972; Arend and Mannik, 1974); this is presumably due to repeating antigenic structures on the albumin molecule. Alternatively, the IgG molecules may appear univalent, such as the incomplete anti-D antibodies that cannot

TABLE I

Some Properties of Human Immunoglobulins

	IgG	IgA	IgM	IgD	IgE
Molecular weight	145,000	160,000 or 320,000	900,000	183,000	190,000
Valence	2	2 or 4	10 or 5	2	2
Complement fixation					
Classic pathway	++	0	+	0	0
Alternate pathway	0	+	0	±	±
Interaction with IgG receptors on phagocyte cells	+	0	0	0	0

For haptens, the measured valence of IgM has been 10, but the valence for large antigen molecules was found to be 5.

cause agglutination due to the steric considerations of the antigenic determinants on the erythrocyte membrane.

The valence of IgM should be 10 on structural basis (see review by Metzger, 1970). The actual measured valence was found to be 10 with small antigenic molecules (haptens). With large antigenic molecules, however, the determined valence was found to be five, with adequate proof that each light and heavy chain pair possess a binding site for the antigen. These observations have been interpreted to result from steric inhibition of the second binding site when the first binding site is occupied by the antigen.

The antigen–antibody interaction is a reversible reaction, and, particularly, the hapten–antibody reaction can be expressed in a simplified manner as

$$\mathrm{Ag} + \mathrm{Ab} \underset{k_2}{\overset{k_1}{\rightleftarrows}} \mathrm{AgAb}$$

and, therefore, according to the principles of mass action the association constant at equilibrium can be expressed as

$$\frac{[\mathrm{Ag\ Ab}]}{[\mathrm{Ag}]\,[\mathrm{Ab}]} = \frac{k_1}{k_2} = K_{12}$$

For this expression, the antigen and the antibody must be homogeneous with respect to the antigenic determinants and the binding sites, respectively. Furthermore, each of the antigenic determinants and antibody-binding sites must be able to interact with each other independently of the other antigenic determinant antibody-binding site interactions. In such systems, the association constants can be determined by knowing the antibody concentration, the concentration of bound antigen, and the concentration of free antigen, as for example by equilibrium dialysis. The interested reader should consult detailed texts such as Kabat and Mayer (1961) or Day (1972) for method and detailed discussion of association constants. The experimentally determined association constants, even for chemically uniform haptens, show heterogeneity due to heterogeneity of antibodies, even though obtained from a single experimental animal in one bleeding. The measurement of association constants between multivalent antigenic molecules and antibodies and between antigenic molecules with several different antigenic determinants and antibodies become complex and are subject to errors. At best, some of the obtained values are approximations. Nevertheless, the approximated association constants, frequently referred to as avidity, express the strength of the bond(s) in immune complex formation. As discussed below, this parameter of antigen–antibody complex formation appears to be related to the pathogenicity of immune complexes.

The biologic properties and pathogenic potential of immune complexes also depend on the class of antibodies in immune complexes (see Sections III,A; III,C; and IV,B,2).

C. Nature of Antigen–Antibody Bond and Lattice Formation

The interaction of an antigenic determinant with the antibody binding site is a noncovalent bond and has been postulated to include hydrophobic, Coulombic, and hydrogen bonds and van der Waals forces. Some experiments suggest that hydrophobic bonds play the major role in forming the bond between an antigenic determinant and the antibody-binding site (Kabat, 1968). Due to these bonds collectively, the free energy of the antigen–antibody bond favors immune complex formation when an antigen and specified antibodies are present together. In immunopathology, it is often desirable to dissociate the antigen–antibody bonds to isolate antibodies for experimentation or for identification of antigens and antibodies in diseased tissues. A variety of molecular perturbants have been employed for this purpose, often quite empirically. Mild perturbants may not suffice to dissociate all antigen–antibody complexes, whereas strong perturbants may lead to denaturation of antibodies (Dandliker *et al.*, 1967; 1968). Low pH, urea, and chaotropic ions are some of the most frequently used perturbants.

Ample evidence has established the valence of antibodies. Therefore, the formation of a network or lattice of immune complexes and the formation of a visible precipitate depend largely on the variables of antigens. Heidelberger and others recognized long ago that multivalence of antigens was essential to precipitation (Heidelberger, 1939). Univalent antigens tend to form Ag_2Ab_1 complexes, whereby each antigen molecule forms a separate antigen–antibody bond with one of the two antigen binding sites on the IgB molecule. Lattice formation and precipitation will not occur with univalent antigens. Bivalent antigens can interact different ways with IgG antibodies, depending on the spacing of the antigenic determinants. If the antigenic determinants are appropriately spaced and located on the three-dimensional molecule, then thermodynamic considerations lead to monogamous bivalent reaction where both antibody-binding sites of one antibody molecule react with the two available antigenic determinants on one antigen molecule, i.e., forming Ag_1Ab_1 molecules (Klimman and Karush, 1967; Crothers and Metzger, 1972). In such a reaction, the association constant is higher than in the alternative reaction of Ag_2Ab_1 (Hornick and Karush, 1972). On the other hand, if the special considerations do not permit a monogamous bivalent reaction, then two antigen molecules might react with two antibody molecules so that both antigen molecules span the binding sites of the two antibody molecules, i.e., forming an Ag_2Ab_2 complex (Schumaker *et al.*, 1973). At high antibody and bivalent antigen concentration, higher polymers may be encountered, but precipitation is unlikely. A complex lattice or precipitate formation requires multivalent antigens, and is often facilitated by presence of several distinct antigenic determinants and presence of antibodies to these determinants. Elegant support of the lattice theory of Marrack (1938) was provided by Pauling *et al.* (1944). They prepared dihaptenic molecules with two separate antigenic determinants and studied the interaction of this material with antibodies directed to the distinct antigenic determinants. With each separate antiserum, no precipitation occurred because the antigenic molecules were univalent with respect to the antibodies. When the dihaptenic substance was added to a mixture of the two antisera, precipitation resulted due to cross-linking with antibodies of two specificities. Furthermore, these complexes were readily soluble in excess of each antigen.

The role of the protein–protein interaction between antibody molecules in immune precipitation has not been fully examined. As an example, partial acetylation of antibodies abrogated precipitability of these molecules, with polyvalent hapten–carrier conjugates, whereas binding to the specific hapten was not altered (Nisonoff and Pressman, 1959). Precipitability was lost presumably due to the increased negative charges induced by acetylation.

In a system of antigen and specific antibodies that are capable of forming a lattice and a precipitate, the degree of lattice formation depends on the relative proportion of antigen and antibody. This is best illustrated by quantitative precipitation curve (Fig. 1). As an example, when increasing

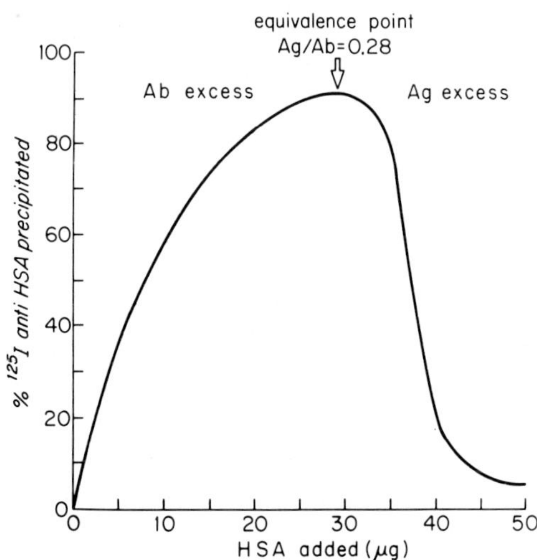

Fig. 1. Precipitin curve. Increasing amounts of antigen (HSA) were added to a standard amount of isolated rabbit antibodies (^{125}I-anti-HSA). The amount of precipitated antibodies increased until the equivalence point with maximum lattice formation was reached. As more antigen was added, the amount of precipitated antibodies was decreased as a result of decreased lattice formation.

amounts of human albumin (HSA) are added to a constant amount of antibodies to HSA, the amount of precipitate increases until the point of optimum proportions is reached; this is called the point of equivalence and signifies maximal lattice formation. If, in this system, more antigen is added to the same amount of antibody, then the amount of precipitate declines and the soluble antigen–antibody complexes with smaller degrees of lattice formation remain in the supernatant. The first evidence for this phenomenon was provided by Pedersen (1936) and by Heidelberger and Pedersen (1937), employing rabbit antibodies to egg albumin in the presence of excess egg albumin. The soluble immune complexes in such a system are polydispersed, depending on the degree of antigen excess. The formation of soluble complexes in the zone of antigen excess was predicted by Goldberg's (1952) theory of antigen–antibody interactions. In such antigen–antibody systems, the formation of soluble complexes in antibody excess require large excesses of antibodies (Nisonoff and Winkler, 1958; Forster and Weigle, 1963).

With large excess of antigen molecules, the bivalent antibody would be expected to form Ag_2Ab_1 complexes, with two separate antigen molecules reacting with each binding site on the antibody. Careful measurement with rabbit antibodies to human serum albumin, or to bovine serum albumin, however, disclosed that, in the presence of 20- to 1000-fold excess antigen, the Ag_2Ab_1 molecular ratio was not achieved and that, at 100-fold antigen excess, both Ag_2Ab_2 and Ag_1Ab_1 complexes existed (Arend *et al.*, 1972; Arend and Mannik, 1974). In these systems, with increasing antigen excess, the polydispersed immune complexes present at fivefold antigen excess, consisting of larger than Ag_2Ab_2 complexes, decreased with increased antigen excess, and the Ag_2Ab_2 and Ag_1Ab_1 complexes increased (Fig. 2). Schematically, immune complexes with varying lattices may be represented as indicated by Fig. 3. If the antigen excess that resulted in formation of small-latticed complexes is removed, then the complexes will reequilibrate and result in large-latticed complexes.

As will be discussed below, the degree of lattice formation of immune complexes significantly influences their biologic properties, as well as their pathogenic potential. Very little work has been done on the actual lattice formation of immune complexes in disease processes. Work on experimental models, however, has shown that variations in lattice of immune complexes influences their pathogenic potential. The majority of these observations have been made on IgG class of antibodies, and very little information is available on lattice formation of other classes of antibodies.

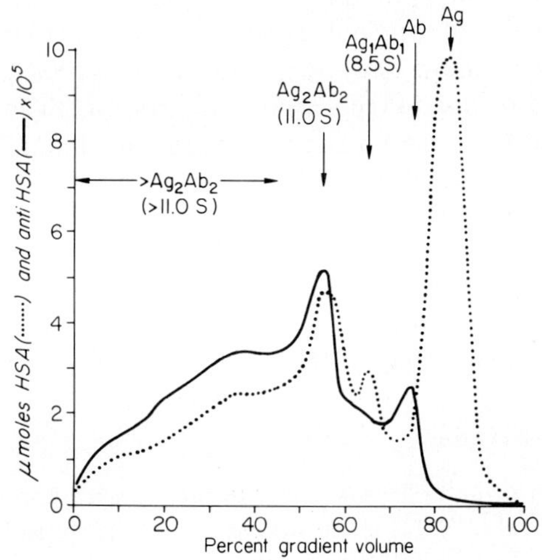

Fig. 2. Sucrose density gradient ultracentrifugation of HSA–rabbit anti-HSA complexes prepared at fivefold antigen excess. The distribution of antigen (μmoles HSA) and antibody (μmoles anti-HSA) are indicated following sucrose density gradient ultracentrifugation (0% is bottom and 100% is top of the 10–30% linear sucrose gradient). The position of various-sized complexes with their sedimentation coefficients, as well as the position of unbound antigen (Ag) and antibody (Ab), are indicated (adapted from Arend *et al.*, 1972).

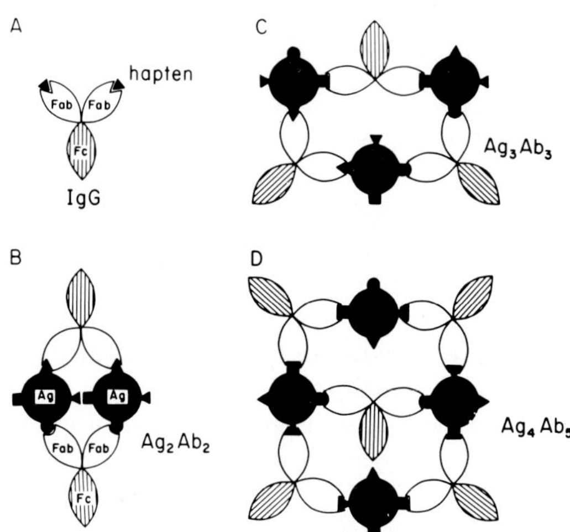

Fig. 3. Schematic representation of the interaction of a univalent hapten with an IgG antibody molecule (A), and of the interaction of a multivalent antigen with antibody molecules to form complexes with varying degrees of lattice structure (B,C,D).

The formation of soluble immune complexes can occur with precipitating systems in presence of antigen excess. In other situations, the limited valence of antigens allows only formation of small-latticed immune complexes, regardless of the antigen–antibody ratio. Small immune complexes (Ag_1Ab_1) can also be formed if due to the spacing of antigenic determinants thermodynamic considerations lead to monogamous bivalent reactions. Finally, low association constants may favor formation of small-latticed complexes.

III. BIOLOGIC PROPERTIES OF IMMUNE COMPLEXES

A. Complement Fixation

The interaction of soluble immune complexes with complement has been examined extensively. Soluble complexes containing rabbit antibodies in antigen excess precipitated following the addition of fresh serum containing complement (Weigle and Maurer, 1957). Soluble aggregates of γ-globulins similarly precipitated with normal human serum (Müller-Eberhard and Kunkel, 1961). The protein responsible for precipitating the soluble aggregates was isolated and is now known as the C1q component responsible for the first step in the fixation of complement by the classical pathway. Cohen (1968) demonstrated that two adjacent rabbit IgG antibody molecules were needed to fix complement in antigen–antibody precipitates formed at equivalence. In this study antibodies with markedly reduced complement-fixing activity, but with normal antigen-binding capacity were prepared by amidation and benzylation of the antibody molecules. When these altered antibodies were mixed with the normal antibodies and reacted together with antigen, complement fixation was suppressed. By evaluating the suppressive effect quantitatively, it was concluded that two adjacent IgG molecules were required for complement fixation.

Hyslop *et al.* (1970) showed that several sizes of complexes were demonstrable by gel filtration when the rabbit antibodies were reacted with a divalent hapten at equivalence. The main 8.7 S peak was examined by electron microscopy and contained predominantly IgG dimers, linked by bivalent hapten molecules, but also some monomers and trimers. The 8.7 S material did not fix complement. Fractions containing complexes definitely larger than the dimers, however, fixed complement efficiently. A dose-response analysis of C1 fixation proved that dimers did not fix C1. Therefore, dimers and probably trimers of rabbit IgG antibodies, linked by bivalent hapten, did not fix complement, whereas higher polymers did fix complement.

Recently, Goers *et al.* (1975) reported that the univalent hapten, nonadecalysyl-ε-DNP-lysine, formed an antigen–antibody complex with a sedimentation coefficient of 6.7 S containing a single antibody molecule. While these complexes fixed complement efficiently, it represents a special situation requiring the presence of the positively charged polylysine chain, which may provide a binding site for C1 and, thus, rendering the complex at least divalent for interaction with C1. The complement-fixing ability of soluble immune complexes prepared with human serum albumin was examined by Mannik *et al.* (1971). Fractions containing complexes exceeding Ag_2Ab_2 (>11 S) were isolated by sucrose density gradient ultracentrifugation and were efficient in complement fixation. Fractions containing Ag_2Ab_2 (11 S) complexes fixed complement with only 10% of the efficiency observed with larger complexes. Since the Ag_2Ab_2 (11 S) complexes were noted after repeated ultracentrifugation to have reequilibrated to form some >11 S complexes and some free 6.6 S antibodies, the ability of Ag_2Ab_2 (11 S) complexes to fix complement was probably overestimated.

Thus, the fixation of complement by soluble immune complexes appears to require an antigen–antibody lattice structure containing more than two and possibly more than three antibody molecules. Since precipitated complexes require two adjacent antibody molecules to initiate complement fixation, soluble complexes may also require similar proximity of adjacent antibody molecules in order to inititate complement fixation. The data of Hyslop *et al.* (1970) would suggest that this conformation may only be achieved with soluble complexes when either large linear or cyclic polymers are formed.

B. Activation of Other Plasma Enzyme Systems

Some evidence suggests that soluble immune complexes can activate other plasma enzyme systems. Simpson *et al.* (1973) suggested that the interaction of immune complexes with Hageman factor (factor XII) accounted for intravascular coagulation and fibrinolysis following the administration of antigen to immunized rabbits. Platelets and fibrinogen levels fell immediately. The platelet levels remained low for several hours, but the fibrinogen levels subsequently increased to greater than normal levels. If Hageman factor were directly activated by immune complexes, then activation of the kinin system could be expected in addition to the coagulation and fibrinolysis systems (Kaplan and Austen, 1972; Magoon *et al.*, 1974; Cochrane *et al.*, 1974). However, Cochrane *et al.* (1972) could find no evidence for direct activation of Hageman factor by immune complexes. Purified, isolated Hageman factor was employed in these studies, and no cleavage of the labeled molecule into its active fragments was observed following incubation with several kinds of immune complexes at varying antigen–antibody ratios. The only preparations found to activate Hageman factor were contaminated with bacteria, which were isolated and found to be potent activators, presumably due to endotoxin. Further studies showed that, although clot-promoting activity could be generated by immune complexes, this activity was not mediated by the intrinsic clotting pathway.

In reviewing the acceleration of blood clotting when whole blood is exposed to immune complexes, Ratnoff (1969) suggested that the discharge of platelet phospholipid (PF3) may be one cause of accelerated clotting, because no acceleration occurs in platelet-poor plasma. The release of platelet constituents following platelet interaction with immune complexes is well documented (Becker and Henson, 1973), and will be discussed below.

C. Interaction of Immune Complexes with Cell Surfaces and Their Biologic Effects

1. *Mononuclear Phagocytes (Macrophages)*

The nature of the interaction of immune complexes with cell-surface membranes and the biologic consequences constitutes a broad subject in itself, and the discussion of this area is necessarily cursory. The various immunoglobulin classes and subclasses differ in their adherence properties with mononuclear phagocytes and other cells and differ in other biologic properties also, as reviewed by Spiegelberg (1974). Immune complexes containing particulate antigens, such as bacteria and red blood cells, were used in early studies to examine the interaction of immune complexes with mononuclear phagocytes (Boyden, 1964; Uhr, 1965; Berken and Benacerraf, 1966; LoBuglio *et al.*, 1967; Huber and Fudenberg, 1968; Huber *et al.*, 1968; Lay and Nussenzweig, 1969; Henson, 1969; Cruchaud and Unanue, 1971). Binding sites specific for the Fc fragment of IgG were found on the cell membrane (Berken and Benacerraf, 1966; LoBuglio *et al.*, 1967; Huber and Fudenberg, 1968). Studies with myeloma proteins indicated human monocytes bound the IgG1 and IgG3 subclasses of human IgG but not IgG2 and IgG4 poorly (LoBuglio *et al.*, 1967; Huber and Fudenberg; 1968; Lawrence *et al.*, 1975). IgM (Huber *et al.*, 1968; Lawrence *et al.*, 1975) and the other immunoglobulin classes (Lawrence *et al.*, 1975) were not bound by human monocytes. Spiegelberg (1974) stated that, following aggregation of the myeloma proteins, monocytes also bound IgG2 and IgG4 in addition to IgG1 and IgG3, but none of the other classes. Thus, it is possible that soluble immune complexes of sufficient lattice structure containing all the subclasses of human IgG may bind to human monocytes, and complexes containing the other human immunoglobulin classes may not bind. However, such data with soluble immune complexes have not been reported.

Similar class and subclass differences in the binding of immunoglobulins to macrophages have been demonstrated in guinea pigs. Guinea pig IgG antibodies to sheep erythrocytes (RBC) bound to macrophages (Boyden, 1964). Uhr (1965) further demonstrated that antigen–antibody complexes containing IgG adhere to macrophages, while complexes containing IgM do not. Finally, Berken and Benacerraf (1966) found that the γ_2G subclass and not the γ_1G subclass of guinea pig IgG adhered to macrophages.

Studies in mice have indicated that sheep RBC sensitized with either mouse 7 S (class?) or 19 S (IgM) antibodies bind to macrophages (Lay and Nussenzweig, 1969). The adherence characteristics of the mouse 7 S immunoglobulins have been examined by Dissanayake and Hay (1975), using IgG1, IgG2a, and IgG2b myeloma proteins. The IgG2a and the IgG2b subclasses bound to mouse peritoneal macrophages with higher affinities than did IgG1. IgG1 did bind at higher concentrations, but, under physiological conditions in competition with the IgG2 subclasses, the binding was relatively low.

The Fc receptor on the mononuclear phagocyte appears to be specific for the $C\gamma_3$ homology region of IgG. Yasmeen *et al.* (1973) demonstrated that the binding of human IgG to guinea pig macrophages is a property of the $C\gamma_3$ region of the molecule. In a similar experiment, the $C\gamma_3$ region of human IgG, particularly from the IgG1 and IgG3 subclasses, mediated binding to human monocytes (Okafor *et al.*, 1974).

The binding characteristics of soluble immune complexes to rabbit macrophages were examined by Phillips-Quagliata *et al.* (1971). Soluble complexes were prepared with rabbit anti-benzylpenicilloyl antibodies and monovalent, divalent, and polyvalent hapten preparations. No increased binding was noted with complexes prepared with monovalent hapten. Enhanced binding of complexes was maximum with complexes prepared with polyvalent hapten; however, the binding with divalent hapten was also increased. Maximum binding occurred with complexes prepared at or near equivalence, while complexes prepared in antigen excess bound poorly or not at all. Thus, conditions favoring the formation of complexes with increased lattice structure were required for maximum binding. The number of Fc receptors was calculated to be approximately 2 million per cell.

Arend and Mannik (1972) further examined the *in vitro* adherence of soluble immune complexes to monocytes. Immune complexes were prepared with human serum albumin (HSA) and rabbit IgG antibodies to HSA at threefold antigen excess. Selective adherence of complexes exceeding Ag_2Ab_2 (>11 S) was observed, while Ag_2Ab_2 (11 S) complexes failed to adhere in the presence of larger complexes. Reduction and alkylation of the antibody molecules used to prepare the complexes resulted in decreased adherence of the complexes to the cells. The average number of alveolar macrophage receptor sites was found to increase from 1.21×10^6 sites per cell on minimally stimulated cells to 2.16×10^6 sites per cell by repeated stimulation with intravenous complete Freund's adjuvant (Arend and Mannik, 1973). The average association constant between the receptors and rabbit monomeric IgG was estimated to be 7.59×10^5 liters/mole on minimally stimulated cells and 9.02×10^5 liters/mole on heavily stimulated cells. Further studies (Arend and Mannik, 1975) indicated that the adherence of these soluble complexes was dependent upon the Fc fragment of the immunoglobulin molecule. The adherence of complexes to macrophages was inhibited by Fc fragments from normal rabbit IgG, but neither by Fab fragments nor by $F(ab')_2$ fragments.

The role of IgM antibodies in the adherence of immune complexes containing particulate antigens has also been examined. Human macrophages do not appear to have a receptor for IgM-sensitized RBC (LoBuglio *et al.*, 1967; Huber and Fudenberg, 1968; Huber *et al.*, 1968; Reynolds *et al.*, 1975). However, the data from rabbits, guinea pigs, and mice are not consistent. Early studies by Uhr (1965) in guinea pigs and by Berken and Benacerraf (1968) in rabbits and mice failed to identify adherence of 19 S IgM-sensitized particulate antigens to isologous macrophages. Henson (1969) found some adherence of IgM sensitized cells to rabbit and guinea pig macrophages, but the activity was less than that seen with IgG. Lay and Nussenzweig (1969) reported that mouse peritoneal macrophages had receptors for mouse IgM-sensitized sheep RBC, but mouse blood monocytes did not.

Adherence studies with soluble complexes containing IgM have not been reported either in humans or in rabbits, guinea pigs, and mice. However, human IgM macroglobulins do not adhere to human monocytes either as monomeric or aggregated protein molecules (Lawrence *et al.,* 1975). Feldman and Pollock (1974) examined the uptake of soluble complexes containing keyhole limpet hemocyanin (KLH) and rat IgG or IgM antibodies to KLH by rat macrophages. Greater uptake was observed with soluble complexes containing IgM antibodies than with soluble complexes containing IgG antibodies. The apparent paradox of this finding may have reflected greater aggregation of the KLH antigen by IgM antibodies than by IgG antibodies, since the uptake of KLH bound to rat erythrocytes was also much greater than the uptake of free KLH. Nevertheless, the above studies with particulate complexes and with aggregated macroglobulins suggest that the adherence of IgM-containing complexes is less efficient than the adherence of IgG-containing complexes.

Of additional interest is a report by Rhodes (1973) that sheep RBC coated with 8 S subunit of guinea pig IgM (19 S) are bound by guinea pig macrophages. The relevance of this finding is uncertain, because the 8 S subunit was prepared by reduction and alkylation of the specific IgM antisera.

Lay and Nussenzweig (1968) had earlier shown that sheep RBC sensitized with herologous rabbit IgM would not adhere to mouse macrophages unless complement factors from mouse serum were added to the antigen–IgM antibody complex. The addition of complement components through C3 was also required for the adherence of sheep RBC coated with rabbit IgM antibodies (Huber *et al.,* 1968). The C3 and IgG receptors on human monocytes were distinct. The adherence of sheep RBC sensitized with rabbit IGM to rabbit macrophages was also enhanced following incubation with rabbit complement (Henson, 1969). The adherence was decreased by treating the serum source of rabbit complement with cobra venom factor, which suggested that C3 was responsible for the adherence activity.

The fate of complexes following their attachment to the macrophage membrane may be determined by the nature of the membrane receptors to which they attach. For example, sheep RBC sensitized with mouse IgG were readily phagocytosed by mouse macrophages, while these same cells sensitized with mouse IgM were not (Lay and Nussenzweig, 1969). Different roles of the macrophage receptor sites for complement (C3) and for IgG during phagocytosis of immune complexes were found by Mantovani *et al.* (1972). The attachment of sheep RBC sensitized with IgG (EA) to macrophages was greatly increased by the addition of complement (EAC), but ingestion was not. The data suggested that particle attachment was mediated primarily by C3 and that ingestion was mediated primarily by IgG. It was suggested that these findings might be relevant to *in vivo* mechanisms of immunization. During a primary immune response, particulate complexes such as EA(IgM) or EA(IgM)C3 would tend to remain on macrophage surfaces and further stimulate immune competent cells. During the secondary response, EA(IgG) or EA(IgG)C3 would tend to be interiorized and degraded by the macrophages.

Recent studies by Wellek *et al.* (1975), by Reynolds *et al.* (1975), and by Rabellino and Metcalf (1975) have demonstrated that macrophages not only have a receptor for the C3b fragment but also for the inactivator-cleaved C3d fragment of the third component of complement. Complexes were prepared with erythrocytes and specific rabbit IgM antibodies and were subsequently exposed to isolated guinea pig complement components to form EAIgMC1423. The adherence and phagocytosis of EAIgMC1423 by guinea pig macrophages was the same, whether or not the complexes had been pretreated with C3b inactivator (Wellek *et al.*, 1975). Similarly, erythrocytes sensitized with rabbit IgM and exposed to C5-deficient mouse serum were negative for C3b, but they were readily phagocytosed by mouse macrophages (Rabellino and Metcalf, 1975). Thus, the adherence was thought to be mediated by C3d. Finally, IgM sensitized sheep erythrocytes were exposed sequentially to individual human complement components; both C3b and C3d binding to human alveolar macrophages was demonstrated (Reynolds *et al.*, 1975). However, when fresh human serum, rather than individual complement components, was used as the complement source, only C3b binding and no C3d binding could be generated. Thus, alveolar macrophages appear to have a receptor site for human C3d, but this site may not be functionally available when whole serum is used as a complement source.

Recent studies by Ross and Polley (1975) have demonstrated that human mononuclear phagocytes will bind IgM-sensitized erythrocytes containing only C1 and C4 (EAC14). The specificity of the C4 binding site was characterized on lymphocytes, and C4 appears to bind to the same membrane site as C3b, but not to the C3d site. While the *in vivo* significance of this observation is not known, the C4 adherence activity may be protected from C3b inactivator and, thus, still available for adherence to the common site for C3b and C4.

The catabolism and fate of IgG-sensitized erythrocytes have been examined following their ingestion by macrophages (Cruchaud and Unanue, 1971; Cruchaud *et al.*, 1975). The erythrocytes were labeled with ^{125}I prior to sensitization with IgG, and, following their ingestion by macrophages, free ^{125}I was released into the supernatant, reflecting catabolism of the antigens. However, small amounts of ^{125}I remained protein bound, both on the macrophage plasma membrane and in the culture supernatants. The nature of the protein-bound ^{125}I was not determined, but it could remain available as an immunogenic moiety. When the IgG antibodies in the ingested complexes were labeled with ^{125}I, a similar rapid release of label from the macrophages occurred. A small amount of material remained attached to the macrophage surface. Approximately 30% of the label released into the supernatant remained protein-bound after 24 hours. The size distribution of this protein-bound material was examined by sucrose density gradient ultracentrifugation. Incompletely degraded IgG was found to increase with time and to contain Fab or $F(ab)_2$ fragments, which would still bind specifically to the erythrocytes. The possibility was suggested that partially degraded molecules may lack the Fc fragment and, thus, combine with an antigen to form a complex which cannot be phagocytosed.

The uptake and fate of immune complexes, prepared with a soluble protein antigen horse radish peroxidase (HRP) and mouse or rabbit anti-HRP, in mouse macrophages was examined by Steinman and Cohn (1972). The uptake of complexes was examined as a function of antigen–antibody interaction, determined by precipitin curves. The maximum uptake of complexes containing either hyperimmune serum from rabbits and mice or purified rabbit IgG antibodies occurred in a zone from fourfold antibody excess to equivalence. The uptake fell off dramatically in antigen excess. The uptake was mediated by the trypsin-resistant Fc receptor. The disappearance of HRP in immune complexes formed at equivalence was exponential by either cell-bound enzyme activity ($t_{1/2}$ = 14–18 hr) or by the disappearance of ^{125}I-HRP radioactivity ($t_{1/2}$ = 30 hr). Furthermore, throughout the study, there was no release of active enzymes into the supernate, and the released radioactivity was soluble in trichloroacetic acid. While the macrophages appeared to interiorize and to completely degrade the HRP, the fate of the antibodies in the immune complexes was not determined.

The release of mediators from the lysosomal granules of macrophages occurs as a result of immunologically induced phagocytosis, as reviewed by Becker and Henson (1973). Weissmann *et al.* (1971) demonstrated that selective extrusion of lysosomal enzymes (β-glucuronidase, arylsulfatase, and acid cathepsin) occurs during phagocytosis of the undigestible particle zymosan; while the release of cytoplasmic enzymes (lactic dehydrogenase) did not occur. Studies by Cardella *et al.* (1974) demonstrated selective release of lysosomal enzymes from mouse macrophages following exposure to immune complexes, prepared at equivalence with either ferritin and rabbit antibodies to ferritin or bovine serum albumin (BSA) and rabbit antibodies to BSA. The maximum release of the lysosomal enzyme, β-glucuronidase, occurred after 6 hours of incubation with the complexes formed at equivalence. The amount of enzyme release was a function of immune complex concentration. The release of lysosomal enzymes by phagocytosis of various soluble immune complexes as a function of lattice or a function of physical size has not been examined.

2. *Neutrophils*

The interaction of immune complexes with neutrophils is similar in nature to that described above for mononuclear phagocytes. Lay and Nussenzweig (1968) showed the existence of IgG and complement receptors on mouse neutrophils, using sheep erythrocytes sensitized with rabbit IgG. Erythrocytes sensitized with IgM antibodies failed to adhere to these cells, unless the sensitized cells were preincubated with fresh serum as a source of complement. Subsequently, Quie *et al.* (1968) provided evidence that the Fc region of IgG was required for this interaction, using bacteria coated with human antibodies of the IgG class. C3 was the complement component needed to promote the interaction of IgM-sensitized cell with neutrophils (Henson, 1969). Messner and Jelinek (1970) demonstrated that the adherence of erythrocytes sensitized with human IgG to neutrophils could be inhibited only by myeloma proteins of the IgG1 and IgG3 subclasses. However, the subclasses of the antibodies used to sensitize the erythrocytes was not determined; thus, neutrophil receptors for the other subclasses may have existed. In fact, Henson *et al.* (1972), as well as Lawrence *et al.* (1975), demonstrated that aggregated human myeloma proteins of all IgG subclasses (IgG1, IgG2, IgG3, and IgG4) and IgA subclasses (IgA1 and IgA2) adhered to human neutrophils.

The mechanism of binding of immune complexes to guinea pig neutrophils was examined by Phillips-Quagliata *et al.* (1969). The binding of ^{131}I-labeled rabbit anti-benzylpenicilloylated antibody was examined in the presence of polyvalent, divalent, and monovalent haptens. The binding of antibody was significantly and consistently increased only in the presence of polyvalent hapten. These results suggest that the polyvalent hapten allowed the formation of soluble complexes with a large-lattice structure, which exhibited greater binding due to increased binding energy from the summation of individual binding sites.

Additional support for this concept was provided by Hawkins and Peeters (1971), who studied the interaction of homologous antigen–antibody complexes with rabbit neutrophils. Neutrophils were exposed to either precipitated complexes (BSA and rabbit antibodies to BSA) or to soluble complexes formed at 20 times or 100 times antigen excess. The neutrophil uptake of soluble complexes containing radiolabeled antibodies was determined. Complexes prepared at 20 times antigen excess, containing some complexes larger than 22 S, were taken into the cell. No neutrophil uptake was observed with complexes prepared at 100 times antigen excess, that only contain small limiting complexes. Ultrastructural studies with precipitated complexes revealed electron-dense material being taken up by the cell. Thus, the size of the immune complex lattice structure determined the uptake of the complexes. In response to the uptake of either precipitated complexes or soluble complexes at 20 times antigen excess, the neutrophils released lysosomal enzymes into the ambient medium. No enzyme release was observed with complexes prepared at 100 times antigen excess. Ward and Zvaifler (1973) pointed out that IgM rheumatoid factor may suppress the phagocytic uptake of antigen–antibody precipitates by neutrophils and the subsequent release of lysosomal enzymes.

Henson (1971a,b) examined the interaction of rabbit neutrophils with zymosan particles coated by rabbit complement or by rabbit antibodies and with nonphagocytosable micropore filters containing BSA–rabbit IgG anti-BSA or ferritin–rabbit IgG anti-ferritin complexes. Lysosomal enzymes were released with both phagocytosable particles and nonphagocytosable surfaces, while minimal release of the cytoplasmic enzyme lactic dehydrogenase (LDH) occurred. Both IgG and C3 were effective in stimulating enzyme release. The amount of antibody required to stimulate enzyme release was less on a nonphagocytosable surface than on a phagocytosable surface. The mechanism of enzyme release during phagocytosis appeared ultrastructurally to occur by degranulation into the phagocytic vacuole and by leakage extracellularly prior to the closure of the phagolysosome (Fig. 4). Enzyme release during the adherence of neutrophils to immune complexes on a nonphagocytosable surface appeared ultrastructurally to occur by direct extrusion of the granules to the exterior of the cell at the sight of the attempted phagocytosis (Fig. 4). Enzyme release from human neutrophils incubated with phagocytosable particles and with nonphagocytosable surfaces containing tetanus toxoid–human IgG anti-tetanus complexes was similar in pattern to that observed with the rabbit system (Henson, 1971c). Immune complexes fixed to collagen polymer membranes were used by Hawkins (1971, 1972) as a nonphagocytosable surface for demonstrating selective release of neutrophil lysosomal enzymes.

The selective release of lysosomal enzymes from human neutrophils was also achieved with aggregated human myeloma proteins of all IgG subclasses (IgG1, IgG2, IgG3, and IgG4) and IgA subclasses (IgA1 and IgA2) while IgM, IgD, and IgE were inactive (Henson *et al.*, 1972). Henson (1973) outlined several mechanisms whereby the extracellular release of lysosomal enzymes may occur following the uptake of aggregates into phagocytic

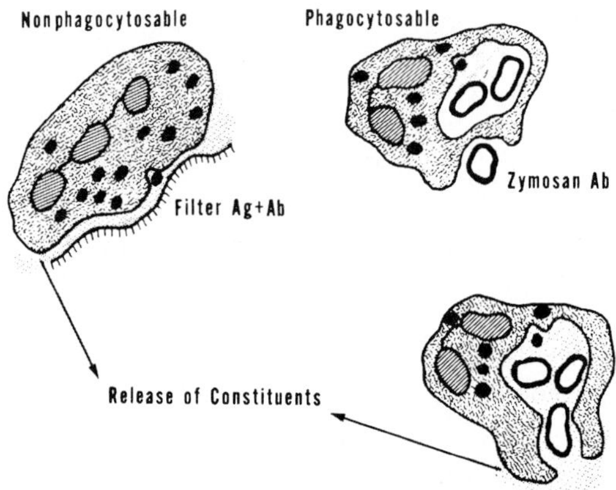

Fig. 4. Two mechanisms of enzyme release from neutrophil granules. Neutrophil degranulation occurred to the exterior of the cell upon interaction with immune complexes on a nonphagocytosable surface (left). Neutrophil degranulation into a phagocytic vacuole after phagocytosis, and subsequent extracellular release of enzymes occurred during phagocytosis of additional particulate immune complexes (right) (from Henson, 1971c).

vacuoles. Granules were extruded into the vacuoles, and extracellular release of enzymes may have occurred when (1) a vacuole opened to take in additional aggregates; (2) a vacuole remained connected to the exterior; (3) a single aggregate was being phagocytosed by two cells; and (4) granule extrusion preceded pseudopod closure around the aggregate.

The above studies on neutrophil interaction with immune complexes point out the mechanisms by which vascular damage may occur. When complexes are deposited along the vasculature (e.g., glomerular capillaries, coronary arteries, etc.) and neutrophils are attracted to the sites by chemotactic mechanisms, enzymes are released during attempted phagocytosis and may, thus, cause damage to surrounding vascular structures.

3. *Eosinophils*

The uptake of immune complexes by eosinophils was established by Litt (1964) in guinea pig peritoneal exudates and by Rappaport (1964) in nasal mucosa of humans with allergies. Following phagocytosis of immune precipitates containing extracts of nematode parasites and immune serum by rat eosinophils, the lysosomal granules appeared to lyse adjacent to the ingested precipitate (Archer, 1969). Ishikawa *et al.* (1974) and Fujita *et al.* (1975) suggested the presence of receptors on eosinophils specific for IgE in immune complexes. Rabellino and Metcalf (1975) demonstrated that eosinophil colony cells derived from mouse bone marrow cultures had receptors for IgG. The specificity of the receptor for the different subclasses of mouse IgG was not determined, and receptors for the other classes of mouse immunoglobulins were not looked for. However, receptors for mouse C3 were looked for on the eosinophils but were not found. Thus, it may be that complexes containing either IgE or IgG antibodies will be found to adhere to eosinophils and to stimulate the release of lysosomal enzymes.

4. *Basophils*

Little emphasis has been placed on the interaction of immune complexes with basophils. Ishizaka *et al.* (1970) and Sullivan *et al.* (1971) demonstrated that human basophils have IgE on their surface and that IgE myeloma proteins would adhere to the surface of basophils but not to the surface of other leukocytes. The receptor on the surface of the basophil was specific for the Fc portion of the IgE molecule (Ishizaka *et al.,* 1970). In the presence of specific antigen or anti-IgE antibodies, basophils will degranulate and release histamine as reviewed by Becker and Henson (1973).

The number of IgE molecules bound per basophil is known to range between 10,000 and 40,000, while the number of receptors ranges from 30,000 to 90,000 (Ishizaka, 1975). A high association constant was found, between 10^8 and 10^9 M^{-1}, which explains the persistent adherence of this cell-bound antibody. Since bridging surface IgE molecules with anti-IgE (or with antigen) is required to initiate histamine release, it would also seem possible that soluble immune complexes containing various allergens and IgE antibodies could adhere to basophils and induce histamine release.

5. *Mast Cells*

In considering the interaction of immunoglobulins and immune complexes with basophilic leukocytes, their interaction with mast cells should also be discussed. The staining properties and chemical composition of basophils and mast cells are similar despite differences in morphology and ultrastructure, and the numbers of mast cells and basophils are inversely related in various species (Dvorak and Dvorak, 1972). Thus rodents, which have extremely few basophils, have increased numbers of mast cells.

Mast cells from rodents, such as mice and rats, not only have receptors for homologous IgE antibodies, but also for the homologous γ_1G subclass of IgG in both rodent species, as noted in several recent reviews (Becker, 1971; Becker and Henson, 1973; Spiegelberg, 1974). The reaginic (IgE) antibody in mice binds firmly to mouse mast cells, whereas the γ_1G antibody binds very weakly unless present as antigen–antibody complexes (Vaz and Prouvost-Danon, 1969). Of interest is the observation that histamine release from mouse mast cells induced by immune complexes prepared at equivalence decreased with time, whereas histamine release by soluble immune complexes prepared in moderate antigen excess remained stable with time (Vaz and Prouvost-Danon, 1969). In addition to receptors for IgE and the IgG_1 subclass of IgG, mouse mast cells also have receptors for the other subclasses of mouse IgG, but no receptors for IgM or IgA (Tigelaar *et al.*, 1971; Cline and Warner, 1972). However, IgG_2 antibodies would not sensitize mouse mast cells for histamine release, and both IgG_{2a} and IgG_{2b} myelomas were able to block passive cutaneous anaphylaxis (PCA) reaction in mice (Ovary *et al.*, 1970). Warner and Ovary (1972) subsequently demonstrated that sheep erythrocytes sensitized with mouse antibodies could be inhibited from forming rosettes with mouse mast cells by IgG_1 myeloma proteins, to a lesser extent by IgG_{2a} and IgG_{2b} myeloma proteins and not by IgA or IgM myeloma proteins. This suggested that IgG_1 and IgG_2 receptors may be different. Furthermore, immune complexes containing DNP_{28}–BGG and mouse anti-DNP antibodies inhibited rosette formation most efficiently when moderate amounts of antigen were mixed with a given amount of antiserum. The inhibition by immune complexes fell off as either high concentrations or low concentrations of antigen were added to the antiserum, which suggested the lattice structure of the complex influenced the degree of inhibition. However, the physical characteristics of the complexes were not discussed. Immune complexes containing heat-sensitive reaginic (IgE) antibodies also inhibited rosette formation as demonstrated by decreased inhibition following heat treatment. Since heating the serum decreased both antibody activity and blocking activity, the reaginic (IgE) and the IgG_1 antibodies were thought to compete for the same site.

The nature of mouse mast cell degranulation was found by Barnett and Justus (1975) to differ, depending on whether the cells had been sensitized with IgG_1 or with IgE antibodies. Cells sensitized with IgG_1 became moderately degranulated as they released relatively few granules extracellularly upon incubation with antigen. Cells sensitized with IgE underwent a more explosive form of degranulation upon incubation with antigen, which resulted in the extracellular release of many granules due to an apparent breakdown of the cell membrane. Thus, immune complexes containing either mouse IgG_1 or mouse IgE antibodies apparently are capable of interacting with mouse mast cells; however, the biologic effects in terms of mediator release may have qualitative differences.

Rats also have two types of homocytotropic antibodies capable of sensitizing rat mast cells, and their interaction with these cells has recently been reviewed by Becker and Henson (1973). Rat IgE and the IgGa subclass of rat IgG both sensitize rat mast cells for histamine release, and the characteristics of this interaction have been examined by Bach *et al.* (1971a,b).

IgE binds firmly to the cells and resists washing, whereas IgGa binds weakly and is easily removed by washing. The release of histamine from IgE-sensitized mast cells occurs rapidly, reaching a maximum within 5 minutes. However, the release from IgGa-sensitized cells occurs more slowly, reaching maximum release at 90 minutes, which suggested to the observers that this mechanism for histamine release required transient interaction of antigen–IgGa antibody complexes with different activation sites on the mast cell. Competitive inhibition studies suggested a common receptor for IgG and IgE on mast cells. The competitive effect of IgE and IgGa antibodies for the mast cell receptor site was more clearly demonstrated in a later study using antigen-specific antibodies isolated by affinity chromatography (Bach *et al.,* 1973). Finally, rat myeloma IgE has a high binding affinity on the order of 10^9 M^{-1} for the receptor sites on rat mast cells, and the number of binding sites per mast cell is approximately 3×10^5 (Conrad *et al.*, 1975).

Mast cells in human skin have been demonstrated to have surface IgE by autoradiography (Callerame and Condemi, 1974). Radioiodinated (^{125}I) antibodies to human IgE identified IgE on the skin mast cells of an atopic patient both before and after the exposure to specific antigen. Radiolabeled (^{125}I) human IgE myeloma protein was also found to adhere to mast cells in human skin by autoradiography (Hubscher *et al.,* 1974). In both studies, mast cell degranulation occurred when a sensitized skin site was challenged with the appropriate allergen. Whether or not immunoglobulins of classes other than IgE can mediate this effect was not determined.

6. *Platelets*

Immune complexes constitute one of the many substances that interact with platelets to cause platelet aggregation and release of platelet constituents. Several reviews exist on this topic (Pfueller and Lüscher, 1972; Osler and Siraganian, 1972; Becker and Henson, 1973; Myllylä, 1973; Mueller-Eckhardt, 1975). The biologic importance of platelets lies in their ability to form dense aggregates upon interaction with a number of substances, including thrombin; other serine esterase enzymes, such as trypsin, collagen, antiplatelet antibodies, immune complexes; and the platelet constituents themselves, such as the adenosine nucleotide ADP. Although immune complexes adhere to platelets of all species, the reaction is mediated by platelet receptors for complement in some species (mouse, rabbit, dog, and horse) and by platelet receptors for the immunoglobulin portion of antigen–antibody complexes in other species (man, baboon, pig, sheep, goat, and ox) (Becker and Henson, 1973). The interaction of immune complexes with platelets has been extensively studied in rabbits and humans.

The interaction of immune complexes with rabbit platelets was recognized some time ago to require complement. Studies with soluble immune complexes demonstrated that the initial interaction or adherence of the complex to the platelet requires that C3 be bound to the complex (Henson and Cochrane, 1969; Henson, 1970; Marney, 1971). Although the initial interaction of complexes containing bound C3 caused aggregation of the platelets, release of platelet constituents did not occur until complement components through C6 were added. Cytoplasmic contents were released, in addition to vasoactive amines, nucleotides, and lysosomal enzymes; the release mechanism was concluded to occur by platelet lysis. The immune complexes used in these studies were most effective when prepared in antibody excess, and results with use of soluble complexes prepared in antigen excess were not reported.

Insoluble complexes containing particulate antigens interact with platelets through a C3 adherence mechanism. Henson and Cochrane (1969) demonstrated that sheep erythrocytes, sensitized with rabbit antibodies (EA), need to react with complement components through C3 to induce platelet aggregation and histamine release. If complement components were added as C6-deficient plasma, aggregation, and histamine release occurred. The same was noted for zymosan particles. Zymosan incubated, however, in the presence of plasma depleted of C3 by cobra venom factor did not produce histamine release. Thus, in contrast to studies with soluble immune complexes, sensitized erythrocytes, and zymosan particles did not require the presence of C6 to stimulate histamine release. Furthermore, the histamine release by such particles was not associated with platelet lysis (Henson, 1970). Immune precipitates prepared at equivalence have also been shown to interact with rabbit platelets to stimulate the release of vasoactive amines (Des Prez and Bryant, 1969).

The interaction of immune complexes with human platelets has also been characterized extensively. Studies by Movat *et al.* (1965) demonstrated that BSA–antiBSA and ferritin–anti ferritin prepared with rabbit antibodies either at equivalence, antigen excess of 2½–5 times, or at twice the antibody excess caused platelet aggregation and release of ADP, serotonin, and histamine during *in vitro* incubation with human platelets. Platelet aggregation and the release of nucleotides were similarly observed following the incubation of human platelets with immune precipitates prepared with horse or sheep antibodies, as well as with heat-aggregated human γ-globulin in absence of complement components (Mueller-Eckhardt and Lüscher, 1968). Other observations indicated that human platelets lacked receptors for complement (Mueller-Eckhardt and Lüscher, 1968; Henson, 1969).

The mechanism of immune complex interaction with human platelets was mediated through the platelet receptor for the Fc fragment of IgG (Israels *et al.*, 1973). Complexes with $F(ab')_2$ fragments failed to cause aggregation, and the preincubation of platelets with Fc fragments blocked the aggregation with complexes.

Penttinen *et al.* (1971) demonstrated that the lattice structure of the immune complex was important in producing platelet aggregation. Complexes were prepared with a hapten–protein conjugate (NIP_{24}–BSA) and rabbit anti-hapten antibodies at varying antigen–antibody ratios. Complexes prepared at eight times antigen excess had a sedimentation coefficient between 7 S and 19 S by sucrose density gradient ultracentrifugation, and gradient fractions containing these complexes did not aggregate platelets. Complexes >19 S were found when they were prepared at either two times antigen excess or two times antibody excess, and, in both cases, fractions containing complexes >19 S caused platelet aggregation. Thus, platelet aggregation appeared to be mediated by large-latticed complexes.

The classes and subclasses of human immunoglobulins responsible for platelet aggregation and release of vasoactive substances was examined by Henson and Spiegelberg (1973). Using both heat and bisdiazotized benzidine aggregated myeloma proteins, IgG1, IgG2, IgG3, and IgG4 caused platelet aggregation and serotonin release. IgA1, IgA2, IgD, IgM, and IgE were all inactive. IgG4 was less active than the other IgG subclasses. After mild reduction and alkylation, the activity of the IgG subclasses was reduced. Isolated Fc fragments of IgG were active, whereas $F(ab')_2$ fragments were not. The release of vasoactive amines was not associated with platelet lysis. Of additional interest was the fact that fresh serum partially inhibited the release by IgG1 and IgG3, but had no effect on the release by IgG2 and IgG4, which suggested that fixation of complement by IgG1 and IgG3 may interfere with binding to the platelet Fc receptor.

The role of complement in the interaction of immune complexes with platelets was further examined by Pfueller and Lüscher (1974). Either bisdiazotized benzidine aggregated human IgG, or ferritin–anti-ferritin (rabbit) complexes were incubated with platelets in the presence of plasma. A biphasic response was noted consisting of an initial rapid release of serotonin, followed by platelet aggregation and a secondary release of serotonin. The first phase could be inhibited by complement components but was unaffected by complement depletion with cobra venom factor (CVF), by EDTA, or by inhibiting ADP action. The second phase required ADP and was inhibited by CVF and EDTA. Thus, the complement system appeared to play a role in modulating both the interaction of complexes with platelets and the release of vasoactive substances.

7. *Lymphocytes*

The interaction of immune complexes with lymphocytes has recently been reviewed by Nussenzweig (1974). The binding of immune complexes to lymphocytes was established by Uhr (1965) and Uhr and Phillips (1966).

Complexes were prepared with flagella from *Salmonella paratyphi B* and guinea pig anti-flagella antibodies. Following the incubation of guinea pig lymphocytes with the complexes, the cells which bound the complexes were detected by adherence of bacteria. Both IgG and IgM antibodies were thought to participate in this phenomenon. The adherence of complexes to lymphocytes was enhanced in the presence of complement but was also noted to a lesser degree in the absence of complement.

LoBuglio *et al.* (1967) demonstrated that human erythrocytes coated with IgG anti-D isoantibodies adhered to some human lymphocytes, whereas IgM antibodies did not mediate such adherence. Since these observations, many studies have been carried out using sensitized erythrocytes for characterizing the interaction of complexes with lymphocytes.

Studies by Bianco *et al.* (1970) on the interaction of mouse lymphocytes with sensitized erythrocytes established the importance of complement in this system. A distinct subpopulation of lymphocytes bound the sheep erythrocytes sensitized with rabbit antibodies (EA) only when components of complement through C3 were added (EAC). The subpopulation of lymphocytes was, thus, designated as "complement receptor lymphocytes" (CRL) and appeared to be B cells by other criteria (Bianco and Nussenzweig, 1971). The split products of C3, presumably C3b, inhibited the binding of EAC (Eden *et al.*, 1973). Ross *et al.* (1973) demonstrated that human lymphocytes have distinctive receptors for C3b and C3d fragments of C3. EAC1-3b reportedly bound to the C3b receptor through the C3c region of uncleaved C3b, as well as to the C3d receptor through the C3d region of uncleaved C3b (Ross and Polley, 1975). EAC1-3d only bound to the C3d receptor. Finally, Ross and Polley (1975) also reported that EAC14 would bind to human lymphocytes through the C3b receptor.

Although erythrocytes sensitized with rabbit antibodies or isoantibodies (EA) did not mediate lymphocyte adherence in the above studies, erythrocytes sensitized with higher concentrations of antibodies adhered to lymphocytes in the absence of complement. Yoshida and Andersson (1972) found that sheep erythrocytes sensitized with the IgG fraction of rabbit anti-sheep erythrocyte antibodies adhered to mouse B cells and T cells. While 5–16% of normal thymic lymphocytes reacted with EA (IgG), this could be increased by examining thymus lymphocytes 4–6 days after cortisone treatment at the time blastoid cells appeared. In addition, EA (IgG) reacted with 60–80% of activated T cells, which were obtained from the lymphoid organs of allogenic mice after reconstitution of irradiated mice with thymus cells. The adherence of EA (IgG) to B cells could be inhibited by preincubating the cells with immune complexes containing BSA and mouse anti-BSA (IgG) in slight antigen excess or with free IgG. On the other hand, the reaction of EA (IgG) with activated T cells was inhibited only by the BSA–anti-BSA complexes and not by free IgG. Thus, B lymphocytes had receptors both for immune complexes containing IgG and for free IgG, whereas activated T cells had receptors only for immune complexes containing IgG and not for free IgG.

Fridman and Golstein (1974) similarly demonstrated a receptor for EA(IgG) on activted mouse T cells and referred to this as immunoglobulin-binding factor (IBF). This factor was released into supernatant during tissue culture; it agglutinated EA(IgG), and it blocked complement-mediated lysis of cells sensitized with intact IgG. The IBF appeared to interact only with the Fc fragment of IgG. In the hand of these investigators, the reaction of EA(IgG) with activated T cells was inhibited by free IgG. Neauport-Sautes *et al.* (1975) further demonstrated that the Fc receptor (IBF) on activated mouse thymocytes was expressed by a subpopulation (30–40%) of the cells. Also, there was no species specificity by the Fc receptor for rabbit, human, or mouse IgG, since they all adhered to the Fc receptor and competitively inhibited each other.

Although mouse thymus cells in previous studies appeared to lack receptors for EA(IgM), T cell receptors for IgM have recently been demonstrated by Moretta *et al.* (1975) and McConnell and Hurd (1976) on human T cells and by Lamon *et al.* (1976) on mouse T cells. In the studies by Moretta *et al.* (1975), ox erythrocytes were sensitized with rabbit IgG or IgM antibodies. EA(IgM) adhered to peripheral blood lymphocytes (PBL) only after the cell suspensions were kept in culture at 37°C for 24 hours with media lacking IgM molecules. Freshly drawn and cultured PBL bound only EA(IgG). EA(IgM) bound almost exclusively to T cells, whereas EA(IgG) appeared to bind to both T and B cells. The binding of EA(IgM) was easily inhibited by free IgM and not by free IgG, and EA(IgG) binding was inhibited by free IgG. McConnell and Hurd (1976) confirmed these results with essentially identical observations. Finally, Lamon *et al.* (1976) demonstrated that sheep erythrocytes sensitized with high concentrations of either mouse IgG or IgM adhered to mouse lymphocytes in the absence of complement. The EA(IgM) adhered to subpopulations of both T and B cells. Lymphocytes with IgM receptors appeared to be exclusive of lymphocytes with IgG and complement receptors. The receptor for IgM was specific for the Fc fragment of IgM, since human IgM $(Fc)_{5\mu}$ fragments completely inhibited the binding of EA(IgM) to thymus cells. Soluble complexes containing dextran and myeloma (MOPC 104E) IgM anti-dextran antibodies also inhibited EA(IgM) binding to thymus cells and did not inhibit EA(IgG) binding. In the same manner, complexes containing IgG were said to inhibit only EA(IgG) binding and not EA(IgM) binding. Thus, the IgM receptor was specific for the Fc fragment of IgM.

The interaction of soluble immune complexes with lymphocytes has been examined, to a limited extent, with preformed antigen–antibody complexes and, to a greater extent, with aggregated γ-globulins.

Basten *et al.* (1972a,b) examined the adherence of three different kinds of immune complexes to mouse thoracic duct lymphocytes (TDL) by autoradiography. The percentage of TDL, which bound complexes, increased with the amount of specific antibody to a range of 15–20% in normal mice. These cells were judged to be B cells, since nearly all TDL from athymic nude mice bound the complexes, and since the proportion of normal TDL which bound complexes could be increased *in vitro* following treatment with anti-θ serum and complement. The greatest binding occurred with IgG_1 class by inhibition studies with myeloma proteins. Some binding was noted with the IgG_{2b} and IgM classes of antibodies, and no binding was observed with IgG_{2a} and IgA classes. The interaction was mediated by the immunoglobulin Fc fragment, since it could not be inhibited by $F(ab')_2$ fragments. Finally, the interaction was complement independent. Similar conclusions were reached by Paraskevas *et al.* (1972) by using other antigen–antibody systems and inhibition of the reverse immune cytoadherence assay. With immunofluorescent techniques, Stout and Herzenberg (1975) further corraborated the existence of the Fc receptors on mouse thymus-derived lymphocytes. Approximately 65% of spleen cells and 15% of thymus cells were labeled by fluoresceinated complexes containing IgG antibodies, whereas less than 5% of spleen cells were labeled with complexes containing either $F(ab')_2$ or IgM antibodies. Mouse spleen and lymph nodes contained 46% and 75% T cells, respectively, with approximately 23% of these T cells having the Fc receptor. Thus, the Fc receptor exists on a subpopulation of T cells.

Studies examining the interaction of aggregated γ-globulins with lymphocytes have produced results similar to those using soluble antigen–antibody complexes. Heat-aggregated human IgG was demonstrated by Brown *et al.* (1970) to adhere to mouse lymphocytes in the absence of complement. Dickler and Kunkel (1972) demonstrated with fluoresceinated, aggregated human IgG the receptor on human and rabbit B lymphocytes. Although the direct detection of lymphocyte binding was optimal with fluoresceinated aggregates larger than 300 S in size, the adherence of smaller complexes could be detected by indirect means. The interaction of human immunoglobulins with human lymphocytes was further examined by Lawrence *et al.* (1975) using myeloma proteins. Unaggregated IgG1 and IgG3 proteins bound to lymphocytes, but unaggregated proteins of the other IgG subclasses, as well as of the other classes did not bind. This binding was mediated through the Fc fragment of IgG. Aggregated IgG of all subclasses and aggregated IgE bound to lymphocytes, whereas aggregated proteins of the other classes did not. Of interest is that C1 on the surface of human B lymphocytes appeared to inhibit the binding of aggregated IgG (Füst *et al.*, 1976).

Receptors for aggregated IgG were demonstrated on mouse lymphocytes by using aggregated mouse myeloma proteins (Anderson and Grey, 1974). Receptors for IgG_{2b} were present on both B and T cells with aggregates binding to 70–80% of spleen cells and 20–45% of thymus cells. The aggregate receptor was found on 80% of B cells, 30% of T cells, and 60% of null cells in the spleen. The binding was mediated by the Fc fragment and was proportional to the size of the aggregates. No binding was observed with monomeric IgG.

Ramasamy *et al.* (1976) essentially confirmed the above observations by using various mouse myeloma proteins to inhibit the Fc rosette formation by lymph node cells with bovine erythrocytes sensitized with mouse antisera. Of particular interest was the observation that an aggregated, mutant IgG_1 myeloma protein lacking the $C\gamma3$ domain did not inhibit rosette formation.

Van Boxel and Rosenstreich (1974) showed that guinea pig thymus cells did not bind the IgG aggregates by immunofluorescence. T lymphocyte preparations activated by antigen *in vivo* or *in vitro* contained cells with receptors for aggregates.

The interaction of antigen–antibody complexes with lymphocytes appeared to be modulated by the complement system in studies carried out by Nussenzweig and colleagues (see review by Nussenzweig, 1974). Miller *et al.* (1973) incubated mouse lymph node lymphocytes, in the presence of fresh mouse serum as a source of complement, with a low concentration of complexes containing radiolabeled bovine serum albumin (^{125}I-BSA) and mouse anti-BSA near equivalence. Under these conditions, 30% of ^{125}IBSA–antiBSA complexes adhere to the lymphocytes (B cells). When the isolated lymphocytes were further exposed to fresh mouse serum, approximately 80% of the bound complexes were rapidly released. The release activity was also present in human, rat, and guinea pig serum, but it was absent in the presence of EDTA and cobra venom factor (CVF). The C3 component seemed to be required for activity, since the activity was absent from genetically C3-deficient human serum and was restored upon the addition of purified human C3. The activity appeared only to require an intact alternate pathway, since C3 and C3b were inactive by themselves, and C3 proactivator (factor B) was required for activity. Both C5-deficient mouse serum and C4-deficient guinea pig serum were active, which suggested the classical pathway and late complement components were unnecessary.

This phenomenon transiently influences the behavior of immune complexes *in vivo*. Miller and Nussenzweig (1974) noted that, within 30 seconds after administration of preformed complexes to mice, some of these materials were bound to lymphocytes and then released into plasma. Similarly, when radiolabeled complexes were bound to lymphocytes *in vitro,* the immune complexes were released into plasma by 3 minutes after injection into mice. Interestingly, the serum of old NZB/W mice was deficient in the ability to release *in vitro* immune complexes bound to lymphocytes (Miller *et al.,* 1975). The decrease in release activity was associated with a decrease in C3 concentration. The role of this phenomenon in disease processes remains to be determined.

D. The Effect of Immune Complexes on the Immune Response

The administration of antigen to experimental animals in the form of an immune complex has long been recognized to modify the response to that antigen (reviewed by Stoner and Terres, 1963; Uhr and Möller, 1968). Although the administration of complexes in antigen excess usually enhanced the antibody response and the administration of complexes in antibody excess suppressed the antibody response, exceptions did exist. Studies by Laissue *et al.* (1971) demonstrated that the enhanced antibody response following immunization with immune complexes is associated with enhanced germinal center formation when compared to immunization with antigen alone. Mice were injected in the footpads with complexes containing tetanus toxoid and mouse anti-toxoid antisera of equivalence or with toxoid alone. The antibody titers rose earlier, and the peak titer was 15-fold higher in mice receiving complexes than in mice receiving antigen alone. The number of germinal centers increased earlier, and their size was larger in the regional lymph nodes of mice receiving complexes than in mice receiving antigen alone. Similar conclusions were reached by Dennert (1971), employing sensitized sheep erythrocytes in mice. A viral vaccine containing formalin-inactivated Venezuelan equine encephalitis virus was also more immunogenic and protective in monkeys, when administered as an immune complex with homologous antibodies at equivalence and in antigen excess, but not in antibody excess (Houston *et al.,* 1974). Thus, the immune response to both soluble and particulate antigens is enhanced when the antigen is presented as an immune complex, except when the complexes are formed with excess IgG antibody.

The kinetics of antibody (anti-BSA) formation in mice receiving immune complexes containing bovine serum albumin (BSA) and rabbit anti-BSA in antigen excess were examined by Terres *et al.* (1972). The anti-BSA production following immunization with complexes resembled a secondary response both qualitatively and quantitatively.

Revoltella *et al.* (1975) examined the *in vitro* differentiation of mouse bone marrow cells into antibody-forming cells following stimulation by immune complexes containing ferritin and isologous antibodies. The binding of complexes to lymphocytes was high in antibody excess and low in antigen excess. The percentage of plasma cells increased progressively to the highest levels in cultures containing complexes in antigen excess at 7 days. In contrast, the number of plasma cells declined in cultures containing complexes in antibody excess. In long-term cultures of synchronized bone marrow cells, which were stimulated by complexes in antigen excess, the concentration of antibodies released into the supernatant reached maximum levels by days 15–16, after which the number of plasma cells declined and the supernatant antibody levels diminished. The addition of free antibody to these cultures at 12 days caused an immediate reduction in the number of plasma cells. The addition of free antigen increased the number of plasma cells and the concentration of supernatant antibodies. Thus, the triggering of lymphocytes and the production of plasma cells in cultures receiving complexes in antigen excess appeared to increase until a state of antibody excess was reached, when antibody production became inhibited.

While the emphasis of the above studies is on the capacity of immune complexes to enhance the humoral immune response, suppression occurred in some instances. In reviewing the regulatory effect of antibody on the immune response, Uhr and Möller (1968) suggested that passively administered antibodies may suppress the immune response when high-affinity antibodies bound the antigen in an immune complex and rendered the antigenic determinant sterically unavailable to the antibody-forming mechanism.

Henny and Ishizaka (1970) found that the humoral response to dinitrophenylated human γ-globulin (DNP–HGG) by guinea pigs was markedly reduced when immunized with immune precipitates containing either excess anti-DNP or anti-carrier (anti-Fc) antibodies. However, such immune complexes in antibody excess did not alter the induction of cell-mediated responses as detected by delayed hypersensitivity skin reactions. Thus, suppression of the immune response by immune complexes appeared to be selective for humoral rather than cellular immunity.

Feldmann and Diener (1970) studied suppression of the immune response by immune complexes *in vitro*. Normal mouse spleen cells were pre-incubated with an immunogenic concentration of polymerized flagellin (POL) and sheep erythrocytes (SRC) in the presence of increasing concentrations of either mouse anti-POL or anti-SRC antisera. The cell cultures were then washed, exposed to antigen alone, washed again, and then assayed for antibody-forming cells. The number of antibody-forming cells was specifically suppressed as the concentration of antibodies in the complexes was increased. When treated spleen cells were transferred to irradiated hosts, no response was detected to subsequent challenge with the immunogen. Thus, the suppression by immune complexes in antibody excess was thought to occur at the level of the immunocompetent cell. An optimum ratio of antigen to antibody in the POL–anti-POL complexes was required during the preincubation to establish tolerance (Diener and Feldmann, 1970). When the concentration of anti-POL antibodies in the complexes was further increased, tolerance induction failed. However, complexes with high antibody concentrations continued to be immunosuppresive when present during the entire culture period. Thus, complexes were thought to suppress the immune response, either at the central level by inducing tolerance in immunocompetent cells, or at the peripheral level by altering the stimulating antigen. Further studies (Feldmann and Diener, 1971) indicated that for tolerance induction, the ratio of antigen to antibody in the complexes was highly important, rather than the absolute amount of either antigen or antibody. The ratio of antigen to antibody required for tolerance induction remained constant over a 10,000-fold range in the concentration of immune complexes. Thus, the lattice structure of the complex may be critical for the induction of tolerance.

Finally, Feldmann and Diener (1972) demonstrated that divalent antibodies were required for antigen cross-linking in order to induce tolerance. In addition, the results suggested that the Fc part of the IgG molecule was not involved in this phenomenon. On the other hand, a study by Sinclair *et al.* (1974) provided evidence that immunosuppression by immune complexes in adoptive transfer experiments required the presence of the Fc portion of antibodies at low doses of the complexes.

It should be pointed out that tolerance has also been broken by immune complexes (Intini *et al.*, 1971). Spleen cells from tolerant mice were first incubated with immune complexes containing the tolerated antigen and heterologous antibodies and were then reinjected into the tolerant donor mice. Tolerance was broken most effectively with complexes prepared in antibody excess and was not broken with antigen alone.

Although the mechanism(s) by which immune complexes may bring about suppression of the immune response has not been precisely defined, it may include the activation of suppressor T lymphocytes. Gershon (1974), in reviewing the evidence for T cell control of antibody production, also cited some evidence that antigen–antibody complexes may work at the T cell level. It was suggested that antigen–antibody complexes, in certain molar ratios, may act as a feedback signal to stimulate suppressor T cells. While Gorczynski *et al.* (1974) also suggested that immune complexes mediate suppression through T cells, a blocking of T lymphocyte receptors by complexes was visualized. Although the evidence for this mechanism is indirect, it was noted in several systems that higher antibody titers can be achieved in irradiated recipients of primed spleen cells than had been achieved in the donors of those cells. It was postulated that the T lymphocytes are inactivated in primed mice because they carry an antigen–antibody complex on their surface. As they are adoptively transferred to an antibody-free environment, the antibody was thought to dissociate and the T lymphocyte to become triggered by the antigen. Also, the antibody response was higher in recipients of primed cells that had been allowed to undergo a period of *in vitro* incubation than it was in recipients of cells not so incubated. The incubation effect can be inhibited with high-titer antibodies. Antigen was thought to be released from the surface of incubated primed cells and, thus, provided self-stimulation, unless antibodies were present, and kept the antigen bound to the cell surface as an immune complex.

The hypothesis that antigen–antibody complexes persisted on T cells of sensitized animals and, thereby, caused suppression of antibody formation was further supported by studies of Kontiainen and Mitchison (1975). The plausibility of this mechanism is consistent with the observations (reviewed in Section III,C,7) that immunoglobulin receptors have been detected on at least a subpopulation of T lymphocytes.

Finally, Taylor and Basten (1976) have recently suggested a sequence of events for the induction of suppressor T cells; immune complexes activate suppressor T cells, which stimulate macrophages to release nonspecific factors capable of suppressing both T and B cells. The macrophage was included to explain the observation that both adherent and nonadherent cell populations were needed in some studies to transfer tolerance dependent on suppressor function.

Less data are available regarding the influence of immune complexes on cellular immunity. However, recent studies by Mackaness *et al.* (1974a,b) and by Lagrange and Mackaness (1975) were interpreted to show that immune complexes interfere with cell-mediated immune responses. Delayed-type hypersensitivity (DTH) reactions in the footpads of mice immunized intravenously with sheep erythrocytes (SRBC) became suppressed after 4 days, associated with an increase in hemagglutinating antibody titer. The administration of small doses of day 4 serum (hemagglutinating titer 1:1024) prior to immunization had no effect on DTH. However, administration of the day 4 serum, which had been adsorbed with SRBC such that the hemagglutinating titer was only 1:32, now markedly inhibited the induction of DTH. Absorbed serum also interrupted the expression of previously established DTH and blocked the adoptive transfer of DTH, whereas the unabsorbed serum did not. Although the presence of antigen–antibody complex was not documented, it was suggested that soluble complexes were responsible for blocking the development of DTH reactions by T cells.

E. The Effect of Immune Complexes on *In Vitro* Functions of Lymphoid Cells

While the above studies have examined the induction of tolerance and immunosuppression of the humoral immune response by immune complexes, considerable evidence suggests immune complexes interfere with cell-mediated cytotoxicity. Serum factors in humans and experimental animals bearing tumors specifically block or suppress the lymphocyte-mediated cytotoxicity to the tumor cells (reviewed by Hellström and Hellström, 1974). Hellström and Hellström (1969) demonstrated that the blocking activity of mouse serum could be removed with anti-mouse γ-globulin and that it could be identified in the 7 S component of fractionated serum. Sjögren *et al.* (1971) then reported some characteristics of the blocking factors, which suggested they may be antigen–antibody complexes. Sera from tumor-bearing mice with blocking activity were absorbed with tumor cells. The cells were washed and eluted with a glycine buffer at pH 3.1. With differential filtration, a fraction with antibodies and a fraction with presumed antigen were obtained. These fractions contained no blocking activity, but upon reconstituting the mixture, blocking activity was recovered, suggesting that immune complexes were involved.

These same methods were used by Wright *et al.* (1973) to characterize serum blocking factors in rats rendered tolerant to skin allografts. These blocking factors specifically block the cytotoxic effect of immune lymphocytes on allogeneic cells. The factors were also specifically removed from tolerant serum by absorption with allogeneic cells and were subsequently eluted at pH 3.1. Further studies suggested that serum blocking factors could be dissociated at low pH into a low molecular weight substance, thought to be the antigen, and into a high molecular weight substance, thought to be the antibodies. However, the exact nature of these substances remains to be identified, and the mechanisms of action in blocking cytotoxicity remain to be clarified.

Baldwin *et al.* (1972,1973) have shown that antigen–antibody complexes block the cytotoxic activity of immune lymphocytes in the rat hepatoma model. As in the above models, sera from tumor-growing animals blocked lymphocyte-mediated cytotoxicity. After tumor excision, blocking activity was lost, and the sera became cytotoxic for tumor cells. Immune complexes were prepared with a solubilized tumor antigen, and the cytotoxic sera and were tested for blocking activity. The target cells were preincubated with complexes containing a standard amount of cytotoxic or blocking sera and increasing amounts of antigen. With increasing amount of the antigen preparation, the blocking activity increased and then declined, presumably due to excess antigen.

The blocking of cell-mediated cytotoxicity is well documented as a phenomenon, but the immunochemical characterization of the immune complexes has not been accomplished. Furthermore, the mechanisms of action of these materials with target cells and effector cells need further clarification.

Immune complexes also inhibit antibody-dependent cell-mediated cytotoxicity (ADCC). MacLennan (1972) demonstrated that soluble immune complexes inhibited lymphocyte cytotoxicity for target cells coated with specific antibodies. Human Chang cells, which were labeled with ^{51}Cr and sensitized with rat anti-Chang antibodies, were examined at the level of maximum killing by normal rat spleen cells. Immune complexes (HSA and rat anti-HSA, dinitrophenylated pig γ-globulin and rat anti-DNP) and heat-aggregated rat IgG inhibited the cytotoxic effect of the spleen cells for the target cells, when added to the cultures. Maximum inhibition of cytotoxicity occurred with soluble complexes prepared in slight antigen excess. Thus, unrelated immune complexes nonspecifically block ADCC.

Lustig and Bianco (1976) similarly examined the role of antigen–antibody complexes on ADCC. Normal mouse spleen cells were cytotoxic for BSA-coupled chicken erythrocytes (chromium labeled) in the presence of mouse anti-BSA (IgG). When BSA–anti-BSA complexes prepared at various antigen–antibody ratios were added to target cells, followed by adding effector spleen cells, cytotoxicity was inhibited by complexes in antigen excess as well as by antigen alone. When effector cells were incubated with complexes and washed prior to being incubated with unsensitized target cells, they became cytotoxic following incubation with complexes in antibody excess, but not with complexes in antigen excess. Thus, some arming of effector cells, rather than blocking, may occur following incubation with complexes in antibody excess.

The arming of effector cells by immune complexes was demonstrated earlier by Perlmann *et al.* (1972) and by Greenberg and Shen (1973). Lymphocytes were rendered more cytotoxic for target cells when they were preincubated with immune complexes containing the target cell antigen than when they were preincubated with antibodies alone (Perlmann *et al.*, 1972). The absorption of specific antibody was 50- to 100-fold greater following incubation with complexes than with antibodies alone. However, the lymphocytes preincubated with complexes became specifically cytotoxic only for target cells not sensitized with specific antibodies, as they were less cytotoxic for sensitized target cells than were lymphocytes preincubated with antibodies alone. Thus, the sensitized target cells and the lymphocyte-bound immune complexes appeared to compete for the lymphocyte receptor required to mediate cytotoxicity.

Mouse spleen cells without phagocytes became cytotoxic when incubated (armed) with immune complexes but not with antigen or antibodies alone (Greenberg and Shen, 1973). Maximum cytotoxicity developed with complexes formed in antibody excess, and arming appeared to be mediated through the effector cells' Fc receptors for mouse IgG.

Recently, Saksela *et al.* (1975) also demonstrated that both human peripheral blood lymphoid cells and mouse spleen cells could be armed with immune complexes or with antibodies alone to become cytotoxic. When mouse spleen cells were preincubated with specific anti-target cell antibodies or with complexes containing the antibodies and increasing amounts of antigen, the cytotoxicity increased markedly with complexes made in antibody excess. As the amount of added antigen in the complex reached equivalence, the cytotoxicity decreased to levels below that seen with antibodies alone. The arming of effector cells also appeared to be mediated by Fc receptors.

Therefore, immune complexes appear to modulate the expression of ADCC depending on the antigen–antibody ratio and the site of interaction. Immune complexes in antibody excess can bind to the surface of lymphocytes, rendering them specific to target cells. Immune complexes at equivalence and in antigen excess block the antibody-dependent cell-mediated cytotoxicity via the interaction with Fc receptors and by occupying the antibody-binding sites on antibody molecules already on the lymphocytes.

In addition to the already discussed functions, immobilized antigen–antibody complexes inhibited the mitogenic response of mouse spleen cells to B cell mitogens (Ryan *et al.*, 1975). The Fc fragments were required for this response, and the inhibition could not be reproduced by suspensions of immune precipitates. The immobilized complexes only minimally inhibited the response to the T cell mitogen, phytohemagglutinin. However, inhibition of concanavalin A mitogenesis was observed. The mechanisms of these phenomena were not explained.

Immune complexes may also alter the immunologic function of other effector cells. Spitler *et al.* (1969) demonstrated that the capillary migration of peritoneal exudate cells from normal guinea pigs could be inhibited in the presence of antigen–antibody complexes (sensitized erythrocytes).

The mechanism of inhibition was not defined, but interaction of complexes with Fc receptors on the exudate cells may have been required, since IgG-sensitized cells, and not IgM-sensitized cells, caused inhibition.

In more recent studies by Rabinovitch *et al.* (1975), immune complexes immobilized on glass cover slips inhibited the phagocytic function of adherent mouse macrophages. The ingestion of sheep erythrocytes sensitized with rabbit IgG antibodies (EA) by macrophages was markedly inhibited on cover slips coated with complexes, in contrast to that observed on cover slips coated with antigen or antibodies alone, but the adherence of EA as well as EAC was not inhibited. Macrophages plated on complexes were still capable of ingesting glutaraldehyde-treated erythrocytes, latex beads, and yeast cell walls, despite their inability to ingest EA. The immobilized complexes appeared to interact with the macrophage Fc receptor to inhibit the ingestion of EA, since complexes prepared with $F(ab')_2$ did not inhibit ingestion of EA.

When complexes were formed on just a limited portion of the cover slip, the ingestion of EA by the cultured macrophages was inhibited only in the limited area where complexes had formed. Thus, inhibition was not mediated by a soluble, diffusible factor. Macrophages cultured with complexes in fluid phase were not inhibited subsequently from ingesting EA, regardless of whether the complexes were prepared at equivalence, in antigen excess, or in antibody excess. The mechanism by which immobilized complexes may have inhibited the ingestion of EA was thought to involve either the loss of Fc receptor function or the failure to transmit a signal for particle ingestion. Since attachment of EA to Fc receptors still occurred, attachment may require fewer Fc receptors than does ingestion.

IV. MODELS OF IMMUNE COMPLEX DISEASES AND THE FATE OF CIRCULATING IMMUNE COMPLEXES

When soluble immune complexes form in the circulation due to the presence of an antigen and endogenous production of antibodies, or when immune complexes are passively introduced into the circulation, biologic consequences that lead to damage of organs occur. Renal injury is a major consequence of these processes, but vasculitis in many organs, arthritis, serositis, skin involvement, central nervous system abnormalities, decrease in circulating platelets and white blood cells are seen, and fever is encountered. Since kidney involvement is a major problem in human immune complex diseases, this process has been studied experimentally in considerable detail. The pathogenic mechanisms by which immune complexes produce disease have been discussed in reviews by Cochrane and Koffler (1973), Germuth and Rodriguez (1973), and in earlier reviews by Weigle (1961) and Unanue and Dixon (1967). Much has been learned about these processes by animal experimentation in rabbits and mice.

In addition to the systemic immune complex diseases, local immune complex diseases exist in humans and can be produced in animals. Thyroiditis induced by immunity to thyroglobulin, as well as antigen-induced arthritis, serve as examples of such problems.

A. Models of Immune Complex Diseases

A variety of models have been used to study the pathogenic events in immune complex diseases by using several antigens in a number of different species. Most of the available information has been obtained in rabbits and in mice. These models can be classified in several ways. (1) Much has been learned from spontaneous animal diseases, such as the disease in New Zealand mice. (2) Some of the pioneering information was obtained by injection of antigens and allowing the immune response of the recipient to provide the antibodies to induce the disease. (3) The pathogenic events could be generated by injection of preformed immune complexes. The spontaneous diseases, particularly the disease in New Zealand black and white mice is discussed elsewhere in this volume. For better understanding of the pathogenic events, the disease models induced by injection of antigen can be categorized as acute and chronic serum sickness (immune complex disease).

1. Acute Experimental Serum Sickness

The majority of information in this category of models has been obtained from studies in rabbits. To induce significant disease, the injection of large quantities of antigen was required; for example 500 mg of bovine serum albumin (BSA) was given intravenously to rabbits weighing 2 kg. The use of radiolabeled antigen allowed easy tracing of the injected material. The injection of BSA into an unimmunized rabbit was followed by rapid equilibration between the intravascular and extravascular spaces and resulted in rapid decline of the serum concentration of BSA. Thereafter, the serum concentration declined gradually due to catabolism of the injected protein. Most of the rabbits developed an immune response, and, when sufficient antibody production evolved, a relatively rapid immune clearance of the radiolabeled BSA occurred.

The rabbits, which developed the most vigorous antibody response and rapidly cleared the antigen, developed glomerulonephritis, vasculitis, synovitis, and heart lesions during the phase of immune clearance. The level of serum complement decreased during this phase, and immune complexes with the radiolabeled antigen were identified in the circulation of rabbits that developed lesions. When the complexes were characterized by sucrose density gradient (SDG) ultracentrifugation, the rabbits with larger (heavier) circulating complexes, approaching a sedimentation coefficient of 19 S, developed more severe glomerular lesions than rabbits with small (light) complexes. An important observation by Cochrane and Hawkins (1968) was that rabbit 19 S complexes, recovered from the SDG fractions, localized in blood vessel walls following their intravenous administration to guinea pigs. However, the guinea pigs had to be treated with high doses of histamine in order to see this effect. The smaller complexes, isolated and administered in a similar manner, did not localize in the blood vessels. These observations suggested that complexes with a large-lattice structure were necessary for vascular deposition.

In the models of acute serum sickness, the peak of disease manifestations was reached shortly after the completion of immune clearance of the antigen from circulation. Thereafter, complement returned to normal levels, and, gradually, the inflammation in kidneys, blood vessels, and elsewhere abated. Thus, when the antigen was exhausted, the pathogenic process subsided.

2. *Chronic Experimental Serum Sickness*

The chronic model of serum sickness in rabbits was achieved by repeated, even daily, intravenous administration of antigen. This was achieved either by injection of a fixed dose or by injection of a dose that was adjusted to the amount of antibodies produced by the rabbit. If the antigen injection was continued for a long period, the experimental animals succumbed to chronic renal failure.

In the induction of chronic serum sickness, any rabbit that mounted an immune response developed chronic glomerulonephritis when the dose of antigen relative to the titer of circulating antibodies was administered in antigen excess. When the same amount of antigen was administered daily (e.g., 12.5 mg of BSA), as emphasized by Germuth and Rodriguez (1973), the development of glomerulonephritis depended on the level of antibody response. Rabbits that mounted a high response or mounted no response had histologically normal glomeruli. Rabbits that mounted a low antibody response developed diffuse glomerulonephritis associated with the deposition of immune complexes in the glomerular capillary loops (see Fig. 10). Following the administration of radiolabeled antigen, circulating immune complexes with a molecular weight (MW) of between 500,000 and 700,000 daltons were detected by SDG ultracentrifugation. These complexes were thought to have a lattice structure between Ag_3Ab_2 and Ag_4Ab_3, and they remained in the circulation up to 24 hours following the administration of antigen. Finally, rabbits that mounted an intermediate level antibody response had deposits of immune complexes in the glomerular mesangium (intercapillary region), associated with mesangial proliferation and normal renal function (see Fig. 11). Larger complexes ranging from 500,000 to several million daltons, but with a predominant size of 1 million daltons, were detected in the circulation of these rabbits. These complexes disappeared from the circulation by 5 hours, in contrast to the persistence of circulating complexes noted above in low responders. The difference in the glomerular distribution of immune complex deposits between the low and intermediate responder groups may have reflected differences in the size or lattice structure of circulating complexes, differences in the duration of time complexes persisted in the circulation, or differences in other factors. Although the precise mechanism for determining the glomerular site of immune complex deposition was not established, circulating complexes with a large-lattice structure were apparently required for deposition.

3. *Serum Sickness Induced by Preformed Immune Complexes*

The acute and chronic forms of experimental serum sickness served to establish the role of immune complexes in inducing pathological lesions. These models, however, were difficult to manipulate to examine the role of lattice formation, dose of antibodies, and other variables for the induction of tissue lesions. For this reason, investigators turned to experimentation with preformed immune complexes. These reagents could be prepared either by solubilizing washed precipitates in antigen excess or by forming soluble complexes with purified antibodies in antigen excess.

The injection of preformed immune complexes into rabbits caused minimal and inconsistent lesions (Cochrane, 1971). The failure to achieve significant lesions in these animals may have been due to the relatively small dosages used or due to other factors. In the one-shot serum sickness of rabbits, on days 8–10, when the immune clearance began, about 200 mg of the injected 500 mg of BSA remained in the rabbit (Dixon *et al.*, 1958). To achieve a rapid immune clearance of this material, the formed immune complexes must be larger than Ag_2Ab_2 (Haakenstad and Mannik, 1974). If one assumes that Ag_2Ab_3 is the minimum lattice formation for rapid clearance, then 350–400 mg of antibody (IgG) would be required for immune clearance. This estimation may explain, in part, the failure to induce significant disease in rabbits with preformed immune complexes.

In mice, however, the intravenous administration of large or repeated doses of immune complexes caused glomerular inflammation, glomerular deposition of immune complexes, and vasculitis (McCluskey and Benacerraf, 1959; McCluskey *et al.*, 1960, 1962; Miller *et al.*, 1960; Mellors and Brzosko, 1962; Okumura *et al.*, 1971). These observations, thus, opened the way to characterize the nature of immune complexes that localized in tissues and caused tissue damage. Furthermore, the lesions induced by injected immune complexes were transient and abated slowly after the immune complexes were cleared from circulation.

4. *Experimental Local Immune Complex Disease*

The basic model of local immune complex disease is the Arthus reaction, induced in actively or passively immunized animals by local injection of antigen. The vasculitis that ensues at the site of antigen injection depends on formation of immune complexes in small vessel walls (Cochrane and Weigle, 1958), complement fixation (Rother *et al.*, 1964; Ward and Cochrane, 1965), and influx of first polymorphonuclear leukocytes and later mononuclear cells (Cochrane *et al.*, 1959; Humphrey, 1955; Cochrane, 1967).

In an analogous manner, local immune complex disease can be produced in any specific organ such as joints, lung, pleural cavity, etc. Of the various body cavities, the antigen-induced arthritis has been examined most extensively. Dumonde and Glynn (1962) showed that by repeated injection of antigen into the joints of rabbits a prolonged synovitis can be induced. Similar inflammation can be produced by the injection of preformed soluble immune complexes (Rawson and Torralba, 1967; Hollister *et al.*, 1973). Of particular interest is that, in these models of synovitis, small amounts of the injected antigen are retained firmly for prolonged periods of time in the superficial areas of the articular cartilage and ligaments (Webb *et al.*, 1971; Cooke *et al.*, 1972; Hollister and Mannik, 1974).

Another example of well-studied local immune complex disease is the thyroiditis induced by injection of heterologous or homologous thyroglobulin. As antibodies are synthesized, immune complexes are formed between thyroglobulin and antibodies in the interstitial spaces (Clagett *et al.*, 1974). Thereafter, acute and chronic inflammatory events follow. The synthesis of thyroglobulin by follicular cells continues, thus providing a source of antigen for continued formation of immune complexes. The key to the production of the disease was the induction of antibody formation by breaking tolerance to thyroglobulin (see review by Weigle, 1973).

B. Fate of Circulating Immune Complexes

Once immune complexes are injected into an animal or form in circulation, their removal by the phagocytic system depends on a number of variables, including the lattice of the immune complexes, the nature of antibodies, the nature of antigen molecules, and the status of the mononuclear phagocyte system. These variables will be discussed in further detail. In human diseases, these parameters have received little attention in relationship to the clinical manifestations and prognosis.

1. The Role of the Lattice of Immune Complexes

To examine the role of lattice of antigen–antibody complexes in the removal of these materials from circulation, endogenously induced models of immune complex disease were not suitable because the degree of lattice formation and the subsequent fate of these materials could not be examined in detail.

Studies by Lightfoot *et al.* (1970) used oligovalent hapten–protein conjugates to prepare immune complexes. The oligovalent antigens were prepared by controlling the number of dinitrophenyl (DNP) haptenic determinants conjugated to the rabbit serum albumin (RSA) carrier molecule. As the number of haptenic substitutions on RSA was increased (e.g., from $DNP_{1.2}$ RSA to $DNP_{1.9}$ RSA), the size distribution of complexes prepared in excess antibody increased by sucrose density gradient ultracentrifugation analysis. The heavier sedimenting complexes were cleared more rapidly, suggesting that the clearance was enhanced as the lattice structure of the complex was increased.

The disappearance kinetics of soluble immune complexes with a defined lattice structure were studied in rabbits by Mannik *et al.* (1971) and Arend and Mannik (1971). Small doses of preformed complexes, which were prepared with several antigens, were administered intravenously. The size distribution of the complexes was followed sequentially by sucrose density gradient (SDG) ultracentrifugation. For example, rabbit antibodies to human serum albumin (HSA) were purified and radioiodinated, and HSA–antiHSA complexes were prepared at fivefold antigen excess. These complexes contained a distinct 6.6 S peak of free antibodies, a partially buried peak of 8.5 S containing Ag_1Ab_1, an 11 S peak of complexes containing two antigen and two antibody molecules (Ag_2Ab_2), and a broad shoulder of larger complexes with a sedimentation coefficient greater than 11 S, containing more than two antigen and two antibody molecules ($>Ag_2Ab_2$) (see Fig. 2). Following injection, the large-latticed ($>Ag_2Ab_2$) complexes were quickly removed from the circulation by the Kupffer cells in the liver, while Ag_2Ab_2 and smaller complexes persisted in the circulation. These findings were further explained by the subsequent finding that the $>Ag_2Ab_2$ complexes selectively adhered to mononuclear phagocytes or macrophages (Arend and Mannik, 1972). The removal of these large-latticed complexes was not mediated by complement components since the removal of immune complexes was altered neither in rabbits depleted of C3 by cobra venom factor nor in rabbits depleted of the early complement components by aggregated γ-globulin. Similar experiments in rhesus monkeys further documented the role of lattice in the removal of immune complexes from circulation (Mannik and Arend, 1971).

Earlier studies in mice had established that small intravenous doses of immune complexes were removed from the circulation by Kupffer cells in the liver (Benacerraf *et al.*, 1959a; Weiser and Laxson, 1962). When small doses of complexes with varying degrees of lattice structure were administered to mice, the complexes were cleared more rapidly from the circulation as the degree of lattice structure was increased (Lightfoot *et al.*, 1970). The above studies in mice were extended by the use of immune com-

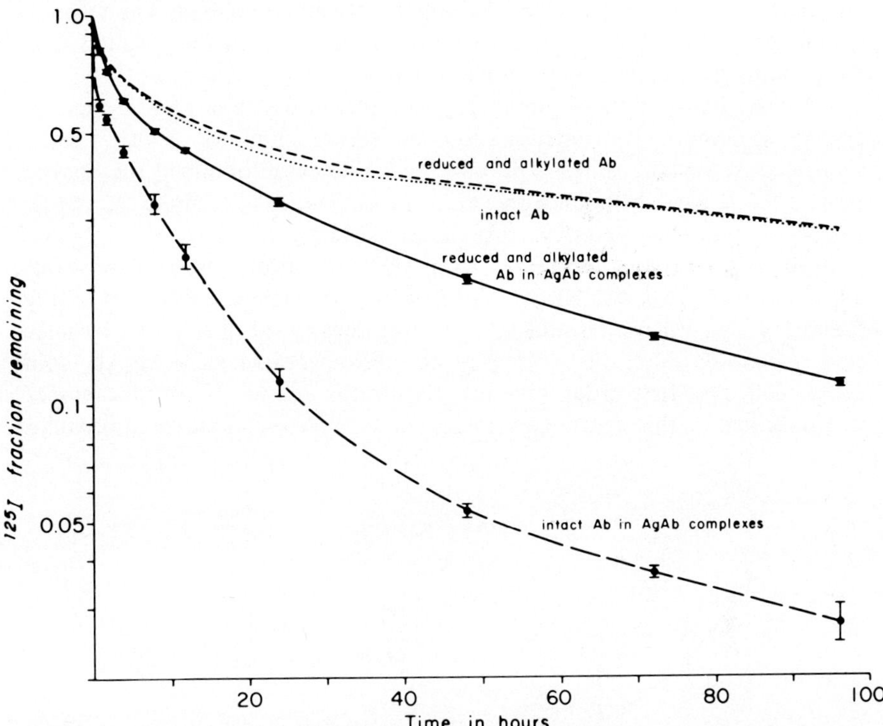

Fig. 5. Disappearance of HSA–rabbit anti-HSA at fivefold antigen excess containing either 5.0 mg of reduced and alkylated antibodies or 5.0 mg of intact antibodies and disappearance of antibodies alone in mice. The disappearance of complexes containing reduced and alkylated antibodies was delayed in comparison to the disappearance of complexes containing intact antibodies, whereas the disappearance of both preparations of antibodies alone was similar (from Haakenstad and Mannik, 1976).

plexes prepared with HSA and rabbit anti-HSA (consisting of IgG), at fivefold antigen excess (Haakenstad and Mannik, 1974). Following the administration of complexes at varying doses, the disappearance of circulating radioactivity was found to be a complicated process. The disappearance of radioactivity was curvilinear over 96 hours when graphed semilogarithmically (Fig. 5). Using both the manual and computer methods of curve peeling, the disappearance was best described statistically by the summation of three exponential components. The first rapid component, with a half-life of 5–10 minutes, was demonstrated in later studies (Haakenstad *et al.,* 1975) to reflect an initial phase of increased vascular permeability. The second component ranged in half-life from 2 to 5 hours and represented the removal of the larger-latticed complexes. The terminal component with a half-life around 40 hours represented the catabolism of the remaining complexes with small lattice.

The size distribution of circulating complexes was analyzed by sucrose density gradient ultracentrifugation of serum obtained from animals sacrificed at various times. The injected complexes contained the characteristic 6.6 S free antibodies, the 11 S peak of Ag_2Ab_2 complexes, and the > 11 S shoulder of > Ag_2Ab_2 complexes as described above (Fig. 2). The removal of > Ag_2Ab_2 complexes from the circulation was relatively fast, whereas the Ag_2Ab_2 (11 S) complexes were removed at a slower rate (Fig. 6 and Fig. 7). When a number of mice were examined in this way by injection of various doses of complexes, the disappearance of > Ag_2Ab_2 complexes followed first-order kinetics. Saturation of this first-order process was observed as the clearance velocity for > Ag_2Ab_2 complexes approached

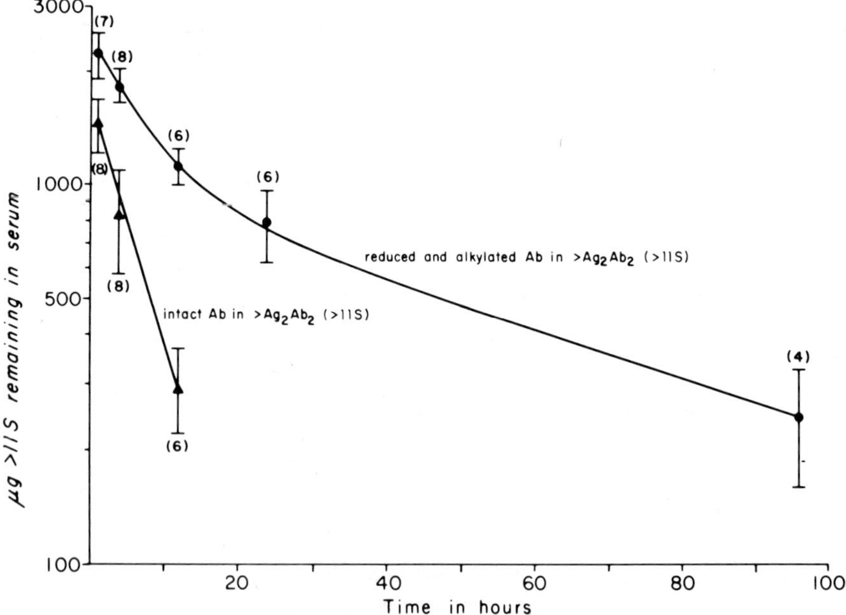

Fig. 6. Disappearance of complexes containing more than two antigen and two antibody molecules (>Ag_2Ab_2) following the administration of complexes as in Fig. 5. The quantity (μg) of >Ag_2Ab_2 (>11 S) remaining in the serum of a number of mice (in parentheses) sacrificed at each time was analyzed by sucrose density gradient ultracentrifugation. The >AG_2Ab_2 persisted longer in mice receiving complexes containing reduced and alkylated antibodies than in mice receiving complexes containing intact antibodies (from Haakenstad and Mannik, 1976).

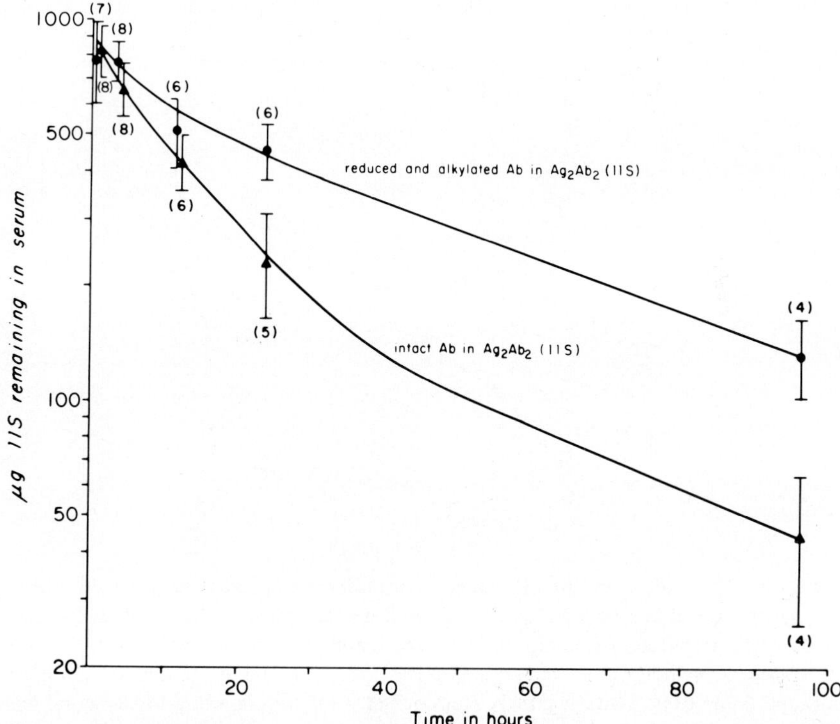

Fig. 7. Disappearance of complexes containing two antigen and two antibody molecules (Ag_2Ab_2) following the administration of complexes as in Fig. 5. The quantity (μg) of Ag_2Ab_2 (11 S) remaining in the serum of a number of mice (in parentheses) sacrificed at each time was analyzed by sucrose density gradient ultracentrifugation. The Ag_2Ab_2 complexes persisted much longer in circulation than the $>Ag_2Ab_2$ complexes with intact antibodies, and the difference between the complexes with intact and with reduced and alkylated antibodies was less than for the $>Ag_2Ab_2$ complexes illustrated in Fig. 6 (from Haakenstad and Mannik, 1976).

a maximum of around 300 μg/hour with doses of complexes containing 2.0 and 5.0 mg of antibodies (Fig. 8). The half-life of $> Ag_2Ab_2$ complexes under steady-state condition was 0.93, 0.96, 1.45, and 3.93 hours for complexes containing 0.1, 1.0, 2.0, and 5.0 mg of antibodies, respectively.

These observations collectively establish that the removal of soluble immune complexes is a function of the lattice of immune complexes. Large-latticed complexes are preferentially removed by the mononuclear phagocyte system, primarily by the Kupffer cells of the liver. Of note is that these cells are intermixed with endothelial cells in liver sinusoids and are

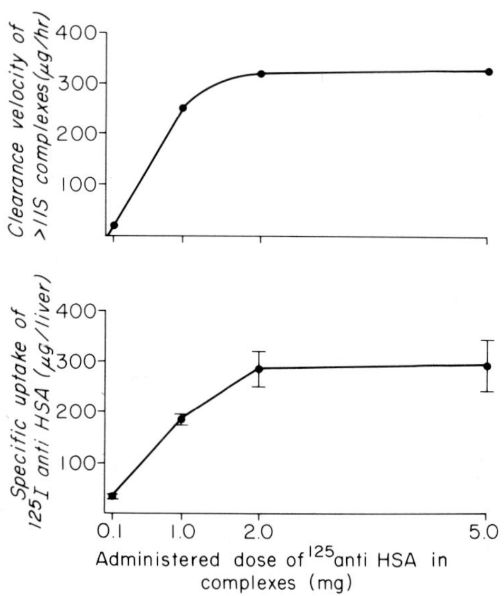

Fig. 8. Saturation of the clearance of immune complexes from the circulation and saturation of the hepatic uptake of immune complexes. HSA–anti-HSA complexes were prepared at fivefold antigen excess and were administered to mice. Both the clearance velocity of $>Ag_2Ab_2$ complexes (top panel) and the hepatic uptake of immune complexes (bottom panel) approached a maximum value at the same dose of complexes (from Mannik *et al.*, 1974).

exposed to the circulating blood (Wisse and Daems, 1970). Furthermore, with a large load of large-lattice complexes, the removal of these materials is decreased, leading to prolonged circulation of this material. Small-latticed complexes (Ag_2Ab_2 and Ag_1Ab_1) persist longer in circulation but are catabolized faster than IgG.

Detailed studies of the role of lattice formation in immune complexes with other classes of immunoglobulins have not been conducted.

The degree of lattice formation is influenced by the molar ratio of antigen to antibody in an *in vitro* mixture of these reagents and, probably, in the *in vivo* setting as well. For example, when HSA-^{125}I-anti-HSA complexes containing 10.0 mg of antibodies per milliliter are prepared at fivefold antigen excess, approximately 60.0% of the antibodies exist as $> Ag_2Ab_2$ complexes. When these same complexes are prepared at 50-fold antigen excess, approximately 10.0% of the antibodies exist as $> Ag_2Ab_2$ complexes (A. O. Haakenstad and M. Mannik, unpublished observation).

Another factor which may influence the lattice of circulating antigen–antibody complexes is the avidity of the antibodies for the antigen. The avidity of antibodies to soluble protein antigens have been shown to vary between inbred strains of mice by Soothill, Steward, and colleagues (Soothill and Steward, 1971; Petty *et al.*, 1972). Mice producing high-affinity antibodies clear the soluble antigen from the circulation at a faster rate than do mice producing low-affinity antibodies (Alpers *et al.*, 1972). Of particular interest was the observation that these two strains of mice, which were prone to nephritis following neonatal lymphocytic choriomeningitis virus infection, produced lower avidity antibodies than did two nephritis-resistant strains (Soothill and Steward, 1971).

2. *The Role of Antibodies*

The nature of antibodies in soluble immune complexes may profoundly alter their fate in circulation. Normal immunoglobulins naturally differ in their avidity for cell-surface receptors on mononuclear phagocytes, neutrophils, etc., depending upon their class and subclass as discussed earlier in Section III,C. It is possible that soluble immune complexes of sufficient lattice structure containing different subclasses of human IgG may have different fate in circulation and, thereby, different pathogenic effects. When immune complexes are experimentally prepared with reduced and alkylated antibodies, many of their biologic properties are altered. Reduced and alkylated antibodies bind antigen and form a lattice structure in the same manner as intact antibodies, but these complexes fix complement inefficiently and adhere poorly to mononuclear phagocytes in comparison to complexes prepared with normal antibodies (Mannik *et al.*, 1971; Arend and Mannik, 1971, 1972). Immune complexes containing reduced and alkylated antibodies have prolonged survival in the circulation of rabbits due to hepatic uptake of large-latticed complexes (Fig. 5) (Mannik *et al.*, 1971; Arend and Mannik, 1972). Two mechanisms contribute to the prolonged survival of complexes containing reduced and alkylated antibodies in mice (Haakenstad and Mannik, 1976). First, the initial phase of enhanced vascular permeability was abrogated. Second, the removal of the large-latticed complexes ($>Ag_2Ab_2$) from the circulation was markedly slowed due to decreased hepatic uptake (see Fig. 6 and Fig. 7). Therefore, these observations seem relevant to human disease, in addition to experimentally induced disease, in view of different biologic characteristics of immunoglobulin classes and subclasses.

3. *The Role of Antigens*

The nature of the antigen may also determine the fate of antigen–antibody complexes. The fate of antigenic materials varies greatly depending on the characteristics of the antigen (Thorbecke and Benacerraf, 1962). Following the intravenous administration of particulate antigens, such as bacteria (Benacerraf *et al.*, 1959b; Howard and Wardlaw, 1958; Biozzi *et al.*, 1960) or viruses (Mims, 1959; Brunner *et al.*, 1960; Uhr and Weissmann, 1965), into unimmunized animals, these materials were rapidly removed from the circulation by the liver. Soluble antigens such as serum proteins (Nakamura *et al.*, 1968; Thorbecke *et al.*, 1960) and dextran molecules (Mayerson *et al.*, 1960) were removed from the circulation by catabolic processes at relatively slow rates. However, denatured or aggregated proteins (Thorbecke *et al.*, 1960; Frei *et al.*, 1965) were cleared rapidly from the circulation by the hepatic mononuclear phagocyte system. The plasma half-life tends to decrease as the molecular weight of the protein increased. In previously immunized animals, of course, the removal of circulating antigen is accelerated (Talmage *et al.*, 1951; Weigle, 1960).

Some native molecules may be cleared very rapidly from the circulation of normal animals. For example, DNA is rapidly cleared from the circulation of mice (Tsumita and Iwanaga, 1963) by the liver. Natali and Tan (1972) also demonstrated that both native DNA and DNA irradiated with ultraviolet light were rapidly cleared from the circulation of nonimmunized rabbits with less than 10% remaining in the circulation after 60 minutes.

The metabolic fate of protein antigens may also be altered by covalently linking haptenic determinants to them. Heavily substituted protein antigens have metabolic characteristics similar to that of particulate antigens, whereas lightly substituted protein antigens behave more like the unsubstituted native molecule (Haurowitz, 1968).

Finally, small-latticed immune complexes, made with antigens that rapidly disappear from circulation, are also quickly removed from circulation (M. Mannik, unpublished observations).

4. *The Role of the Mononuclear Phagocyte System*

The characteristics of the mononuclear phagocyte system, including the Kupffer cells in the liver, can alter the removal of circulating immune complexes.

As already discussed, the clearance kinetics of immune complexes from the circulation of mice showed saturation with the large-latticed ($>Ag_2Ab_2$) complexes when varying doses of preformed complexes were injected (Fig. 8) (Haakenstad and Mannik, 1974). During the same experiments, the specific hepatic uptake of complexes was examined at 1 hour following each dose. Saturation of the hepatic uptake was demonstrated (Fig. 8), approaching a maximum of around 300 μg of antibodies in complexes during the experiment with the high doses. The saturation of hepatic uptake of complexes thus resulted in prolonged circulation of large-latticed complexes and enhanced glomerular deposition (Haakenstad and Mannik, 1974; Haakenstad *et al.*, 1976) as discussed below (Fig. 14).

Wilson and Dixon (1971) postulated that an alteration in the function of the mononuclear phagocyte system may occur in the rabbit model of chronic immune complex disease. They measured the clearance rate of radiolabeled, heat-aggregated rabbit serum albumin (RSA) in rabbits receiving daily injections of BSA. No changes in the function of the mononuclear phagocyte system could be demonstrated by this technique 24 hours after a previous injection of BSA. In further studies, the disappearance of aggregated RSA was examined 10 minutes after the daily injection of BSA. These experiments suggested that depression in the function of the mononuclear phagocyte system occurs after prolonged exposure to circulating immune complexes.

The concept of saturation of the mononuclear phagocyte system was established for the clearance of carbon particles by Biozzi *et al.* (1953). Since that time, the physiology and pathophysiology of the mononuclear phagocyte (reticuloendothelial) system has been studied extensively (see review by Saba, 1970). The mononuclear phagocyte system participates in the phagocytic clearance of foreign particulate matter, bacteria, viruses, colloidal substances, denatured proteins, endotoxins, lipid emulsions, etc. Functional alterations of the system occur under many natural or experimentally induced conditions including the various shock syndromes, bacterial infections, viral infections, radiation injury, and tumor growth. Norman (1974) compared the clearance kinetics of carbon particles, aggregated albumin, lipid emulsion, foreign red cells, and latex particles in rats. In each case, the removal of the substance from the circulation was subject to saturation kinetics. In addition, competitive inhibition and a retardation of clearance rate was observed when two different substances were administered simultaneously. Benacerraf *et al.* (1959a) demonstrated that the administration of antigen–antibody complexes 10 minutes after the administration of carbon particles interfered with the subsequent clearance of the carbon in both mice and rabbits. Therefore, it is reasonable to speculate that conditions may occur in which the host is susceptible to immune complex disease because of functional alterations of the mononuclear phagocyte system.

The removal from circulation of antibody-coated particles may differ somewhat from removal of soluble immune complexes, as a function of antibody density on the particle. As an example, the *in vivo* clearance of guinea pig erythrocytes sensitized with either rabbit IgM or IgG antibodies was examined in guinea pigs by Schreiber and Frank (1972a,b). IgM-sensitized cells with 60 complement-fixing sites per cell were initially cleared rapidly by the liver and then released back into the circulation, where they survived normally. The initial clearance depended on complement, as demonstrated by the lack of clearance in C4-deficient or cobra venom factor-treated guinea pigs. Inactivation of the complement-dependent mechanism of liver uptake was thought to be responsible for release of the IgM-sensitized cells back into the circulation. IgG-sensitized cells with 17 complement-fixing sites per cell were also removed quickly by the liver but later sequestered predominantly in the spleen. When the IgG-sensitized cells contained more than 90 complement-fixing sites per cell, the liver uptake remained predominant. However, the hepatic uptake of IgG-sensitized cells with more than 90 complement-fixing sites per cell was apparently mediated by complement receptors, since, in C4-deficient guinea pigs, these cells were sequestered predominantly in the spleen. When the cells were sensitized with greater amounts of IgG to provide 511 sites per cell, liver sequestration predominated even in C4-deficient animals. Nevertheless, the *in vivo* data are generally consistent with the above *in vitro* data (Mantovani *et al.*, 1972) in suggesting that the attachment of particulate antigen–antibody complexes is mediated by complement receptors, while ingestion requires IgG receptor function.

Atkinson and Frank (1974) subsequently demonstrated that the initial hepatic uptake of IgM-sensitized erythrocytes, which had been exposed to fresh serum, was apparently mediated by the C3b receptor on hepatic macrophages. After exposure to C3b inactivator, these sensitized erythrocytes had C3d on their surface, and these cells had normal survival.

C. Factors That Influence Localization of Immune Complexes

Experimentally induced immune complex disease have involvement of a number of organs. In the endogenous disease induced by antigen injection, acute inflammatory lesions occur in the joints, on the heart valves, and in the medium-sized arteries at major branch points, such as the coronary arteries at the point of branching from the aorta and the pulmonary, mesenteric, splenic, pancreatic, gastric, and renal arteries (Cochrane and Koffler, 1973; Germuth and Rodriguez, 1973). In the rabbit model of chronic immune complex disease, glomerulonephritis predominates (Cochrane and Koffler, 1973; Germuth and Rodriguez, 1973). In a recent study, Brentjens *et al.* (1974) found that pulmonary lesions occurred following the induction of chronic immune complex disease with injections of BSA. Membranous and/or proliferative pulmonary lesions occurred with glomerulonephritis in rabbits having a rise in antibody titer to levels requiring 100–150 mg of BSA per day in order to keep the ratio of antigen to antibody in the circulation at equivalence or in slight antigen excess. Thickening of the alveolar capillary wall and intestitium was due to the accumulation of electron-dense deposits, which contained BSA, rabbit IgG, and C3 by immunofluorescence and immunoelectron microscopy. Rabbits requiring low doses of BSA (e.g., 12.5 mg) to maintain the above ratio of antigen to antibody developed no or only slight pulmonary lesions despite the development of proteinuria with glomerular changes of variable degree. Thus, extraglomerular lesions can occur in the chronic immune complex disease model and probably reflects the formation of larger amounts of circulating complexes. Acute immune complex disease was also induced in a group of rabbits, and some of the rabbits that developed proteinuria and granular glomerular deposits also had deposits in the interstitium and capillary walls of the lung. Detailed studies have not been conducted on the factors that may influence the development of extraglomerular lesions in these models. Thus, the marked variability of clinical presentation and course of immune complex diseases cannot be adequately explained on experimental basis. The deposition of immune complexes in glomeruli has been extensively examined.

1. Types of Glomerular Localization of Immune Complexes

On the basis of immunofluorescence microscopy and transmission electron microscopy, the deposition of immune complexes can be divided into subendothelial, mesangial, and subepithelial patterns (see Fig. 9). In the subendothelial deposition of immune complexes, the immunoglobulins are deposited in granular manner along the peripheral capillary loops (Fig. 10), and by electron microscopy deposits are identified in subendothelial area on the capillary side of the basement membrane. Along with these deposits, mesangial deposits are seen as well. Routine histology may show profound increase of cellularity endothelial swelling, necrosis, and decrease in capillary lumen. By immunofluorescence microscopy, the mesangial distribution of complexes shows immunoglobulins in a central branching pattern (Fig. 11). Ultrastructural studies show electron dense deposits in the mesangium, primarily in the mesangial matrix (Fig. 12). By routine histology, these kidney sections may appear normal or with increased mesangial cellularity and increased extracellular mesangial material. In the subepithelial deposition of immune complexes marked, granular immunoglobulin deposits are noted by immunofluorescence microscopy in the peripheral glomerular loops (Fig. 10). The electron-dense deposits by electron microscopy are localized in the subepithelial area on the urinary space side of the basement membrane (Fig. 13). By routine histology, the capillary lumens are patent, the basement membrane is thickened, and the Bowman's capsule may show increased cellularity and fibrosis. Similar patterns of immunoglobulin deposition have been noted in human immune complex disease (Cochrane and Koffler, 1973; Germuth and Rodriguez, 1973). A number of investigations have been carried out to explain these differences in glomerular localization of immune complexes. The final answer to this problem, however, is not available.

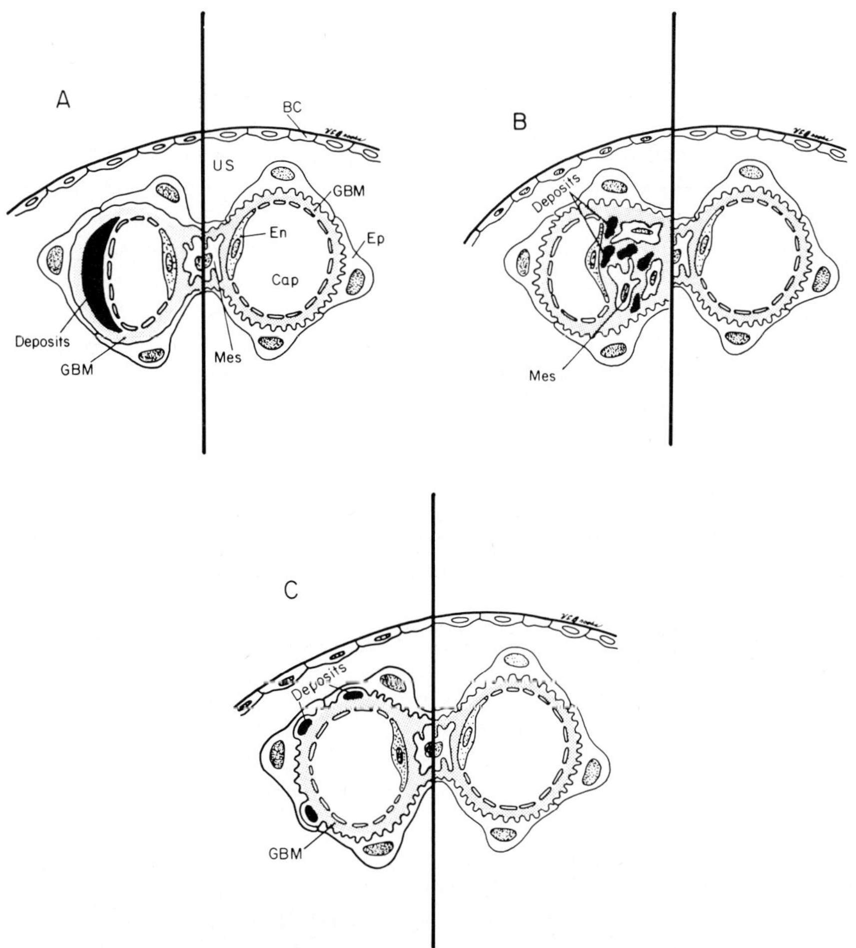

Fig. 9. Schematic representation of immune complex deposits within the glomerular capillary. (A) Subendothelial deposition pattern. (B) Mesangial deposition pattern. (C) Subepithelial deposition pattern. Abbreviations: BC, Bowman's capsule; Cap, capillary; En, endothelial cell; Ep, epithelial cell; GBM, glomerular basement membrane; Mes, mesangial cell; and US, urinary space. (Adapted from Striker *et al.*, 1976.)

2. *Role of Lattice and Other Features of Immune Complexes*

The experimental models discussed above (Section IV,A) provided evidence that the deposition of antigen–antibody complexes in the glomeruli is associated with the persistence of large-latticed circulating complexes, while glomerular lesions and proteinuria were specifically correlated with the presence of heavy sedimenting complexes (Cochrane and Hawkins, 1968).

Germuth and Rodriguez (1973) developed a hypothesis about the mechanisms controlling the site of immune complex localization on the basis of their observations on experimental models. The site of glomerular deposition in the chronic model of immune complex disease, following the daily administration of 12.5 mg of BSA, depended on the size characteristics of the circulating complexes, as demonstrated by sucrose density gradient ultracentrifugation. The presence of small complexes was associated with deposits in the glomerular capillary loops (Fig. 10), while large complexes were associated with deposits in the mesangium (Fig. 11).

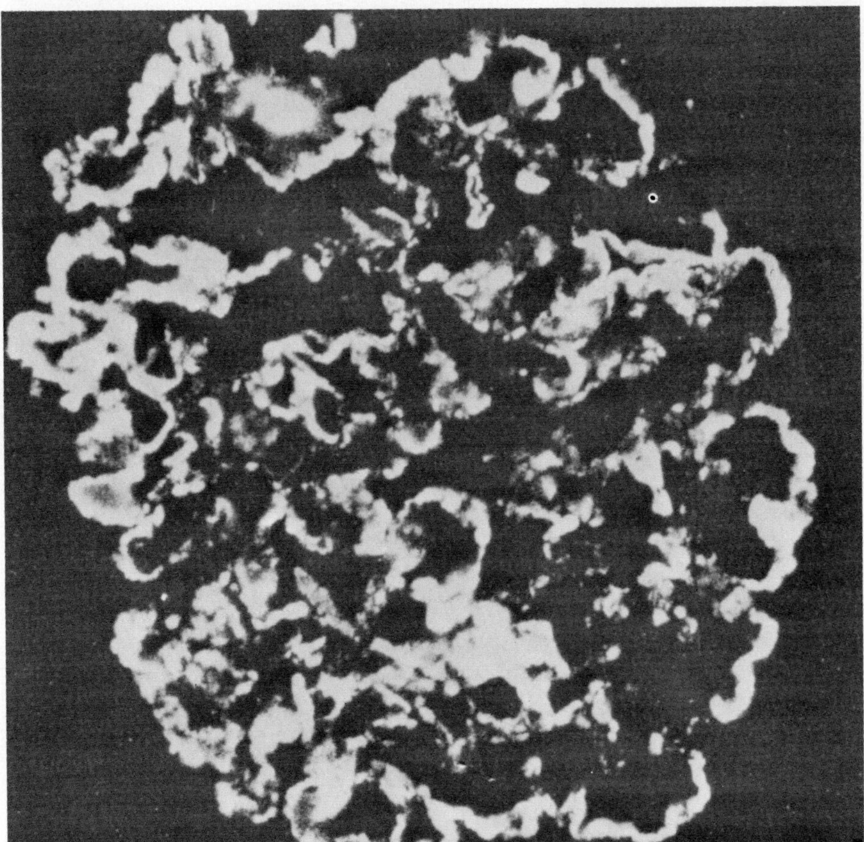

Fig. 10. Deposition of immune complexes in the glomerular peripheral capillary loops of a rabbit responding with low levels of antibodies following the chronic (daily) administration of 12.5 mg BSA. Complexes with a molecular weight of 5–7 $\times 10^5$ daltons were detected in the circulation by sucrose density gradient ultracentrifugation (from Germuth *et al.*, 1972).

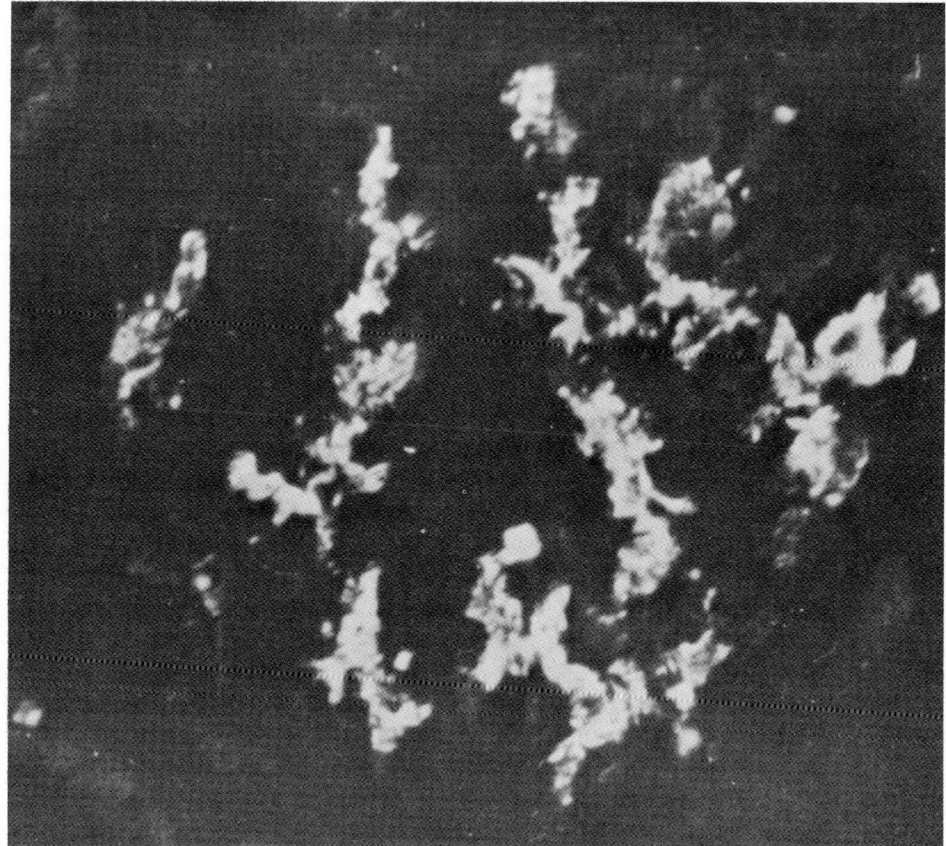

Fig. 11. Deposition of immune complexes in the glomerular mesangium of a rabbit responding with intermediate levels of antibodies following the chronic (daily) administration of 12.5 mg BSA. Complexes with a molecular weight of approximately 1×10^6 daltons were detected in the circulation by sucrose density gradient ultracentrifugation (from Germuth *et al.*, 1972).

During the injection of preformed, soluble immune complexes into mice, several points became apparent on the localization of complexes in glomeruli (Haakenstad *et al.*, 1976). First, only large-latticed complexes were localized in the glomeruli, since immunoglobulin deposits and electron-dense deposits were present only during the latter part of the disappearance of circulating, large-latticed complexes. The deposited material disappeared from glomeruli, while small-latticed (Ag_2Ab_2) complexes remained in circulation. Furthermore, when reduced and alkylated antibodies were used to prepare the complexes, as already pointed out in Sec-

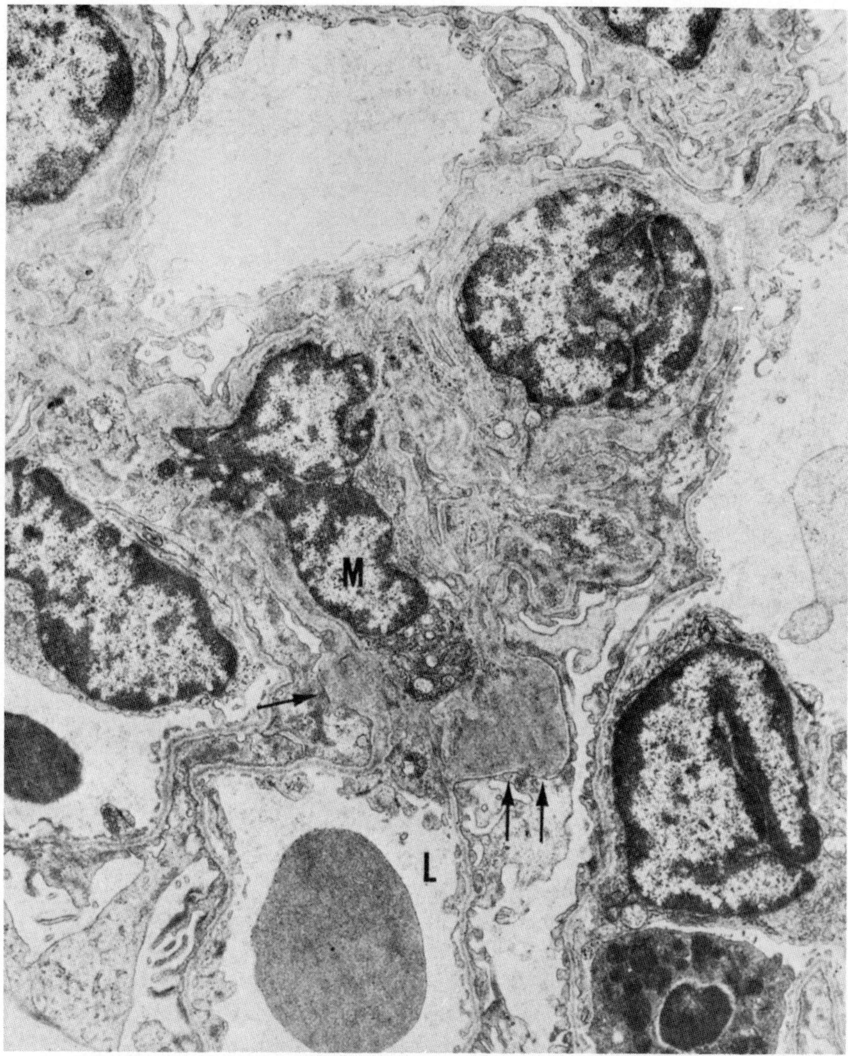

Fig. 12. Mesangial (M) deposits (arrows) of immune complexes by electron microscopy (original × 6000). Deposits existed in the junction between the mesangium and the glomerular capillary loop (L), but they were absent from the peripheral capillary loop proper. This pattern was characteristic of rabbits mounting an intermediate level antibody response to the chronic administration of BSA (from Germuth and Rodriguez, 1973).

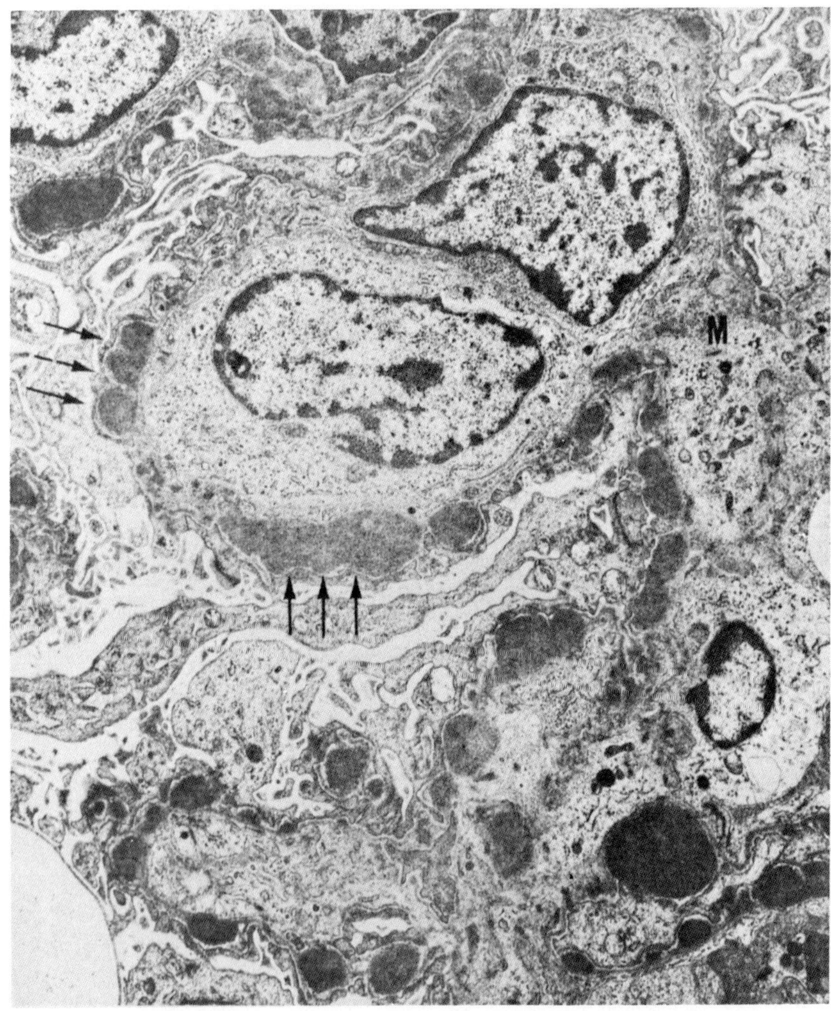

Fig. 13. Subepithelial deposits (arrows) of immune complexes in the glomerular capillary loop by electron microscopy (original × 6300). The mesangium (M) was free of deposits. This distribution of deposits was characteristic of rabbits responding with a low-level antibody response to the chronic administration of BSA (from Germuth and Rodriguez, 1973).

tion IV,B,2, the large-latticed complexes persisted longer in circulation because of decreased removal of complexes by the hepatic mononuclear phagocyte system. In these experiments, enhanced deposition of complexes and persistence of complexes in glomeruli were noted (Fig. 14). Second, during these experiments, the electron-dense deposits were seen early in the course after injection in the subendothelial area and later in the mesangial (matrix). In these acute experiments, the subendothelial deposits disappeared within 24 hours after the large-latticed complexes were cleared from the circulation, whereas, the deposits in the mesangium persisted longer. No complexes were seen in the subepithelial area, even though large-latticed ($>Ag_2Ab_2$) and small-latticed (Ag_2Ab_2) complexes were injected. This observation casts doubt on the possibility of circulating immune complexes reaching the subepithelial area. In the endogenous disease, therefore, other factors must be operable that alter the glomerular basement membrane. Alternatively, the subepithelial complexes could be formed locally between antigens that have reached the area and antibodies that follow later. Obviously, rearrangement of lattice must occur in this area, to result in the large electron-dense deposits, if these are predominantly composed of deposits or precipitates of immune complexes. Of note is that deposits in this area were decreased by administration of large doses of antigen (Wilson and Dixon, 1971).

The nature of the antigen may also be important in determining the site of immune complex localization. The recent observations by Nydegger *et al.* (1975) and Izui *et al.* (1976) suggested that DNA administered to mice appeared to accumulate within the renal glomerulus where it might subsequently interact with antibody to form a complex *in situ*. In addition, *in vitro* experiments demonstrated physical attachment of DNA to isolated glomerular basement membrane and to collagen. This mechanism may possibly be important in the glomerular localization of DNA–anti-DNA complexes, which is found in the glomerulonephritis of human SLE (Koffler *et al.*, 1967) and of NZB/W mice (Lambert and Dixon, 1968).

Another mechanism by which antigen may localize within the glomerulus was described experimentally by Mauer *et al.* (1973). Aggregated foreign proteins were administered to rabbits and were observed to localize within the glomerular mesangium. These kidneys were transplanted to normal rabbits who then received an injection of rabbit antibodies specific for the aggregated antigen. The circulating antibody reacted with the antigen localized in the glomerular mesangium resulting in severe glomerulonephritis. The relevance of this mechanism to natural disease mechanisms is not yet determined.

The glomerulonephritis in spontaneous murine leukemia has been demonstrated by Pascal *et al.* (1973) to be associated with immune complex

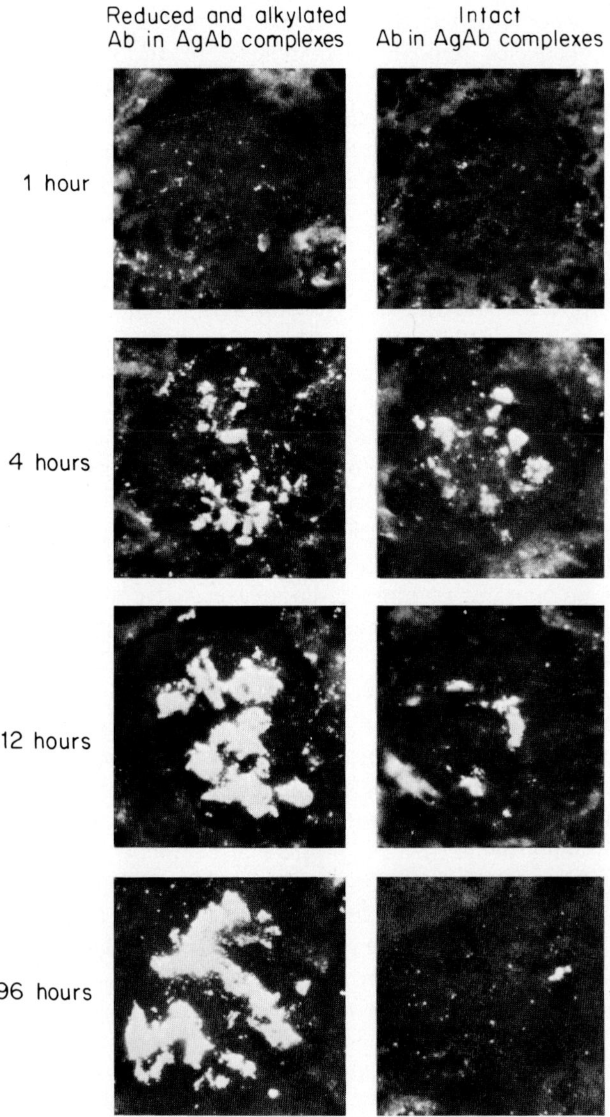

Fig. 14. Glomerular deposition of complexes in mice by immunofluorescence microscopy. The complexes were prepared as in Fig. 5. The rabbit IgG deposits were detected with fluorescein-conjugated goat antibodies to rabbit IgG. The deposits were greater in intensity and persisted longer following the administration of complexes containing reduced and alkylated antibodies than following the administration of complexes containing intact antibodies (from Haakenstad *et al.*, 1976).

deposits. The presence of deposits correlated well with the presence of C-type viral particles. Of particular interest was the observation that mesangial cells were surrounded by C-type viral particles, which were budding from the cell's plasma membrane. In this instance, the local production of antigen may have been responsible for the *in situ* formation of immune complex deposits.

The biologic properties of the antibodies in the antigen–antibody complex may be important in the fate of the deposited complexes. As discussed above under factors influencing the fate of soluble immune complexes, the immunoglobulin classes and subclasses differ in their capacity to interact with phagocyte surface receptors (Spiegelberg, 1974). The complexes may remain at the site of deposition unless they interact with phagocyte surface receptors and initiate mechanisms for attracting phagocytes to the site of deposition.

3. The Role of Vascular Permeability

The degree of vascular permeability may be important in determining the site of immune complex deposition. Cochrane (1963a,b) first used the intravenous administration of preformed antigen–antibody complexes to guinea pigs to demonstrate that the localization of complexes within vessel walls in this model required a state of increased vascular permeability. The vascular localization of complexes was achieved by inducing systemic anaphylaxis shortly after the administration of preformed complexes. Anaphylaxis was induced by the intravenous administration of an antigen to which the animal had been previously sensitized. The same effect could also be achieved with histamine administration, which was concluded to be the important mediator of increased vascular permeability.

The studies in guinea pigs were extended by Cochrane and Hawkins (1968). They demonstrated that complexes failed to localize in blood vessels if more than 2 minutes elapsed before the histamine was administered, since the large-latticed complexes were largely removed prior to that time. Furthermore, complexes prepared at 20-fold antigen excess produced vascular localization, whereas complexes prepared at 100-fold antigen excess did not. Analysis of these preparations on sucrose density gradients indicated that the heavier sedimenting complexes, larger than 19 S, were absent from the 100-fold antigen excess preparation. Only those fractions containing complexes larger than the 19 S marker protein localized in tissues. Therefore, the guinea pig experiments provided additional evidence that a large-latticed structure was required for vascular localization. However, it was necessary to administer lethal doses of histamine in order to see this effect.

The role of vasoactive amines in the localization of complexes in the acute rabbit model of experimental immune complex disease was examined by Kniker and Cochrane (1968). Rabbits treated with antiplatelet antibodies had marked decrease of arterial and cardiac lesions. Glomerular lesions and proteinuria were also inhibited, and the glomerular localization of antigen–antibody complexes was reduced. The decrease in cardiovascular and glomerular lesions was maximal in rabbits treated with both histamine and serotonin antagonists, while the suppression of lesions was only partial in rabbits receiving either antagonist alone. Thus, when either the platelet reservoir of vasoactive amines was removed by antiplatelet antibodies or the rabbits were treated with antagonists of the vasoactive amines, suppression of the arterial and glomerular lesions occurred.

The mechanisms by which vasoactive amines can be released from platelets have been reviewed by Cochrane and Koffler (1973). The described mechanisms included (1) immune complexes incubated with platelets in the presence of plasma resulted in lysis of the platelet and histamine release; this release was complement dependent and did not occur in C6-deficient plasma; (2) the addition of neutrophils to immune complexes and platelets in the presence of C6-deficient plasma resulted in the release of histamine and serotonin; (3) particulate antigens in the presence of platelets and the early complement components through C3 resulted in release of histamine and serotonin; (4) antigen in the presence of sensitized leukocytes and platelets resulted in the release of vasoactive amines. The first three mechanisms required complement activation at least through C3, whereas complement activation was not required for the fourth mechanism.

The fourth mechanism noted above, i.e., the leukocyte-dependent mechanism of histamine release, correlated well with the induction of glomerulonephritis in acute immune complex diseases in rabbits (Henson and Cochrane, 1971). Rabbits depleted of C3 with cobra venom factor still developed glomerulonephritis with glomerular and arterial deposition of complexes. Therefore, the fourth mechanism may be more important functionally than the first three mechanisms in the deposition of circulating immune complexes. It should be added, however, that complement depletion altered the characteristics of the arterial lesions. Both neutrophil infiltration and necrosis were found in the arterial lesions of control rabbits, but these findings were absent in the complement-depleted rabbits.

The important cell in the leukocyte-dependent mechanism was identified as the basophil by Siraganian and Osler (1971). Benveniste *et al.* (1972) discovered that the leukocyte-dependent histamine release (LDHR) from platelets could be transferred from sensitized rabbits to normal rabbits with serum. The serum factor was identified as the IgE class of antibodies. They also demonstrated that the basophil was responsible for the LDHR. During the *in vitro* study of this reaction by electron microscopy, the degranulation of basophils and the subsequent aggregation of platelets in association with basophils was observed following exposure of the sensitized cells to the specific antigen. Thus, IgE-sensitized basophils appeared to release their histamine content and a platelet-activating factor (PAF). The PAF, in turn, caused aggregation of platelets and further histamine release. Whether the LDHR mechanism is the most important mechanism for releasing vasoactive amines in the other experimental models of immune complex disease or in human immune complex disease has not been determined. However, an increase in vascular permeability mediated by the release of vasoactive amines appears to play a role in the deposition of circulating complexes.

V. DETECTION OF IMMUNE COMPLEXES

In recent years, many different methods have been developed for detecting the presence of immune complexes in serum and other biologic fluids. Many of the developed techniques for detection of antigen–antibody complexes rely on the biologic properties, such as complement fixation, interaction with cell receptors for IgG, and interaction with cell receptors for complement components. The exact nature of the detected complexes has not been defined in terms of the lattice required for detection. Furthermore, the employed tests do not detect immunoglobulins of all classes that may participate in the formation of immune complexes. Nevertheless, the assays for immune complexes represent a new approach to the diagnosis and management of diseases, even though their utility in clinical practice remains to be determined.

A. Physical Methods

Immune complexes in early studies of patients with rheumatoid arthritis were detected by the relatively insensitive method of analytical ultracentrifugation. Complexes with a sedimentation coefficient of 22 S were identical by Franklin *et al.* (1957) in the sera of selected patients with rheumatoid arthritis. These high molecular weight complexes could be dissociated in urea or at low pH into IgM and IgG. Some patients with rheumatoid arthritis and some with hyperglobulinemic purpura were demonstrated to have intermediate-sized complexes with sedimentation rates between 9 S and 17 S (Kunkel *et al.*, 1961). The intermediate-sized complexes were dissociated into 7 S material in urea or under acid conditions.

Immune complexes have also been identified in serum and other fluids by their sedimentation characteristics or sucrose density gradient ultracentrifugation. Hannestad (1967) demonstrated that the synovial fluid of some patients with rheumatoid arthritis contained fast-sedimenting IgG that was identified immunochemically in fractions obtained by sucrose density gradient ultracentrifugation. Bombardieri *et al.* (1973) identified fast-sedimenting IgG in the serum of patients with systemic lupus erythematosus (SLE) following centrifugation of serum samples on discontinuous sucrose gradients. The sequential fractions were tested for IgG by a solid-phase radioimmunoassay, which employed inhibition of binding of radioiodinated IgG by specific antibodies to human IgG, coupled to polyaminopolystyrene particles. Some patients with active SLE contained an increased concentration of aggregated IgG in the pellet. Microgram quantities of aggregates were detected by this method. Ludwig and Cusumano (1974) similarly examined the distribution of IgG in the serum of patients with tumors. Radiolabeled, ^{125}I-Fab′ fragments of antibodies to human IgG were mixed with the serum samples prior to sucrose density gradient ultracentrifugation. The distribution of IgG was detected by the radioactivity in the gradient fractions. As little as 13 μg of IgG in immune complexes could be detected by this technique. Finally, circulating immune complexes have also been detected by Eardley and Tempelis (1975), with comparable techniques in the sera of chickens tolerant to bovine serum albumin by sucrose density gradient ultracentrifugation. The complexes were detected by adding agarose beads coupled with rabbit anti-BSA to the gradient fractions. The immunoadsorbent beads were then washed and incubated with radioiodinated antibodies to chicken γ-globulin. The radioactivity bound to the beads, thus, reflected the presence of BSA-chicken anti-BSA complexes. The complexes were detected in the bottom third of linear 10–40% sucrose gradients, and they sedimented at 22.8 S by analytical ultracentrifugation.

Immune complexes have been identified by their heavier molecular weight as detected by gel filtration. Jewell and MacLennan (1973) found suggestive evidence for immune complexes in the sera of patients with ulcerative colitis or Crohn's disease. Fractions that eluted between the IgM and monomeric IgG peaks on Sepharose 6B inhibited antibody-dependent cell-mediated cytotoxicity. Since these inhibitory eluates also contained high molecular weight IgG by immunodiffusion, the inhibitory factors were thought to be composed of immune complexes containing IgG. Gel filtration on Sephadex G-200 and sucrose density gradient (SDG) ultracentrifugation techniques were used by Norberg (1974) to detect IgG complexes in sera of patients with rheumatoid arthritis. Evidence for complexes was demonstrated by the presence of IgG within the IgM peak and between the IgM and IgG peaks following gel filtration or SDG ultracentrifugation. The immunoglobulins in the fractions were detected by radial immunodiffusion. Gel filtration techniques were similarly used by Wiik (1975) to demonstrate intermediate-sized complexes between the IgM and IgG peaks in patients with rheumatoid arthritis and with Felty's syndrome. Finally, gel filtration on Sephadex G-200 was used by Amlot *et al.* (1976) to detect an increase in the apparent molecular weight of the C3 component of complement due to presumed binding to immune complexes. The C3 was measured with a sensitive microhemagglutination inhibition assay. C3 was found in the high molecular weight fractions of plasma from patients with Hodgkin's disease but not in these fractions from normal plasma. These observations suggested that immune complexes were present in the plasma of patients with Hodgkin's disease.

B. Interaction with C1q

The interaction of immune complexes with the C1q component of complement has been used by a number of investigators to detect immune complexes (Agnello *et al.*, 1971; Nydegger *et al.*, 1974; Sobel *et al*, 1975; Johnson *et al.*, 1975; Farrel *et al.*, 1975; Svehag, 1975; Zubler *et al.*, 1976a,b; Hay *et al.*, 1976; Svehag and Burger, 1976). Agnello *et al.* (1970) described a gel diffusion method in agarose for demonstrating the precipitation reaction between C1q and aggregated IgG larger than 19 S. C1q also formed a precipitin reaction with soluble immune complexes prepared in 2- to 20-fold antigen excess. This method detected complexes in hypocomplementemic sera from patients with systemic lupus erythematosus (SLE) and in hypocomplementemic joint fluids from patients with rheumatoid arthritis. Further studies (Agnello *et al.*, 1971) on the nature of C1q precipitins in SLE sera demonstrated both high (>19 S) and low (approximately 7 S) molecular weight material by SDG ultracentrifugation, which reacted with C1q. IgG was present in both fractions and the low molecular weight contained no biologic polyanions such as DNA and endotoxin.

More sensitive methods of detecting the interaction of C1q with immune complexes have been devised. Nydegger *et al.* (1974) employed the use of polyethylene glycol (PEG) precipitation of soluble complexes, which had bound radiolabeled ^{125}I-C1q. Concentrations of PEG were used that did not precipitate free ^{125}I-C1q. As little as 10 μg of heat-aggregated human IgG was detected by this method. However, the detection of complexes containing BSA and rabbit anti-BSA by PEG precipitation of bound ^{125}I-C1q was enhanced at equivalence and at mild degrees of antigen excess. This assay was positive with sera of SLE patients with low complement levels, but not in the sera of SLE patients with normal complement levels. This assay was also positive with sera of hepatitis patients carrying HB-Ag, but not with sera of healthy carriers of HB-Hg. Zubler *et al.* (1976a) modified the C1q binding assay for detection of immune complexes in unheated sera by adding EDTA prior to adding ^{125}I-C1q and PEG. This prevented ^{125}I-C1q from forming the C1qrs complex. Thus, unbound ^{125}I-C1q remained soluble and ^{125}I-C1q bound to immune complexes precipitated in PEG. Intrinsic C1q as well as DNA and endotoxin interferred very little in the modified test. The ^{125}I-C1q binding was elevated in 91% of patients with SLE. Sera and synovial fluids from patients with rheumatoid arthritis and other disorders were assayed for the presence of complexes by this technique (Zubler *et al.*, 1976b). Immune complexes were identified in the sera and synovial fluid of both seropositive and seronegative rheumatoid arthritis. SDG ultracentrifugation studies demonstrated the highest binding activity in the 10 S to 22 S molecular weight fractions and may have represented the intermediate complexes.

Sobel *et al.* (1975) described a more sensitive method, known as the C1q deviation test, for detecting the presence of C1q binding material in sera and other fluids. The detection of immune complexes was based on their ability to competitively inhibit the binding of ^{125}I-C1q to sheep erythrocytes sensitized with rabbit IgG. Heat-aggregated IgG could be detected at a concentration of 5 μg/ml of serum. Experimentally prepared soluble immune complexes containing BSA and rabbit anti-BSA in antigen excess were also detected by the C1q deviation test. Patients with dengue hemorrhagic fever contained C1q binding material in their sera. The greatest amount of inhibitory material was seen in patients with severe shock, and the least amount of inhibitory material was seen in patients with mild disease.

Johnson *et al.* (1975) found that C1q bound to complexes in pathological sera remained soluble in the pseudoglobulin fraction prepared under mildly alkaline conditions at low ionic strength, whereas the C1q in normal sera is precipitated in the euglobulin fraction. The C1q was detected in the pseudoglobulin fraction by rocket electrophoresis in many patients with immune complex-type vascular disease, but only rarely in healthy adults.

Aggregated IgG and immune complexes containing IgG were detected by their ability to bind C1q in an assay that used C1q-coated polystyrene tubes and ^{32}P-labeled protein A-rich *Staphylococcus aureus* (Farrell *et al.*, 1975). Heat-aggregated IgG or immune complexes containing either HSA–rabbit anti-HSA or BSA–rabbit anti-BSA were detected, when added to the C1q-coated tubes followed by the addition of labeled staphylococcal cells. Aggregated IgG in the 19 S–25 S range was detected at a concentration of 8 μg/ml. This solid-phase C1q-binding assay was further modified (Svehag, 1975) by using heat-aggregated, ^{125}I-labeled IgG as the indicator molecule in the radioimmunoassay. The binding of aggregated ^{125}I-IgG could be inhibited by as little as 2–5 ng of unlabeled, aggregated IgG. Less than 50 ng of IgG in preformed immune complexes was detected by this assay. C1q-coated tubes were used by Ahlstedt *et al.* (1976) to detect human IgG aggregates, which were identified by enzyme-linked anti-human IgG. Less than 10 ng/ml of sample were detected by this method. C1q-coated tubes were used by Hay *et al.* (1976) to detect immune complexes in 12 of 31 patients with SLE. Radioiodinated rabbit anti human IgG was utilized to detect the immune complexes bound to C1q; as little as 1 μg of aggregated IgG could be detected. Recently, Svehag and Burger (1976) covalently coupled C1q to agarose for affinity chromatography. Preformed virus–antibody complexes were recovered by this method. The 22 S complexes and the intermediate complexes were isolated from sera of patients with rheumatoid arthritis.

C. Interaction with Rheumatoid Factors

Immune complexes have been detected in sera and joint fluids of patients with rheumatoid arthritis and other disorders by their ability to react with rheumatoid factors. Monoclonal rheumatoid factors, isolated from patients with lymphoproliferative disorders, formed a precipitin line by immunodiffusion with 57% of sera and 70% of joint fluids from patients with rheumatoid arthritis (Winchester *et al.*, 1971). Only 8% of the sera from patients with systemic lupus erythematosus (SLE) and none of the joint fluids from patients with SLE, gonococcal infections, Reiter's syndrome, degenerative joint disease, or traumatic injury were positive. Joint fluids that precipitated with C1q also precipitated with monoclonal rheumatoid factor, but many joint fluids reacted only with monoclonal rheumatoid factor. The monoclonal rheumatoid factors precipitated small-sized heat aggregates of IgG that were not precipitated by C1q. Thus, smaller aggregates of γ-globulin appeared to be detected by precipitation with monoclonal rheumatoid factors than with C1q.

Luthra *et al.* (1975) increased the sensitivity of detecting immune complexes with monoclonal rheumatoid factor by developing a solid-phase radioimmunoassay. Immune complexes were detected in the sera and synovial fluids of patients with rheumatoid arthritis by their ability to inhibit the interaction of ^{125}I-aggregated IgG (20–30 S) with monoclonal rheumatoid factor conjugated to microcrystalline cellulose. Unlabeled, aggregated IgG was easily detectable by this assay at a concentration range of 2–7 μg/ml. Fifty micrograms of monomeric IgG was required to produce the same inhibition as produced by about 1 μg of aggregated IgG. The presence of polyclonal rheumatoid factor did not interfere in this assay. However, heating sera at 56°C for 60 minutes to inactivate complement appeared to produce inhibitory aggregates. The inhibitory activity in rheumatoid sera was localized in both intermediate (approximately 11 S) and heavier (19 S and larger) sedimenting fractions by sucrose density gradient ultracentrifugation. The inhibitory activity in normal human sera was less than that seen with 25 μg of aggregated IgG. Twenty-six percent of sera and 22% of synovial fluids from patients with rheumatoid arthritis contained inhibitory activity above the normal range. Similar inhibitory activity was rarely detected in the sera of patients with systemic lupus erythematosus and other disorders.

A radioimmunoassay, which used polyclonal rheumatoid factor for detecting immune complexes was devised by Cowdery *et al.* (1975). The assay used a standard serum containing IgM–rheumatoid factor and ^{125}I-heat aggregated IgG, which was then precipitated by sheep anti-human IgM to determine the amount of radiolabeled material bound by the rheumatoid factor. Preformed complexes containing tetanus toxoid and human anti-toxoid antibodies were detected in this assay by their ability to inhibit the 50% binding of the rheumatoid factor to 150 ng of ^{125}I-aggregated IgG. Maximum inhibition of binding was detected with complexes at equivalence, but complexes in antibody excess and low levels of antigen excess also inhibited binding. As little as 125 ng of soluble immune complexes could be detected with this assay. When clinical specimens were tested for the presence of immune complexes, they were readily detected in the sera of patients with SLE, polymyositis, and hepatitis. However, complexes were only rarely detected in the sera and joint fluids of patients with rheumatoid arthritis because the additional rheumatoid factor in these specimens produced an apparent increase in ^{125}I-aggregated IgG binding, rather than inhibition. Thus, in contrast to the above studies using monoclonal rheumatoid factors, the method using polyclonal rheumatoid factors detected complexes better in patients with other forms of vasculitis than in patients with rheumatoid arthritis.

D. Platelet Aggregation

The aggregation of human platelets by immune complexes, which was discussed in Section III,C,6, is mediated by the platelet receptor for the Fc fragment of IgG. Penttinen *et al.* (1969) established that aggregation of human platelets was a sensitive method for detecting IgG-containing soluble immune complexes. However, complexes with a sedimentation coefficient greater than 19 S were needed to induce platelet aggregation (Penttinen *et al.*, 1971). The platelet aggregation technique was 100-fold more sensitive in detecting the presence of aggregated IgG (1 μg/ml) than was the precipitation technique of detecting aggregated IgG (100 μg/ml) with IgM–rheumatoid factor (Wager *et al.*, 1973). IgM–rheumatoid factors, isolated from dissociated IgM–IgG cryoglobulins, inhibited platelet aggregation by immune complexes containing rabbit antibodies or human antibodies. This observation was used by Penttinen *et al.* (1973) to differentiate three types of platelet aggregation. The "immune complex" type of platelet aggregation activity was identified in unheated serum fractions sedimenting faster than 19 S and was inhibitable by IgM–rheumatoid factors. The "antibody type" platelet aggregation was induced by antiplatelet antibodies with 7 S and 19 S sedimentation coefficients; it was present in unheated serum and was not inhibitable by IgM–rheumatoid factors. Finally, the "aggregated IgG type" of platelet aggregations was produced by sera with high IgG levels (and low albumin levels) by heating the sera at 56°C for 30 minutes, and the activity was localized in the greater than 19 S gradient fractions and was inhibitable by IgM–rheumatoid factors. This last type probably reflected unusual sensitivity to heat-induced aggregation of IgG in these sera. Examples of each type of reactions were identified in patients with hepatitis and other disorders. Norberg (1974) found that 24% of 146 rheumatoid factor-positive sera (unheated) produced platelet aggregation due to the presence of 19 S or larger complexes, whereas 56% of 40 of these sera, selected randomly for gel filtration studies, had intermediate IgG complexes. Immune complexes have been similarly identified by platelet aggregation in 41% of sera from patients (39) with acute respiratory illness due to *Mycoplasma pneumoniae* (Biberfeld and Norberg, 1974) and in 6 of 26 patients with sarcoidosis (Hedfors and Norberg, 1974).

E. Interaction with Receptors on Lymphoid Cells

Immune complexes readily bind to B lymphocytes via Fc and C3 receptors as discussed in Section III,C,6. Continuous lymphoblastoid cell lines with B cell characteristics were examined by Theofilopoulos *et al.* (1974a,b) for the presence of Fc and complement receptors in order to seek indicator system for the detection of immune complexes. The Raji human cell line, which had receptors for Fc, C3b, and C3d but lacked detectable membrane bound immunoglobulin, was selected as an indicator cell. Aggregated human IgG (AHG) bound to these cells in the presence of normal serum or IgG only when complement was available, i.e., the binding occurred via the complement receptors. Also, the binding of AHG was eightfold greater in the presence of complement than in the absence of complement. The binding of AHG in the presence of complement involved the receptors for both C3–C3b and C3d. Up to 40% of AHG containing complement could be released from the Raji cell surface by the subsequent addition of more fresh serum, purified C3 or C3b, comparable to the results of Miller *et al.* (1973) and Miller and Nussenzweig (1974), as discussed earlier in Section III,C,6.

The Raji cells were used to detect immune complexes in several clinical conditions (Theofilopoulos *et al.,* 1974c). Binding of soluble immune complexes was detected by an immunofluorescence assay. The sensitivity of the assay was examined by first incubating FITC-labeled AHG with the Raji cells in the presence of fresh or heated serum followed by the addition of unfluoresceinated anti-human IgG. Binding of AHG in fresh serum was detected at a concentration of 200 ng/ml, whereas AHG in heated serum required a concentration of 200–300 μg/ml for detection. Marked adherence was observed only with aggregates larger than 19 S by SDG ultracentrifugation. The adherence of HSA–rabbit anti-HSA complexes at threefold antigen excess were detected at a similar concentration by first incubating the complexes with the Raji cells in fresh serum followed by the addition of FITC-labeled anti-rabbit IgG. The adherence of soluble HSA–anti-HSA complexes was maximum at two- to sixfold antigen excess, but adherence was not detected in antibody excess or beyond 30-fold antigen excess. Rabbits with acute serum sickness contained complexes in their sera during the phase of immune clearance by this assay. Mice infected with LCM virus also contained virus–IgG complexes by this system, using an FITC-labeled antiserum to mouse immunoglobulins.

The Raji cell test for detecting complexes in human sera was modified by first incubating the cells with 1 mg of human IgG and then with Fab′ fragments of rabbit anti-human IgG to reduce the binding of monomeric IgG to Fc receptors. The cells were then incubated with patient or normal sera, followed by FITC-labeled rabbit anti-human IgG. Complexes were, thus, detected in sera of patients with immune complex diseases.

Finally, the above methods were further modified to quantify immune complexes by radioimmunoassay (Theofilopoulos *et al.,* 1976). After the test serum was added to the Raji cells, a ^{125}I-labeled rabbit anti-human IgG was added. The amount of ^{125}I–rabbit anti-human IgG bound to the cells was determined and compared to a standard curve of ^{125}I–rabbit anti-human IgG uptake by cells incubated with increasing amounts of aggregated human IgG. As little as 6 μg/ml of 35–95 S-aggregated IgG could be detected. The 19–34 S aggregates of IgG were detected at 25 μg/ml, and the 11–18 S aggregates were detected at a concentration of 50 μg/ml. Sera from patients with several different disorders were assayed for the presence of immune complexes. Immune complex-type material equivalent to more than 12 μg of aggregated human IgG (exceeding the upper limit in normal sera) was found in 52.9% of patients with serum hepatitis, 100% of patients with SLE, 56% of selected patients with other forms of vasculitis, and in patients with malignant tumors. The sera from patients with HB_s-Ag-positive hepatitis and a positive assay for immune complexes contained HB_s-Ag, C3, and IgG in the lower (heavy) fractions following SDG ultracentrifugation. Sera from asymptomatic carriers negative for immune complexes contained HB_s-Ag, C3, and IgG in the middle portion of the gradient. The amount of immune complexes correlated directly with disease activity and inversely with complement levels in patients with SLE. Thus, the Raji cell radioimmunoassay was both sensitive and quantitative for detecting immune complexes in human sera.

An assay for detecting circulating immune complexes was developed using macrophages from guinea pig peritoneal exudates (Onyewotu *et al.*, 1974). Macrophages obtained 3–5 days after intraperitoneal injection with liquid paraffin were incubated simultaneously with test sera and ^{125}I-labeled aggregated human IgG in a competitive assay. Complexes were detected in the serum by inhibiting the uptake of the ^{125}I-aggregated IgG. As little as 25 ng of HSA–rabbit anti-HSA complexes formed at 50-fold antigen excess inhibited the uptake of ^{125}I-aggregated IgG. Complexes were demonstrated in 88% of randomly selected SLE sera. SLE sera also inhibited the macrophage uptake of HSA–^{125}I–rabbit anti-HSA complexes prepared in a range from 50-fold antigen excess to 50-fold antibody excess with the uptake of complexes at 50-fold antigen excess being subject to the greatest inhibition. It was subsequently pointed out (Onyewotu *et al.*, 1975) that only 6 of 62 selected sera from seropositive patients with rheumatoid arthritis inhibited the uptake of radioiodinated human aggregated IgG, but that 28 of the sera actually enhanced the uptake of aggregates. The enhanced uptake was thought to be due to rheumatoid factors that bound to immune complexes or altered IgG.

The method of Onyewotu *et al.* (1974) was employed by Stühlinger *et al.* (1976) to test sera from patients with various types of glomerulonephritis for the presence of circulating immune complexes. The uptake of radiolabeled aggregates was inhibited by as little as 62 ng of cold aggregates. Significant inhibition was found in the sera of patients with various types of glomerulonephritis, as well as in experimental rabbits with acute serum sickness during the phase of immune elimination.

F. Other Methods

A method for detecting DNA:anti-DNA complexes in sera of patients with systemic lupus erythematosus was developed by Harbeck *et al.* (1973). Antibodies to DNA were measured in sera by the DNA-binding assay before and after digestion with deoxyribonuclease (DNase). An increase in binding of native DNA after DNase digestion suggested that the anti-DNA antibodies were blocked with DNA in the form of an immune complex prior to digestion. Complexes were detected in 11 of 15 SLE sera with active nephritis, whereas they were not detected in patients with either in-

TABLE II

Established Human Immune Complex Diseases[a]

Diseases	Identified antigens	Selected references
	Administered Antigens[b]	
Serum sickness	Animal antitoxins and antiserums, and other animal proteins, or hormones	
	Drugs	
	Microbial Antigens	
Poststreptococcal glomerulonephtitis	Plasma membrane antigens of β-hemolytic streptococci	Andres *et al.*, 1966; Michael *et al.*, 1966; Treser *et al.*, 1970
Glomerulonephritis of bacterial endocarditis	Bacterial antigens	Gutman *et al.*, 1972; Levy and Hong, 1973; Perez *et al.*, 1976
Glomerulonephritis of infected ventriculoatrial shunts	*Staphylococcus epidermidis* antigen	Dobrin *et al.*, 1975
Glomerulonephritis of syphilis	Treponemal antigen	Gamble and Reardan, 1975; Tourville *et al.*, 1976
Glomerulonephritis of thyphoid fever	*Salmonella* Vi antigen	Sitprija *et al.*, 1974
Immune complex disease of hepatitis B infection	Hepatitis B antigen	Gocke *et al.*, 1970; Combes *et al.*, 1971; Brzosko *et al.*, 1974; Kohler *et al.*, 1974
Glomerulonephritis of toxoplasmosis	*Toxoplasma* antigen	Ginsburg *et al.*, 1974

Glomerulonephritis of quartan malaria	*Plasmodium malariae* antigen	Hendrickse *et al.*, 1972
Glomerulonephritis of schistosomiasis	*Schistosoma mansoni* antigen	Falcão and Gould, 1975
	Autologous antigens	
Systemic lupus erythematosus	DNA, nucleoprotein	Koffler *et al.*, 1967
	C-type viral antigens	Panem *et al.*, 1976
Rheumatoid arthritis	IgG as antigen for rheumatoid factor	Hannestad, 1967; Winchester *et al.*, 1970; Pope *et al.*, 1975
Mixed cryoglobulinemia	IgG as antigen	Meltzer *et al.*, 1966; Druet *et al.*, 1973
Glomerulonephritis due to renal tubular antigen	Renal tubular antigen	Naruse *et al.*, 1973
Thyroiditis with thyroid carcinoma	Thyroglobulin	Kalderon *et al.*, 1975
	Tumor antigens	
Colonic carcinoma with nephritis	Specific tumor antigen	Couser *et al.*, 1974
	Carcinoembryonic antigen	Costanza *et al.*, 1973
Bronchogenic carcinoma with nephritis	Specific tumor antigen	Lewis *et al.*, 1971
Clear cell renal carcinoma with nephritis	Antibodies to RTE (proximal tubule brush border antigen)	Ozawa *et al.*, 1975

[a] See also reviews Roy *et al.* (1972) and Wilson and Dixon (1974).

[b] The development of immune complex diseases in humans due to heterologous proteins and drugs was established primarily by the close association of clinical abnormalities and the administered antigens and not by identification of the antigen and antibodies in target organs.

active SLE or non-SLE nephritis. In a subsequent report on a larger series of SLE patients, 78% of patients with overt nephritis had detectable complexes (Bardana *et al.*, 1975).

The presence of immune complexes was also detected by histamine release from perfused guinea pig lung preparations (Baumal and Broder, 1968; Gordon *et al.*, 1969). This method was used in particular to detect immune complexes in the serum and synovial fluid of patients with rheumatoid arthritis (Gordon *et al.*, 1975).

VI. OVERVIEW OF HUMAN IMMUNE COMPLEX DISEASES

In recent years, an increasing number of human diseases have been identified as immune complex diseases. The manifestations of these disorders have one or more clinical features that include glomerulonephritis, arthritis, skin eruptions, vasculitis, pleuritis, pericarditis, and fever. In some patients, only one or a few of these manifestations are present. The basic reasons for the variability of symptoms and signs of the immune complex diseases have not been established. The deposition or formation of immune complexes in target tissues is an underlying mechanism of these disorders, but since the immune response is not necessarily confined to the production of antibodies, cell-mediated immunity may also contribute to the disease process.

In the strict sense, a human disease should be classified as an immune complex disease when the specific antibodies and antigens are identified that participate in the genesis of inflammation. Among the established immune complex diseases, this identification was at times achieved by eluting the specific antibodies and antigens from one or more target organs and the subsequent immunochemical identification of the recovered materials. In other instances, the specific antigens were identified by immunofluorescent techniques using specific antibodies for the identification of antigens in situations where the immunoglobulins were distributed in glomeruli or blood vessel walls in a manner characteristic of immune complex diseases. With the improvement of techniques for the identification of soluble immune complexes, in biologic fluids, as described in the preceding section, new approaches have become available for identifying suspected immune complex diseases. Once complexes are identified in a biologic fluid, the constituent antibodies and antigens can be defined.

As discussed in the preceding section, an experimentally induced one-shot serum sickness or immune complex disease is a self-limited disease. The immunologically induced inflammation abates when the antigen is

TABLE III

Possible Human Immune Complex Diseases

Glomerulonephritis of unknown etiology with granular deposits of immunoglobulins on glomerular basement membrane
Glomerulonephritis in various diseases (sarcoidosis, visceral abscesses, varicella, mononucleosis and other viral diseases, retroperitoneal lymphomas and other tumors)
Drug-induced glomerulonephritis (gold salts, penicillamine)
Scleroderma renal disease
Diabetic glomerulosclerosis
Renal tubular immune complex disease
Various forms of vasculitis (periarteritis nodosa, small vessel vasculitis)
Wegener's granulomatosis
Childhood dermatomyositis and polymyositis
Anaphylactoid purpura (Schönlein–Henoch syndrome)
Erythema nodosum loprosum
Chronic thyroiditis
Hypersensitivity pneumonitis
Dengue hemorrhagic fever
Subacute sclerosing panencephalitis
Amyotrophic lateral sclerosis
Periodontal disease

eliminated from the circulation or from the target organ. The presence of antibodies alone causes no harm. Repeated administration of the antigen can convert the experimentally induced lesions to chronic inflammation that persists as long as the administration of antigens is continued. Similarly, human immune complex diseases can be self-limited or chronic disorders, depending on the transient or continued presence of antigens. Serum sickness due to the administration of a heterologous antitoxin serves as an example of a limited human illness that abates when the heterologous proteins are cleared from the host. Similarly, a transient immune complex disease results from a treatable infection with microorganisms. Subacute bacterial endocarditis serves as an excellent example. The glomerulonephritis and other manifestations abate when the bacteria as a source of antigens are eradicated by appropriate antibiotics. On the other hand, when the antigens for an immune complex disorder are present continuously or in recurrent episodes, the disease becomes chronic, disabling, and even fatal. Such persistence of antigens occurs when the antigen is a component of the host, elaborated from a persistent microbial organism, synthesized by a tumor, or administered to the patient for a therapeutic purpose.

The discussion of the identified immune complex diseases in humans is beyond the scope of this chapter. Some of these disorders are covered in other chapters of this volume. Table II provides a list of established immune complex disease in humans with selected references to original work and reviews. This list will undoubtedly grow as antigens are identified in certain drug-induced lesions, as the nature of more tumor antigens are elucidated and as viral or other microbial antigens are recognized in lesions.

In several human diseases, the clinical manifestations resemble the findings in established immune complex diseases and deposits of immunoglobulins and complement components have been identified in renal glomeruli, blood vessel walls, or other target organs. Specific antibodies or antigens have not been identified in these sites. Therefore, these disorders should be categorized as possible immune complex diseases (Table III). Further investigations on these diseases should establish the involved antigens and antibodies and, thus, elucidate the etiology of these diseases.

ACKNOWLEDGMENT

The preparation of this manuscript was aided in part by a postdoctoral fellowship to Alan O. Haakenstad and a Clinical Research Center Grant, both from the Arthritis Foundation and by the NIH Research Grant AM 05602.

REFERENCES

Agnello, V., Winchester, R. J., and Kunkel, H. G. (1970). *Immunology* **19,** 909.

Agnello, V., Koffler, D., Eisenberg, J. W., Winchester, R. J., and Kunkel, H. G. (1971). *J. Exp. Med.* **134,** 228 s.

Ahlstedt, S., Hanson, L. Å., and Wadsworth, C. (1976). *Scand. J. Immunol.* **5,** 293.

Alpers, J. H., Steward, M. W., and Soothill, J. F. (1972). *Clin. Exp. Immunol.* **12,** 121.

Amlot, P. L., Slaney, J. M., and Williams, B. D. (1976). *Lancet* **1,** 449.

Anderson, C. L., and Grey, H. M. (1974). *J. Exp. Med.* **139,** 1175.

Andres, G. A., Accinni, L., Hsu, K. C., Zabriskie, J. B., and Seegal, B. C. (1966). *J. Exp. Med.* **123,** 399.

Archer, G. T. (1969). *Pathology* **1,** 133.

Arend, W. P., and Mannik, M. (1971). *J. Immunol.* **107,** 63.

Arend, W. P., and Mannik, M. (1972). *J. Exp. Med.* **136,** 514.

Arend, W. P., and Mannik, M. (1973). *J. Immunol.* **110,** 1455.

Arend, W. P., and Mannik, M. (1974). *J. Immunol.* **112,** 451.

Arend, W. P., and Mannik, M. (1975). *In* "Mononuclear Phagocytes in Immunity, Infection and Pathology" (R. van Furth, ed.), p. 303. Blackwell, Oxford.

Arend, W. P., Teller, D. C., and Mannik, M. (1972). *Biochemistry* **11,** 4063.

Atkinson, J. P., and Frank, M. M. (1974). *J. Clin. Invest.* **54,** 339.

Bach, M. K., Bloch, K. J., and Austen, K. F. (1971a). *J. Exp. Med.* **133,** 752.
Bach, M. K., Bloch, K. J., and Austen, K. F. (1971b). *J. Exp. Med.* **133,** 772.
Bach, M. K., Brashler, J. R., and Stechschulte, D. J. (1973). *Immunochemistry* **10,** 305.
Baldwin, R. W., Price, M. R., and Robins, R. A. (1972). *Nature (London), New Biol.* **238,** 185.
Baldwin, R. W., Price, M. R., and Robins, R. A. (1973). *Br. J. Cancer* **28,** 37.
Bardana, R. M., Harbeck, R. J., Hoffman, A. A., Pirofsky, B., and Carr, R. I. (1975). *Am. J. Med.* **59,** 515.
Barnett, J. B., and Justus, D. E. (1975). *Infect. Immun.* **11,** 1342.
Basten, A., Miller, J. F. A. P., Sprent, J., and Pye, J. (1927a). *J. Exp. Med.* **135,** 610.
Basten, A., Warner, N. L., and Mandel, T. (1972b). *J. Exp. Med.* **135,** 627
Baumal, R., and Broder, J. (1968). *Clin. Exp. Immunol.* **3,** 525.
Becker, E. L. (1971). *Adv. Immunol.* **13,** 267.
Becker, E. L., and Henson, P. M. (1973). *Adv. Immunol.* **17,** 93.
Benacerraf, B., Sebestyen, M., and Cooper, N. S. (1959a). *J. Immunol.* **82,** 131.
Benacerraf, B., Sebestyen, M. M., and Schlossman, S. (1959b). *J. Exp. Med.* **110,** 27.
Benveniste, J., Henson, P. M., and Cochrane, C. G. (1972). *J. Exp. Med.* **136,** 1356.
Berken, A., and Benacerraf, B. (1966). *J. Exp. Med.* **123,** 119.
Berken, A., and Benacerraf, B. (1968). *J. Immunol.* **100,** 1219.
Bianco, C., and Nussenzweig, V. (1971). *Science* **173,** 154.
Bianco, C., Patrick, R., and Nussenzweig, V. (1970). *J. Exp. Med.* **132,** 702.
Biberfeld, G., and Norberg, R. (1974). *J. Immunol.* **112,** 413.
Biozzi, G., Benacerraf, B., and Halpern, B. N. (1953). *Br. J. Exp. Pathol.* **34,** 441.
Biozzi, G., Howard, J. G., Halpern, B. N., Stiffel, C., and Mouton, D. (1960). *Immunology* **3,** 74.
Bombardieri, S., Lightfoot, R. W., Jr., and Christian, C. L. (1973). *Proc. Soc. Exp. Biol. Med.* **144,** 148.
Boyden, S. V. (1964). *Immunology* **7,** 474.
Brentjens, J. R., O'Connell, D. W., Pawlowski, I. B., Hsu, K. C., and Andres, G. A. (1974). *J. Exp. Med.* **140,** 105.
Brown, J. C., De Jesus, D. G., and Holborow, E. J. (1970). *Nature (London)* **228,** 367.
Brunner, K. T., Hurez, D., McCluskey, R. T., and Benacerraf, B. (1960). *J. Immunol.* **85,** 99.
Brzosko, W. J., Krawczynski, K., Nazarewicz, T., Morzycka, M., and Nowoslawski, A. (1974). *Lancet* **2,** 7879.
Callerame, M. L., and Condemi, J. J. (1974). *Am. J. Clin. Pathol.* **62,** 823.
Cardella, C. J., Davies, P., and Allison, A. C. (1974). *Nature (London)* **247,** 46.
Clagett, J. A., Wilson, C. B., and Weigle, W. O. (1974). *J. Exp. Med.* **140,** 1439.
Cline, M. J., and Warner, N. L. (1972). *J. Immunol.* **108,** 339.
Cochrane, C. G. (1963a). *J. Exp. Med.* **118,** 489.
Cochrane, C. G. (1963b). *J. Exp. Med.* **118,** 503.
Cochrane, C. G. (1967). *Prog. Allergy* **11,** 1.
Cochrane, C. G. (1971). *J. Exp. Med.* **134,** 75s.

Cochrane, C. G., and Hawkins, D. (1968). *J. Exp. Med.* **127,** 137.
Cochrane, C. G., and Koffler, D. (1973). *Adv. Immunol.* **16,** 185.
Cochrane, C. G., and Weigle, W. O. (1958). *J. Exp. Med.* **108,** 591.
Cochrane, C. G., Weigle, W. O., and Dixon, F. J. (1959). *J. Exp. Med.* **110,** 481.
Cochrane, C. G., Wuepper, K. D., Aiken, B. S., Revak, S. D., and Spiegelberg, H. L. (1972). *J. Clin. Invest.* **51,** 2736.
Cochrane, C. G., Revak, S. D., Wuepper, K. D., Johnston, A., Morrison, D. C., and Ulevitch, R. (1974). *Adv. Biosci.* **12,** 237.
Cohen, S. (1968). *J. Immunol.* **100,** 407.
Combes, B., Stastny, P., Shorey, J., Eigenbrodt, E. H., Barrera, A., Hull, A. R., and Carter, N. W. (1971). *Lancet* **2,** 234.
Conrad, D. H., Bazin, H., Sehon, A. H., and Froese, A. (1975). *J. Immunol.* **114,** 1688.
Cooke, T. D., Hurd, E. R., Ziff, M., and Jasin, H. E. (1972). *J. Exp. Med.* **135,** 323.
Costanza, M. E., Pinn, V., Schwartz, R. S., and Nathanson, L. (1973). *N. Engl. J. Med.* **289,** 520.
Couser, W. G., Wagonfeld, J. B., Spargo, B. H., and Lewis, E. J. (1974). *Am. J. Med.* **57,** 962.
Cowdery, J. S.,Jr., Treadwell, P. E., and Fritz, R. B. (1975). *J. Immunol.* **114,** 5.
Crothers, D. M., and Metzger, H. (1972). *Immunochemistry* **9,** 341.
Cruchaud, A., and Unanue, E. R. (1971). *J. Immunol.* **107,** 1329.
Cruchaud, A., Berney, M., and Balant, L. (1975). *J. Immunol.* **114,** 102.
Dandliker, W. B., Alonso, R., deSaussure, V. A., Kierszenbaum, F., Levison, S. A., and Schapiro, H. C. (1967). *Biochemistry* **6,** 1460.
Dandliker, W. B., deSaussure, V. A., and Levandoski, N. (1968). *Immunochemistry* **5,** 357.
Day, E. D. (1972). "Advanced Immunochemistry," Williams & Wilkins, Baltimore, Maryland.
Dennert, G. (1971). *J. Immunol.* **106,** 951.
Des Prez, R. M., and Bryant, R. E. (1969). *J. Immunol.* **102,** 241.
Dickler, H. B., and Kunkel, H. G. (1972). *J. Exp. Med.* **136,** 191.
Diener, E., and Feldmann, M. (1970). *J. Exp. Med.* **132,** 31.
Dissanayake, S., and Hay, F. C. (1975). *Immunology* **29,** 1111.
Dixon, F. J., Vazquez, J. J., Weigle, W. O., and Cochrane, C. G. (1958). *AMA Arch. Pathol.* **65,** 18.
Dobrin, R. S., Day, N. K., Quie, P. G., Moore, H. L., Vernier, R. L., Michael, A. F., and Fish, A. J. (1975). *Am. J. Med.* **59,** 660.
Druet, P., Letonturier, P., Contet, A., and Mandet, C. (1973). *Clin. Exp. Immunol.* **15,** 483.
Dumonde, D. C., and Glynn, L. e. (1962). *Br. J. Exp. Pathol.* **43,** 373.
Dvorak, H. F., and Dvorak, A. M. (1972). *Hum. Pathol.* **3,** 454.
Eardley, D. D., and Tempelis, C. H. (1975). *J. Immunol.* **115,** 719.
Eden, A., Bianco, C., Nussenzweig, V., and Mayer, M. M. (1973). *J. Immunol.* **110,** 1452.
Falcão, H. A., and Gould, D. B. (1975). *Ann. Intern. Med.* **83,** 148.

Farrell, C., Søgaard, H., and Svehag, S.-E. (1975). *Scand. J. Immunol.* **4,** 673.
Feldman, J. D., and Pollock, E. M. (1974). *J. Immunol.* **113,** 329.
Feldmann, M., and Diener, E. (1970). *J. Exp. Med.* **131,** 247.
Feldmann, M., and Diener, E. (1971). *Immunology* **21,** 387.
Feldmann, M., and Diener, E. (1972). *J. Immunol.* **108,** 93.
Forster, O., and Weigle, W. O. (1963). *J. Immunol.* **90,** 935.
Franklin, E. C., Holman, H. R., Müller-Eberhard, H. J., and Kunkel, H. G. (1957). *J. Exp. Med.* **105,** 425.
Frei, P. C., Benacerraf, B., and Thorbecke, G. J. (1965). *Proc. Natl. Acad. Sci. U.S.A.* **53,** 20.
Fridman, W. H., and Golstein, P. (1974). *Cell. Immunol.* **11,** 442.
Fujita, Y., Rubinstein, E., Greco, D. B., Reisman, R. E., and Arbesman, C. E. (1975). *Int. Arch. Allergy Appl. Immunol.* **48,** 577.
Füst, G., Erdei, A., Sármay, G., Medgyesi, G. A., and Gergely, J. (1976). *Clin. Immunol. Immunopathol.* **5,** 377.
Gamble, C. N., and Reardan, J. B. (1975). *N. Engl. J. Med.* **292,** 449.
Germuth, F. G., Jr., and Rodriguez, E. (1973). "Immunopathology of the Renal Glomerulus." Little, Brown, Boston, Massachusetts.
Germuth, F. G., Jr., Senterfit, L. B., and Dreesman, G. R. (1972). *Johns Hopkins Med. J.* **130,** 344.
Gershon, R. K. (1974). *Contemp. Top. Immunobiol.* **3,** 1.
Ginsburg, B. E., Wasserman, J., Huldt, G., and Bergstrand, A. (1974). *Br. Med. J.* **3,** 664.
Gocke, D. J., Hsu, K., Morgan, C., Bombardieri, S., Lockshin, M., and Christian, C. L. (1970). *Lancet* **2,** 1149.
Goers, J. W., Schumaker, V. N., Glovsky, M. M., Rebek, J., and Müller-Eberhard, H. J. (1975). *J. Biol. Chem.* **250,** 4918.
Goldberg, R. J. (1952). *J. Am. Chem. Soc.* **74,** 5715.
Gorczynski, R., Kontiainen, S., Mitchison, N. A. and Tigelaar, R. E. (1974). *In* "Cellular Selection and Regulation in the Immune Response" (G. M. Edelman, ed.), p. 143. Raven, New York.
Gordon, D. A., Bell, D. A., Baumal, R., and Broder, I. (1969). *Clin. Exp. Immunol.* **5,** 57.
Gordon, D. A., Koehler, B. E., Russell, M. L., Urowitz, M. B., and Broder, I. (1975). *Ann. N.Y. Acad. Sci.* **256,** 338.
Greenberg, A. H., and Shen, L. (1973). *Nature* (*London*), *New Biol.* **245,** 282.
Gutman, R. A., Striker, G. E., Gilliland, B. C., and Cutler, R. E. (1972). *Medicine* (*Baltimore*) **51,** 1.
Haakenstad, A. O., and Mannik, M. (1974). *J. Immunol.* **112,** 1939.
Haakenstad, A. O., and Mannik, M. (1976). *Lab. Invest.* **35,** 283.
Haakenstad, A. O., Case, J. B., and Mannik, M. (1975). *J. Immunol.* **114,** 1153.
Haakenstad, A. O., Striker, G. E., and Mannik, M. (1976). *Lab. Invest.* **35,** 293.
Hannestad, K. (1967). *Clin. Exp. Immunol.* **2,** 511.
Harbeck, R. J., Bardana, E. J., Kohler, P. F., and Carr, R. I. (1973). *J. Clin. Invest.* **52,** 789.

Haurowitz, F. (1968). "Immunochemistry and the Biosynthesis of Antibodies." Wiley, New York.

Hawkins, D. (1971). *J. Immunol.* **107,** 344.

Hawkins, D. (1972). *J. Immunol.* **108,** 310.

Hawkins, D., and Peeters, S. (1971). *Lab. Invest.* **24,** 483.

Hay, F. C., Nineham, L. J., and Roitt, I. M. (1976). *Clin. Exp. Immunol.* **24,** 396.

Hedfors, E., and Norberg, R. (1974). *Clin. Exp. Immunol.* **16,** 493.

Heidelberger, M. (1939). *Bacteriol. Rev.* **3,** 49.

Heidelberger, M., and Pedersen, K. O. (1937). *J. Exp. Med.* **65,** 393.

Hellström, I., and Hellström, K.-E. (1969). *Int. J. Cancer* **4,** 587.

Hellström, K.-E., and Hellström, I. (1974). *Adv. Immunol.* **18,** 209.

Hendrickse, R. G., Glasgow, E. F., Adeniyi, A., White, R. H. R., Edington, G. M., and Houba, V. (1972). *Lancet* **1,** 1143.

Henney, C. S., and Ishizaka, K. (1970). *J. Immunol.* **104,** 1540.

Henson, P. M. (1969). *Immunology* **16,** 107.

Henson, P. M. (1970). *J. Immunol.* **105,** 476.

Henson, P. M. (1971a). *J. Immunol.* **107,** 1535.

Henson, P. M. (1971b). *J. Immunol.* **107,** 1547.

Henson, P. M. (1971c). *J. Exp. Med.* **134,** 114 s.

Henson, P. M. (1973). *Arthritis Rheum.* **16,** 208.

Henson, P. M., and Cochrane, C. G. (1969). *J. Exp. Med.* **129,** 167.

Henson, P. M., and Cochrane, C. G. (1971). *J. Exp. Med.* **133,** 554.

Henson, P. M., and Spiegelberg, H. L. (1973). *J. Clin. Invest.* **52,** 1282.

Henson, P. M., Johnson, H. B., and Speigelberg, H. L. (1972). *J. Immunol.* **109,** 1182.

Hollister, J. R., and Mannik, M. (1974). *Clin. Exp. Immunol.* **16,** 615.

Hollister, J. R., Liang, G. C., and Mannik, M. (1973). *Arthritis Rheum.* **16,** 10.

Hornick, C. L., and Karush, F. (1972). *Immunochemistry* **9,** 325.

Houston, W. E., Pedersen, C. E., Jr., Cole, F. E., Jr., and Spertzel, R. O. (1974). *Infect. Immun.* **10,** 437.

Howard, J. G., and Wardlaw, A. C. (1958). *Immunology* **1,** 338.

Huber, H., and Fudenberg, H. H. (1968). *Int. Arch. Allergy Appl. Immunol.* **34,** 18.

Huber, H., Polley, M. J., Linscott, W. D., Fudenberg, H. H., and Müller-Eberhard, H. J. (1968). *Science* **162,** 1281.

Hubscher, T., Bootello, A., and Eisen, A. H. (1974). *J. Allergy Clin. Immunol.* **53,** 150.

Humphrey, J. H. (1955). *J. Exp. Pathol.* **36,** 283.

Hyslop, N. E., Dourmashkin, R. R., Green, N. M., and Porter, R. R. (1970). *J. Exp. Med.* **131,** 783.

Intini, C., Segré, D., Segré, M., and Myers, W. L. (1971). *J. Immunol.* **107,** 1014.

Ishikawa, T., Wicher, K., and Arbesman, C. E. (1974). *Int. Arch. Allergy Appl. Immunol.* **46,** 230.

Ishizaka, K., Tomioka, H., and Ishizaka, T. (1970). *J. Immunol.* **105,** 1459.

Ishizaka, T. (1975). *Int. Arch. Allergy Appl. Immunol.* **49,** 129.

Israels, E. D., Nisli, G., Paraskevas, F., and Israels, L. G. (1973). *Thromb. Diath. Haemorrh.* **29,** 434.

Izui, S., Lambert, P.-H., and Miescher, P. A. (1976). *J. Exp. Med.* **144,** 428.
Jewell, D. P., and MacLennan, I. C. M. (1973). *Clin. Exp. Immunol.* **14,** 219.
Johnson, A. H., Mowbray, J. F., and Porter, K. A. (1975). *Lancet* **1,** 762.
Kabat, E. A. (1968). "Structural Concepts in Immunology and Immunochemistry." Holt, New York.
Kabat, E. A., and Mayer, M. M. (1961). "Experimental Immunochemistry," 2nd ed. Thomas, Springfield, Illinois.
Kalderon, A. E., Bogaars, H. A., and Diamond, I. (1975). *Clin. Immunol. Immunopathol.* **4,** 101.
Kaplan, A. P., and Austen, K. F. (1972). *J. Exp. Med.* **136,** 1378.
Klinman, N. R., and Karush, F. (1967). *Immunochemistry* **4,** 387.
Kniker, W. T., and Cochrane, C. G. (1968). *J. Exp. Med.* **127,** 119.
Koffler, D., Schur, P. H., and Kunkel, H. G. (1967). *J. Exp. Med.* **126,** 607.
Kohler, P. F., Cronin, R. E., Hammond, W. S., Olin, D., and Carr, R. I. (1974). *Ann. Intern. Med.* **81,** 448.
Kontiainen, S., and Mitchison, N. A. (1975). *Immunology* **28,** 523.
Kunkel, H. G., Müller-Eberhard, H. J., Fudenberg, H. H., and Tomasi, T. B. (1961). *J. Clin. Invest.* **40,** 117.
Lagrange, P. H., and Mackaness, G. B. (1975). *J. Exp. Med.* **141,** 82.
Laissue, J., Cottier, H., Hess, M. W., and Stoner, R. D. (1971). *J. Immunol.* **107,** 822.
Lambert, P. H., and Dixon, F. J. (1968). *J. Exp. Med.* **127,** 507.
Lamon, E. W., Andersson, B., Whitten, H. D., Hurst, M. M., and Ghanta, V. (1976). *J. Immunol.* **116,** 1199.
Lawrence, D. A., Weigle, W. O., and Spiegelberg, H. L. (1975). *J. Clin. Invest.* **55,** 368.
Lay, W. H., and Nussenzweig, V. (1968). *J. Exp. Med.* **128,** 991.
Lay, W. H., and Nussenzweig, V. (1969). *J. Immunol.* **102,** 1172.
Levy, R. L., and Hong, R. (1973). *Am. J. Med.* **54,** 645.
Lewis, M. G., Loughridge, L. W., and Phillips, J. M. (1971). *Lancet* **2,** 134.
Lightfoot, R. W., Jr., Drusin, R. E., and Christian, C. L. (1970). *J. Immunol.* **105,** 1493.
Litt, M. (1964). *Ann. N.Y. Acad. Sci.* **116,** 964.
LoBuglio, A. F., Cotran, R. S., and Jandl, J. H. (1967). *Science* **158,** 1582.
Ludwig, F. J., and Cusumano, C. L. (1974). *J. Natl. Cancer Inst.* **52,** 1529.
Lustig, H. J., and Bianco, C. (1976). *J. Immunol.* **116,** 253.
Luthra, H. S., McDuffie, F. C., Hunder, G. G., and Samayoa, E. A. (1975). *J. Clin. Invest.* **56,** 458.
McCluskey, R. T., and Benacerraf, B. (1959). *Am. J. Pathol.* **35,** 275.
McCluskey, R. T., Benacerraf, B., Potter, J. L., and Miller, F. (1960). *J. Exp. Med.* **111,** 181.
McCluskey, R. T., Benacerraf, B., and Miller, F. (1962). *Proc. Soc. Exp. Biol. Med.* **111,** 764.
McConnell, I., and Hurd, C. M. (1976). *Immunology* **30,** 835.
Mackaness, G. B., Lagrange, P. H., and Ishibashi, T. (1974a). *J. Exp. Med.* **139,** 1540.

Mackaness, G. B., Lagrange, P. H., Miller, T. E., and Ishibashi, T. (1974b). *J. Exp. Med.* **139,** 543.

MacLennan, I. C. M. (1972). *Clin. Exp. Immunol.* **101,** 275.

Magoon, E. H., Spragg, J., and Austen, K. F. (1974). *Adv. Biosci.* **12,** 225.

Mannik, M., and Arend, W. P. (1971). *J. Exp. Med.* **134,** 19s.

Mannik, M., Arend, W. P., Hall, A. P., and Gilliland, B. C. (1971). *J. Exp. Med.* **133,** 713.

Mannik, M., Haakenstad, A. O., and Arend, W. P. (1974). *Prog. Immunol., Int. Congr. Immunol., 2nd, 1974* Vol. 5.

Mantovani, B., Rabinovitch, M., and Nussenzweig, V. (1972). *J. Exp. Med.* **135,** 780.

Marney, S. R., Jr. (1971). *J. Immunol.* **106,** 82.

Marrack, J. R. (1938). *Med Res. Counc. (G.B.), Rep. Ser.* **SRS-230.**

Mauer, S. M., Sutherland, D. E. R., Howard, R. J., Fish, A. J., Najarian, J. S., and Michael, A. f. (1973). *J. Exp. Med.* **137,** 553.

Mayerson, H. S., Wolfram, C. G., Shirley, H. H., Jr., and Wasserman, K. (1960). *Am. J. Physiol.* **198,** 155.

Mellors, R. C., and Brzosko, W. J. (1962). *J. Exp. Med.* **115,** 891.

Meltzer, M., Franklin, E. C., Elias, K., McCluskey, R. T., and Cooper, N. (1966). *Am. J. Med.* **40,** 837.

Messner, R. P., and Jelinek, J. (1970). *J. Clin. Invest.* **49,** 2165.

Metzger, H. (1970). *Adv. Immunol.* **12,** 57.

Michael, A. F., Jr., Drummond, K. N., Good, R. A., and Vernier, R. L. (1966). *J. Clin. Invest.* **45,** 237.

Miller, F., Benacerraf, B., McCluskey, R. T., and Potter, J. L. (1960). *Proc. Soc. Exp. Biol. Med.* **104,** 706.

Miller, G. W., and Nussenzweig, V. (1974). *J. Immunol.* **113,** 464.

Miller, G. W., Saluk, P. H., and Nussenzweig, V. (1973). *J. Exp. Med.* **138,** 495.

Miller, G. W., Steinberg, A. D., Green, I., and Nussenzweig, V. (1975). *J. Immunol.* **114,** 1166.

Mims, C. A. (1959). *Br. J. Exp. Pathol.* **40,** 533.

Moretta, L., Ferrarini, M., Durante, M. L., and Mingari, M. C. (1975). *Eur. J. Immunol.* **5,** 565.

Movat, H. Z., Mustard, J. F., Taichman, N. S., and Uriuhara, T. (1965). *Proc. Soc. Exp. Biol. Med.* **120,** 232.

Müller-Eberhard, H. J., and Kunkel, H. G. (1961). *Proc. Soc. Exp. Biol. Med.* **106,** 291

Mueller-Eckhardt, C. (1975). *Klin. Wochenschr.* **53,** 889.

Mueller-Eckhardt, C. and Lüscher, E. F. (1968). *Thromb. Diath. Haemorrh.* **20,** 155.

Myllylä, G. (1973). *Scand. J. Haematol., Suppl.* **19,** 1.

Nakamura, R. M., Speigelberg, H. L., Lee, S., and Weigle, W. O. (1968). *J. Immunol.* **100,** 376.

Naruse, T., Kitamura, K., Miyakawa, Y., and Shibata, S. (1973). *J. Immunol.* **110,** 1163.

Natali, P. G., and Tan, E. M. (1972). *J. Clin. Invest.* **51,** 345.

Neauport-Sautes, C., Dupuis, D., and Fridman, W. H. (1975). *Eur. J. Immunol.* **5,** 849.
Nisonoff, A., and Pressman, D. (1959). *J. Immunol.* **83,** 138.
Nisonoff, A., and Winkler, M. H. (1958). *J. Immunol.* **81,** 65.
Norberg, R. (1974). *Scand. J. Immunol.* **3,** 229.
Norman, S. J. (1974). *Lab. Invest.* **31,** 161.
Nussenzweig, V. (1974). *Adv. Immunol.* **19,** 217.
Nydegger, U. E., Lambert, P. H., Gerber, H., and Miescher, P. A. (1974). *J. Clin. Invest.* **54,** 297.
Nydegger, U. E., Izui, S., Zubler, R., Lambert, P. H., and Miescher, P. A. (1975). *In* "The Immunological Basis of Connective Tissue Disorders," (Silvestri, L. G., ed.) p. 85. Am. Elsevier, New York.
Okafor, G. O., Hay, F. C., and Turner, M. W. (1974). *Nature* (*London*) **248,** 228.
Okumura, K., Kondo, Y., and Tada, T. (1971). *Lab. Invest.* **24,** 383.
Onyewotu, I. I., Holborow, E. J., and Johnson, G. D. (1974). *Nature* (*London*) **248,** 156.
Onyewotu, I. I., Johnson, P. M., Johnson, G. D., and Holborow, E. J. (1975). *Clin. Exp. Immunol.* **19,** 267.
Osler, A. G., and Siraganian, R. P. (1972). *Prog. Allergy* **16,** 450.
Ovary, Z., Vaz, N. M., and Warner, N. L. (1970). *Immunology* **19,** 715.
Ozawa, T., Pluss, R., Lacher, J., Boedecker, E., Guggenheim, S., Hammond, W., and McIntosh, R. (1975). *Q. J. Med.* **44,** 523.
Panem, S., Ordóñez, N. G., Kirstein, W. H., Katz, A. I., and Spargo, B. H. (1976). *N. Engl. J. Med.* **295,** 470.
Paraskevas, F., Lee, S.-T., Orr, K. B., and Israels, L. G. (1972). *J. Immunol.* **108,** 1319.
Pascal, R. R., Koss, M. N., and Kassel, R. L. (1973). *Lab. Invest.* **29,** 159.
Pauling, L., Pressman, D., and Campbell, D. H. (1944). *J. Am. Chem. Soc.* **66,** 330.
Pedersen, K. O. (1936). *Nature* (*London*) **138,** 363.
Penttinen, K., Myllylä, G., Mäkelä, O., and Vaheri, A. (1969). *Acta Pathol. Microbiol. Scand.* **77,** 309.
Penttinen, K., Vaheri, A., and Myllylä, G. (1971). *Clin. Exp. Immunol.* **8,** 389.
Penttinen, K., Wager, O., Räsänen, J. A., Myllylä, G., and Haapanen, E. (1973). *Clin. Exp. Immunol.* **15,** 409.
Perez, G. O., Rothfield, N., and Williams, R. C. (1976). *Arch. Intern. Med.* **136,** 334.
Perlmann, P., Perlmann, H., and Biberfeld, P. (1972). *J. Immunol.* **108,** 558.
Petty, R. E., Steward, M. W., and Soothill, J. F. (1972). *Clin. Exp. Immunol.* **12,** 231.
Pfueller, S. L., and Lüscher, E. F. (1972). *Immunochemistry* **9,** 1151.
Pfueller, S. L., and Lüscher, E. F. (1974). *J. Immunol.* **112,** 1201.
Phillips-Quagliata, J. M., Levine, B. B., and Uhr, J. W. (1969). *Nature* (*London*) **222,** 1290.
Phillips-Quagliata, J. M., Levine, B. B., Quagliata, F., and Uhr, J. W. (1971). *J. Exp. Med.* **133,** 589.
Pope, R. M., Teller, D. C., and Mannik, M. (1975). *J. Immunol.* **115,** 365.

Quie, P. G., Messner, R. P., and Williams, R. C. (1968). *J. Exp. Med.* **128,** 553.
Rabellino, E. M., and Metcalf, D. (1975). *J. Immunol.* **115,** 688.
Rabinovitch, M., Manejias, R. E., and Nussenzweig, V. (1975). *J. Exp. Med.* **142,** 827.
Ramasamy, R., Richardson, N. E., and Feinstein, A. (1976). *Immunology* **30,** 851.
Rappaport, B. Z. (1964). *J. Immunol.* **93,** 792.
Ratnoff, O. D. (1969). *Adv. Immunol.* **10,** 145.
Rawson, A. J., and Torralba, T. P. (1967). *Arthritis Rheum.* **10,** 44.
Revoltella, R., Pediconi, M., Bertolini, L., and Bosman, C. (1975). *Cell. Immunol.* **20,** 117.
Reynolds, H. Y., Atkinson, J. P., Newball, H. H., and Frank, M. M. (1975). *J. Immunol.* **114,** 1813.
Rhodes, J. (1973). *Nature* (*London*) **243,** 527.
Ross, G. D., and Polley, M. J. (1975). *J. Exp. Med.* **141,** 1163.
Ross, G. D., Polley, M. J., Rabellino, E. M., and Grey, H. M. (1973). *J. Exp. Med.* **138,** 798.
Rother, K., Rother, U., and Schindera, F. (1964). *Z. Immunitaetsforsch.* **126,** 473.
Roy, L. P., Fish, A. J., Michael, A. F., and Vernier, R. L. (1972). *Prog. Clin. Immunol.* **1,** 1.
Ryan, J. L., Arbeit, R. D., Dickler, H. B., and Henkart, P. A. (1975). *J. Exp. Med.* **142,** 814.
Saba, T. M. (1970). *Arch. Intern. Med.* **126,** 1031.
Saksela, E., Imir, T., and Mäkel, O. (1975). *J. Immunol.* **115,** 1488.
Schreiber, A. D., and Frank, M. M. (1972a). *J. Clin. Invest.* **51,** 575.
Schreiber, A. D., and Frank, M. M. (1972b). *J. Clin. Invest.* **51,** 583.
Schumaker, V. N., Green, G., and Wilder, R. L. (1973). *Immunochemistry* **10,** 521.
Simpson, J. G., Robertson, A. J., and Stalker, A. L. (1973). *In* "Clinical Aspects of Microcirculation" (J. Ditzel and D. H. Lewis, eds.), p. 260. Karger, Basel.
Sinclair, N. R. StC., Lees, R. K., Abrahams, S., Chan, A. P. L., Fagan, G., and Stiller, C. R. (1974). *J. Immunol.* **113,** 1493.
Siraganian, R. P., and Osler, A. G. (1971). *J. Immunol.* **106,** 1252.
Sitprija, V., Pipatanagul, V., Boonpucknavig, V., and Boonpucknavig, S. (1974). *Ann. Intern. Med.* **81,** 210.
Sjögren, H. O., Hellström, I., Bansal, S. C., and Hellström, K.-E. (1971). *Proc. Natl. Acad. Sci. U.S.A.* **68,** 1372.
Sobel, A. T., Bokisch, V. A., and Müller-Eberhard, H. J. (1975). *J. Exp. Med.* **142,** 139.
Soothill, J. F., and Steward, M. W. (1971). *Clin. Exp. Immunol.* **9,** 193.
Spiegelberg, H. L. (1974). *Adv. Immunol.* **19,** 259.
Spitler, L., Huber, H., and Fudenberg, H. H. (1969). *J. Immunol.* **102,** 404.
Steinman, R. M., and Cohn, Z. A. (1972). *J. Cell Biol.* **55,** 616.
Stoner, R. D., and Terres, G. (1963). *J. Immunol.* **91,** 761.
Stout, R. D., and Herzenberg, L. A. (1975). *J. Exp. Med.* **142,** 611.
Striker, G. E., Quadracci, L. J., and Cutler, R. E. (1976). *In* "Major Problems in Pathology" (J. Bennington, ed.). Saunders, Philadelphia, Pennsylvania (in press).

Stühlinger, W. D., Verroust, P. J., and Morel-Maroger, L. (1976). *Immunology* **30,** 43.

Sullivan, A. L., Grimley, P. M., and Metzger, H. (1971). *J. Exp. Med.* **134,** 1403.

Svehag, S.-E. (1975). *Scand. J. Immunol.* **4,** 687.

Svehag, S.-E., and Burger, D. (1976). *Acta Pathol. Microbiol. Scand., Sect. C* **84,** 45.

Talmage, D. W., Dixon, F. J., Bukantz, S. C., and Dammin, G. J. (1951). *J. Immunol.* **67,** 243.

Taylor, R. B., and Basten, A. (1976). *Br. Med. Bull.* **32,** 152.

Terres, G., Morrison, S. L., Habicht, G. S., and Stoner, R. D. (1972). *J. Immunol.* **108,** 1473.

Theofilopoulos, A. N., Bokisch, V. A., and Dixon, F. J. (1974a). *J. Exp. Med.* **139,** 696.

Theofilopoulos, A. N., Dixon, F. J., and Bokisch, V. A. (1974b). *J. Exp. Med.* **140,** 877.

Theofilopoulos, A. N., Wilson, C. B., Bokisch, V. A., and Dixon, F. J. (1974c). *J. Exp. Med.* **140,** 1230.

Theofilopoulos, A. N., Wilson, C. B., and Dixon, F. J. (1976). *J. Clin. Invest.* **57,** 169.

Thorbecke, G. J., and Benacerraf, B. (1962). *Prog. Allergy* **6,** 559.

Thorbecke, G. J., Maurer, P. H., and Benacerraf, B. (1960). *Br. J. Exp. Pathol.* **41,** 190.

Tigelaar, R. E., Vaz, N. M., and Ovary, Z. (1971). *J. Immunol.* **106,** 661.

Tourville, D. R., Byrd, L. H., Kim, D. U., Zajd, D., Lee, J., Reichman, L. B., and Barkin, S. (1976). *Am. J. Pathol.* **82,** 479.

Treser, G., Semar, M., Ty, A., Segal, I., Franklin, M. A., and Lange, K. (1970). *J. Clin. Invest.* **49,** 762.

Tsumita, T., and Iwanaga, M. (1963). *Nature* (*London*) **198,** 1088.

Uhr, J. W., (1965). *Proc. Natl. Acad. Sci. U.S.A.* **54,** 1599.

Uhr, J. W., and Möller, G. (1968). *Adv. Immunol.* **8,** 81.

Uhr, J. W., and Phillips, J. M. (1966). *Ann. N.Y. Acad. Sci.* **129,** 793.

Uhr, J. W., and Weissmann, G. (1965). *J. Immunol.* **94,** 544.

Unanue, E. R., and Dixon, F. J. (1967). *Adv. Immunol.* **6,** 1.

Van Boxel, J. A., and Rosenstreich, D. L. (1974). *J. Exp. Med.* **139,** 1002.

Vaz, N. M., and Prouvost-Danon, A. (1969). *Prog. Allergy* **13,** 111.

Wager, O., Penttinen, K., Räsänen, J. A., and Myllylä, G. (1973). *Clin. Exp. Immunol.* **15,** 393.

Ward, P. A., and Cochrane, C. G. (1965). *J. Exp. Med.* **121,** 215.

Ward, P. A., and Zvaifler, N. J. (1973). *J. Immunol.* **111,** 1777.

Warner, N. L., and Ovary, Z. (1972). *Scand. J. Immunol.* **1,** 41.

Webb, F. W. S., Ford, P. M., and Glynn, L. E. (1971). *Br. J. Exp. Pathol.* **52,** 31.

Weigle, W. O. (1960). *In* "Mechanisms of Antibody Formation" (M. Holub and L. Jarošková, eds.), p. 283. Academic Press, New York.

Weigle, W. O. (1961). *Adv. Immunol.* **1,** 283.

Weigle, W. O. (1973). *Pathol. Annu.* **8,** 329.

Weigle, W. O., and Maurer, P. H. (1957). *J. Immunol.* **79,** 223.

Weiser, R. S., and Laxson, C. (1962). *J. Infect. Dis.* **111,** 55.

Weissmann, G., Dukor, P., and Zurier, R. B. (1971). *Nature* (*London*), *New Biol.* **231,** 131.

Wellek, B., Hahn, H. H., and Opferkuch, W. (1975). *J. Immunol.* **114,** 1643.

Wilk, A. (1975). *Acta Pathol. Microbiol. Scand., Sect. C* **83,** 354.

Wilson, C. B., and Dixon, F. J. (1971). *J. Exp. Med.* **134,** 7 s.

Wilson, C. B., and Dixon, F. J. (1974). *Kidney Int.* **5,** 389.

Winchester, R. J., Agnello, V., and Kunkel, H. G. (1970). *Clin. Exp. Immunol.* **6,** 689.

Winchester, R. J., Kunkel, H. G., and Agnello, V. (1971). *J. Exp. Med.* **134,** 286 s.

Wisse, E., and Daems, W. T. (1970). *In* "Mononuclear Phagocytes" (R. van Furth, ed.), p. 200. Davis, Philadelphia, Pennsylvania.

Wright, P. W., Hargreaves, R. E., Bansal, S. C., Bernstein, I. D., and Hellström, K.-E. (1973). *Proc. Natl. Acad. Sci. U.S.A.* **70,** 2539.

Yasmeen, D., Ellerson, J. R., Dorrington, K. J., and Painter, R. H. (1973). *J. Immunol.* **110,** 1706.

Yoshida, T. O., and Andersson, B. (1972). *Scand. J. Immunol.* **1,** 401.

Zubler, R. H., Lange, G., Lambert, P. H., and Miescher, P. A. (1976a). *J. Immunol.* **116,** 232.

Zubler, R. H., Nydegger, U., Perrin, L. H., Fehr, K., McCormick, J., Lambert, P. H., and Miescher, P. A. (1976b). *J. Clin. Invest.* **57,** 1308.

Part III

VIRAL ASPECTS

Chapter 12

H-2 Restriction of Cell-Mediated Virus-Specific Immunity and Immunopathology: Self-Recognition, Altered Self, and Autoaggression

ROLF M. ZINKERNAGEL

I. INTRODUCTION

Cell-mediated autoimmunity, defined as thymus-derived lymphocyte (T cell) mediated reactivity against cells expressing solely "normal" self, is poorly defined in mice, and its existence is hard to prove. Detection and analysis of autoimmunity are complicated by the fact that mice often have ongoing viral infections and nonspecific responses to them. Also, most cultured cell lines used as targets for measuring autoimmunity and mice used for the same purpose possess endogenous viruses that are "activated" during experimentation. Thus, reasonable controls for "normal" cells or "normal" mice are difficult to find.

However, cell-mediated immune damage of cells expressing viral antigens (Zinkernagel and Doherty, 1974a,b; Doherty *et al.*, 1976a) or chemically modified (Shearer, 1974; Shearer *et al.*, 1975) has been well defined *in vitro* and *in vivo*. Although this T cell reactivity is not against normal self but, rather, against self in association with a foreign antigen, it may well represent many of the so-called cell-mediated autoimmune phenomena. Therefore, this report describes mainly the evidence of immune and autoimmune or autoaggressive phenomena resulting from virus infections without attempting to review the field comprehensively.

The fundamental mechanisms of self–nonself discrimination are discussed in other chapters. However, it may be appropriate to outline some speculations that impinge on the specific function of cell-mediated immunity (CMI) and on its role in immune surveillance.

The idea that CMI is directed against intracellular pathogens and that this activity may represent a sort of graft versus host reaction against infected tissue was formulated soon after the discovery that CMI is critically involved in allograft rejection (Table I). Mitchison (1954) speculated on the similarities between alloreactivity and CMI of an individual animal to chemicals or to tuberculin. Thus, tissue antigens are slightly altered when associating with these exogenous antigens, comparable to the slight difference from one alloantigen to another. The H-2 antigens were given a more direct biologic function by Thomas (1959), who proposed that this cell-surface marker system prevents horizontal spreading of tumor cells (see also Burnet, 1970). This idea was developed further by Lawrence (1959) into a most fascinating model of universal T cell reactivity to self + X. This hypothesis described prophetically in 1959 what we accidentally discovered experimentally in 1973/1974 to be the specificity of cytotoxic T cells and T cells quite generally. Since I became aware of the Lawrence hypothesis, my co-workers and I can only apologize humbly and rather tardily for never having referred to these reports. We used the term "altered self" to describe that T cells are specific for both virus and self major transplantation antigens, much as Lawrence used the same definition. In the same sense, we attempted to state that T cells are probably primarily preoccupied with recognizing altered self as different from normal self, rather than with distinguishing self from nonself as originally formulated by Burnet (see Burnet, 1959; Burnet and Fenner, 1949).

TABLE I

The Targets of T Cell-Mediated Immunity Other Than in Transplanation Reactions: A Selected History of Interpretations

T cell function	Target	Role of H-2	References
Rejection of contact allergens	Slightly altered self in contrast to vastly different from self	Discussion of similarity of graft rejection and DTH to chemicals	Mitchison, 1954
Tumor immune surveillance	Tumor cell mutation of self	Prevents horizontal spread of tumors	Thomas, 1959
General immune surveillance	Self + X	Self-marker?	Lawrence, 1959
Tumor immune surveillance	Tumor cell	Prevents horizontal spread of tumors	Burnet, 1970
Immune surveillance T and B cells	Before immuno-competence is reached self, thereafter mainly alloantigens	Self-marker which drives somatic generation of diversity	Jerne, 1971
T helper	Macrophage–B cell	Physiological interaction	Katz and Benacerraf, 1975, 1976; Erb and Feldman, 1974; Taussig *et al.*, 1975
Virus specific cytotoxicity general immune surveillance	"Altered self" (virus + self or modification of self) or "dual interaction"	Self-marker Self-marker	Zinkernagel and Doherty, 1974b; Doherty and Zinkernagel, 1975b

Support for the concept of H-2 restriction of T cell-mediated effector functions brought rather direct evidence for a role of major transplantation antigens in syngeneic CMI. This phenomenon has been interpreted with two basic models as will be discussed in a later section. The altered self concept and the dual recognition model both incorporate ideas of self + X (Zinkernagel and Doherty, 1974a,b; Doherty *et al.*, 1976a; Katz and Benacerraf, 1975, 1976) and assign a fundamental biologic role for H-2 antigens as self-markers in immunologic surveillance.

The aim here is to try to summarize some evidence which demonstrates that the basic mechanism resulting in antiviral immunity and/or T cell-mediated immunopathology are similar, i.e., both are caused by cell destruction. Further, we examine whether cell-mediated reactivity to normal self exists alone or only in association with concurrent recognition of a foreign antigen or whether such reactivity is against altered self (reviewed in Doherty *et al.*, 1976a; Zinkernagel and Doherty, 1976).

II. THE TARGETS OF T CELL-MEDIATED IMMUNITY

The targets for T cell-mediated immunity are, probably exclusively, cells. This seems obvious from the fact that all T cell-mediated phenomena studied so far are strongly associated with cell-surface structures coded for by the major murine histocompatibility (H-2) complex (Table IIA,B). Thus, T cells are simultaneously specific for a particular antigen and for a particular K, I, or D region product of the H-2 gene complex. The evidence for this contention and speculation on its biologic significance have been reviewed recently (Doherty and Zinkernagel, 1975b, Zinkernagel and Doherty, 1976; Katz and Benacerraf, 1976; Klein, 1975, 1976; Doherty *et al.*, 1976a; Blanden *et al.*, 1976a). For most of these T cell functions, the role of the H-2 gene complex in defining T cell specificity has been shown for induction, as well as for primary and secondary effector cell specificity (Katz and Benacerraf, 1975; Dunlop *et al.*, 1976; M. B. C. Dunlop and R. V. Blanden, unpublished).

The example of cell-mediated cytotoxicity against virus-infected target cells may appropriately serve to demonstrate T cell reactivity from the viewpoint of autoimmunity for several reasons. First, CMI is crucial in overcoming most primary virus infections in mammals (Blanden, 1974; Bloom and Rager-Zisman, 1975; Notkins, 1975). Clearly, immune mechanisms other than direct T cell-mediated cytotoxicity also play an important role in a host's recovery from a primary virus infection. T cell-dependent lymphokine-mediated effector functions are of great importance, i.e., migration inhibition factor, immune interferon, and macrophage activation (reviewed by Blanden, 1974; Bloom and Rager-Zisman, 1975; Blanden *et al.*, 1976a).

Second, the murine models of lymphocytic choriomeningitis virus (LCMV) infections ideally demonstrate the spectrum of both beneficial, i.e., immunoprotective and damaging (therefore, immunopathological) effects of CMI. In fact, the distinction between immunoprotection and immunopathology is made only with respect to clinical outcome, since the causal immune mechanisms are probably the same. The symptoms depend mainly on the animal's anatomic characteristics of the organs preferentially infected by the virus, susceptibility to the virus in question, extent of infection, and the host's capability to mount an immune response (Hotchin, 1971; Doherty and Zinkernagel, 1974; Cole and Nathanson, 1975). Antibodies may participate, although their main importance is probably to prevent late spreading of virus and secondary infections. Antibody-mediated immunity also can be protective or can cause immunopathology, dependent mainly on antigen persistance and host factors. Immune complex glomerulonephritis is a classical example (reviewed in Wilson and Dixon, 1974).

III. MURINE LYMPHOCYTIC CHORIOMENINGITIS VIRUS INFECTIONS

LCMV is a budding RNA virus of the arenavirus group and is not harmful to many kinds of cells (Lehmann-Grube, 1971; Melnick, 1973). Thus, pathology is not, as in most virus infections, caused by the destructive activity of virus itself but by the host's immune response to it. The clinical manifestations of LCMV infections in mice depend on virus strain, mouse strain, route of infection, virus dose, and immunocompetence of the host (Fig. 1) and have been comprehensively reviewed (Hotchin, 1971; Doherty and Zinkernagel, 1974; Cole and Nathanson, 1975). In immunologically competent mice, intravenous (i.v.) injection of LCMV causes mild systemic disease and parallel immunity. CMI is central for virus elimination (Blanden, 1974; Mims and Blanden, 1972; Zinkernagel and Welsh, 1976). However, immunologically competent mice injected intracerebrally (i.c.) with LCMV die about 6–8 days later of an acute lymphocytic choriomeningitis (LCM), classically described by Armstrong and Lillie (1934), Traub (1936), Haas (1954), Hotchin (1971), and Cole and collaborators (1972). The many reports describing T cell-mediation of acute LCM (Doherty and Zinkernagel, 1974; Cole and Nathanson, 1975) need be summarized here only briefly. Infection i.v. or i.c. at times before immunocompetence is reached and/or all means of reducing the immunocompetent T cells in adult mice [i.e., thymectomy (Rowe *et al.*, 1963), lethal irradiation (Rowe, 1956),

TABLE IIA

Role of H-2 Gene Complex in Defining Specificity of T Cells

T cell function	Antigen	H-2 gene region antigen involved at effector and/or induction level	References
Helper	DNP–KLH	I-A, I-B	Kindred and Shreffler, 1972; Katz *et al.*, 1973, 1975; Katz and Benacerraf, 1975, 1976; Erb and Feldman, 1975
DTH	Fowl γ-globulin	I-A, I-B	Miller *et al.*, 1975
	LCMV	K, D	Zinkernagel, 1976b
	DNFB	K, I, D	Vadas *et al.*, 1976
Cytotoxicity	Alloantigen	K, (I), D	Brondz *et al.*, 1975; Shreffler, 1974; Cerottini and Brunner, 1974; Klein, 1975, 1976
	Virus	K, D	Zinkernagel and Doherty, 1974a,b; Table IIb
	TNP		Shearer, 1974; Shearer *et al.*, 1975
	Minor H		Bevan, 1975
	H–Y		Gorden *et al.*, 1975
Proliferation		I region equivalent in guinea pigs	Rosenthal and Shevach, 1973, 1976
		I	Schwartz and Paul, 1976
Immunopathology	LCMV	K, D	Doherty *et al.*, 1976
Antiviral protection	Ectromelia	K, D	Kees and Blanden, 1976
	LCMV	K, D	Zinkernagel and Welsh, 1976
Macrophage activation	Listeria monocytogenes	K?, I	Zinkernagel, 1974

TABLE IIB

H-2K and D Restriction of Virus-Specific Cytotoxicity

Virus	Classification	Nucleic acid	Envelope	Budding	References
LCMV	Arena	RNA	+	+	Zinkernagel and Doherty, 1974a,b
Ectromelia	Pox	DNA	+	–	Blanden *et al.*, 1975
Vaccinia	Pox	DNA	+	–	Koszinowski and Thomssen, 1975
Sendai	Paramyxo	RNA	+	+	Doherty and Zinkernagel, 1976
Friend	Oncorna	RNA	+	+	Blank *et al.*, 1976
MSV	Oncorna	RNA	+	+	Ortiz de Landazuri and Herberman, 1972; Herbermann *et al.*, 1973 Gomard *et al.*, 1976; Plata, 1976
SV40	Papova	DNA	–	–	Trinchieri *et al.*, 1976
Influenza	Myxo	RNA	+	+	Yap and Ada, 1976
Coxsackie B-3	Picorna	RNA	–	–	Wong *et al.*, 1977
Rabies	Rhabdo	RNA	+	+	Doherty *et al.*, 1976

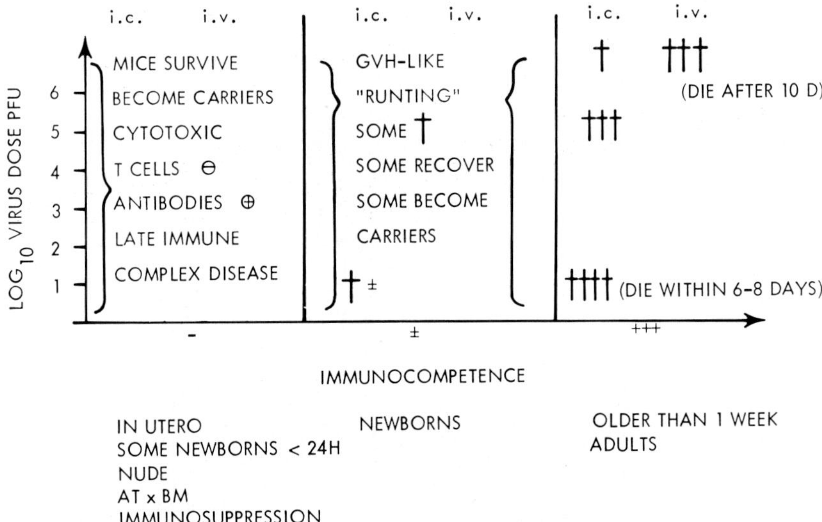

Fig. 1. Clinical symptoms and course of disease after LCMV infection in mice depend on route of infection, virus dose, and degree of immunocompetence. The less virus that is injected i.c. and the greater the immunocompetence of the host, the greater the morbidity and mortality of LCM. Immunoincompetent mice will become carrier mice; they will not generate cytotoxic T cells but will develop antibodies to LCMV. This may lead to immune complex disease. Mice that are about to become immunocompetent may become carrier mice or may develop a runt disease or alternatively die of LCM or become immune. The outcome in all cases depends on virus strain and mouse strain.

and bone marrow reconstitution (Cole and Nathanson, 1975; Doherty and Zinkernagel, 1974), cyclophosphamide treatment at the time of or soon after infection (Cole *et al.*, 1972), anti-lymphocyte serum treatment (Hirsch *et al.*, 1967), use of genetically thymus-deprived mice (nude) (Cole and Nathanson, 1975)] have two major consequences: (1) mice cannot eliminate LCMV and, thus, become virus carriers, and (2) they do not develop fatal LCM. Thus, virus elimination and acute LCM are predominantly T cell-mediated phenomena.

More direct evidence for this contention has been obtained. First, T cell-dependent accumulation of mononuclear inflammatory cells in cerebrospinal fluid, generation of virus-specific cytotoxic T cells in lymphoid tissue and clinical symptoms all develop in parallel (Fig. 2; Zinkernagel and Doherty, 1973; Doherty and Zinkernagel, 1974). Second, cerebrospinal fluids of clinically affected mice contain a high percentage of LCMV-specific cytotoxic T cells. Third, the capacity of LCMV immune spleen cells to transfer to naive mice antiviral protection as measured by (1) reduction of plaque-forming units in preinfected recipients (Zinkernagel and Welsh, 1976), (2) delayed-type hypersensitivity reactions in footpads (Zinkernagel, 1976b), and (3) acute LCM in i.c. preinfected and immunosuppressed recipient mice (Doherty *et al.*, 1976a) develops in parallel with the cytolytic capacity measured *in vitro*. All these properties of LCMV immune cells have identical specificities, kinetics, and cellular parameters (Table III, Zinkernagel and Doherty, 1976). The kinetics of the developing cellular immune responses after i.v. or i.c. infection can then be monitored *in vitro* by using ^{51}Cr assays to measure the capacity of spleen cells to lyse specifically LCMV-infected target cells (Oldstone and Dixon, 1970; Marker and Volkert, 1973; Zinkernagel and Doherty, 1973; Gardner *et al.*, 1974). Cytolytic activity reaches a peak around 5–9 days after infection depending on virus dose and injection route (Marker and Volkert, 1973; Gardner *et al.*, 1974; Doherty and Zinkernagel, 1974).

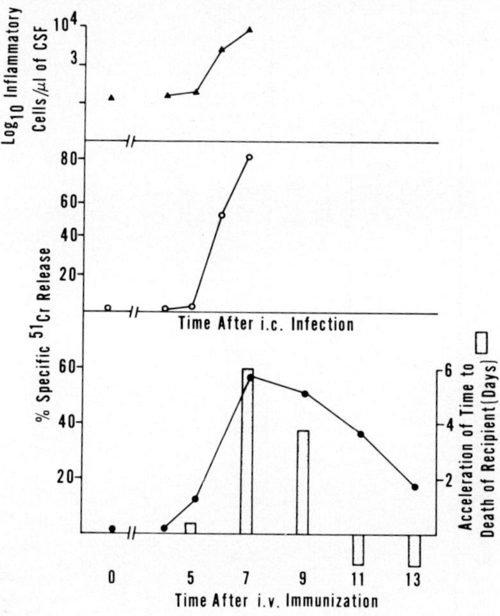

Fig. 2. Kinetics of generation of virus-specific cytotoxic T cells after i.v. (●) or i.c. (○) infection with LCMV. In the uppermost panel, the kinetics of concentration of inflammatory white blood cells in cerebrospinal fluid (CSF) are recorded. In the lowest panel, cytotoxicity after i.v. infection is compared with the capacity of the same cells to adoptively transfer acute LCMV to i.c. infected, immunosuppressed recipients. Modified from Doherty and Zinkernagel (1974) and Doherty and Zinkernagel (1975b).

TABLE III

Parameters of LCMV Immune T Cells

	In Vitro	*In Vivo*		
	Cytotoxicity ^{51}Cr release assay	Adoptive induction of acute LCM	Adoptive transfer of antiviral protection	Adoptive transfer of DTH
Specificity versus other viruses	+	+	+	+
Anti-θ + C sensitive	+	+	+	+
Peak activity	7–9 d	7–9 d	7–9 d	7–9 d
H-2 regions coding for self-marker involved				
K, D	+	+	+	+
I	–	–	–	–
Cross-reactivity between wild type H-2K^{b} and mutant H-2K^{ba}	–	–	–	–

Adapted from Zinkernagel and Doherty, 1976.

IV. H-2 RESTRICTION OF CMI TO VIRUS INFECTION

We discovered quite fortuitously that the specificity of cytolytic T cells is not for the virus alone, but also for the cell surface marker coded by the major histocompatibility complex in H-2K and H-2D present in the animal in which the T cells were sensitized (Zinkernagel and Doherty, 1974a,b, 1976). The analysis of this H-2 restriction phenomenon can be summarized as follows:

Only the H-2 genes and none of the non-H-2 genes are involved (Doherty and Zinkernagel, 1975a).

Of the various gene regions of H-2, only the K and D regions, which code for the major transplantation antigens, are relevant (Blanden *et al.*, 1975; Zinkernagel and Doherty, 1975). The I region of H-2, which codes for immune response genes and Ia cell-surface structures, is not involved in virus-specific cytolytic interactions.

The private specificities, but not the public ones are important (Zinkernagel and Doherty, 1976).

T cell recognition of antigen associated with only one of the four specificities in H-2 heterozygotes, possibly different K or D alleles, is sufficient (Zinkernagel *et al.*, 1975).

Infected target cells that do not express H-2K and D antigens are not lysed by cytotoxic T cells (Zinkernagel and Oldstone, 1976).

Virus-immune T cells from some H-2K^b mutant mice (which differ from wild type mice by a mutation of the gene coding for the K^b structure and which because of this reject skin grafts of wild type H-2K^b) fail to lyse infected H-2K^b wild type targets. The structure defined by these mutants is, therefore, recognized by T cells for virus-specific cytolysis (Klein, 1975, 1976; Zinkernagel, 1976b). This structure is either the "alterable" self-structure or the self-marker that is recognized by the self-recognitive structure.

The H-2 restriction reflects T cell specificity, but not the absolute need for T cells and infected target cells to be H-2 compatible. Thus, a virus-specific cytotoxic T cell is specific for only one K or D allele (Zinkernagel and Doherty, 1975). In an infected mouse of H-2^k type, T cells of H-2^k type, are exposed to viral antigen only in association with H-2^k self-structures. Therefore, they only can lyse infected H-2^k cells, since they have not been sensitized to H-2^d plus virus. In chimeric mice, whose lymphoreticular system has been manipulated, H-2^k cells can be sensitized to virus plus a foreign H-2^d antigen. Thus, T cells of one parental (P_1) H-2 type can develop in irradiated hybrid F_1 mice, which were reconstituted with P_1 bone marrow cells, which now can be sensitized to virus plus H-2 of P_1 or virus plus

H-2 of the other P_2 type. Distinct virus immune T cells from $P_1 \rightarrow F_1$ bone marrow chimeras lyse specifically either infected P_1 or infected P_2 target cells, but not infected target cells of an unrelated P_3 type (von Boehmer *et al.*, 1975; Zinkernagel, 1976c; Pfizenmaier *et al.*, 1976). Since here immune T cells and target cells do not share H-2K or D products, the "self" marker on the target must be recognized unidirectionally.

There is no obvious trivial explanation for this H-2 restriction, such as allogeneic inhibition or suppression (Hellström and Möller, 1965), for the following reasons. First, admixture of allogeneic third party cells *in vitro* (or *in vivo*) has no negative effect on H-2K or D compatible activities (Zinkernagel and Welsh, 1976). Second, F_1 hybrid offspring $\rightarrow$ parent combinations or compatibility at one out of four in heterozygotes different K and D regions are as efficient as syngeneic combinations (Zinkernagel and Doherty, 1976).

V. IS VIRUS-SPECIFIC CYTOTOXICITY DIRECTED AGAINST "ALTERED SELF" OR AGAINST VIRUS AND SELF INDEPENDENTLY?

In an attempt to explain the H-2 restriction of virus-specific T cell cytotoxicity two models have been proposed (Fig. 3; Zinkernagel and Doherty, 1974a,b; reviewed and discussed in Doherty *et al.*, 1976a; Zinkernagel, 1976a,b; Katz and Benacerraf, 1975; Lawrence, 1959).

The dual recognition model was originally proposed as "the physiological interaction" model by Katz and Benacerraf (1975; Katz *et al.*, 1973, 1975) to explain H-2 restriction of T–B cell collaboration; this model has been adapted to explain the experimental results when responses to virus infection are evaluated. Accordingly, virus-specific cytotoxic T cells express two independently clonally expressed specificities, one for a self-marker and one for a viral antigen (Zinkernagel and Doherty, 1975). The specificity of the recognition structure for viral antigen is probably defined by an immunoglobulin variable region (V) gene equivalent (Ramseier and Lindenmann, 1969, 1972; Binz and Wigzell, 1975a,b; Doherty *et al.*, 1976c; Zinkernagel and Doherty, 1976). The self-recognizer would have to be a structure expressed to recognize H-2 structures on hemopoietic stem cells and lymphocytes when a host reaches immunologic competence (Bechtol *et al.*, 1974; Katz and Benacerraf, 1975, 1976; Zinkernagel and Doherty, 1976). Whether the V gene equivalent specific for self is identical to the one on alloreactive cells that specifically recognizes major transplantation antigen is unknown (Doherty *et al.*, 1976c). Alternatively, a completely different, but very specific, mechanism such as glycosyltransferases could serve as a self-recognition system, as discussed by Blanden *et al.* (1976b). The two different V gene structure equivalents or receptors could form one composite receptor that recognizes a complex of self plus virus, much like the heavy and light chains of immunoglobulins that have distinct V gene-coded structures. This variant of the dual recognition model brings it close to the alternative model. The dual recognition model implies that multiple self-recognition alone or multiple antigen recognition alone is of much lower avidity than when both occur together. For this reason, both receptors would have to be linked somehow, and the self-marker and antigen would have to be close together or complexed. Operationally, this composite model is, so far, not distinguishable from the altered-self model.

The altered-self model proposes that T cells possess only one single V gene structure equivalent that recognizes a complex of self plus virus or a modification of the self-marker, i.e., either changes in tertiary structure by membrane disturbance, expression of neoantigens, direct modification (see Doherty *et al.*, 1976a; Zinkernagel and Doherty, 1976), or derepression of

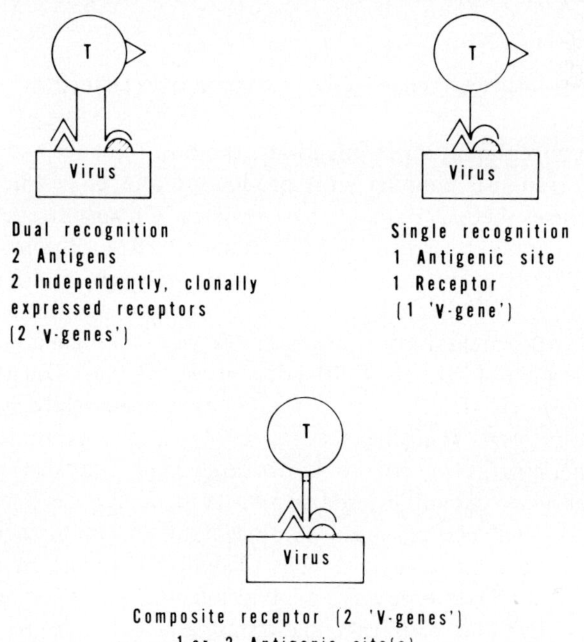

Fig. 3. The models for T cell recognition: dual recognition, composite receptor, and single recognition (altered self). For details see text.

regulatory genes that control expression of multigenically coded major transplantation antigens (Bodmer, 1973; Invernizzi and Parmiani, 1975; Garrido *et al.*, 1976). Within the altered-self model, foreign transplantation antigens (alloantigens) are just one form of altered self.

The various experimental analyses can be explained with both models (reviewed in Doherty *et al.*, 1976a; Blanden *et al.*, 1976a; Zinkernagel and Doherty, 1976). Open to further challenge, the situation can be summarized as follows: None of the experimental evidence would allow exclusion of one or the other of the two models. Evidence from different experimental models is, however, more easily compatible with the dual recognition or the composite receptor model. Bevan (1975) and Gorden *et al.* (1975) have shown that cytotoxic activity against minor transplantation antigens is also restricted by the major transplantation antigens. These findings suggest that other cell surface antigens are only recognized when the self-marker is recognized as well.

The critical question raised by these models is that of T cell specificity. Only the isolation and characterization of the T cell receptor and/or of the antigenic entity recognized by T cells will settle the issue.

VI. IMMUNE PROTECTION AND IMMUNOPATHOLOGY

In most conventional virus infections, the host's recovery depends upon his immune response stopping virus production and/or cell destruction by cytolytic viruses before damage has reached dimensions beyond which homeostasis cannot be reestablished (Blanden, 1974; Bloom and Rager-Zisman, 1975). It is difficult to differentiate between virological damage and immune lysis of infected cells, since both cause cell death. One of the best studied experimental infections is mouse pox or vaccinia virus infection of mice (Blanden, 1971, 1974; Blanden *et al.*, 1976a). During pox virus infection, cytotoxic T cells are generated that specifically lyses infected target cells *in vitro* (Gardner *et al.*, 1974). Such cytotoxic activity is probably meaningful *in vivo* only if target cells can be lysed before infectious progeny assemble (Ada *et al.*, 1976; Zinkernagel and Althage, 1977; Fig. 4). Evidence has been obtained that this is, in fact, a possible effector function for cytotoxic T cells (Table IV). In this *in vitro* model, target cells of the H-2^d type were acutely infected with vaccinia virus and, after 1 hour, overlaid with vaccinia immune spleen cells for 5 hours at 37°C. Immune cells from H-2 compatible mice lysed infected targets. Where lysis occurred, virus titers were significantly lower than in wells where targets were overlaid with normal spleen cells or H-2 incompatible immune spleen cells. This strongly suggests that virally induced cell surface antigens can be recognized by T cells before infectious progeny are assem-

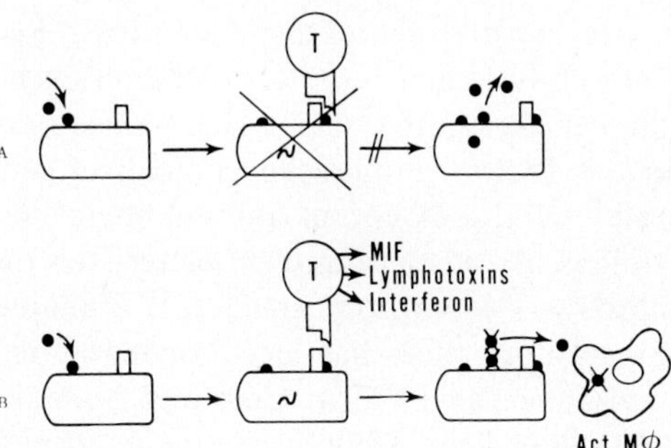

Fig. 4. Two ways in which virus-immune T cells control virus growth and spreading: (A) cytotoxic T cells may lyse freshly infected target cells before infectious virus progeny are assembled and/or released; (B) T cells recognize the relevant self plus viral antigens then release lymphokines like immune interferon or migration inhibitory factor (MIF), which may inactivate free virus by decreasing the efficiency of infection or by preventing it from infecting surrounding cells or macrophages (act MØ = activated macrophage). Zinkernagel and Althage, 1977.

TABLE IV

T Cell Dependence of Antiviral Effect of Cytotoxic Spleen Cells *In Vitro*[a]

Spleen[a] cells	Cell treatment	J774 (H-2[d]) targets 5 hours after infection[a] with vaccinia virus: $\log_{10}$ PFU/well	^{51}Cr release
B10.D2 (H-2[d])			
Immune	AKR anti-θ C3H + C[b]	4.66 ± 0.10[c]	21.1 ± 0.7[c]
	Normal AKR + C	2.73 ± 0.09	101.3 ± 2.2
	None	2.78 ± 0.10	97.5 ± 1.9
B10.D2		±	±
Normal	None	4.79 ± 0.02	25.2 ± 1.0
B10.BR (H-2[k])		±	±
Immune[d]		4.60 ± 0.15	21.0 ± 0.8
Normal	None	4.85 ± 0.10	18.7 ± 0.7

[a] Target cells, immune spleen cells, PFU determination, and ^{51}Cr release test were performed as described (Doherty *et al.*, 1976b; Zinkernagel and Doherty, 1976).

[b] AKR anti-θ C3H (purchased from Bionetics, Kensington, Md.; Cat. No. 8301-01, Lot No. 231-61-5) at a 1:10 dilution and rabbit complement (C) at a 1:6 dilution lyse spleen cells (5×10^7/ml) to 43%.

[c] Means ± SEM of triplicates. Significantly greater or smaller ($p < 0.01$) as normal AKR + C or no treatment, but not different from normal spleen cells.

[d] B10.BR immune spleen cells lysed vaccinia-infected L929 (H-2[k]) target cells to 40.5 ± 0.8%, as compared to 10.9 ± 0.3 by B10.D2 immune spleen cells (from Zinkernagel and Althage, 1977).

bled. Infections with poorly cytopathogenic virus, i.e., LCMV, cause minimal virological cytolysis and most cell destruction is caused by CMI. In both models, the beneficial effect of CMI is gained only via cell destruction. However, in the LCMV model the clinical outcome is determined, probably exclusively, by the extent of immunologic damage and by the critical pathophysiological and anatomic characteristics of the target organ.

Acute LCM, although a laboratory artifact, is a unique example of cell-mediated immunopathology that has been reviewed in detail (Hotchin, 1971; Doherty and Zinkernagel, 1974; Cole and Nahtanson, 1975). After i.c. injection, LCMV localizes predominantly in ependyma and choroid plexus and systemically in lymphoid tissues (Hotchin, 1971; Mims, 1960; Mims and Tosolini, 1969). Cytotoxic T cells generated under these circumstances are presumably, with some preference,recruited to the infected ependyma and choroid plexus where they destroy the liquor–blood barrier and, thus, cause lethal brain edema. Because of the rigidity of the skull, the anatomic situation becomes limiting (Doherty and Zinkernagel, 1974). The degree of clinical symptoms depends, probably critically, on the relative antigen distribution in ependyma versus viscera (Fig. 5). Most of the virus injected i.c. gets disseminated systemically. Thus, if high doses of virus are used for i.c. infection, the cytotoxic T cells are recruited more extensively to sites other than the brain, and the overall incidence of acute LCM and death is decreased. This phenomenon has been described by Hotchin (1971) as high-dose immune paralysis. The same target cell destruction in the liver does not usually end in death, since sufficient functional tissue remains. However, this may not be true if all of the liver is infected and is virtually completely destroyed by T cells, as happens after infections with high doses of LCMV.

What happens when immunocompetent cells become infected with virus and, thus, become targets for virus-specific immune attack themselves?

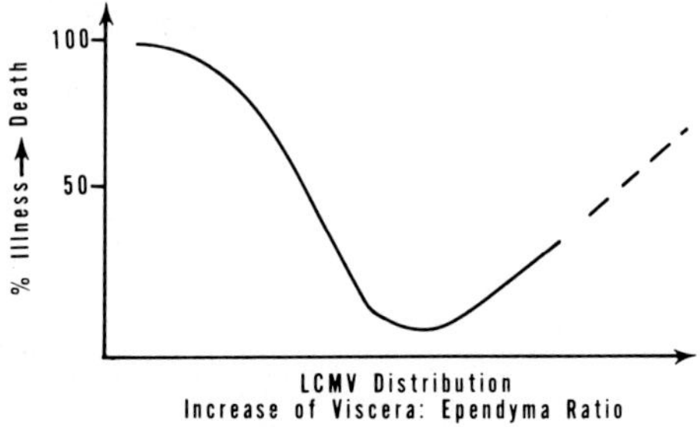

Fig. 5. T cell-mediated immune pathological disease and death by acute LCM or systemic autoaggressive disease depends on the relative distribution of viral antigen in ependyma and choroid plexus versus viscera.

Direct experimental evidence is lacking, but the following consequences are possible. (1) Cytotoxic T cells lyse T cells or their precursors, thus, decreasing or eliminating specific immune responses. (2) Noncytolytic, virus-immune T cells could induce infected B cells to produce antibodies abnormally (Bretscher, 1973; Lafferty and Cunningham, 1975). Many antibody responses depend on some "help" to B cells provided by T cells. Normally poorly detectable levels of anti-self antibodies are produced and, virtually no T help for such anti-self antibody production exists. If, however, virus-specific T cells recognize viral antigens on infected B cells, such an interaction could provide abnormal "help" and could induce B cells to produce higher levels of anti-self antibodies. This abnormal induction of self-reactive antibody-producing cells could explain the high frequency with which autoantibodies are found during and after some virus infections.

VII. IS THERE EVIDENCE FOR CYTOTOXICITY AGAINST "NORMAL" SELF DURING VIRUS INFECTIONS?

With both models, but particularly with the altered-self model, one could expect that generation of specifically reactive T cells to self plus virus or virally altered self could result in T cells "cross-reacting" with normal self. The evidence produced in favor of such a notion is incomplete. Blanden and Gardner (1976) found cytotoxic activity against uninfected target cells in spleens soon after infection with ectromelia virus. It is difficult to explain why this activity is not detectable on infected targets. Pfizenmayer *et al.* (1975) have shown that, during LCMV infection, some cytotoxicity against presumably uninfected normal targets can be measured. It is not known whether virus carryover in the spleen cell population infecting the normal targets could explain part or all of this effect. In the LCMV model, activity against normal targets was never greater than against infected targets. In our hands, this effect against normal targets was variable and depended very much on the mouse strain and the target cell used. When significant levels were reached, cytotoxicity was usually nonspecific (Table V) and demonstrable across H-2 and species barriers. At least part of this nonspecific activity seemed to be caused by T cells as described by Blanden and Gardner (1976). In our hands, this nonspecific activity is not anti-θ sensitive and, therefore, not directly mediated by T cells. The conclusion that T cells directed against normal self are generated early during virus infection is, therefore, unlikely to be the correct or sole explanation for this phenomenon. It has to be stressed also that this cytotoxicity was about 50–100 times smaller than peak activity on infected syngeneic targets a few days later. Nevertheless, if these preliminary data should be confirmed,

TABLE V

Nonspecific Early Cytotoxic Activity of Spleen Cells from Virus-Infected Mice

Uninfected target cell	H-2 type or species	Percent ^{51}Cr Release by 4 days LCMV or 3 days vaccinia virus immune[a] spleen cells tested at 100:1 for 6 hours at 37°C					
		C3H (H-2^k)			B10.BR (H-2^k)		
		Normal	LCMV	Vaccinia	Normal	LCMV	Vaccinia
L929	k	29.0	50.7	31.1	27.9	35.0	31.5
J774	d	32.1	78.4	41.9	24.9	49.0	37.0
P815	d	22.3	20.9	20.8	16.9	20.8	20.5
60A	d	8.6	55.3	31.1	16.1	12.9	29.4
EL4	b	26.4	86.6	40.3	19.9	36.3	29.7
Raji	Human	14.6	57.3	33.5	22.4	17.3	23.9
WIL 2	Human	7.0	58.3	31.9	11.7	23.9	30.5

[a] Mice were infected i.v. with 5×10^6 PFU of WE LCMV or 1×10^7 PFU of WR vaccinia virus (a generous gift of Dr. Joklik, Duke University, Durham, N.C.) (R. M. Zinkernagel, unpublished).

what could be their mechanistic explanation? If it is a T cell function, can its generation be explained by polyclonal activation, by inaccurate specificity, i.e., cross-reactivity with normal self, or by other mechanisms? The analysis of these phenomena may well bring a better understanding of autoimmune processes caused by virus infections.

VIII. SUMMARY

Although it is unclear as yet which model, altered self or dual recognition, explains the apparently universal H-2 restriction of murine T cell-mediated immune functions, the evidence is very strong that all such immune reactions compare self with modified self (and not with nonself). For example, virus-specific cell-mediated cytotoxicity is directed against infected self-cells. Although this self is altered, such destruction is clinically and phenomenologically not distinguishable from destruction of normal self and may well explain a large part of cell-mediated auto-aggressiveness. Quite possibly, polyclonal activation, abnormal induction, or other mechanisms induce, in addition, T cells or B cells against normal self—events which could explain the high frequency of autoantibodies induced by virus infections.

ACKNOWLEDGMENTS

This is publication No. 1190 from the Department of Cellular and Developmental Immunology, Scripps Clinic and Research Foundation, La Jolla, Calif. 92037. Part of this research was supported by USPHS Grant AI-07007.

REFERENCES

Ada, G. L., Jackson, D. C., Blanden, R. V., Thahla, R., and Bowern, N.A. (1976). *Scand. J. Immunol.* **5,** 23–30.

Armstrong, C., and Lillie, R. D. (1934). *Public Health Rep.* **49,** 1019–1027.

Bechtol, K. B., Freed, J. H., Herzenberg, L. A., and McDevitt, H. O. (1974). *J. Exp. Med.* **140,** 1660–1675.

Bevan, M. J. (1975). *Nature* (*London*) **256,** 419–420.

Binz, H., and Wigzell, H. (1975a). *J. Exp. Med.* **142,** 197–211.

Binz, H., and Wigzell, H. (1975b). *J. Exp. Med.* **142,** 1218–1230.

Blanden, R. V. (1971). *J. Exp. Med.* **133,** 1074–1084.

Blanden, R. V. (1974). *Transplant. Rev.* **19,** 56–88.

Blanden, R. V., and Gardner, I. D. (1976). *Cell. Immunol.* **22,** 271–282.

Blanden, R. V., Doherty, P. C., Dunlop, M. B. C., Gardner, I. D., Zinkernagel, R. M., and David, C. S. (1975). *Nature* (*London*) **254,** 269–270.

Blanden, R. V., Hapel, A. J., Doherty, P. C., and Zinkernagel, R. M. (1976a). *In* "Immunobiology of the Macrophage" (D. S. Nelson, ed.), pp. 367–400. Academic Press, New York.

Blanden, R. V., Hapel, A. J., and Jacks, M. D. (1976b). *Immunochemistry* **13,** 179–191.

Blank, K. J., Freedman, H. A., and Lilly, F. (1976). *Nature* (*London*) **260,** 250–252.

Bloom, B. R., and Rager-Zisman, B. (1975). *In* "Viral Immunology and Immunopathology" (A. L. Notkins, ed.), pp. 113–136. Academic Press, New York.

Bodmer, W. F. (1973). *Transplant. Proc.* **5,** 1471–1475.

Bretscher, P. (1973). *Cell. Immunol.* **6,** 1–11.

Brondz, B. D., Egordov, I. K., and Drizlikh, G. I. (1975). *J. Exp. Med.* **141,** 11–26.

Burnet, F. M. (1959). "The Clonal Selection Theory of Acquired Immunity." Cambridge Univ. Press, London and New York.

Burnet, F. M. (1970). "Immunological Surveillance." Pergamon, Oxford.

Burnet, F. M., and Fenner, F. (1949). "The Products of Antibodies." Macmillan, Melbourne, New York.

Cerottini, J. C., and Brunner, K. T. (1974). *Adv. Immunol.* **18,** 67–132.

Cole, G. A., and Nathanson, N. (1975). *Progr. Med. Virol.* **18,** 94–115.

Cole, G. A., Nathanson, N., and Prendergast, R. A. (1972). *Nature* (*London*) **238,** 335–337.

Doherty, P. C., and Zinkernagel, R. M. (1974). *Transplant. Rev.* **19,** 89–120.

Doherty, P. C., and Zinkernagel, R. M. (1975a). *J. Exp. Med.* **141,** 502–507.

Doherty, P. C., and Zinkernagel, R. M. (1975b). *Lancet* **1,** 1406–1409.

Doherty, P. C., and Zinkernagel, R. M. (1976). *Immunology* **31,** 27–32.

Doherty, P. C., Blanden, R. V., and Zinkernagel, R. M. (1976a). *Transplant. Rev.* **29,** 89–124.

Doherty, P. C., Dunlop, M. B. C., Parish, C. R., and Zinkernagel, R. M. (1976b). *J. Immunol.* **117,** 187–190.

Doherty, P. C., Trinchieri, G., Götze, D., and Zinkernagel, R. M. (1976c). *Immunogenetics* **3,** 517–529.

Dunlop, M. B. C., Blanden, R. V., Zinkernagel, R. M., and Doherty, P. C. (1976). *Immunology* **311,** 181–186.

Erb, P., and Feldman, M. (1975). *J. Exp. Med.* **142,** 460–472.

Gardner, I., Bowern, N. A., and Blanden, R. V. (1974). *Eur. J. Immunol.* **4,** 64–68.

Gardner, I., Bowern, N. A., and Blanden, R. V. (1975). *Eur. J. Immunol.* **5,** 122–180.

Garrido, F., Schirrmacher, V., and Festenstein, H. (1976). *Nature* (*London*) **259,** 228–230.

Gomard, E., Duprez, V., Henin, Y., and Levy, J. P. (1976). *Nature* (*London*) **260,** 707–708.

Gorden, R. D., Simpson, E., and Samelson, L. E. (1975). *J. Exp. Med.* **142,** 1108–1120.

Haas, V. H. (1954). *J. Infect. Dis.* **94,** 187–198.

Hellström, K. E., and Möller, G. (1965). *Prog. Allergy* **9,** 158–245.

Herbermann, R. B., Nunn, M. E., Lavrin, D. H., and Asotsky, R. (1973). *J. Natl. Cancer Inst.* **51,** 1509–1512.

Hirsch, M. S., Murphy, F. A., Russe, H. P., and Hicklin, M. D. (1967). *Proc. Soc. Exp. Biol. Med.* **125,** 980–983.

Hotchin, J. (1971). *Virol. Mongr.* **3,** 1–71.

Invernizzi, G., and Parmiani, G. (1975). *Nature* (*London*) **254,** 713–714.

Jerne, N. K. (1971). *Eur. J. Immunol.* **1,** 1–19.

Katz, D. H., and Benacerraf, B. (1975). *Transplant. Rev.* **22,** 175–195.

Katz, D. H., and Benacerraf, B. (1976). *In* "The Role of Products of the Histocompatibility Gene Complex in Immune Response" (D. H. Katz and B. Benacerraf, eds.), pp. 355–385. Academic Press, New York.

Katz, D. H., Hamoka, T., Dorf, M. E., and Benacerraf, B. (1973). *Proc. Natl. Acad. Sci. U.S.A.* **70,** 2624–2628.

Katz, D. H., Graves, M., Dorf, M. E., Dimuzio, H., and Benacerraf, B. (1975). *J. Exp. Med.* **141,** 263–268.

Kees, U., and Blanden, R. V. (1976). *J. Exp. Med.* **143,** 450–456.

Kindred, B., and Shreffler, D. C. (1972). *J. Immunol.* **109,** 940–943.

Klein, J. (1975). "Biology of the Mouse Histocompatibility Complex." Springer-Verlag, Berlin and New York.

Klein, J. (1976). *Curr. Top. Immunobiol.* **5** (in press).

Koszinowski, U., and Thomssen, R. (1975). *Eur. J. Immunol.* **5,** 245–251.

Lafferty, K. J., and Cunningham, A. J. (1975). *Aust. J. Exp. Biol. Med. Sci.* **53,** 27–42.

Lawrence, H. S. (1959). *Physiol. Rev.* **39,** 811–859.

Lehmann-Grube, F. (1971). *Virol. Monogr.* **10,** 1–173.

Marker, O., and Volkert, M. (1973). *J. Exp. Med.* **137,** 1511–1525.

Melnick, J. l. (1973). *Prog. Med. Virol.* **16,** 337–342.

Miller, J. F. A. P., Vadas, M. A., Whitelaw, A., and Gamble, J. (1975). *Proc. Natl. Acad. Sci. U.S.A.* **72,** 5095–5060.

Mims, C. A. (1960). *Br. J. Exp. Pathol.* **41,** 52–59.

Mims, C. A., and Blanden, R. V. (1972). *Infect. Immun.* **6,** 695–698.

Mims, C. A., and Tosolini, F. A. (1969). *Br. J. Exp. Pathol.* **50,** 584–592.

Mitchison, N. A. (1954). *Proc. R. Soc. London, Ser. B* **142,** 72–87.

Notkins, A. L. (1975). *In* "Viral Immunology and Immunopathology" (A. L. Notkins, ed.), pp. 149–166. Academic Press, New York.

Oldstone, M. B. A., and Dixon, F. J. (1970). *Virology* **112,** 505–513.

Ortiz de Landazuri, M., and Herberman, R. B. (1972). *Nature* (*London*), *New Biol.* **238,** 18–19.

Plala, F., Jongeneel, V., Cerottini, J. C., and Brunner, K. T. (1976). *Europ. J. Immunol.* **6,** 823–829.

Pfizenmaier, K., Trostmann, H., Röllingholf, M., and Wagner, H. (1975). *Nature* (*London*) **298,** 238–240.

Pfizenmaier, K., Starzinski-Powitz, A., Rodf, H., Röllingholf, M., and Wagner, H. (1976). *J. Exp. Med.* **143,** 999–1004.
Ramseier, H., and Lindenmann, J. (1969). *Pathol. Microbiol.* **34,** 379–387.
Ramseier, H., and Lindenmann, J. (1972). *Transplant. Rev.* **10,** 57–96.
Rosenthal, A. S., and Shevach, E. M. (1973). *J. Exp. Med.* **138,** 1194–1212.
Rosenthal, A. S., and Shevach, E. M. (1976). *In* "The Role of Products of the Histocompatibility Gene Complex in Immune Response" (D. H. Katz and B. Benacerraf, eds.), pp. 335–350. Academic Press, New York.
Rowe, W. P. (1956). *Proc. Soc. Exp. Biol. Med.* **92,** 194–198.
Rowe, W. P. (1963). *Proc. Soc. Exp. Biol. Med.* **114,** 248–256.
Schwartz, R. N., and Paul, W. E. (1976). *J. Exp. Med.* **143,** 529–540.
Shearer, G. M. (1974). *Eur. J. Immunol.* **4,** 527–533.
Shearer, G. M., Rehn, T. G., and Garbarino, C. A. (1975). *J. Exp. Med.* **141,** 1348–1364.
Taussig, M. J., Munro, A. J., Campbell, R., David, C. S., and Staines, N. A. (1975). *J. Exp. Med.* **142,** 694–700.
Thomas, L. (1959). *In* "Cellular and Humoral Aspects of the Hypersensitive States" (H. S. Lawrence, ed.), pp. 529–532. Harper (Hoeber), New York.
Traub, E. (1936). *J. Exp. Med.* **63,** 533–546.
Trinchieri, G., Aden, D. P., and Knowles, B. B. (1976). *Nature* **261,** 312–314.
Vadas, M. A., Miller, J. F. A. P., Whitelaw, A. M., and Gamble, J. R. (1976). *Proc. Natl. Acad. Sci. U.S.A.*
von Bohmer, H., Hudson, L., and Sprent, J. (1975). *J. Exp. Med.* **142,** 989–997.
Wilson, C. B., and Dixon, F. J. (1974). *Annu. Rev. Med.* **25,** 83–98.
Wiktor, T. J., Doherty, P. C., and Koprowski, H. (1977). *Proc. Natl. Acad. Sci. U.S.A.* **74,** 334–338.
Wong, C. Y., Woodruff, J. J., and Woodruff, J. F. *J. Immunol.* (in press).
Yap, K. L., and Ada, G. L. *Immunology* (1977). **32,** 151–160.
Zinkernagel, R. M. (1974). *Nature (London)* **251,** 230–233.
Zinkernagel, R. M. (1976a). *In* "Germinal Centers and Lymphatic Tissue" (M. Feldmann and A. Globerson, eds.), pp. 527–530. Academic Press, New York.
Zinkernagel, R. M. (1976b). *J. Exp. Med.* **143,** 437–443.
Zinkernagel, R. M. (1976c). *Nature (London)* **261,** 139–141.
Zinkernagel, R. M., and Althage, A. (1977). *J. Exp. Med.*
Zinkernagel, R. M., and Doherty, P. C. (1973). *J. Exp. Med.* **138,** 1266–1269.
Zinkernagel, R. M., and Doherty, P. C. (1974a). *Nature (London)* **248,** 701–702.
Zinkernagel, R. M., and Doherty, P. C. (1974b). *Nature (London)* **251,** 547–548.
Zinkernagel, R. M., and Doherty, P. C. (1975). *J. Exp. Med.* **141,** 1427–1436.
Zinkernagel, R. M., and Doherty, P. C. (1976). *Contemp. Top. Immunobiol.* **7** (in press).
Zinkernagel, R. M., and Oldstone, M. B. A. (1976). *Proc. Natl. Acad. Sci. U.S.A.*
Zinkernagel, R. M., and Welsh, R. M. (1976). *J. Immunol.*
Zinkernagel, R. M., Dunlop, M. B. C., and Doherty, P. C. (1975). *J. Immunol.* **115,** 1613–1616.

Chapter 13

Viruses, Autoimmunity, and Murine Lymphoma

MAX R. PROFFITT, MARTIN S. HIRSCH, AND PAUL H. BLACK

I. INTRODUCTION

Autoimmune phenomena frequently occur in association with viral diseases (for review, see Hirsch and Proffitt, 1975). Some of these diseases involve extensive lymphoproliferation, which may culminate in frank lymphoma. Type-C oncornaviruses have been associated with the development of lymphoreticular tumors in a variety of experimental animals. Although many studies have strongly suggested a similar association of viruses (RNA oncornaviruses as well as DNA herpesviruses) with human neoplastic diseases, firm documentation of their role as etiologic agents has been elusive. Nevertheless, viruses may be involved in the initiation of some of the autoimmune diseases discussed in other chapters of this volume.

The mechanisms by which viruses could initiate autoimmune disorders are many and varied. Most of these mechanisms involve some type of alteration, by the virus, of host target cells that results in normal host lymphocytes reacting against autoantigens. However, it is also possible that virus infection could lead to the activation of lymphoid cells having autoimmune potential (Hirsch and Proffitt, 1975; Bretscher, 1973). Recently, we have been studying a murine model that closely links type-C oncornavirus infection, autoimmune reactivity, and lymphoma development (Proffitt *et al.*, 1973b, 1975a,b). This model may provide a clearer understanding of the pathogenesis of some lymphoproliferative diseases.

II. T CELL-MEDIATED AUTOREACTIVITY IN A MODEL OF MURINE LYMPHOMAGENESIS

Mice infected as neonates with murine leukemia virus of the Moloney strain (MuLV-M carriers) develop disseminated lymphomas of thymic origin and most die within approximately 4–6 months. Prior to the appearance of lymphoma, a severe, premature, bilateral, but asynchronous, involution of the thymus occurs. This is accompanied by pronounced intrathymic cell destruction and proliferation of lymphoblastic cells. Eventually, the thymus enlarges with malignant lymphoblasts that subsequently disseminate to peripheral lymphoid tissues and other organs (Dunn *et al.*, 1961; Metcalf, 1966; Siegler, 1968). Similar events occur spontaneously in AKR mice that are congenital carriers of endogenous MuLV of the Gross strain (MuLV-G) (Siegler, 1968).

In order to study the relationship of the immune response to the pathogenesis of lymphoma, we established a colony of C3H/He mice carrying MuLV-M by injecting mice with the virus MuLV-M during the first 24 hours after birth. These mice reached breeding age and bore at least one litter before the onset of lymphoma. Thereafter, all subsequent generations have transmitted the virus to their offspring. The incidence of lymphoma in mice from this colony approaches 90% by approximately 6 months.

C3H/He mice carrying the WE strain of lymphocytic choriomeningitis virus (LCMV carriers) or lactic dehydrogenase virus (LDHV carriers) since birth also were used in some studies. These two viruses are similar to type-C oncornaviruses in that their nucleic acid is RNA and they replicate by budding from the host cell plasma membrane. However, they are not known to be oncogenic. LCMV is pathogenic and depending upon the age and susceptibility of the mice may cause either a severe, immunologically mediated neurological disease or a chronic immune-complex glomerulonephritis (Lehmann-Grube, 1971); it also may lead to the activation of endogenous oncornaviruses and, thence, to the development of lymphomas in certain strains of mice (Oldstone *et al.*, 1971). LDHV is not overtly pathogenic, although mild glomerulonephritis is evident in some infected mice (Oldstone and Dixon, 1971; Porter and Porter, 1971).

In all of our studies, age- and sex-matched normal C3H/He mice served as controls. Target cells for the detection of cell-mediated immune reactions by microcytotoxicity assay consisted of normal syngeneic, allogeneic, and xenogeneic fibroblasts, as well as syngeneic fibroblasts infected with MuLV-M, MuLV-G, LCMV, or transformed *in vitro* by the chemical carcinogen 3-methylcholanthrene (Reznikoff *et al.*, 1973a,b; Proffitt *et al.*, 1976). Procedures for the establishment of virus carrier mice, target cells, and a transplantable, MuLV-M-induced lymphoma have been described, as have methods for preparing thymocyte and lymphoma cell suspensions for microcytotoxicity assays (Proffitt *et al.*, 1973a, 1975a,b).

III. AUTOREACTIVITY OF THYMOCYTES FROM MuLV-M CARRIER MICE

During the course of lymphomagenesis in MuLV-M carriers, thymocytes become vigorously reactive against normal syngeneic target cells, whereas they spare identically derived target cells infected with MuLV-M. The autoaggressive cells are detectable during both the preneoplastic and frankly neoplastic periods. They may appear in the thymus as early as 4 weeks of age, but are not readily detectable in the peripheral lymph nodes and spleen until the time the lymphoma cells begin to disseminate from the thymus (approximately 16–20 weeks of age). Lymphoma cells *in situ* or derived from MuLV-M carriers and transplantable subcutaneously into normal young adult mice, also exhibit autoaggressive behavior, thereby linking the malignancy to the proliferation of functionally aberrant lymphoid cells.

We have noted further that some young MuLV-M carriers (8–10 weeks old) have lymphocytes and thymocytes with reactivity against MuLV-associated antigens (Proffitt *et al.*, 1973a). Occasional normal C3H/He mice also show similar reactivity (unpublished observations by the authors); this may reflect natural autogenous immunity to endogenous MuLV (Ihle *et*

TABLE I

Summary of *In Vitro* Reactivity of Lymphoid Cells from Normal or Virus-Carrier Mice against Syngeneic Normal, Virus-Infected, or Chemically Transformed Target Cells

	Target cells[a]				
Effector cells	Uninfected	MuLV-M infected	MuLV-G infected	LCMV infected	MCA transformed
Thymocytes[b]					
Normal	−	±	±	−	−
MuLV-M carrier	+	−	−	+	+
LCMV carrier[b]	−	−	NT	−	NT
LDHV carrier[b]	−	−	NT	NT	NT
Lymphoma					
In situ	+	−	NT[c]	NT	NT
Transplantable[d]	+	−	NT	NT	NT
Lymphocytes					
MuLV-M carrier (early)[e]	−	+	NT	NT	NT
MuLV-M carrier (late)[f]	+	−	NT	NT	NT

[a] C3H/HeJ embryo cells either uninfected or infected with Moloney (MuLV-M), Gross (MuLV-G), or lymphocytic choriomeningitis (LCMV) viruses, or transformed by 3-methylcholanthrene (MCA).

[b] C3H/He mice, either uninfected, or persistently infected with MuLV-M, LCMV, or LDHV (lactic dehydrogenase virus) since birth.

[c] Not tested.

[d] Derived from MuLV-M carrier.

[e] 8–10 weeks old.

[f] 16–24 weeks old.

al., 1974; Hirsch *et al.*, 1975; Herberman *et al.*, 1975; Zarling *et al.*, 1975). These observations are summarized in Table I.

Thus, it appears that autoaggressive cells, as well as cells with reactivity against MuLV-associated antigens, may be simultaneously present for some time in MuLV-M carriers, with subsequent waning of antiviral (or antitumor) activity. In this regard, it has been shown that mice infected neonatally with MuLV of the Rauscher strain (MuLV-R) develop immune responsiveness to MuLV-R-associated antigens; however, this responsiveness wanes rapidly as the mice mature (McCoy *et al.*, 1972). Similar results indicate that in AKR mice, a spontaneous antileukemic reaction that appears during the preleukemic period disappears with the development of lymphoma (Gomard *et al.*, 1974).

IV. CHARACTERIZATION OF AUTOAGGRESSIVE THYMOCYTES FROM MuLV-M CARRIER MICE

Autoaggressive thymocytes from MuLV-M carriers have been characterized (Proffitt *et al.*, 1975b). They are infected with MuLV, and they belong to a light buoyant density, nonadherent, θ-antigen-positive population of thymocytes (T cells). These cells bear the histocompatibility marker (H-2^k) of C3H/He mice, but do not have readily detectable murine immunoglobulin (IgG) on their surfaces. Procedures for the physical removal of macrophages do not eliminate the autoaggressive cells (unpublished observations by the authors). The presence of increased numbers of hydrocortisone-resistant thymocytes in MuLV-M carriers and the failure of hydrocortisone treatment to eliminate the autoaggressive cells suggests that they are part of an expanded population of functionally mature, autoreactive T cells. The salient characteristics of these cells are summarized in Table II.

V. SPECIFICITY OF VIRUS-ASSOCIATED AUTOREACTIVITY

Our studies indicate that the activation of autoaggressive T cells in MuLV-M carriers is specific for MuLV. Thymocytes from mice persistently infected with LCMV or LDHV since birth are not autoaggressive (Table I) (Proffitt *et al.*, 1976). However, LCMV may be able to activate autoreactive T cells transiently. In contrast to our findings in persistent LCMV carriers, it was recently reported that infection of adult mice with LCMV led to the appearance of autoreactive splenic T cells

TABLE II

Characteristics of Autoreactive MuLV-M Carrier Thymocytes

Cell type		Sensitivity to treatment with	
Lymphoid morphology	Yes	Anti-θ-C3H	Yes
Light buoyant density	Yes	Anti-mouse IgG	No
Nonadherent	Yes	Anti-H-2^k	Yes
Macrophage	No		
Hydrocortisone resistant	Yes		
MuLV infected	Yes		

within 3 days after infection (Pfizenmaier *et al.,* 1975). In this case, however, the autoreactivity waned rapidly with the appearance of T cells having cytotoxic reactivity against LCMV-infected syngeneic target cells. In view of our findings in MuLV-M carriers and those of Oldstone *et al.* (1971) indicating that LCMV may activate endogenous MuLV, it would be of interest to determine whether activated endogenous type-C oncornaviruses might be involved in this transient appearance of autoreactivity after LCMV infection.

VI. SPECIFICITY OF THE PROTECTIVE EFFECT CONFERRED ON SYNGENEIC TARGET CELLS BY INFECTION WITH MuLV-M 038

The previously mentioned sparing of target cells following their infection with MuLV-M also is seen after infection of the target cells with a related oncornavirus, MuLV-G. However, identically derived target cells infected with LCMV (which, like MuLV, buds from the host cell plasma membrane during replication) are not spared. Moreover, the sparing is not simply the result of transformation of target cells. This is indicated by the fact that syngenic fibroblasts transformed by the chemical carcinogen 3-methylcholanthrene, but negative for readily detectable MuLV infections (Reznikoff *et al.,* 1973b, and observations by the authors) are as susceptible to reduction by MuLV-M carrier thymocytes as are normal, uninfected syngeneic target cells (Table I).

Thymus cells are intimately involved in the recognition and control of reactivity to self-antigens (Burnet, 1969; Weigle *et al.,* 1972; Allison, 1973; Bretscher, 1973; Greaves *et al.,* 1974). Thus, the specific manner in which MuLV-M infection appears to alter normal recognition of self-antigens and results in the sparing of MuLV infected cells suggests that this alteration may play a significant role in the persistence of virus infection and in the evolution of lymphomas in MuLV-M carrier mice.

VII. SPECIFICITY OF TARGET CELL KILLING BY AUTOAGGRESSIVE MuLV-M CARRIER THYMOCYTES

Specificity studies employing syngeneic, allogeneic, and xenogeneic target cells have shown that thymocytes from MuLV-M carriers are reactive against cells of all mouse strains so far tested except AKR (Table III). Reactivity against DBA/2 target cells was minimal. When xenogeneic cells were used as targets, in only two experiments was there slight reactivity against monkey cells. There was no reaction against human, rat, or hamster cells. In fact, significantly enhanced numbers of rat and hamster target cells were found at the conclusion of the assays even though, in the same experiments, there was a dramatic reduction of syngeneic target cells. It remains to be determined whether the reactivity by MuLV-M carrier thymocytes is monoclonal and directed against one antigen common to most mouse strains, or whether there is restricted reactivity directed against a variety of murine, but not xenogeneic, antigens.

It is not apparent why the reactivity of MuLV-M carrier thymocytes is directed primarily against syngeneic and allogeneic, rather than against xenogeneic cells. However, in the normal mouse, there may be many more lymphoid cells with receptors for alloantigens than for xenoantigens (Jerne, 1971). We have previously proposed that MuLV might directly or indirectly

TABLE III

Summary of Reactivity of Normal and MuLV-M Carrier C3H/HeJ Thymocytes against Syngeneic, Allogeneic, and Xenogeneic Target Cells

	Target cell reduction by thymocytes from			
Target cells	MuLV-M carrier C3H/He	Mean reduction[a] (%)	Normal C3H/He	Mean reduction (%)
Mouse				
C3H/He (H-2^k)	(17/17)[b]	57	(0/17)	−20
BALB/c (H-2^d)	(7/7)	47	(2/7)	9
C57BL/6 (H-2^b)	(3/3)	40	(0/3)	5
SWR (H-2^q)	(3/3)	39	(0/3)	−15
DBA/2 (H-2^d)	(1/4)	25	(0/4)	−4
AKR (H-2^k)	(0/3)	−8	(0/3)	2
Human	(0/1)	4	(0/1)	8
Monkey	(2/3)	15	(0/3)	3
Rat	(0/3)	−36	(0/3)	−43
Hamster	(0/3)	−29	(0/3)	−22

[a] Mean of percentage reduction for all experiments. For each experiment, the percentage reduction was calculated as follows:

$$1 - \frac{\text{Number of target cells remaining after reaction with effector cells}}{\text{Number of target cells remaining after growth in culture medium alone}} \times 100$$

The number of target cells remaining in each experiment was based on the mean value of counts of at least 16 replicate wells at the end of a 48-hour assay period (Proffitt *et al.*, 1975a).

[b] No. of experiments with significant target cell reduction ($p < 0.01$)/total No. of experiments.

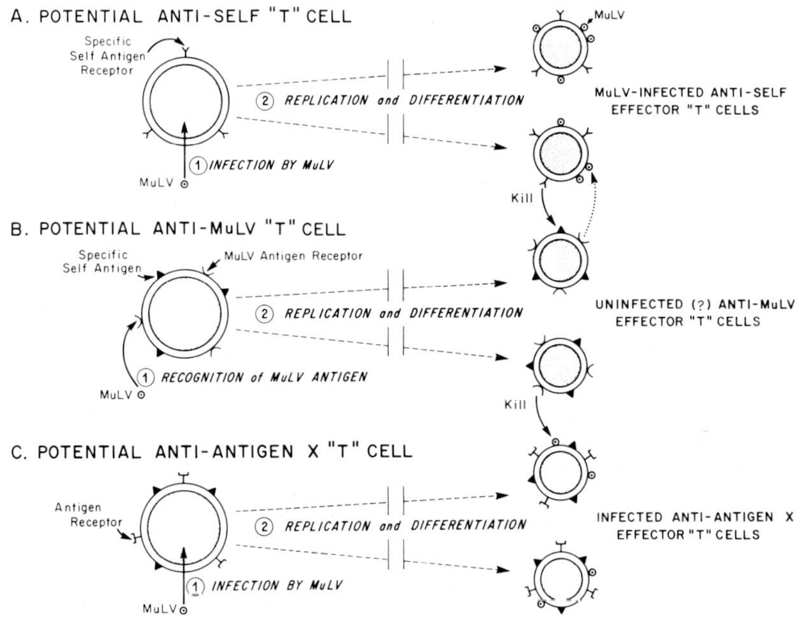

Fig. 1. Hypothetical model of intrathymic cellular interactions in mice infected with MuLV-M. Represented are antigen-reactive thymocytes with varied capabilities to respond to different antigens. Thymocyte (A) has potential reactivity against certain specific self-antigens; ordinarily this self-reactivity is unexpressed (see Proffitt *et al.,* 1975b). Upon infection by MuLV, cell (A) might be stimulated to divide and to express its autoreactive potential. Other thymic cells have different reactive potentials: cell (B) against MuLV-M-associated antigens, and cell (C) against a hypothetical antigen *X*. Upon recognition of MuLV-associated antigens, cell (B) would divide and proliferate into a clone able to react against MuLV-infected cells. If anti-self cells were to destroy anti-MuLV cells, the infected clones of anti-self cells would selectively replicate; if anti-MuLV cells were to destroy infected anti-self cells, the infection and autoaggressive reactivity would be contained. Cell (C) also might be infected by MuLV, resulting in the expansion of cell clones with varied immunologic capabilities (e.g., reactivity against certain other nonself antigens or perhaps abnormal expression of immunoregulatory T cells). [Figure reprinted from the *International Journal of Cancer,* **15**;230–245 (1975) with the permission of The International Union Against Cancer, Geneva, Switzerland.]

cause abnormal "activation" of potentially autoreactive thymocytes or thymocytes with other potential reactivities (Fig. 1) (Proffitt *et al.*, 1975b). If T cells with alloreactive potential are present in great numbers in relation to T cells with xenoreactive potential, then one might expect to see a broad range of reactivities against allogeneic but not against xenogeneic cells.

The failure of MuLV-M carrier thymocytes to react against AKR cells may simply reflect sparing, due to the presence of endogenous MuLV-G (Rowe *et al.*, 1971), similar to that seen when C3H cells were exogenously infected with MuLV-G (Table I) (Proffitt *et al.*, 1976). Whether differential expression of endogenous viral genetic information in other allogeneic cells could be related to their decreased susceptibility to killing by MuLV-M carrier thymocytes is presently being investigated. There is evidence for noncoordinant expression of certain MuLV proteins in normal mice. For example, DBA/2 mice normally show a low incidence of spontaneous leukemia. Nevertheless, moderate levels of the viral core protein, p30, and high levels of the viral envelope glycoprotein, gp69/71, are present in their cells (Strand *et al.*, 1975). It may be the expression of a virus-induced cell surface protein, even in the absence of infectious virus, that accounts for the partial sparing of DBA/2 target cells by MuLV-M carrier thymocytes.

Specificity studies, employing transplantable lymphoma cells derived from MuLV-M carriers as effector cells in reactions against syngeneic and selected allogeneic and xenogeneic target cells, gave results similar to those obtained with thymocytes from preleukemic MuLV-M carriers (Table I) (Proffitt *et al.*, 1976), thus providing a further link between autoreactivity and lymphoma.

VIII. DISCUSSION

Our results suggest one means by which autoreactivity induced by a virus can culminate in lymphoma. Furthermore, they may provide an explanation for the persistence of certain chronic virus infections. We have proposed that, in newborn mice, infection by MuLV-M of a subpopulation of thymus cells having potential anti-self reactivity (Proffitt *et al.*, 1975b) might activate and/or fix this function during subsequent differentiation of those cells, thus allowing a clone(s) of mature, virus-infected, autoaggressive T cells to arise (Fig. 1). The autoaggressiveness of infected T cells would be particularly crucial where uninfected lymphocytes, including those with potential or actual anti-viral reactivity were available as potential target cells. Since lymphocytes capable of responding to MuLV-associated antigens are present in young MuLV-M carriers (Proffitt *et al.*, 1973a) as well as in some normal mice (Ihle *et al.*, 1974; Hirsch *et al.*, 1975;

Herberman *et al.*, 1975; Zarling *et al.*, 1975), a "civil war" could ensue. In fact, this might explain much of the cellular destruction and premature thymic involution in MuLV-M infected mice. The outcome of such a "civil war" would determine the subsequent course of lymphoma development. If immunocompetent anti-viral cells were able to keep autoaggressive cells expressing virus-associated antigens under control, lymphoma development could be delayed or prevented. On the other hand, if normal immunocompetent cells, including those involved in anti-viral or anti-tumor immune surveillance were compromised, the autoaggressive cells could replicate freely, culminating in disseminated lymphoma. The persistence of high levels of virus in carrier mice would be aided by a waning immune response to virus-associated antigens and by the autoaggressive cells' sparing of other cells infected with the virus. The persistence of virus in other carrier states such as congenital rubella in man, where lymphocyte populations are both infected with and functionally altered by rubella virus (Dent *et al.*, 1968; Rawls, 1974) also may be accounted for in this way.

We have further suggested that T cells other than those having autoreactive potential could be activated during the course of a MuLV-M infection (Fig. 1). Thus, one might expect a variety of aberrant immune reactivities to develop in infected mice. In addition to T cells having autoreactive and alloreactive potential, certain suppressor T cells may become activated during MuLV-M infection. Normal immune responses to antigens, such as sheep erythrocytes (SRBC), or to mitogens, such as phytohemagglutinin (PHA), decline in aging MuLV-M carriers. The decline precedes the appearance of overt lymphoma and is accompanied by an increase in suppressor T cell activity (Cerny *et al.*, 1977). Whether this represents the virus-induced, aberrant expression of a subpopulation of immunoregulatory T cells must be further studied.

Our findings may have broader application to other animal models in which virus infection, autoimmune reactivity, and lymphoreticular neoplasia are present. In certain strain combinations of mice undergoing a graft versus host reaction (GVHR) (Elkins, 1971), endogenous type-C oncornaviruses may become activated (Hirsch *et al.*, 1970, 1972; Armstrong *et al.*, 1973). Immunosuppression may develop with defects in both T cell and B cell functions (Solnik *et al.*, 1973). Coombs'-positive autoimmune hemolytic anemia can occur as well (Oliner *et al.*, 1961; Simonsen, 1962), and malignant lymphoreticular tumors frequently arise in these animals (Datta and Schwartz, 1976; Gleichmann *et al.*, 1976). Thus, in both MuLV-M carrier mice and in GVHR mice, virus-induced alterations of lymphocytes may account for immune dyscrasias that culminate in lymphoreticular malignancies, although other pathogenetic mechanisms may be operative (Datta and Schwartz, 1976).

Several parallels exist between the disease that evolves in MuLV-M carrier mice and the spontaneous autoimmune disease of NZB mice (for review, see Levy, 1974); similar mechanisms may be involved in the evolution of disease in both. In NZB mice, there is early hyperimmune activity toward certain antigens, followed by a decline of some normal immune responses, presumably related to defective T cell functions (Barthold *et al.*, 1974). These animals also develop autoantibodies, immune-complex deposition (Levy, 1974), and lymphocyte-mediated autoreactivity (Stiller *et al.*, 1973); thymic abnormalities (DeVries and Hijmans, 1967) analogous to those observed in mice infected with MuLV-M are seen also (Dunn *et al.*, 1961; Metcalf, 1966; Siegler, 1968). According to some workers, many NZB mice eventually develop lymphoreticular neoplasia (East, 1970; Levy, 1974). Most of the defects observed in NZB mice have been linked to the presence of high titers of xenotropic, type-C oncornavirus, although the role of this virus as an oncogenic agent is still unclear (Levy, 1974).

Autoimmune phenomena also accompany infection of mice or rats with other murine oncornaviruses (Cox and Keast, 1973; Kuzumaki *et al.*, 1974). We have preliminary evidence that autoaggressor thymocytes may be operative in aging AKR mice where a high incidence of spontaneous lymphoma is seen. Likewise, similar reactivity has been noted in mice infected with MuLV of the Abelson strain (MuLV-A) (M. Sklar and W. P. Rowe, personal communication). This virus, closely related to MuLV-M, causes lymphomas predominantly of B cell, rather than T cell, origin (Sklar *et al.*, 1975). As do thymocytes from MuLV-M carriers, lymphocytes from MuLV-A-infected mice react against uninfected syngeneic cells, but they spare cells infected with MuLV-A.

It would be of great interest to know whether the pathogenesis of lymphoma in cats infected with feline leukemia virus (FeLV) (Essex, 1975) involves the expression of autoreactivity. Immunosuppression associated with aberrant T cell function is certainly a feature of this disease (Cockerell *et al.*, 1976), as is thymic pathology and abnormal involution of the thymus (Anderson *et al.*, 1971; Perryman *et al.*, 1972).

Although a direct relationship among virus infection, autoimmune reactivity and neoplasia has not been documented in human disease states, certain features are similar to those evident in the animal models discussed. In benign lymphoproliferative diseases, such as heterophile-positive infectious mononucleosis (IM) induced by Epstein-Barr virus (EBV) or heterophile-negative IM induced by cytomegalovirus (CMV), autoimmune sequelae may be seen (Epstein and Achong, 1973; Editorial, 1973; Klein, 1975; Weller, 1971a,b). Whether infection of lymphoid cells by either EBV or CMV is related to this phenomenon must remain conjectural at present. Although EBV can infect and replicate in lymphocytes (Epstein and

Achong, 1973; Klein, 1975), it has not been established whether this is true for CMV in man. However, the presence of copies of CMV DNA in human lymphoid cells has been reported (Joncas *et al.*, 1975), and infectious CMV has been found in association with leukocyte-rich fractions from the blood of heterophile-negative IM patients (Lang *et al.*, 1968; Fiala *et al.*, 1975).

Certain connective tissue disorders are characterized by immune dyscrasias, including autoimmunity, that may eventuate in lymphoreticular neoplasia. In patients with Sjögren's syndrome (SS) or systemic lupus erythematosus (SLE), there is evidence for both cell-mediated and humoral reactivity to autoantigens (Bloch *et al.*, 1965; Berry *et al.*, 1972; Abe *et al.*, 1973; Podleski and Podleski, 1973; Tannenbaum and Schur, 1974). Defects of certain immune functions are common (Leventhal *et al.*, 1967; Tannenbaum and Schur, 1974; Suciu-Foca *et al.*, 1974). Sjögren's syndrome is characterized by an increase in lymphoreticular hyperplasia, and infiltration of salivary gland ductal tissue by reactive T and B cells probably accounts for much of the damage to those tissues (Talal *et al.*, 1974). Not infrequently, lymphoreticular hyperplasia in SS patients progresses to immunoblastic sarcoma (Anderson and Talal, 1972; Lukes and Collins, 1974). As in SS, the incidence of lymphoreticular neoplasia also may be increased in SLE patients (Canoso and Cohen, 1975), and thymic abnormalities are seen frequently (Hare and Mackay, 1969). Although evidence for the association of viruses with SS is unclear (Cremer *et al.*, 1974), ultrastructural evidence for viruslike particles in the cells (including lymphocytes) of SS patients has been presented (Györkey *et al.*, 1972; Grimley *et al.*, 1973). Immunochemical, immunofluorescent, and ultrastructural studies all have indicated an increased expression of primate type-C oncornavirus markers in SLE patients (Strand and August, 1974; Lewis *et al.*, 1974; Dixon, 1974). In both SS and SLE, infection by exogenous viruses or activation of endogenous oncornaviruses might lead to proliferation of virus-altered T or B lymphocytes, some of which exhibit autoimmune reactivity. If partially controlled by normal immunoregulatory or immune surveillance mechanisms, recurrent, persistent autoimmune phenomena could ensue; however, ineffective regulation might account for uncontrolled lymphoid hyperplasia advancing to B or T cell immunoblastic lymphomas.

Myasthenia gravis (MG) is another human disorder with autoimmune features that sometimes progresses to lymphoma. A variety of autoantibodies is found in MG patients (Beutner *et al.*, 1962; van der Geld and Strauss, 1966). An important role for the thymus in this disease is well documented (Castleman, 1966; Abdou *et al.*, 1974; Goldstein and Schlesinger, 1975). Functional alteration of thymocytes and peripheral lymphocytes in MG patients is apparent. In mixed leukocyte reactions, MG patients' thymus cells may stimulate peripheral lymphocytes from the same patient and vice versa (Abdou *et al.*, 1974). There is histological evidence for thymitis in many patients with this disease (Goldstein, 1966), and thymomas may develop in 10% or more of MG patients (Castleman, 1966). Although a viral etiology for MG has not been demonstrated, virus infection of thymus cells in MG patients is possible and should be further explored.

Our findings also may have relevance to the pathogenesis of other virus-induced syndromes. Studies have indicated that lymphocytes infiltrating into the liver may be responsible for much of the tissue damage associated with chronic active hepatitis (Vischer, 1971; Dudley *et al.*, 1973). Although a part of this damage is probably the result of immunocompetent lymphocytes reacting against hepatitis virus-associated antigens on liver cells, reactivity against normal liver cells also is expressed. Recent studies have shown that peripheral lymphocytes from patients having chronic active hepatitis are reactive against normal autochthonous liver cells or liver cell lines maintained in tissue culture (Thomson *et al.*, 1974; Wands and Isselbacher, 1975; Paronetto and Vernace, 1975). Likewise, humoral autoantibodies also are found in conjunction with hepatitis virus infections (Dudley *et al.*, 1973). Although these phenomena could be indirectly induced by hepatitis virus via any of several mechanisms (Hirsch and Proffitt, 1975), it would be of interest to know whether lymphoid cells in hepatitis patients are ever infected with the virus.

In conclusion, we have attempted to show how virus infection of lymphoid cells may alter those cells and cause aberrant expression of their functional capabilities. Different viruses may have unique tropisms for different subpopulations of lymphoid cells. We have described a model wherein an oncogenic murine virus (MuLV-M), upon infecting T cells, causes some of those cells to become autoaggressive and, subsequently, to acquire malignant potential. Other viruses may have similar pathogenetic effects; however, the expression of the effects may depend upon the lymphotropism and oncogenic potential of the inducing virus.

ACKNOWLEDGMENT

We gratefully acknowledge the advice and contributions made by Dr. Beatriz Gheridian and Dr. Ian McKenzie during the course of the studies we have reported. The expert technical assistance of Bernice Allito, David Ellis, and John Landsberg is also appreciated. We wish to thank Linda Parlee and Maudlyn Wright for their assistance in the preparation of this manuscript. Our studies were supported in part by USPHS Grants 1 R01 CA161677-01 and CA12464-04, and by Contract TVP

43222 from the Virus Cancer Program of the National Cancer Institute. Max R. Proffitt was a Special Fellow of the Leukemia Society of America during the course of these studies.

REFERENCES

Abdou, N. I., Lisak, R. P., Zweiman, B., Abrahamsohn, I., and Penn, A. S. (1974). *N. Engl. J. Med.* **291,** 1271–1275.

Abe, T., Hara, M., Yamesaki, K., and Homma, M. (1973). *Arthritis Rheum.* **16,** 688–694.

Allison, A. C. (1973). *Ann. Rheum. Dis.* **32,** 283–293.

Anderson, L. G., and Talal, N. (1972). *Clin. Exp. Immunol.* **10,** 199–221.

Anderson, L. J., Jarrett, W. F. J., Jarrett, O., and Laird, H. M. (1971). *J. Natl. Cancer Inst.* **47,** 807–817.

Armstrong, M. Y. K., Ruddle, N. H., Lipman, M. B., and Richards, F. F. (1973). *J. Exp. Med.* **137,** 1163–1179.

Barthold, D. R., Kysela, S., and Steinberg, A. D. (1974). *J. Immunol.* **112,** 9–16.

Berry, H., Bacon, P. A., and Davis, J. D. (1972). *Ann. Rheum. Dis.* **31,** 298–302.

Beutner, E. H., Witebsky, E., Ricken, D., and Adler, R. H. (1962). *J. Am. Med. Assoc.* **182,** 46–58.

Bloch, K. J., Buchanan, W. W., Wohl, M. J., and Bunim, J. J. (1965). *Medicine (Baltimore)* **44,** 187–231.

Bretscher, P. (1973). *Cell. Immunol.* **6,** 1–11.

Burnet, F. M. (1969). "Cellular Immunology." Melbourne Univ. Press, Melbourne.

Canoso, J. J., and Cohen, A. S. (1975). *Arthritis Rheum.* **17,** 383–390.

Castleman, B. (1966). *Ann. N.Y. Acad. Sci.* **135,** 496–504.

Cerny, J., Proffitt, M. R., and Black, P. H. (1977). Manuscript in preparation.

Cockerell, G. L., Krakowka, S., Hoover, E. A., Olsen, R. G., and Yohn, D. S. (1976). *In* "Comparative Leukemia Research 1975," Bibliotheca Hematologica No. 43 (J. Clemmesen and D. S. Yohn, eds.), pp. 81–83. Karger, Basel.

Cox, K. O., and Keast, D. (1973). *J. Natl. Cancer Inst.* **50,** 941–946.

Cremer, N. E., Daniels, T. E., Oshiro, L. S., Marcus, F., Claypool, R., Sylvester, R. A., and Talal, N. (1974). *Clin. Exp. Immunol.* **18,** 213–224.

Datta, S. K., and Schwartz, R. S. (1976). *Transplant. Rev.* **31,** 44–78.

Dent, P. B., Olson, G. B., Good, R. A., Rawls, W. E., South, M. A., and Melnick, J. L. (1968). *Lancet* **1,** 291–293.

DeVries, M. J., and Hijmans, W. (1967). *Immunology* **12,** 179–196.

Dixon, F. (1974). *Lancet* **2,** 1302 (as quoted in Lancet editorial).

Dudley, F. J., Oshea, M. G., and Sherlock, S. (1973). *Clin. Exp. Immunol.* **13,** 367–372.

Dunn, T. B., Moloney, J. B., Green, A. W., and Arnold, B. (1961). *J. Natl. Cancer Inst.* **26,** 189–221.

East, J. (1970). *Prog. Exp. Tumor Res.* **13,** 85–134.

Editorial. (1973). *Lancet* **2,** 712–714.

Elkins, W. L. (1971). *Prog. Allergy* **15,** 78–187.

Epstein, M. A., and Achong, B. G. (1973). *Annu. Rev. Microbiol.* **27,** 413–436.

Essex, M. (1975). *Adv. Cancer Res.* **21,** 175–248.

Fiala, M., Payne, J. E., Berne, T. V., Moore, T. C., Henle, W., Montgomerie, J. Z., Chatterjee, S. N., and Guze, L. B. (1975). *J. Infect. Dis.* **132,** 421–433.

Gleichmann, E., Gleichmann, H., and Wilke, W. (1976). *Transplant. Rev.* **31,** 156–224.

Goldstein, G. (1966). *Lancet* **2,** 1164–1167.

Goldstein, G., and Schlesinger, D. H. (1975). *Lancet* **2,** 256–259.

Gomard, E., Leclerc, J. C., and Levy, J. P. (1974). *Nature* (*London*) **250,** 671–673.

Greaves, M. F., Owen, J. J. T., and Raff, M. C. (1974). "T and B Lymphocytes: Origins, Properties and Roles in Immune Responses," pp. 215–224. Am. Elsevier, New York.

Grimley, P. M., Decker, J. L., Michelitch, H. J., and Frantz, M. M. (1973). *Arthritis Rheum.* **16,** 313–323.

Györkey, F., Sinkovics, J. G., Min, K. W., and Györkey, P. (1972). *Am. J. Med.* **53,** 148–158.

Hare, W. J., and Mackay, I. R. (1969). *Arch. Intern. Med.* **124,** 60–63.

Herberman, R. B., Nunn, M. E., and Lavrin, D. H. (1975). *Int. J. Cancer* **16,** 216–229.

Hirsch, M. S., and Proffitt, M. R. (1975). *In* "Viral Immunology and Immunopathology" (A. L. Notkins, ed.), pp. 419–434. Academic Press, New York.

Hirsch, M. S., Black, P. H., Tracy, G. S., Leibowitz, S., and Schwartz, R. S. (1970). *Proc. Natl. Acad. Sci. U.S.A.* **67,** 1914–1917.

Hirsch, M. S., Phillips, S. M., Solnik, C., Black, P. H., Schwartz, R. S., and Carpenter, C. B. (1972). *Proc. Natl. Acad. Sci. U.S.A.* **69,** 1069–1072.

Hirsch, M. S., Kelly, A. P., Proffitt, M. R., and Black, P. H. (1975). *Science* **187,** 959–961.

Ihle, J. N., Hanna, M. G., Jr., Roberson, L. E., and Kenney, F. T. (1974). *J. Exp. Med.* **139,** 1568–1581.

Jerne, N. K. (1971). *Eur. J. Immunol.* **1,** 1–9.

Joncas, J. H., Menezes, J., and Huang, E. S. (1975). *Nature* (*London*) **258,** 432–434.

Klein, G. (1975). *N. Engl. J. Med.* **293,** 1353–1357.

Kuzumaki, N., Kodama, T., Takeichi, N., and Kobayashi, H. (1974). *Int. J. Cancer* **14,** 483–492.

Lang, D. J., Scolnick, E. M., and Willerson, J. T. (1968). *N. Engl. J. Med.* **278,** 1147–1149.

Lehmann-Grube, F. (1971). "Lymphocytic Choriomeningitis Virus." Springer-Verlag, Berlin and New York.

Leventhal, B. G., Waldorf, D. S., and Talal, N. (1967). *J. Clin. Invest.* **46,** 1338–1345.

Levy, J. A. (1974). *Am. J. Clin. Pathol.* **62,** 258–280.

Lewis, R. M., Tannenberg, W., Smith, C., and Schwartz, R. S. (1974). *Nature (London)* **252,** 78–79.

Lukes, R. J., and Collins, R. D. (1974). *Cancer* **34,** 1488–1503.

McCoy, J. L., Fefer, A., Ting, R. C., and Glynn, J. P. (1972). *Cancer Res.* **32,** 1671–1678.

Metcalf, D. (1966). "The Thymus," pp. 100–117. Springer-Verlag, Berlin and New York.

Oldstone, M. B. A., and Dixon, F. J. (1971). *J. Immunol.* **106,** 1260–1266.

Oldstone, M. B. A., Aoki, T., and Dixon, F. J. (1971). *Science* **174,** 843–845.

Oliner, H., Schwartz, R. S., and Dameshek, W. (1961). *Blood* **17,** 20–44.

Paronetto, F., and Vernace, S. (1975). *Clin. Exp. Immunol.* **19,** 99–104.

Perryman, L. E., Hoover, E. A., and Yohn, D. (1972). *J. Natl. Cancer Inst.* **49,** 1357–1365.

Pfizenmaier, K., Trostmann, H., Röllinghoff, M., and Wagner, H. (1975). *Nature (London)* **258,** 238–240.

Podlesli, W. K., and Podleski, V. G. (1973). *Nature (London)* **241,** 278–279.

Porter, D. D., and Porter, H. G. (1971). *J. Immunol.* **106,** 1264–1266.

Proffitt, M. R., Hirsch, M. S., and Black, P. H. (1973a). *J. Immunol.* **110,** 1183–1188.

Proffitt, M. R., Hirsch, M. S., and Black, P. H. (1973b). *Science* **182,** 821–823.

Proffitt, M. R., Hirsch, M. S., Gheridian, B., McKenzie, I. F. C., and Black, P. H. (1975a). *Int. J. Cancer* **15,** 221–229.

Proffitt, M. R., Hirsch, M. S., McKenzie, I. F. C., Gheridian, B., and Black, P. H. (1975b). *Int. J. Cancer* **15,** 230–240.

Proffitt, M. R., Hirsch, M. S., Ellis, D. H., Gheridian, B., and Black, P. H. (1976). *J. Immunol.* **117,** 11–15.

Rawls, W. E. (1974). *Prog. Med. Virol.* **18,** 273–288.

Reznikoff, C. A., Brankow, D. W., and Heidelberger, C. (1973a). *Cancer Res.* **33,** 3231–3238.

Reznikoff, C. A., Bertram, J. S., Brankow, D. W., and Heidelberger, C. (1973b). *Cancer Res.* **33,** 3239–3249.

Rowe, W. P., Hartley, J. W., Lander, M. R., Pugh, W. E., and Teich, N. (1971). *Virology* **46,** 866–876.

Siegler, R. (1968). *In* "Experimental Leukemia" (M. A. Rich, ed.), pp. 51–98. Appleton, New York.

Simonsen, M. (1962). *Prog. Allergy* **6,** 349–388.

Sklar, M. D., Shevach, E. M., Green, I., and Potter, M. (1975). *Nature (London)* **253,** 550–552.

Solnik, C., Gleichmann, H., Kavanah, M., and Schwartz, R. S. (1973). *Cancer Res.* **33,** 2068–2077.

Stiller, C. R., Russell, A. S., McConnachie, P., Dossetor, J. B., and Diener, E. (1973). *Clin. Exp. Immunol.* **15,** 445–450.

Strand, M., and August, J. T. (1974). *J. Virol.* **14,** 1584–1596.

Strand, M., Lilly, F., and August, J. T. (1975). *Cold Spring Harbor Symp. Quant. Biol.* **39,** 1117–1122.

Suciu-Foca, N., Buda, J. A., Thiem, T., and Reemtsma, K. (1974). *Clin. Exp. Immunol.* **18,** 295–301.

Talal, N., Sylvester, R. A., Daniels, T. E., Greenspan, J. S., and Williams, R. C., Jr. (1974). *J. Clin. Invest.* **53,** 180–189.

Tannenbaum, H., and Schur, P. H. (1974). *J. Rheumatol.* **1,** 392–412.

Thomson, A. D., Cochrane, M. A. G., McFarlane, I. G., Eddleston, A. L. W. F., and Williams, R. (1974). *Nature* (*London*) **252** 721–722.

van der Geld, H. W. R., and Strauss, A. J. L. (1966). *Lancet* **1,** 57–60.

Vischer, T. L. (1971). *Prog. Allergy* **15,** 268–327.

Wands, J. R., and Isselbacher, K. J. (1975). *Proc. Natl. Acad. Sci. U.S.A.* **72,** 1301–1303.

Weigle, W. O., Chiller, J. M., and Habicht, G. S. (1972). *Transplant. Rev.* **8,** 3–25.

Weller, T. H. (1971a). *N. Engl. J. Med.* **285,** 203–214.

Weller, T. H. (1971b). *N. Engl. J. Med.* **285,** 267–274.

Zarling, J. M., Nowinski, R. C., and Bach, F. H. (1975). *Proc. Natl. Acad. Sci. U.S.A.* **72,** 2780–2784.

Chapter 14

C-TYPE RNA VIRUSES AND AUTOIMMUNE DISEASE

JAY A. LEVY

I. INTRODUCTION

A. Viruses and Human Autoimmune Disease

Viruses have been frequently associated with autoimmune phenomena in mans (Table I). Polyarteritis and arthritis can be observed after infection with rubella and serum hepatitis viruses (Williams *et al.*, 1968; Gocke *et al.*, 1970; Alpert *et al.*, 1971; Popper and Mackay, 1972). Coombs'-positive hemolytic anemia accompanies cytomegalovirus (CMV), Epstein-Barr virus, and viral pneumonia (Ziff, 1971; Zuelzer *et al.*, 1966; Dacie, 1955; Thomas, 1964). Anti-nuclear antibodies are observed during hepatitis and CMV infections (Andersen and Andersen, 1975; Plotz, 1975) and immune complex nephritis has been seen with serum hepatitis and coxsackie virus infections (Burch and Colcolough, 1969; Myers *et al.*, 1973).

A connection between virus infection and autoimmune disease in man was originally suggested by Goodpasture in 1919 when he observed a patient

TABLE I

Viruses Associated with Human Autoimmune Disorders[a]

Virus	Autoimmune symptoms[b]
Rubella	Polyclonal gammopathy
Cytomegalovirus	CHA, ANF
Serum hepatitis	ANF, polyarteritis, arthritis, ICN
Epstein-Barr (infectious mononucleosis)	Thrombocytopenia, CHA
Influenza, viral pneumonias	CHA
Coxsackievirus	ICN

[a] For references, see Levy (1974).

[b] CHA, Coombs + hemolytic anemia; ICN, immune complex nephritis; LE, presence of LE cells; ANF, anti-nuclear factor.

with pulmonary and glomerular lesions following an influenza virus infection. Although not all patients with Goodpasture's syndrome have a history of influenza, other reports on this association have appeared (Wilson and Smith, 1972).

The list of viruses associated with human autoimmune syndromes is increasing, and this fact raises the important question whether all autoimmune diseases can be attributed to infectious agents acquired by horizontal transmission or inherited through the germ cell (vertical transmission). In light of recent evidence suggesting integration of certain viruses in mammalian cells without replication of the virus (Zhdanov, 1975), the inability to find infectious viruses in tissues of patients with autoimmune disease cannot be considered proof of their playing no role in the disease.

B. Animal Model Systems

For obvious reasons, investigative studies of the relationship of viruses to autoimmune disease are best conducted using animal systems which share common characteristics with the disease in humans (Table II).

Animal models of autoimmunity include thyroiditis observed in obese white leghorn chickens (OS) (Witebsky *et al.*, 1969; Wick *et al.*, 1974), Aleutian disease of mink (Porter *et al.*, 1969), the autoimmune disease of New Zealand Black (NZB) mice (Talal and Steinberg, 1974; Bielschowsky *et al.*, 1959), equine infectious anemia (EIA) (Henson and McGuire, 1971; Squire, 1968), and canine lupus erythematosus (Lewis *et al.*, 1965). The Coombs'-positive hemolytic anemia in the X strain of rabbits (Fox *et al.*, 1971), the paraproteinemia occurring in the SJL/J mouse strain (Wanebo *et al.*, 1966) and the anti-nuclear antibodies noted in the SWAN mice (Monier *et al.*, 1969, 1971) are other examples of autoimmunelike findings in animal systems.

A viral etiology for these immune disorders has been established in the Aleutian mink in which an infectious small DNA virus is involved (Porter *et al.*, 1969) and in EIA in which a transmissible agent resembling a C-type virus, induces the hemolytic anemia syndrome (Nakajima *et al.*, 1969). Canine lupus may also be caused by an exogenously acquired (i.e., horizontal transmission) C-type virus (Lewis and Schwartz, 1971). OS thyroiditis appears linked to a genetic defect in the chickens, although branched tubular structures suggestive of a viral infection have been observed in the thyroid glands of these animals (Wick *et al.*, 1974). No viral studies of X rabbits have been reported.

In mouse strains with autoimmunelike syndromes, infectious C-type RNA viruses are detected, but are not necessarily responsible for the disorders. These endogenous (i.e., inherited through the germ cell), C-type

TABLE II

Animal Model Systems for Autoimmune Disease[a]

Animal	Strain	Associated virus	Disease characteristics[b]
Chicken	White leghorn obese	?[c]	Thyroiditis Hypothyroidism
Mouse	NZB	+	CHA, ICN, LE, A-DNA, ANF
	NZW	+	Milder form of NZB disease
	(NZB × NZW)F_1	+	More severe form of NZB disease
	SJL/J	+	Paraproteinemia, ANF
	SWAN	?	ANF, ICN
Mink	Aleutian	+	CHA, ICN, LE, A-DNA, ANF
Rabbit	X	?	CHA
Dog	German shepherd, Poodle	?	CHA, ICN, LE, A-DNA, ANF
Horse	Not specified	+	CHA, hypergammaglobulinemia Lymphoid hyperplasia, ICN

[a] Adapted from Levy (1974).

[b] CHA, Coombs + hemolytic anemia; ICN, immune complex nephritis; LE, presence of LE cells; A-DNA, anti-DNA antibody. ANF, antinuclear factor.

[c] Branched tubular structures suggesting a virus infection have been seen in the thryoid. (Wick *et al.*, 1974).

viruses are expressed at various times during the life of all mice (see below). In the inbred NZB mice, however, they are produced in high titers by all cells from embryos to adulthood (Levy *et al.*, 1975b). The SJL/J mice expresses, at 2–4 months of age, a C-type virus which can induce lymphomas and reticulum cell sarcomas in certain recipient mice (Haran-Ghera and Kotler, 1968; Haran-Ghera *et al.*, 1973; Chang *et al.*, 1974). Its role in the paraproteinemia of this strain, however, is unknown. A viral etiology for the SLE-like syndrome in the SWAN mice has been considered, but a genetic cause has been generally accepted (Monier *et al.*, 1969, 1971). Nevertheless, since all mouse strains probably contain integrated endogenous C-type viruses, the possibility that these viruses play a role in the autoimmune disorder in SWAN mice should be considered.

In examining the possibility that viruses are responsible for autoimmunity, we shall concentrate on three animal models in which a C-type virus may be the etiologic agent: NZB mice, EIA, and canine lupus. In the NZB mouse, the virus is endogenous, i.e., inherited vertically through the species. In the horse and perhaps the dog, the autoimmune disease is linked to viruses horizontally acquired after birth.

II. C-TYPE VIRUSES

A. History and Background

The discovery of C-type RNA viruses occurred at the turn of this century when Ellerman and Bang (1908) noted that lymphomas in chickens could be produced by a filterable agent. Only 3 years later in the same animal species, Peyton Rous (1911) described the well-known Rous sarcoma virus, an agent which caused solid tumor development in susceptible chickens. The intense research on these RNA viruses, however, did not receive its impetus until 1951 when Ludwik Gross showed that similar viruses could be isolated from mammals. He recovered the Gross virus from the inbred AKR mouse strain (Furth *et al.*, 1933; Gross, 1951). Within 25 years, new C-type viruses were described in various animal species including snakes and fish (Table III) (Papas, *et al.*, 1976 for other references, see Levy, 1976a). Many of these viruses were recognized only with the aid of the electron microscope (EM). This instrument was first used by Claude *et al.* in 1947 to examine the C-type viruses discovered by Rous.

B. Classification

Because of the existence in 1960 of several viruses with oncogenic properties, Bernhard (1960) devised his well-accepted system of classification which identified RNA viruses by their size, morphology by EM, and manner of replication. The letter A was used to describe 75-mμ doughnut-shaped particles which are found in the cytoplasm and do not bud from the cell surface. They have an electron translucent center and double membranes and are still considered by many to be precursors of other viruses. The letter B was given to the 105-mμ budding mammary tumor virus, first reported by Bittner (1936). Its eccentric electron-dense nucleoid and double membranes distinguished it readily from the third class of RNA viruses, the type C. These latter viruses are 100 mμ in diameter and characterized by a central electron-dense nucleus, surrounded by an inner core of nucleoproteins and a lipoprotein envelope coat. Like the B-type, they bud from cell membranes. Immature B- and C-type particles have electron-translucent nucleoids.

Six to seven proteins with molecular weights (MW) ranging between 10,000 and 80,000 daltons make up the C-type virion structure. Each contain three classes of antigenic determinants: type specific, group specific, and interspecies. A major viral structural component is a core protein of about 30,000 daltons, referred to as the p30 (Strand and August, 1974a). This protein has strong antigenic reactivity and contains the major

TABLE III

Animal Vertebrate Species in Which C-Type Viruses Have Been Detected

Mammalian	Pisces
Cat	Fish
Cow	
Deer	
Dog	Reptilia
Guinea pig	Viper
Chinese hamster[a]	
Syrian gold hamster	Aves
Horse	Chicken
Mouse	Duck
Pig	Pheasant
Rabbit[b]	Quail[c]
Rat	Turkey
Sheep	
Primates	
Baboon	
Chimpanzee	
Gibbon	
Human	
Marmoset	
Rhesus	
Woolly	

[a] Tihon and Green (1973).

[b] A. Hellman, personal communication.

[c] Y. C. Chang, personal communication. Further references for this table are found in Levy (1976a).

Animals listed above are those in which viruses with C-type morphology have been described. In some cases, the isolation of the virus has not been achieved; in others, the classification of the viruses as C-type is not conclusive.

group-specific (gs) antigen, common to type-C viruses of the same species (Gregoriades and Old, 1969). This protein also carries strong interspecies antigens that are cross-reactive with other known mammalian type-C viruses (Geering *et al.*, 1968; Gilden *et al.*, 1971; Strand and August, 1973, 1974a). Another important virion constituent is a glycoprotein of about 70,000 daltons which is part of the virion envelope and is present as well on the cell surface (Strand and August, 1973). This protein, referred to as gp70, contains the principal type-specific antigens which characterize individual C-type viruses of a particular animal species and are recognized by virus neutralization (Steeves *et al.*, 1974). It also carries group-specific determinants. Other murine C-type virus proteins carrying type, group, and interspecies determinants identified as viral specific include gp45, p15, p15(E), p12, and p10. In this review, we shall concentrate on the p30 and gp70 antigenic determinants.

Since the B- and C-type viruses bud from the cell surface without lysing the cells, they differ from other RNA and DNA viruses, which usually kill the cell in which they replicate. For this reason, these RNA viruses, in contrast to other cancer viruses, have an enhanced transforming capacity. Oncogenic DNA viruses, for instance, generally lyse the cell they might otherwise have transformed.

Infection with B- and C-type viruses also leads to production of cells with new (e.g., viral) antigens on their cell surface (McCoy *et al.*, 1972). All cells infected by one kind of C-type virus, therefore, contain common antigens. Such a characteristic has been helpful in distinguishing virus-induced tumors from the chemically induced types which have distinctive antigenic properties (Baldwin, 1973). These latter tumors, however, often carry viral antigens as well. The antigens appearing on the surface of virus-infected cells may promote an immune reaction of the host and lead to enhanced tumor rejection (Barbieri *et al.*, 1971; Greenberger and Aaronson, 1973). This property of virus-infected cells will be discussed later in reference to the induction of autoantibodies.

An important constituent of the C-type viruses, as well as certain other RNA viruses, is an enzyme which permits the copying of their RNA into DNA (Batimore, 1970; Temin and Mitzutani, 1970). By this RNA-dependent DNA polymerase (reverse transcriptase) the virus is able to integrate as DNA into the chromosome of the host cell and pass latently to subsequent generations (Temin, 1971; Huebner and Todaro, 1969). By such a mechanism, cells can exist with little or no evidence of C-type virus infection. They may spontaneously, or after external stimulation, produce the virus by transcribing DNA → RNA → protein. The intracellular milieu of the infected cell regulates the ultimate production of this integrated C-type virus genome.

C. Murine Endogenous C-Type Viruses

Biologic evidence presented by Gross (1954, 1974), Huebner and Todaro (1969), and Huebner and Igel (1971), as well as data from more recent genetic studies (Rowe, 1973), have established the fact that C-type virus genomes are inherited by different animal species (Table IV). They are endogenous, i.e., passed to the progeny through the germ cell. At least three different classes of murine C-type viruses (MuLV) have been defined,

TABLE IV

Classes of Endogenous C-Type Virus

1. Ecotropic (Gr. *oikos,* home, one's environment; Gr. *tropos,* turning); Viruses that infect and replicate efficiently in cells from their own host species

2. Xenotropic (Gr. *xenos,* foreigner): Viruses that infect and replicate efficiently *only* in cells from an animal species foreign to the host

3. Amphotropic (Gr. *amphos,* both): Viruses that infect and replicate efficiently both in cells from their own host species and in cells from heterologous species

according to their host range. Some of these classes are found in other animals and may have counterparts in humans.

1. Ecotropic Viruses

The discovery of C-type viruses in mice by Gross was aided by the development in the early 1920's of an inbred strain of mice with a high incidence of leukemia. Using the AKR mouse derived by Jacob Furth (1933), Gross was able to demonstrate a filterable agent, which was inherited through the genome of the mouse cells and which, when inoculated into susceptible mice, gave rise to leukemia (Gross, 1951). Subsequent studies by Gross and other researchers confirmed the presence of this inherited virus with oncogenic properties. They further demonstrated that the susceptibility of mice to infection by this murine leukemia virus varied from strain to strain. Recent evidence suggests that multiple genes determine the ability of a leukemia virus to infect and cause tumors in a mouse strain (Rowe, 1973). In particular, the Fv-1 locus which has two dominant alleles, N and B, regulates susceptibility of the cell to virus infection (Lilly and Pincus, 1973).

Because these mouse tumor viruses preferably infect cells from their own species we have called them descriptively ecotropic from the Greek word *oikos,* which means "home or one's environment" (Levy, 1974). Their host range is limited to mouse and rat cells. They are recovered from many, but not all mouse strains. After infection, they can cause leukemias and lymphomas in susceptible hosts. They are readily detected in tissue culture by the induction of syncytia with XC cells (Rowe *et al.,* 1970).

2. Xenotropic Viruses

While Furth provided a mouse strain for the eventual recovery of the ecotropic mouse leukemia virus, Marianne Bielschowsky provided a species of mice for the eventual recognition of a different class of endogenous mouse viruses. Dr. Bielschowsky arrived in New Zealand in 1948 and was encouraged by her husband to develop inbred strains of mice at the medical school in Dunedin, since only random-bred strains obtained from England were available at the Cancer Institute. She selected a pair of agouti-colored mice and began a series of inbreeding experiments in which she selected for black coat color. After 20 generations of brother–sister matings, she established the inbred strain of New Zealand Black (NZB) mice (Bielschowsky *et al.*, 1959). She and her colleagues were the first to describe in these mice an autoimmune syndrome characterized by hypergammaglobulinemia, antibodies to red blood cells and nucleic acids, and immune complex nephritis (Bielschowsky *et al.*, 1959). If this strain of mouse did not succumb to nephritis, it frequently developed reticulum cell sarcomas (East *et al.*, 1967; Mellors, 1966). The disease complex resembled autoimmune disease and, particularly, systemic lupus erythematosus in humans. The inherited susceptibility of this strain to autoimmune disease became well established by the studies of Bielschowsky and others (Bielschowsky *et al.*, 1959; Ghaffar and Playfair, 1971; Helyer and Howie, 1963; East *et al.*, 1965; Mellors, 1966; Holmes and Burnet, 1964).

In the mid-1960's, several laboratories reported detecting, by electron microscopy, C-type virus particles budding from the cell surface of NZB tissues (Yumoto and Dmochowski, 1967; Mellors and Huang, 1966, East *et al.*, 1967). This spontaneous virus production occurred concomitantly with the genetic transmission of the disease (East *et al.*, 1967). Mellors and East were among the first to suggest that these murine C-type viruses might be responsible for the autoimmune disease and neoplasia developed by this New Zealand strain. Attempts to isolate and characterize the virus, however, were not successful, and, for a period of time, it was considered a defective virus, i.e. noninfectious.

In 1970, we demonstrated that the C-type virus associated with NZB mice was not defective and could infect rat cells (Levy and Pincus, 1970). Subsequent studies have defined the NZB virus as a prototype for a second class of endogenous viruses common to the *Mus musculus* (house mouse) species. We have called it descriptively xenotropic (Gr. *xenos,* foreign; *tropos,* turning) (Levy, 1973a, 1974) because this C-type virus cannot exogenously infect mouse cells, but it can productively infect cells from a wide variety of foreign species. Xenotropic viruses are infectious for cells from species as varied as mongoose and anteater and even cells of a different animal class such as pigeons and turkeys (Levy, 1974, 1975a, Oie *et al.*, 1976) (Table V). While sharing p30 with other MuLV, the X-tropic virus has a distinct type-specific gp70 envelope antigen as demonstrated by neutralization studies (Levy, 1973a; 1974). It is, therefore, easily distinguished serologically from the ecotropic MuLV.

The xenotropic viruses have been recovered from many different strains

TABLE V

Animal Cell Lines Susceptible to Infection by Mouse Xenotropic Virus

Mammalian	
Anteater	Human
Armadillo	Lion
Bat	Marmoset
Bear	Mink
Cat	Miopithicus
Chimpanzee	Mongoose (African water)
Cow	Mongoose (black-footed)
Deer (black-footed)	Muntjac
Dog	Orangutan
Gazelle	Rabbit
Gorilla	Racoon
Guinea pig	Rat
Horse	Rhesus monkey
Avian	
Duck	Pheasant
Quail	Pigeon
Parakeet	Turkey

of house mice including wild mice from Japan and San Francisco (Table VI) (Arnstein *et al.,* 1974; Todaro *et al.,* 1973; Aaronson and Stephenson, 1973; Benveniste *et al.,* 1974; Levy, 1975b). Biochemical studies suggest that all mouse strains contain the same number of structural genes for this class of virus (~6–9) (Chattopadhyay *et al.,* 1974). Each mouse strain, however, differs in its extent of X-tropic virus expression. They were first identified in the NZB strain since all cells from this mouse spontaneously produce large quantities of the virus (Levy *et al.,* 1975b). Other strains express X-tropic virus at less frequency and titer (Table VI) and their cells vary in the extent of virus production during the lifetime of the mouse. The intracellular milieu appears to regulate the ultimate production of the virus by a cell.

Ecotropic viruses have been recovered from many but *not all* strains of house mice. Tissues from NZB, NIH Swiss, C57/Leaden, and 129/J strains, for instance, have been extensively studied, and no ecotropic viruses have been detected (Levy, 1973a, 1974, 1975b). Molecular studies have also supported this observation, since the AKR–Gross type genome has not been detected by hybridization studies in the above strains (Chattopadhyay *et al.,*

1974, personal communication). When present, usually 1–2 copies of the AKR genome are detected in mice (Chattopadhyay *et al.*, 1974).

3. *Amphotropic Viruses*

Recently, a third class of endogenous viruses has been identified in wild mice captured in regions around Los Angeles (Rasheed *et al.*, 1976; Hartley and Rowe, 1976). These viruses have the host range of both the xenotropic and ecotropic classes. They productively infect mouse cells as well as cells from a variety of heterologous species. Similar to X-tropic viruses (Levy, 1974; Levy *et al.*, 1975b), they are not effective in inducing syncytia with XC cells. Because of this dual tropism, they have been called descriptively amphotropic (Gr. *amphos,* both). The wild mice, recovered from Lake Casitas and Bouquet Canyon, also contain ecotropic and xenotropic viruses. The amphotropic virus, therefore, may represent the progenitor for the other two classes of endogenous viruses or may represent a recombinant virus. The relationship of this class of viruses to the lymphomas and neurologic disease observed in the wild mice (Officer *et al.*, 1973) is presently under study.

D. C-Type Viruses as Agents of Autoimmunity

Since C-type viruses can be inherited by a species, and can also horizontally infect susceptible animals, they represent good candidates for agents

TABLE VI

Relative Levels of Spontaneous X-Tropic Virus Production in Mouse Strains

High	Moderate
NZB	NIH Swiss (Micro)
NZB × NZW	C57BL
NZB × C57BL	C57BL/10Sn
NZB × SWR	C57BL/58N
NZB × 129	*Mus molossinus*
	Nude (Swiss)
Low	Very low
BALB/c	129
SJL/J	SWR
A/J	Wild mice (San Francisco)
NZW	
C3H	
AKR	
C58BL	

of autoimmune disease. Their endogenous expression in embryos supports defining them as self-antigens (Levy, 1975b, 1976a). Host responses against the viral antigens would qualify then, as autoantibodies. Virus expression, endogenous or after exogenous infection, however, could mediate the processes leading to autoimmune disease if the viral proteins induced an anti-viral reaction of the host. The NZB mouse offers a model system to study the potential role of endogenous (inherited) C-type viruses (vertical transmission) in this disease. The EIA virus and possibly the canine agent are examples of exogenously acquired virus infections (horizontal transmission) which might give rise to autoantibodies. Evidence that these latter two viruses are C-type, however, is not yet conclusive.

III. AUTOIMMUNE DISEASE OF NEW ZEALAND BLACK MICE

A. Clinical Findings

The inherited disease complex of NZB mice has been described in many reports (Talal and Steinberg, 1974; Bielschowsky *et al.*, 1959; Helyer and Howie, 1963; Holmes and Burnet, 1963, 1964). Similar to observations in humans, this murine form of lupus erythematosus is most prevalent and severe in females (Table VII).

In brief, the mice develop normally until 3 months of age when they begin to show signs of immunologic injury; generalized lymphoid hyperplasia occurs, and their thymuses become infiltrated with B cells (Burnet and Holmes, 1964; Greenspan *et al.*, 1974). Anti-erythrocyte antibodies first appear at 3 months of age and are of the incomplete warm antibody type. By 5 months of age, this IgG antibody is found in high titer in the serum. The mice have by then a generalized hypergammaglobulinemia. Anemia and reticulocytosis develop in most animals by 15 months of age.

Anti-thymic antibodies are produced as early as 2 weeks of age and reach a peak when the mice are 6–9 months old (Shirai and Mellors, 1971). Lupus erythematosus (LE) cells and positive anti-nuclear and anti-nucleic acid antibodies are also detected in high titer by that time.

Splenomegaly and severe membranous immune complex (IC) glomerulonephritis are often sequelae of the autoimmune process. Proteinuria usually precedes other signs of kidney disease. Antigens identified in immune complexes include DNA and viral proteins (Dixon *et al.*, 1971; Mellors *et al.*, 1969, 1971). If the mice do not succumb to the IC nephritis and anemia, up to 20% develop lymphoid neoplasias of the immunoblastic type (Mellors, 1966; De Vries and Hijmans, 1967).

TABLE VII

Similarities between the Disease Complex of NZB Mice and Human Autoimmune Disease

Genetic predisposition
Female predominance
Thymic injury
Coombs'-positive hemolytic anemia
Splenomegaly and lymphoid hyperplasia
Hypergammaglobulinemia
Enhanced autoantibody production
Anti-lymphocyte antibodies
Anti-nucleic acid antibodies
Anti-erythrocyte antibodies
Hypocomplementemia
LE phenomenon
Impairment of cell-mediated immunity
Immune-complex glomerulonephritis
Neoplasia

Revised from Levy (1975b).

An arteritis similar to human polyarteritis nodosa has been reported in 10% of the mice (Hicks, 1966). Moreover, enlargement of salivary and lacrimal glands with infiltration by lymphocytes, reminiscent of Sjögren's syndrome, is frequently observed.

B. Virus Studies

Our studies of New Zealand Black mice have demonstrated that xenotropic C-type viruses are spontaneously produced by all cells of the NZB mouse throughout its life. Clones of cells cultured from adult tissues as well as from early developing embryos produce high titers of X-tropic virus (Levy *et al.*, 1975b). No ecotropic MuLV is detected in this mouse strain.

This hyperproduction of virus by NZB mice contrasts with that of other strains which produce very little virus and at a low incidence. As noted in Table VI, the SWR and 129/J strains have almost no detectable infectious virus produced during their lifetime, although they contain up to nine copies of X-tropic virus in their genome. When these strains or other mice are bred with New Zealand Black mice, the F_1 generations show dominance for the production of xenotropic virus [Levy, 1973a; Levy, J., Joyner, J., Nayar, K., Kouri, R. (1977). *Amer. Assoc. Micro.* (abst.) p. 294.] (Table VIII).

TABLE VIII

Expression of X-Tropic C-Type Virus in Adult Tissue from NZB Mice and F_1 Hybrids[a]

Mouse strain	Thymus	Spleen	Liver	Kidney	Tumors[b]
NZB	9/9	12/12	2/2	50/50	1/1
C57BL/6	1/2	6/11		4/9	
NZW	1/3	2/3		1/2	
SWR/J	1/7	1/9		0/8	
129/J	1/9	0/9		0/9	
(NZB × C57BL/6)F_1		2/2		4/4	
(NZB × NZW)F_1	4/4	2/2	3/3	4/4	4/4
(NZB × SWR)F_1	4/4	4/4		4/4	
(NZB × 129)F_1	4/4	4/4		4/4	

[a] Figures represent the number of animals from whom infectious xenotropic virus was recovered over the number of animals tested.

[b] Reticulum cell sarcoma.

Macrophage cultures established from (NZB × C57BL/6)F_1 mice, however do not spontaneously produce the virus (Levy, 1974). Recovery of xenotropic viruses only occurs after exposure of the cells to iododeoxyuridine. This unique difference in virus production by the macrophage may be significant (Section VIII).

C. Host Response to C-Type Viruses

1. *Immunoglobulins*

Because of the high incidence of immune complex disease in some mouse strains and the possibility that the mouse might mount a response against its endogenous viruses, various studies have concentrated on anti-viral activity in mouse serum. By radioimmune precipitation assays, Ihle and his co-workers have demonstrated the presence in normal mouse sera of immunoglobulins of the IgG and IgM class that bind to ecotropic viruses (Ihle *et al.*, 1973; Lee and Ihle, 1975; Lee *et al.*, 1974). Recent evidence suggests that there are no immunoglobulins that bind selectively to xenotropic viruses (J. N. Ihle, personal communication). Since ecotropic C-type viruses are inherited in the host genome as normal components of the mouse, it is surprising that antibodies to these viruses are found regularly. The antibodies could be considered natural circulating autoantibodies, but their function or effect is not yet understood. They do not efficiently neutralize C-type viruses *in vitro,* although they may serve that function *in vivo.* Moreover, some studies suggest they have cytotoxic activity (Nowinski and Klein, 1975).

2. *Neutralizing Factor*

We and others have shown the ability of mouse sera to neutralize xenotropic but not ecotropic viruses (Levy, 1973b, 1975b,c; Aaronson and Stephenson, 1974). This selective ability of mouse sera to inactivate xenotropic viruses, but not ecotropic viruses, was at first considered a difference in the affinity of binding antibodies to a particular class of endogenous viruses. Recent evidence from our laboratory, however, has shown that the neutralization of xenotropic viruses is not due to an immunoglobulin. It results from the interaction of xenotropic viruses with a factor associated with serum lipoproteins (Levy, 1975b,c; Levy *et al.*, 1975a; Leong *et al.*, 1977). Purified immunoglobulin classes have no neutralizing activity against xenotropic viruses, and mouse serum that has been depleted of immunoglobulins maintains its ability to neutralize X-tropic viruses at the same titer as untreated serum (Table IX) (Levy *et al.*, 1975a). Moreover, only absorption with concentrated preparations of xenotropic virus eliminates this neutralizing activity from mouse serum. This observation suggests that direct interaction of the X-tropic virus with the factor results in virus neutralization.

Because NZB mice have antibodies to normal thymic (T) tissues we have attempted to compare neutralizing activity against xenotropic virus with this anti-thymic activity of the serum. As demonstrated in Table X, no correlation between the anti-T activity and anti-viral activity could be demonstrated. These two kinds of "anti-self reactions" and the regulation of their production are obviously different.

The possible role of neutralizing factor in the eventual development of autoimmune disease is not clear, but it is present in highest titer in New Zealand Black mice—levels as high as 1:10,000 (Levy, 1975b; Levy *et al.*, 1975a). Studies are in progress to determine the effect of inoculating high levels of this factor into other mouse strains.

D. Xenotropic Viruses and Autoimmune Disease

This coexistence in NZB mice of the predisposition to autoimmune disease and a persistent and enhanced expression of the endogenous xenotropic virus from embryo to adult life has suggested that a basic genetic defect in the strain is linked with a derepression of this viral genome and the development of autoimmunity. If not directly causative, the virus

TABLE IX

Comparison of Levels of Binding Antibodies to Neutralizing Factor in Mouse Sera

Strain	Age (months)	RIP	NF
$(B6C3)F_1$	3	+	1000[a]
	3	−	≥1000
	4	+	≥1000
	4	−	1000
C3H	2	+	≥1000
	2	−	≥1000
	4	+	1000
	4	−	1000

[a] Figures represent the end titer of serum that gave effective neutralization.

Mouse sera were tested for binding immunoglobulins to AKR-MuLV by radioimmune precipitation (RIP) techniques by J. Ihle *et al.*, 1973). Neutralizing factor (NF) levels were measured by neutralization of the infectivity of xenotropic viruses for rat cells. Data indicates no correlation between the presence of serum anti-viral immunoglobulins and the factor responsible for X-tropic virus inactivation.

may contribute significantly to the disease simply because of its enhanced expression and the presence of anti-viral factors in mouse sera.

1. Animal Inoculation

Since xenotropic viruses are not infectious for cells of their own species, it is difficult to assess directly their relationship to murine autoimmune disease. Mellors and Huang (1967) had reported the transfer of certain characteristics of NZB disease to random-bred Swiss mice with cell-free extracts and filtrates of NZB spleens. Their results, however, have not been confirmed (Braverman, 1968; Russell *et al.*, 1970; Schaap *et al.*, 1975). We inoculated high-titered X-tropic virus preparations into newborn NIH, BALB/c and C57 mice and noted no pathology after 18 months (J. A. Levy and P. Arnstein, unpublished observations).

Recognizing the limitation of extrapolating results obtained from other animal hosts, we have, nevertheless, experimented with heterologous species. Rats and ducks were inoculated at birth and in embryo (ducks) with X-tropic virus, but no apparent effect on embryogenesis nor development was noted in these animals. Anti-X-tropic virus antibodies and the virus were detected, however, in the infected ducks. Two ducks, inoculated at birth with a xenotropic virus pseudotype of a murine sarcoma virus, developed multiple fibrosarcomas (Levy, 1977a). This result indicated that known oncogenic genomes enveloped in another virus coat can affect heterologous hosts. It further demonstrated that X-tropic virus infection of heterologous species can occur *in vivo*. Up to now, no signs of autoimmune disease have been noted in any infected animal.

2. *Significance of Host Humoral Response*

The identification of at least two different types of response of the host to endogenous viruses raises interesting questions about the interrelationship of the host reaction to the virus and the development of autoimmune disease. Some studies have suggested that the binding anti-viral antibodies in the presence of complement can be cytotoxic to cells producing the virus (Nowinski and Klein, 1975). Direct inoculation in tissue culture of serum containing neutralizing factor has not, however, shown any cytopathic effects. Eluates of kidneys from New Zealand Black mice have low levels of anti-X-tropic virus neutralizing activity as well as anti-viral Ig (Dixon *et al.*, 1971; J. A. Levy, unpublished data). More complete studies of these immune complexes must obviously be performed before any conclusions can be made about the role of these antiviral factors in the IC nephritis.

Conceivably, the production of infectious X-tropic virus could be atavistic, and only viral antigen expression on the surface of the cell should be coded for by the integrated viral genome. We, as well as other investigators, have noted X-tropic virus antigen on the outer membrane of cells free of budding viruses (Oshiro *et al.*, 1977; Kennel and Feldman, 1976, see p. 437). Considering the host response to these antigens, one might expect the anti-viral reaction to destroy the cells producing the virus. The neutralizing factor, however, may interact with the viral antigen on the cell surface and

TABLE X

Relationship of Anti-T Antibody to Anti-X-Tropic Virus-Neutralizing Activity

Serum	Anti-T	Anti-X-tropic		Anti-Ecotropic
NZB POOL-5 (17–19 mo.)	1:1024	>10,000	>20,000	<10
NZB POOL-7 (8–10 mo.)	1:16	>10,000	>20,000	<10

Anti-thymocyte antibodies were measured by Shirai and Mellors (1971). Anti-xenotropic and ecotropic virus activity was determined by neutralization tests using the NZB and Rauscher MuLV, respectively.

assist in normal cell function (Levy, 1976a) (see Section VIII). Overproduction of either virus or these factors may lead to autoimmune disease.

3. *Immune Complex Nephritis*

One characteristic of autoimmune disease is the circulating immune complexes, which precipitate out in the tissues, especially in the kidney. Immune complex nephritis, is not necessarily a sign of autoimmunity since many mice show this pathology without the more generalized characteristics of the disease such as anti-native DNA antibodies. Immune complex glomerulonephritis, has been associated with infection of mice with several C-type virus isolates (Dunn and Green, 1966; Hirsch *et al.*, 1969; Pascal *et al.*, 1973; Recher *et al.*, 1966; Crocker *et al.*, 1974; Oldstone *et al.*, 1972).

C-type virus antigens and anti-viral antibodies have been reported in the kidneys of NZB mice (Dixon *et al.*, 1971; Mellors *et al.*, 1969, 1971; Tonietti *et al.*, 1970; Yoshiki *et al.*, 1974). DNA–anti-DNA complexes are also present, but which IC produces the kidney pathology needs to be determined. Because X-tropic virus is the only endogenous virus of NZB mice, the anti-viral antibodies must be directed against this virus class. Since, no immunoglobulins that bind to X-tropic viruses have been detected in mouse sera, the identity of the antibodies needs to be resolved. Neutralizing factor(s) may be involved. Whether the IC nephritis in other mouse strains results from similar anti-X-tropic virus reactions requires further study (Levy, 1975b, see p. 442).

In general, the C-type viruses are probably promotors, rather than initiators, of this IC disease. Immunologic factors, regulated genetically, appear to be the key determinants.

4. *Phenotypic Mixing among Xenotropic and Ecotropic Viruses*

The xenotropic and ecotropic classes of endogenous mouse C-type viruses do not interfere with infection of a cell by one another (Levy, 1974, 1977a,b; Levy *et al.*, 1975b). A mouse cell which is spontaneously producing xenotropic virus can be superinfected with an ecotropic virus and produce both classes of viruses. Rat cells that are susceptible to infection by both classes of C-type virus can be simultaneously infected by both and give rise to progeny of the two parental types. During this concurrent infection, the viral genomes can interchange their envelope coats so that xenotropic viruses emerge with an ecotropic coat and vice versa (Fig. 1). One can superinfect mouse cells with xenotropic virus in an ecotropic coat and these mouse cells now spontaneously produce progeny xenotropic and ecotropic viruses (Levy, 1977b). This exchanging of envelope coats is called phenotypic mixing, since the genome which directs the replication of the virus is not changed; only its outside surface is modified. These experiments enable one to put an ecotropic virus genome into cells that were previously resistant to this class of viruses

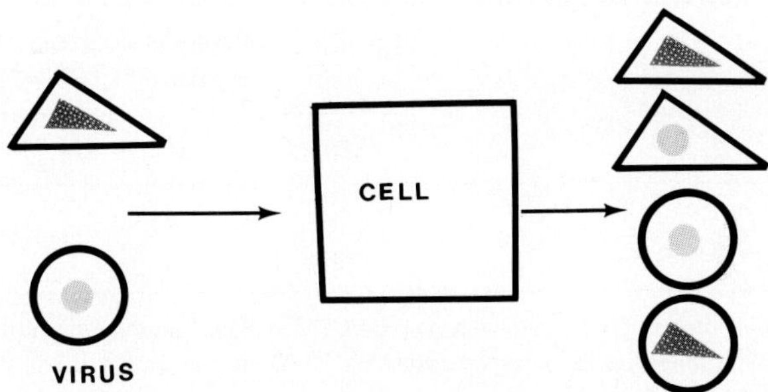

Fig. 1. Phenotypic mixing. A cell infected by two viruses produces progeny that consist of the original parental types and viruses that have exchanged their outside envelope coats.

(Table XI). The infected cell will now express ecotropic virus and its antigens.

This phenomenon may account for enhanced symptoms of autoimmune disease. If a cell spontaneously producing xenotropic viruses is infected by or starts producing ecotropic virus as well, phenotypic mixing will occur. If the host mounts an immune response against the xenotropic virus, the ecotropic virus enveloped in a xenotropic coat will also be affected. Since ecotropic virus is produced by mouse cells in much higher quantity (>6 logs) than X-tropic virus (~3 logs) (Levy *et al.*, 1975b) phenotypic mixing will be substantial. The number of antigenically changed ecotropic viruses may surpass the amount of xenotropic virus itself. IC nephritis may then develop. This kind of phenotypic mixing among these two mouse classes is involved in the enhanced immune complex nephritis observed with ecotropic virus infection of NZB mice (Talal *et al.*, 1971) or the IC nephritis noted in other mouse strains (Levy, 1975b).

In a more specific example, (NZB × NZW)F_1 mice differ from their NZB parent in that they contain an endogenous ecotropic virus. This virus is passed to the hybrid by the NZW mouse strain (Levy, 1974). One reason this hybrid may have a more severe IC disease than NZB mice could be the degree of phenotypic mixing of endogenous viruses that occurs in this mouse strain. The significance of this possibility will become more apparent when the type and quantity of virus–anti-virus complexes in the kidney are known.

Phenotypic mixing has also been observed between C-type viruses and other RNA viruses such as vesicular stomatitis virus (Zavada, 1972;

TABLE XI

Phenotypic Mixing of Xenotropic and Ecotropic MuLV

	Progeny ecotropic virus recovered (PFU/0.5 ml)		
	Mink	Marmoset	Mongoose
AKR-MuLV	0	0	0
AKR-MuLV (NZB-MuLV)	>300	92	102

The AKR-ecotropic murine leukemia virus (MuLV) is unable to infect cultured mink, marmoset, and mongoose cells. After infecting NZB mouse embryo cells (producing NZB-MuLV) with the AKR-MuLV, phenotypic mixing occurs and an AKR-MuLV(NZB-MuLV) virus is produced. This virus contains the ecotropic genome with the xenotropic envelope coat. It can now infect the heterologous cells and produce parental AKR-MuLV.

Krontiris *et al.*, 1973). The increase in immunologic reactions observed in NZB mice infected with lymphochoriomeningitis (LCM) virus (Oldstone and Dixon, 1969) perhaps results from phenotypic mixing of this virus with endogenous X-tropic virus.

5. *Graft Versus Host Reaction*

NZB mice have a syndrome resembling a graft versus host reaction (GVHR). Their lymphocytes are autoreactive and cytotoxic; late in life immunoblastic lymphomas occur. De Vries and Hijmans (1967) have suggested that the NZB thymus is the target of their GVHR-like disease. Studies by Schwartz and his colleagues have demonstrated that mice undergoing GVHR have a higher incidence of leukemias and lymphomas (Schwartz and Beldotti, 1965; Gleichmann *et al.*, 1972). Some studies suggested that this GVHR specifically activated ecotropic C-type viruses and these viruses were responsible for the lymphomas (Hirsch *et al.*, 1970, 1972). The induction of neoplasia in PH mice undergoing a GVHR-like syndrome (Stanley and Walters, 1966) has been explained by the presence of AKR-MuLV in the spleen cells inoculated (Levy and Huebner, 1970). Studies from other laboratories, including our own have indicated that GVHR can occur without the induction of ecotropic viruses (Sherr *et al.*, 1974; Levy *et al.*, 1977). In our studies, 10–30% of spleens from BALB/c mice and (BALB/c × A/J)F_1 (CAF_1) mice normally produced low levels of endogenous xenotropic but not ecotropic virus. With the induction of GVHR, the frequency of xenotropic virus expression reached 100%. We believe the recovery of ecotropic virus in other studies resulted from the presence of this virus in the spleen cell inoculum or in the recipient mice.

GVHR then increased the production of xenotropic virus by lymphoid cells. Stimulation of B cells by lipopolysaccharides has given similar results (Moroni *et al.*, 1975). The possibility of this enhanced viral expression causing autoimmunity needs further evaluation. One can envision in NZB mice a vicious cycle in which enhanced virus expression and anti-virus reactions lead to increased virus expression, and so forth.

In GVHR experiments, using strains of mice which do not have ecotropic viruses, e.g., C57/L and NZB, Datta and Schwartz (1976) noted lymphoma production in the absence of detectable ecotropic virus.

These studies, taken in view of our own studies with CAF_1 mice, indicate that lymphoma production resulting from GVHR is not necessarily linked to the production of infectious ecotropic virus. Since reticulum cell sarcoma is a common malignancy in NZB mice, the chronically expressed xenotropic virus, if not a direct transforming particle, may act as a constant antigenic stimulus. It may thereby place a rapidly proliferating population of cells in the reticuloendothelial system at risk of malignant change (Levy, 1975b, 1976a). A relationship between antigenic stimulation and lymphoma development in mice has been described (Kruger, 1971; Kouttab and Jutila, 1972; Metcalf, 1961).

IV. EQUINE INFECTIOUS ANEMIA VIRUS

We have discussed murine endogenous xenotropic C-type viruses and their possible relationship to the autoimmune disorders in mice. Equine infectious anemia permits us to examine an autoimmune disorder linked to an exogenously (horizontally) acquired infection.

A. History

Equine infectious anemia (EIA) was first described as a distinct disease in horses in 1843. In 1904, Vallee and Carre published the initial report showing that the etiologic agent was infectious and filterable. In fact, EIA was one of the first filterable agents identified which caused disease in animals (Henson and McGuire, 1974; Ishitani, 1970).

B. Clinical Findings

EIA is a viral disease of horses characterized by infection throughout the lifetime of the horse, intermittent fevers, loss of weight, anemia, and progressive weakness. It is readily transmitted to horses by inoculation of blood or serum.

Histopathologically, it is a condition in which mononuclear and lymphoid cells proliferate in or infiltrate the reticuloendothelial organs, particularly liver, bone marrow, and spleen (Henson and McGuire, 1971). Enhanced phagocytosis by these mononuclear round cells is characteristic of the disease. Because of this marked increase in lymphoreticular tissue, some pathologists have considered EIA an autoimmune disease with characteristics of leukemia (Ishitani, 1970). Specific symptoms include the following.

1. *Fever*

Experimentally-infected horses develop fever within 8–15 days after virus inoculation. The animals are ill for as long as a month, lose weight, and die at various time periods after virus infection (Henson and McGuire, 1971, 1974). If the animal survives this acute disease, it often develops repeated attacks of clinical illness, which alternate with intervals of clinical normalcy. A few infected horses become asymptomatic carriers for months or years after infection. When the animals show signs of clinical disease, they are always viremic.

2. *Anemia*

During EIA virus infection, various hemaglutinins can be identified in the horse plasma. These are predominantly IgM and react with horse red cells and not with red cells from other animal species. It was originally thought that the hemolysis of horse red cells encountered during EIA was associated with complement-coating of the erythrocytes and not an immunoglobulin (McGuire *et al.*, 1969). Henson and McGuire (1971), however, noted immunoglobulins on the horse red blood cell surfaces in low concentration. Following the technique of Gilliland *et al.* (1970), they showed that the quantity of Ig was below the threshold of detectability by the Coombs' test.

The warm hemagglutinins have no hemolytic activity but enhance the phagocytosis of the horse erythrocytes by macrophages. This reaction is probably one of the principal causes of the anemia, since free ferritin appears in the blood of horses during EIA virus infection. The measurement of this circulating ferritin has been developed into one technique for detecting virus infection (Oki, 1961).

Some reports indicate that anemia results as well from reduced erythropoietic activity during EIA virus infection (Obara and Nakajima, 1961).

3. *Glomerulitis and Hepatitis*

The glomerulitis observed in EIA virus infected horses does not appear to be caused primarily by a direct immunologic injury to kidney tissue but is related to the deposition of immune complexes and complement in the glomeruli (Henson *et al.*, 1973). In contrast, the liver disease probably results from direct immunologic injury. Pathologic examination suggests an inflammatory response of the host to the liver macrophages and Kupffer's cells containing viral antigen is involved (Henson *et al.*, 1973).

C. Virus

1. Characteristics

Although EIA was described nearly 75 years ago, characterization of the causative agent of EIA was delayed because of the lack of an adequate virus assay. All virus studies had to be performed with horses. With the development by Kobayashi and Kono (1967) of a virus assay using horse leukocyte cultures, the EIA agent could be easily measured. The EIA virus is quantitated by cytopathic changes which occur in cultured leukocytes (Kobayashi and Kono, 1967; Kono and Kobayashi, 1967). The appearance of viral antigen in horse kidney cell cultures as detected by immunofluorescence can also be used as a biologic assay (Kono and Yoshino, 1974).

Characteristics of the EIA agent include the following (Table XII): The virus buds from horse leukocytes and is primarily infectious for only white cells of this animal species. Macrophages appear to be the most susceptible cells to infection. By electron microscopy, a heterogeneity of viruslike particles is noted. A typical type measures between 100 and 120 nm in size and has a nucleoid of about 45 nm (Tajima *et al.*, 1969; Nakajima *et al.*, 1969a). The density of the particles varies between 1.13 and 1.16 gm/ml (Nakajima *et al.*, 1969b; Nakajima, 1973; Charman *et al.*, 1976). This virus

TABLE XII

Physicochemical and Biologic Properties of Equine Infectious Anemia Virus

1. Nucleic acid type: high molecular weight RNA (~70 S); DNA is required for virus replication
2. Capsidal symmetry: unable to see structural detail but probably different from helical components observed in myxoviruses
3. Envelope: possesses a lip-containing-envelope, approximately 9 nm in thickness
4. Particle size and shape: considerable variation; approximately 90–140 nm in diameter; predominantly spherical
5. Possesses surface projections but not as prominent as those seen in myxoviruses
6. Sensitive to ether
7. Buoyant density: mainly 1.15 gm/ml but shows considerably broad distribution
8. Released from plasma membrane by the process of budding
9. Contains internal virion reverse transcriptase

[a] Adapted from Nakajima (1973).

therefore resembles C-type RNA tumor viruses. Particles with characteristics of both A- and B-type viruses have also been seen. Studies using ^{3}H-uridine showed conclusively that the EIA agent has RNA as its nucleic acid core (Nakajima *et al.*, 1970).

The propagation of the virus appears to be DNA dependent and it may contain DNA as a minor component (Nakajima, 1973). Most recently, the EIA virus has been shown to have a high molecular weight RNA (~70S) and an internal virion reverse transcriptase—properties similar to those of C-type viruses (Charman *et al.*, 1976).

2. *Distribution*

The EIA virus localizes in several tissues of the horse after infection (Kono *et al.*, 1971; McGuire *et al.*, 1971). Viral antigen is present primarily in the cytoplasm of mononuclear cells, particularly macrophages. Immunofluorescent testing demonstrated it as early as 6 days after infection in horses with clinical signs of infection. The virus can be detected in the serum of infected horses as early as day 5. It persists in the circulation and reaches its highest titers in the bone marrow, which is most likely its original site of infection. (Nakajima *et al.*, 1974). The virus titers fluctuate in direct correlation with the severity of the clinical disease in the horse (Henson *et al.*, 1973). Over 95% of the infectious virus in the serum circulates complexed with anti-viral antibodies which are nonneutralizing (Henson *et al.*, 1973). Rabbit anti-equine γ-globulin, added to horse serum, reduces by over 2 logs the viral infectivity of the serum. This circulation of virus–antibody complexes in the blood resembles that observed with other chronic virus infections, such as lactic dehydrogenase (LDH), lymphochoriomeningitis (LCM), and Aleutian mink disease viruses (Notkins, 1971).

3. *Immunology*

The EIA virus has both type-specific and group-specific antigens which can be recognized by serologic tests. As with C-type viruses, the group-specific antigens refer to those components of the virus which are shared by all members of the EIA virus group. The type-specific antigens, identified by virus neutralization, refer to those proteins which separate the EIA viruses into individual isolates.

Complement-fixing antibody, usually detected for only a short period of time after the first febrile reaction (Kono and Kobayashi, 1966), detects a group-specific antigen which corresponds to the p30 of RNA C-type viruses. For the diagnosis of EIA, however, immunodiffusion is the most helpful test since precipitating antibodies to the group-specific antigen remain positive in the blood of infected horses for long periods of time (Kono, 1969; Nakajima *et al.*, 1971; Henson *et al.*, 1971).

In demonstrating the specificities for two serologic tests, eight different strains of the EIA virus were investigated by means of complement fixation and neutralization tests. All strains shared a common complement-fixing antigen as demonstrated by cross-reactivity with CF antibody. Cross-neutralization tests, however, revealed that each strain was only neutralized by its own homologous antiserum (Kono *et al.*, 1971).

4. *Antigenic Modification of the Virus*

The presence of immune complexes in the circulation of the horse has been one means by which the EIA virus persists in the animal. The immunoglobulins that bind to the virus do not neutralize it. They may, however, block the effectiveness of neutralizing antibody. Another mechanism for virus persistence was described by Kono *et al.* (1973). They noted that infectious viruses in the circulation of a horse could not be neutralized by antiserum against the original inoculated virus. After infection with an EIA virus, modifications in the envelope coat of that virus occurred so that the neutralizing antibodies, which were raised against the parental virus, were no longer effective in inactivating the progeny virus. The isolates could be differentiated from one another by neutralizing but not complement-fixing or precipitating antibodies. Their work supported the idea that the persistence of the virus in the blood of infected horses occurred by the development of antigenically distinct virus populations which were not susceptible to neutralizing antibody produced against a preceding virus. This antigenic drift resembles that of influenza virus, but it occurs more rapidly with EIA virus infection.

D. Role of the Immune System in Control of EIA Virus Infection

In studies using vaccines prepared against EIA virus, Kono *et al.* (1970) noted differences in the type of protection provided against subsequent infection by EIA. Horses inoculated repeatedly with an avirulent EIA virus acquired perfect resistance to infection with the highly virulent homologous virus. This resistance, however, was not maintained against virulent heterologous viruses. In contrast, horses clinically recovering from infection with a highly virulent virus, when challenged with an immunologically different virus, remained completely free of symptoms of infection. Kono (1973) concluded that humoral immunity prevented reinfection by homologous virus, and cellular immunity offered protection against infection by other EIA isolates. This cellular immunity only resulted when significant replication of virulent viruses occurred. The importance of cellular immunity was further indicated by the appearance of fever in asymptomatic horses following the administration of anti-lymphocyte serum or corticosteroids (Kono, 1973). Apparently lymphocytes eliminate those cells which express viral antigens on their surface and, thereby, prevent spread of the virus. If an infected cell escapes from this immune surveillance, viremia with antigenic shifts can result in enhanced propagation of the virus.

E. Interaction of the Virus and Immune System in the Pathogenesis of EIA

The immune system in horses is an important factor in the pathogenesis of EIA (Perryman *et al.,* 1971). Studies of humoral and cellular responses suggest that EIA-infected horses are not immunosuppressed (Henson and McGuire, 1974). The hypergammaglobulinemia is similar to the polyclonal response observed in other persistent viral infections. The identity of predominantly anti-EIA antibodies, however, requires further study.

Horses infected with EIA have reduced levels of complement (C3) during active hemolytic disease. Their erythrocytes bear C3 on their surface, and the glomeruli contain deposits of either immunoglobulins or C3 (Henson and McGuire, 1971). The attachment of C3 on red blood cells (RBC) presumably reflects the viral antigen–antibody reaction at the surface of the cell. Although no EIA viral antigen has been detected in bone marrow cells belonging to the erythrocyte maturation series, conceivably the viral antigen binds to circulating erythrocytes and, subsequently, interacts with specific antibodies.

The anemia of EIA is predominantly hemolytic and results from all or one of three factors: (1) viral antigen on the erythrocyte binds to anti-viral antibodies leading to C3 activation and hemolysis; (2) RBC coated with C3 have a shortened life span due to an increased osmotic fragility; and (3) the virus induces the production of RBC hemagglutinins by a carrier–hapten mechanism (see Section VI,B).

There is also some indication that viral propagation in macrophages may lead to generalized bone marrow suppression and impaired reticuloendothelial cell function.

The lesions noted in the liver and kidney of infected horses are primarily caused by enhanced cellular immunity to virus-containing cells. When Henson and his co-workers (1973) treated horses infected with the EIA virus with the anti-lympholytic and immunosuppressive agent, cyclophosphamide, these horses did not develop hepatitis and glomerulonephritis.

Finally, the immune response as noted above, permits persistence of the virus in the circulation. Viruses, coated with precipitating or CF antibodies, are protected from neutralizing antibody. Moreover, when the virus–antibody complexes are phagocytized by macrophages, the viruses can replicate in these cells and spread. In contrast, other viruses such as herpes and pox, are inactivated by macrophages.

V. CANINE SYSTEMIC LUPUS ERYTHEMATOSUS

Another animal model of autoimmunity whose cause may be linked to a C-type virus is canine lupus erythematosus. This disease complex in dogs is not rare and does not appear to be genetically linked (Lewis *et al.*, 1965). Because of its sporadic nature, it is a good model for human autoimmune disease.

A. History

In 1965, Lewis and his co-workers reported the clinical pathological features of a multisystemic canine disease that resembled human systemic lupus erythematosus (SLE). Its cardinal features were autoimmune hemolytic anemia, thrombocytopenia, and membranous glomerulonephritis. Positive lupus cells and other serologic abnormalities indicated that this disorder was immunologic. The cases they reported involved two poodles, a cocker spaniel, a fox terrier, a wire-haired fox terrier, a German Shepherd, and one mongrel. The dogs ranged in age from 4 to 6 years (roughly equivalent to 30–40 years of age in man). Four of them were female, two of which received ovariohistorectomies. No one breed appeared more susceptible to development of this SLE, and no environmental stimuli, including medicines, that could induce the disease was identified.

B. Clinical Findings

The disease first became clinically evident as a result of hematologic abnormalities, although three animals initially presented with proteinuria. Other abnormalities included intermittent lameness in two dogs, alopecia in two, and an eruption in a butterfly distribution on the face of one dog. One dog exhibited the sequential development of arthritis, butterfly rash, autoimmune hemolytic anemia, thrombocytopenia, and, finally, nephritis within a period of approximately 1 year (Lewis *et al.*, 1965). Hemolytic anemia was the most prominent feature of the disease and was accompanied by reticulocytosis, normoblastemia, urobilinuria, and hyperplasia of the erythroid elements of the bone marrow. In each case, the direct antiglobulin test of dog erythrocytes was positive (1–3+) (Lewis *et al.*, 1965; Lewis and Schwartz, 1971).

Thrombocytopenia was found in six of the animals, accompanied by easy bruising, ecchymosis, petechiae, and active bleeding from mucous membranes. A normal number of megakaryocytes was found in the bone marrow, and this finding, along with the appropriate response to corticosteroids, suggested the disorder was analogous to the idiopathic (ITP) type in humans. Four dogs eventually underwent splenectomy because of recurrent manifestations of the hematologic components of the disease. Although hypergammaglobulinemia was not observed in these initial seven dogs described, three out of eight dogs with SLE subsequently studied had hypergammaglobulinemia (Lewis *et al.*, 1965).

The diagnosis of SLE in these dogs was substantiated by the detection of LE cells, anti-nuclear antibodies, complement-fixing antibodies to DNA–histone complexes, positive antiglobulin tests, and rheumatoid factor. Antithyroid and anti-red blood cell antibodies were also consistently detected in the dogs.

C. Genetic Studies

Inbreeding experiments were conducted with three different sets of dogs: two groups of German Shepherds (line A and B) and a C line of French poodles (Lewis and Schwartz, 1971). These animals, by brother–sister matings, produced 480 animals. The progeny had excessively high neonatal mortality, multiple serological abnormalities, and thymic lesions. At the time of the published report, the animals were too young (3 years) to have developed clinical SLE.

LE cells were noted in all of the first generation animals from the A and C lines in which the original female parent had SLE and the males were normal. The cells were also present in 87% of the F_2 generation in the A line and 68.4% of the F_2 progeny in the C line. When F_2 brother–sister matings were made in the C line, 75% of the F_3 puppies developed positive LE tests.

A second abnormal finding, anti-nuclear antibody (ANA), was detected in the sera of 31% of the inbred dogs in the colony. Forty-eight of these 55 animals had positive LE cells. The lack of correlation between the two tests suggested the development of ANA was not related to the LE cell phenomenon. A third abnormal antibody, rheumatoid factor, was detected in the sera of 13 members of the colony although none of these animals had arthritis.

Postmortem examination revealed lesions of the thymus in 36.6% of the colony dogs over 6 months of age. In one thymus, lymphoid follicles and active germinal center formation was observed as an expanding mass of pleomorphic reticulum cells. This mass was confirmed to one lobule of the affected organ and was similar to the type B reticulum cell tumor described in mice (Lewis and Schwartz, 1971).

D. Virus Studies

These breeding results with dogs were most consistent with the transmission of the disease by a nongenetic mechanism, such as a virus. In attempts to isolate the responsible agent, cell-free filtrates were prepared from the spleens of SLE dogs and injected into newborn dogs, mice, and rats (Lewis *et al.*, 1973). Anti-nuclear antibody and positive LE cells were noted in the canine recipients. In one dog with lupus nephritis, murine leukemia virus p30 was detected in the diseased glomeruli (F. Quimby, personal communication). Some also developed antibody to double-stranded DNA. ANA and, in some cases, antibodies to double-stranded DNA were produced as well in the murine recipients (Lewis *et al.*, 1973; Schwartz, 1975). No abnormalities were detected in the rats. When extracts were prepared from spleens of two normal beagle dogs that were housed in the same quarters as the SLE colony, these filtrates also induced ANA in the CAF_1 mouse recipients. In contrast, filtrates prepared from the spleens of three dogs that had never been in contact with the colony did not induce this ANA in mice. As further controls, filtrates were prepared from the spleens of normal cats, rabbits, guinea pigs, rats, and mice and injected into newborn CAF_1 mice. This procedure did not lead to ANA production within the 1 year period of observation. Since CAF_1 mice, unlike other mice, do not develop positive ANA before the age of 1 year (Lewis *et al.*, 1973), the induction of ANA in recipient mice with canine lupus extracts indicated a modification in the serologic response in this strain.

Some of the mice which received the dog spleen filtrates developed malignant lymphomas. Murine leukemia viruses were identified in these tumors by electron microscopic, biologic, and serologic techniques. Puppies inoculated with extracts of these lymphomas developed ANA and positive LE tests within 4 months. In contrast, tumor cells and cell-free filtrates from two transplantable lymphoid tumors of mice that were not induced by the canine filtrate but contained MuLV, failed to elicit ANA production in newborn puppies. The canine filtrate-induced tumors that developed in the mouse colonies were transplantable and were populated by cells that ranged from undifferentiated reticulum types to immature plasma cells. One tumor (SP104) produced a monoclonal IgA(K) protein that had anti-native DNA activity (Schwartz, 1975; Dixon *et al*, 1975).

The virus associated with this tumor was a B-tropic C-type virus with an AKR envelope coat (Schwartz, 1975; J. A. Levy, unpublished data). Its ecotropic nature was confirmed by its inability to infect cells of a heterologous species. No xenotropic virus production was detected in these tumor cells. The SP104 virus had a low oncogenicity in animals and induced antinuclear antibodies in inoculated mice. No homology was noted between canine cellular RNA and a cDNA probe made from the SP104 virus, using reverse transcriptase (F. Quimby, personal communication). These results suggest that the SP104 virus is an endogenous virus of the CAF_1 mouse and contains no genetic material of dogs. While the SP104 virus does not appear to be different from other ecotropic viruses the induction in mice of a plasmacytoma with anti-DNA activity is intriguing. These observations, however, must be confirmed in other laboratories. It is conceivable, for instance, that some factor (not necessarily a virus) in the canine filtrates induced a latent murine endogenous C-type virus which was responsible for the tumor and the ANA production. Nevertheless, this tumor induction in mice, filtrate transmission to other dogs, and serologic signs of SLE induced with spleen extracts from dogs raised near the SLE colony but not from dogs kept separate, suggest that a transmissible agent could be involved.

VI. OTHER CHARACTERISTICS OF C-TYPE VIRUS INFECTION WHICH MAY BE INVOLVED IN THE PATHOGENESIS OF AUTOIMMUNITY

A. Effect on the Immune System

Autoimmunity has been primarily considered a result of circulating humoral autoantibodies; their production may be linked to deranged T or B cell function (see below). T cell cytotoxicity and abnormal macrophage function (see Section VIII) may also be involved in the disorder. The effect of C-type viruses on these immune responses must be considered. C-type virus infection can reduce humoral and cellular immunity and, thereby, contribute to the development of abnormal immune responses (Notkins *et al.*, 1970). This suppression, however, has been primarily demonstrated with the FMR laboratory strains of MuLV, and other MuLV, such as endogenous AKR-MuLV, may not be immunosuppressive (J. N. Ihle, personal communication).

Cremer (1967) found that rats infected with Moloney leukemia virus had a reduced ability to make antibodies to sheep red blood cells. Friend virus infection in young mice also reduces the ability of their lymphocytes to react in the Jerne test to sheep red blood cells. Adult mice infected with Friend or Rauscher leukemia virus, and chickens infected with avian leukosis virus become immunodepressed. The degree of this immunodepression is related to the dose of the infecting virus (Notkins *et al.*, 1970).

The effect of C-type virus infection on the T-cell response is discussed in other chapters in this book. In brief, it has been reported that during the course of infection with Moloney MuLV, peripheral lymphocytes (presumably T cells) are cytotoxic for cells producing C-type virus (Proffitt *et al.*, 1973). Later, when most thymocytes become infected, the specificity of this reaction changes, and these lymphocytes become cytotoxic only for normal cells; virus-infected cells are protected. Proffitt and his co-workers (1973), on one hand, believe this modification in the response of the T cell results in autoimmune disease (see Chapter 13). On the other hand, the results of Zinkernagel and Doherty (1974) and of Schrader *et al.* (1975) suggest the cytotoxicity for virus-infected cells causes autoimmunity, and, in some cases, is monitored by histocompatability loci. A T cell responds to an H-2 receptor altered directly by the virus or modified by association with a viral antigen. This latter effect of the virus relates to its ability to uncover or produce new antigens on the cell surface.

B. Induction of New Antigens on the Cell Surface

Infection of a cell with a C-type virus usually leads to productive infection. Since the cell is not lysed, virus particles continually bud from the cell and place new proteins on its surface. These "new" antigens may affect the immune response of the host.

Many research groups have noted that rejection of tumor cells is enhanced after infection or induction of C-type viruses on the cell surface (Barbieri *et al.*, 1971; Greenberger and Aaronson, 1973). Silagi *et al.* (1972) have reported a melanoma cell line that became nontumorogenic when exposed to BUDR. This halogenated pyrimidine activated endogenous C-type viruses in the melanoma line.

This enhanced antigenicity of virus-infected cells may result from two general phenomena.

1. *Heterogenization*

Coined by Svet-Moldafsky *et al.* (1968), this term describes the appearance on a cell of new antigens coded for by an infecting virus (Fig. 2). The host immune system recognizes the viral antigens as foreign and mounts a reaction against them. During this immune response, the infected cell is destroyed.

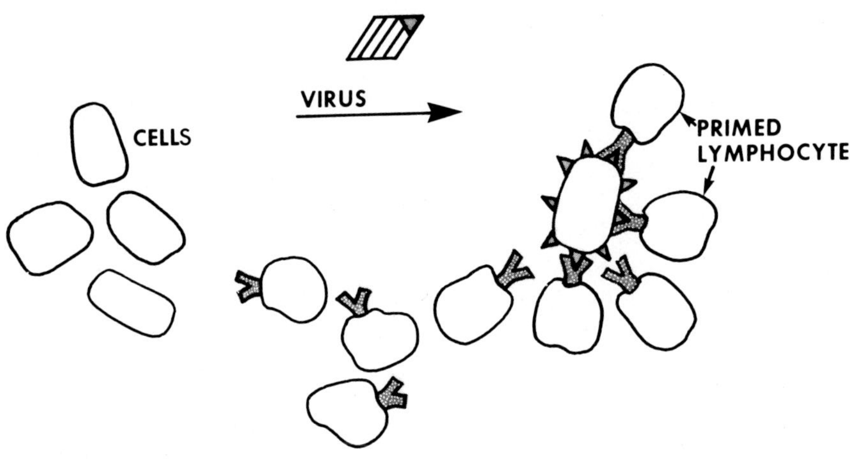

Fig. 2. By heterogenization a virus places new antigens on the cell surface. Lymphocytes are primed to react directly or make antibody to the viral proteins. In the process of this immune interaction with the virus, the cell is destroyed. [From Svet-Moldavsky *et al.* (1968).]

2. *Lindenmann Effect*

Van Loghem (1965) was among the first to suggest that autoantibodies might result from structural alteration of cell antigens due to viral infection. Lindenmann (1974) demonstrated experimentally that cells, after infection by enveloped viruses, become more antigenic. He noted that Ehrlich ascites cells, usually nonantigenic in mice, become highly immunogenic after infection with influenza virus (Lindenmann and Klein, 1967). The tumor cells, their extracts, or the progeny virus itself induced an immune response against the infected and noninfected tumor cells. Lindenmann reasoned that the virus acted as a carrier for cell components, which as haptens, were not antigenic (Fig. 3).

By either of these two mechanisms, an enhanced expression of C-type viruses would lead to new "antigen" formation on the cell surface and could induce an autoimmune reaction of the host. The virus uncovers or places these antigens on the cell surface, which the host immune system views as foreign. A reaction of the host against the virus directly, or against the normal cell components linked as haptens to the virus, results in autoimmunity. Following MuLV infection, mouse erythrocytes acquire viral antigens and can have C-type viruses budding from their surface (Reilly and Schloss, 1971; Wollmann *et al.*, 1970; Levy, 1975b). Sensitized lymphocytes from mice infected by Friend or Rauscher leukemia viruses, react both with virus-infected erythrocytes and with erythrocytes from noninfected animals (Cox and Keast, 1973). The hemolytic anemias observed in autoimmune disease may result from a similar mechanism. This phenomenon could be involved in the appearance of embryonic antigens on tumors or on cells transformed by viruses. The embryonic antigens are uncovered self-proteins, which may be viewed as foreign by the host. Since C-type viruses have been observed and isolated from early developing embryos (Levy, 1975b, 1976a,b; Chase and Piko, 1973; Vernon *et al.*, 1973) some of these embryonic antigens may actually represent endogenous viruses.

Finally, a reaction against the virus or the virus-infected cell may, in itself, cause sensitization of the host to particular subcellular organelles that are released into the circulation secondary to cell destruction. Such a mechanism for production of "anti-self" antibodies was proposed by Weir

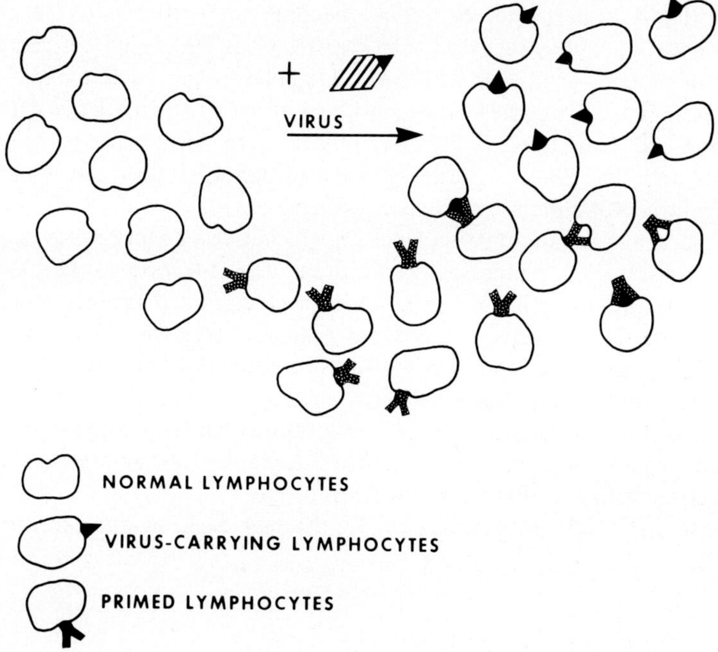

Fig. 3. Carrier–hapten (Lindenmann effect): by this mechanism, a replicating virus or the expression of its antigens on the cell surface increase the immunogenicity of the cell. Lymphocytes are primed to react or make antibody to the virus, to the virus-modified antigen or to normal cell components made antigenic by their association with viral proteins. Both humoral and cellular immune responses are involved. (Adapted from Levy, 1974.)

(1967) when he showed that chemical destruction of liver induces the production of anti-liver antibodies in certain strains of rats.

C. Integration of Other Viruses Using C-Type Virus Enzymes

The preceding examples dealt with productive C-type virus infections. It is apparent, however, that viral protein expression does not necessarily require virus replication.

We have discussed the ability of C-type viruses to transcribe their RNA into DNA through the help of an RNA-dependent DNA polymerase. This method of reverse transcription permits them to integrate into the cell genome, even without replication, and pass vertically to the progeny. Recently, Zhdanov (1975) has suggested that other RNA viruses, such as measles virus or arborviruses, could use the reverse transcriptase of endogenous C-type viruses, or of cells, and transcribe their RNA genome into a DNA. They, thereby, could become integrated into the cellular genomes. He also has reported that measles virus DNA and antigen can be found in tissues of patients with SLE. He believes this finding explains the high titers of anti-measles virus antibody in sera from patients with SLE (Phillips and Christian, 1973). His observations have not yet been confirmed, and the measles antibody levels probably reflect the generalized hypergammaglobulinemia associated with SLE.

Simpson and Iinuma (1975) have shown that respiratory syncytial virus, which causes flulike illnesses in children, can integrate as DNA in the genome of infected cells. When DNA extracted from the infected cells was added to permissive cells, the original parental virus was recovered. These observations introduce the idea that autoimmune disease could result from the integration of one specific virus or any of several viruses into the genome of the host cells. Without being replicated, they could produce, on the cell surfaces, antigens which induce immunologic responses of the host. The susceptibility to this virus integration may be a genetic determinant in the host and could be responsible for finding SLE in only certain individuals.

VII. C-TYPE VIRUSES AND HUMAN AUTOIMMUNE DISEASE

While attempts to isolate an infectious virus from patients with autoimmune disease continue, researchers are also looking at tissues from patients with these diseases for signs of C-type virus infection. Their studies in humans are modeled after investigations in mice.

A. Virus Antigens: *Mouse Studies*

Observations in mice indicate that C-type virus antigens may be concentrated in the renal glomeruli or present on the surface of normal cells. Mellors and co-workers (1969; 1971; Yoshiki *et al.*, 1974), using immunofluorescent techniques, noted a high concentration of viral antigen in the kidneys of NZB mice. Dixon *et al.* (1971) also identified murine C-type virus antigens and antibodies in the immune complexes of these mice. These antigens must correspond to the xenotropic virus associated with this strain.

Work in several laboratories have indicated that the MuLV gp70 may be present on the surface of cells without production of detectable infectious virus (Ikeda *et al.*, 1974; Del Villano *et al.*, 1975; Kennel and Feldmann, 1976). By immunofluorescent techniques, Lerner and his co-workers (1976) found that a protein similar or identical to the MuLV gp70 major envelope glycoprotein is on the surface of 129/J thymocytes, in lymphoid tissues, and in murine epithelial lining cells (particularly in the testes). Because we have recovered xenotropic viruses regularly from mouse tissues, both malignant and benign, we believe these immunofluorescent tests could be detecting either X-tropic virus or its antigen on the cell surface.

In collaboration with L. Oshiro we have detected xenotropic C-type virus antigens on the surface of infected heterologous cells without the presence of budding virus particles (Oshiro *et al.*, 1977). This antigen was demonstrated by immunoelectron microscopy, using rabbit antiserum prepared against the type-specific antigen of the X-tropic virus.

B. Virus Antigens: *Human Studies*

Following these observations in the murine lupus model and because several protein components of mammalian C type viruses have interspecies determinants, investigators have begun to look at tissues from humans with systemic lupus erythematosus for virus-related antigens. Strand and August (1974b) were the first to report that tissues from patients with SLE contained proteins related to those of mammalian C-type viruses. By competition radioimmunoassay, they suggested that SLE tissues contain two of the principal structural components of type-C RNA viruses: the major core protein (p30) and the major envelope glycopeptide (gp70). They extracted from the kidney and placenta of certain patients with SLE a substance that had the same apparent affinity for antibody binding as that of the purified viral proteins. This competitor was partially purified on phosphocellulose. By size fractionation during gel filtration and immunoprecipitation tests, it appeared similar to the p30 viral protein. Strand and August, moreover, noted some competition with extracts from certain human tumors and normal spleens. Work from other laboratories has also demonstrated viral proteins similar to those of mammalian C-type viruses associated with certain human cancers: p30 (Sherr and Todaro, 1974) and reverse transcriptase (Todaro and Gallo, 1973; Gallagher *et al.*, 1974; Gallo *et al.*, 1973). Sutherland and Mardiney (1973) reported the detection by immunofluorescence of an antigen related to the interspecies determinant of the p30 of mammalian C-type viruses in kidneys from two patients with acute myelocytic leukemia and IC nephritis. These results with human tissues need further confirmation. In particular, those obtained by competition assay must be reevaluated since extracts of human tissues might contain substances which interfere with the radioimmunoprecipitation assays and might not be true competitor molecules.

In other studies of SLE, Lewis *et al.* (1974) noted the presence of an antigenic determinant shared by MuLV on the surface of certain peripheral lymphocytes from patients with SLE. Using antiserum prepared against the SP104 virus (see Section V,D), they observed bright areas of fluorescence on about 1% of the SLE lymphocytes, but not on control cells.

Mellors and Mellors (1976) reported immunopathologic studies on autopsy material from a patient with systemic lupus erythematosus. In the kidney of the afflicted patient, they noted the presence of an antigenic determinant related to the p30 interspecies antigen of the murine, feline, RD114/baboon, and the woolly/gibbon C-type viruses.

Sections of lupus kidney were treated with goat and rabbit antisera prepared against the p30 of mouse, cat, and primate viruses. Immunofluorescence was noted diffusely and focally in the peripheral capillary wall and mesangium of the glomeruli. The involvement included at least 10% of all glomeruli in the sections studied, whereas none of the kidneys from control patients showed any reaction with the anti-p30 sera. Lupus and control kidneys showed no reaction either with fluoresceinated anti-goat or anti-rabbit immunoglobulin sera at the dilutions used. The specificity of the immunofluorescent reaction was confirmed by absorbing the goat anti-p30 serum with viral proteins and testing the residual antibody activity on lupus kidney sections. No residual antibody activity was observed after absorbing the antiserum with sonicates of any one of the four viruses listed above. Moreover, whereas as little as 3 μg of protein from lupus spleens completely eliminated the antibody activity of the serum, 24 times this amount of control spleen protein did not absorb out the antibody activity of the anti-p30 sera. More specifically, the lupus spleen extract competed as an absorbing antigen in the intraspecies-specific antigen assay system, in which goat anti-RD114-p28 serum was tested on cells infected with the feline RD114 virus.

These studies suggested a relationship of the lupus antigen to the RD 114 endogenous primate virus group. The Mellors' concluded that an antigen related to the interspecies determinants of the mammalian p30 virus protein was selectively located, along with the autologous-bound immunoglobulins, in the peripheral capillary wall and mesangium of the SLE renal glomeruli.

Recently, Panem and her co-workers (1976; S. Panem, personal communication) detected, by indirect immunofluorescence, the presence of C-type virus antigens in kidney biopsies of 18 patients with SLE. The antiserum they used was prepared against a virus (HEL-12) that they recovered from culture fluids of diploid human embryonic lung cells (Panem *et al.*, 1975). This HEL-12 virus shares biologic and serologic properties with C-type RNA viruses from both the gibbon/woolly monkey group and the baboon. Its identity as a true human virus has not yet been determined.

In the studies by Panem *et al.* (1976), the intensity of immunofluorescence with the anti-HEL-12 virus antiserum correlated with the extent of immune complex deposition along the glomerular basement membrane. It was eliminated by absorption of the serum with cytoplasmic proteins from cells infected with HEL-12 virus or with lupus kidney eluates. Immunoglobulins eluted from the lupus kidneys mediated cytoplasmic immunofluorescence in HEL-12-infected fibroblasts. The same sections prepared from kidneys of patients with SLE were examined by immunofluorescence using reagents against RD114 p28, woolly monkey, herpes simplex, influenza, mumps, and vaccinia viruses. In all cases, no staining of the specimens occurred. It was interesting that high-filtered woolly monkey and RD114 antisera did not give fluorescence, since the reverse transcriptase of the HEL12 virus shares serologic properties with these primate viruses (S. Panem, personal communication).

Viral antigens were not detected in 15 specimens from patients with nonlupus immune complex glomerulonephritis and other renal diseases, regardless of the extent of immunoglobulin deposition (Panem *et al.*, 1976; S. Panem, personal communication).

These results confirmed those of others cited above, particularly the Mellors, since the RD114 virus intraspecies antigen cross-reacts with that of the baboon virus. Different viral proteins, however, may be measured. The Mellors' assay detects p30 reactivity, whereas Panem *et al.* (1976) may be viewing an antigenic determinant of gp70. Their studies need further investigation with sera prepared against other C-type viruses, particularly those cultivated in human cells, and against other antigens.

All these observations open up the very exciting and interesting possibility that C-type viruses are involved in human SLE. C-type viruses have been observed in normal placentas (Kalter *et al.*, 1973; Vernon *et al.*, 1974) and those from patients with SLE (Imamura *et al.*, 1976; Levy, 1975b). Further studies of placental tissue for the possible presence of the HEL-12, primate or other C-type virus antigens are awaited.

VIII. DISCUSSION

Three animal model systems of autoimmunity associated with a C-type virus infection have been reviewed. In the NZB mouse, the virus is part of the genome of the cells and is inherited as an endogenous agent. Its spontaneous release from the cell appears regulated genetically so that virus expression varies from strain to strain, although the number of integrated virus genes in all strains is probably the same. In the equine and canine models, the virus is exogenously acquired and gives rise to clinical findings once it has established itself in the host. In the horse, symptoms of virus infection can occur as early as 5–6 days; in dogs, the time interval is much longer. Adequate virus expression appears to be the major determinant in the development of autoimmunity. The interesting observation has been made that human autoimmune syndromes associated with infectious viruses are often short-lived and disappear once virus expression has diminished. This fact suggests that persistent viral expression induces and maintains the autoimmune responses; once the virus is lost, the disease process is arrested (Pisciotta and Hinz, 1957; Zuelzer *et al.*, 1966). Such an explanation fits well into the syndromes that result from exogenous virus expression. Once the virus is suppressed, autoimmunity disappears. In EIA, the control of virus infection is complicated by its capacity for antigenic modification. One wonders whether some of these changes could be due to phenotypic mixing of EIA isolates with endogenous horse viruses.

With endogenous, integrated viruses, a balance between normal and enhanced virus expression may be the deciding factor in the development of autoimmunity. The xenotropic virus is common in house mice where it is expressed in developing embryos, placentas, uteri, and in many normal organs throughout the lifetime of the mouse (Levy, 1975b, 1976a). Since this virus is found in high frequency and titer in the NZB mouse, its enhanced expression, on the one hand, may be the cause of NZB autoimmune disease. Limited expression of xenotropic virus, on the other hand, as in embryos, may be important for normal development and function of the cell. We have proposed that the endogenous C-type viruses represent one of the regulators of maturation (embryogenesis and differentiation) and the aging processes (autoimmune disease and cancer) (Fig. 4) (Levy, 1976a). The neutralizing factor, associated with mouse lipoproteins, would affect these natural life processes by interacting with xenotropic virus antigen on the cell

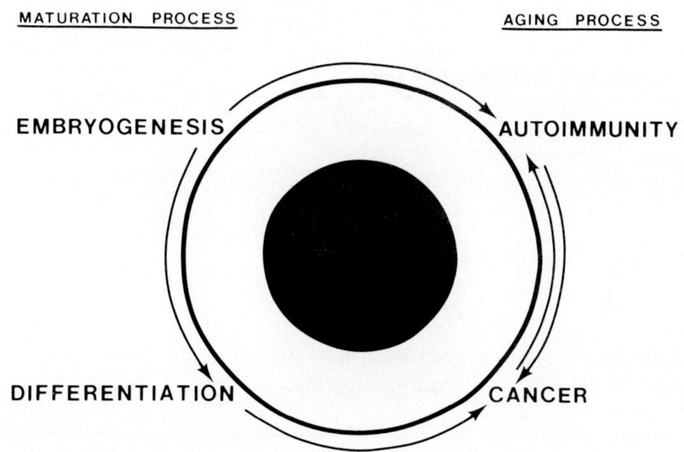

Fig. 4. Endogenous C-type viruses may be positive regulators in early and late stages of development. They may be involved in normal maturation (e.g., embryogenesis, differentiation) as well as aging processes such as autoimmune disease and cancer.

surface. A similar mechanism has been suggested for the influence of protein hormones on cell function (Robinson *et al.*, 1971). It is interesting that lipoproteins with biologic activity at the cell surface have been described in human systems. Goldstein and Brown (1974) reported the ability of a low-density lipoprotein to interact with normal cultured human cells and stop cholesterol synthesis. Cells from subjects with inherited hypercholesterolemia lack receptors for this specific lipoprotein. Chisari and Edgington (1975) have described a rosette-inhibiting factor which attaches to thymocytes and prevents E-rosette formation and diminishes the response of these cells in mixed lymphocyte reactions. This factor is associated with β-lipoproteins found in sera of adult men with acute viral hepatitis B infection. These lipoproteins may be interacting with virus receptors on the cell surfaces.

Studies of animal models suggest three general mechanisms for induction of autoimmunity by C-type viruses: (1) T cell enhancement, (2) T cell suppression, and (3) neoantigen expression on the cell surface (Table XIII). In the first situation, infection of T cells by the virus enhances its cytotoxicity for cells expressing the virus (Proffitt *et al.*, 1973; Zinkernagel and Doherty, 1974; Schrader *et al.*, 1975). In the second situation, T cells infected by virus are suppressed, leading to enhanced autoantibody production by the B cells (Allison *et al.*, 1971; Van Loghem, 1965). Neonatal thymectomy in mice and rabbits has demonstrated that early loss of T function can lead to

TABLE XIII

C-Type Viruses and the Immune System

Mechanism	Immune reaction	Effect
1. Infection of T cells	Enhancement of T cell response	Cytotoxicity
2. Infection of T cells	Suppression of T cell response; Enhancement of B cell response	Increased autoantibody production
3. Virus antigen expression on cell surface	Enhanced cellular and humoral response	Cytoxicity and increased production

autoantibody production (Sutherland *et al.*, 1965; Yunis *et al.*, 1969). Neonatal thymectomy also increases autoimmune thyroiditis and autoantibody production in obese strain (OS) chickens (Wick *et al.*, 1974). However, T cell dysfunction does not always give rise to autoimmunity. In certain diseases with depressed T cell function, such as sarcoidosis, no increase in circulating autoantibodies has been observed (James *et al.*, 1975).

The third mechanism can be summarized by the following steps (Fig. 5): exogenous infection or a genetic predisposition for increased endogenous production of C-type viruses places virus antigens on the cell surface (step 1). By heterogenization, or the Lindenmann effect, the host mounts an anti-viral and anti-cell response, illustrated by cellular and humoral responses, as well as by increased levels of neutralizing factor (step 2). Increased T cell cytotoxicity results (step 3) and leads to tissue destruction (step 4) (see mechanisms 1 and 2, Table XIII). A thymectomy-like syndrome would result (step 5). As noted above, B cells would be released from suppressor T cell control and produce increased levels of autoantibodies (step 6). Anti-thymic antibodies observed, may result from the cellular or humoral response. The hypergammaglobulinemia (step 6) includes antibodies to nucleic acids (step 7) and viruses (step 13). The former may represent a reaction to intermediate steps in the replication of the C-type virus (Talal *et al.*, 1971); viruses may also initiate these anti-nucleic acid autoantibodies secondary to cell destruction (steps 8, 15). LE cells become evident (step 9), and circulating immune complexes accumulate in the kidney (step 10), producing IC nephritis (step 11).

Some of the renal lesions might even result from a direct action of antiviral factors with kidney cells producing the virus. Since all mouse strains probably contain xenotropic viruses, we have raised the question whether most pathogenic viral immune complexes result from reaction of the host to enhanced endogenous xenotropic and not ecotropic virus expression. By phenotypic mixing, the ecotropic virus may increase the xenotropic virus antigen load and give rise to IC nephritis.

The hemolytic anemia observed in all these animal models, as well as the thrombocytopenia in canine lupus, could result from virus expression on these cells (steps 12–14). As noted previously, Rauscher virus antigens on mouse erythrocytes induced generalized anti-RBC antibodies. In EIA, the presence of a virus antigen on red cells appears related to the enhanced hemolysis resulting from either C3 attachment to virus–antibody complexes or to increased phagocytosis.

Autosensitization to particulate cell fragments released during tissue destruction may also induce autoantibody production and its pathological effects (steps 8, 15). Finally, the neutralizing factor in increased titer may contribute to this autoimmune disease by enhanced interaction with virus-producing cells (step 16) and with the virus itself (step 17).

One should consider as well the possible role of the macrophage in autoimmunity. Several viral diseases, in which circulating immune complexes and autoantibodies are found, involve viruses which replicate in macrophages. These include Aleutian disease virus of mink, lactic dehydrogenase virus, EIA, and perhaps, LCM. It is interesting that xenotropic virus is not spontaneously produced by macrophages from NZB hybrid mice

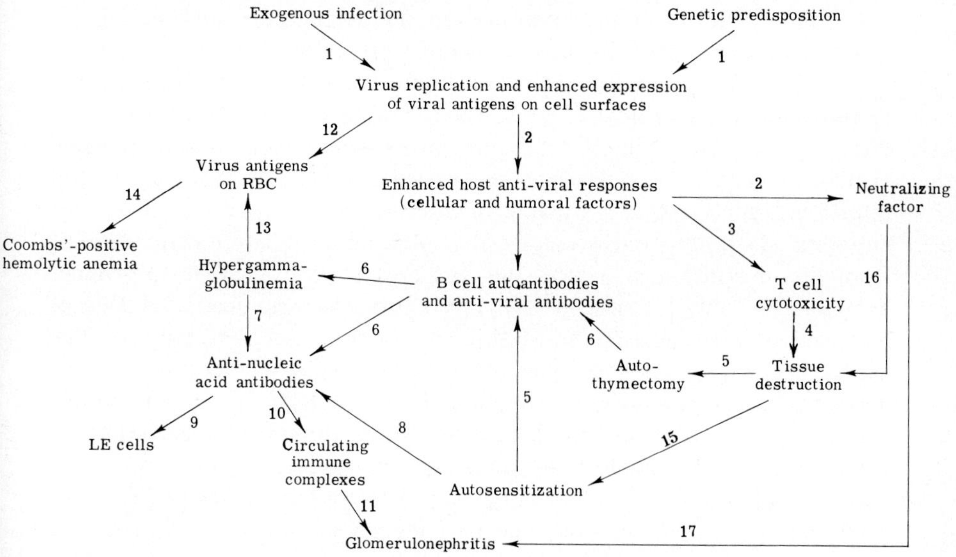

Fig. 5. Possible role of C-type viruses in autoimmune disease.

(Levy, 1974). Greenwood (1968) ascribed the low incidence of SLE in the tropics, compared to the black population in the United States, to the ubiquity of malaria. He and co-workers have shown a significant delay in the NZB disease by infecting the animals early in life with murine malaria (Greenwood *et al.*, 1970). While malaria may have a protective effect by enhancing phagocytosis of the reticuloendothelial system (Gabrielsen, 1974), it seems most likely that the parasite suppresses this macrophage function. Recently, we have studied the effect of low calorie and low phenylalanine diet on the immune complex nephritis of (NZB $\times$ NZW)F_1 mice (Gardner *et al.*, 1977). As has been reported (Dubois and Strain, 1973; Fernandes *et al.*, 1976), the experimental mice had significantly less IC disease than the controls. What was surprising was the lack of effect these diets had on virus production, levels of virus-neutralizing factor, and titers of anti-viral immunoglobulins and anti-nucleic acid antibodies. Humoral antibodies did not appear to be the chief factor in the pathogenesis of nephritis. Diet deficiencies have been shown to affect macrophage function (Coovadia and Soothill, 1976). Conceivably, the etiology of IC nephritis resides in the macrophages which are modified by viral infection. Further work with this cell population seems warranted.

IX. CONCLUSIONS AND SUMMARY

Chronic viral infection, abnormal immunoregulation, and permissive genes have been cited as factors leading to autoimmunity (Datta and Schwartz, 1974). Autoantibodies in limited quantity can be found in disease-free men and mice (Peterson and Makinodan, 1972); they may, in fact, be important in normal life processes. Since autoimmunelike symptoms develop in patients recovering from viral disease, several infectious agents may be capable of altering the immune system so this autoantibody production is enhanced. Autoimmune syndromes may result from the integration of a virus into the host genome and the subsequent expression of only its antigens. Thymic injury and structural alteration of host cell antigens caused by viral infection may also be involved. The genetic makeup of the host, however, would be the key determinant to the development of this disease complex. If the animal is not susceptible genetically to enhanced virus expression or horizontal virus infection, or cannot respond immunologically to a virus antigen or virus-modified host antigens, autoimmunity would not occur. The sporadic cases of SLE suggest that if a common infectious or endogenous agent is involved, the response of an individual to this agent varies. The correlation of certain HLA antigens with autoimmune syndromes supports the conclusion that genetic factors determine the susceptibility of individuals to the development of these diseases (McDevitt and Bodmer, 1974; Feltkamp *et al.*, 1974; Goldberg *et al.*, 1976).

Observations in animal model systems suggest that chronic C-type virus infection may be responsible for autoimmune disease in many animal species including human. These viruses may enter exogenously or be inherited as endogenous agents as illustrated in mice. In mouse strains, in fact, limited virus expression, may be necessary for normal development, whereas abnormally high production may lead to autoimmunity. Proper balance in the intracellular regulation of this virus and/or virus antigen expression would, therefore, be a means of prevention of the murine-type disease.

C-type viruses have been observed in the trophoblast layer of human placentas (Kalter *et al.*, 1973; Vernon *et al.*, 1974; Imamura *et al.*, 1976; Levy, 1975b), particularly in multiparous women (M. L. Vernon, personal communication). The developing embryo is very similar to a grafted tissue. Recognition of C-type viruses at the trophoblast layer may be indicative of a mild GVHR in this tissue between maternal and fetal antigens. Production of murine xenotropic virus is selectively enhanced in the spleens of mice undergoing a GVHR, and after lymphocyte stimulation (Sherr *et al.*, 1974; Levy *et al.*, 1977; Moroni *et al.*, 1975). The placental viruses, such as mouse X-tropic viruses, may represent immunologic agents or results of cell–cell interactions that are needed for embryogenesis and normal development (Levy, 1976a). Autoimmune disease, then, would represent an extreme of this natural process in which an enhanced reaction with self-antigens (e.g., endogenous viruses) occurs. Since the human placental virus is seen in small quantity and does not spread through the tissue, we believe it represents the human xenotropic virus. The observations in NZB mice, therefore, may be very applicable to man.

Epidemiologic data suggest that, similar to NZB mice, genetic factors are involved in human SLE. Family and twin studies confirm the inherited nature of this disease, but environmental factors such as a virus could also be involved (Phillips, 1975; Siegel and Lee, 1973; Block *et al.*, 1975). Antinuclear factors and anti-lymphocyte antibodies have been found in patients with SLE (Pincus *et al.*, 1969; Terasaki *et al.*, 1970). The high incidence of lymphocytotoxic antibodies in close household contacts of SLE patients (De Horatius and Messner, 1975) suggests exogenous transmission of an infectious agent. Double-stranded RNA, as well as nucleic acid antibodies, have been recovered from SLE kidneys which show the pathological changes of immune complex nephritis (Tan *et al.*, 1966). Moreover, the branched tubular structures observed in cells from patients with SLE (Chou, 1967; Fresco, 1970; Goodman *et al.*, 1973; Gyorkey *et al.*, 1969;

Kawano *et al.*, 1969), though not actual virus particles (Pincus *et al.*, 1970), are often found in cells infected by viruses.

The clarification of these observations and their interpretation lies in further research, primarily in animal model systems, where manipulation of the experimental design is possible and the genetic makeup of the host is well understood. Despite the failure thus far to isolate a C-type virus from tissues of patients with SLE (Phillips, 1975; Phillips *et al.*, 1976; J. A. Levy, unpublished data), the findings cited above, as well as the detection of viral antigens in SLE kidneys (see Section VII,B), encourages us to continue to consider that a C-type virus is involved in this disease.

ACKNOWLEDGMENTS

Research by the author cited in this chapter was supported by NCI USPHS Grant CA 13086, NCI Contract N01 CP 43381 and a grant from the Council for Tobacco Research. The author is recipient of Research Career Development Award No. 5 K04 CA 70990 from the National Cancer Institute.

REFERENCES

Aaronson, S. A., and Stephenson, J. R. (1973). *Proc. Natl. Acad. Sci. U.S.A.* **70,** 2055–2058.

Aaronson, S. A., and Stephenson, J. R. (1974). *Proc. Natl. Acad. Sci. U.S.A.* **71,** 1957–1961.

Allison, A. C., Denman, A. M., and Barnes, R. D. (1971). *Lancet* **2,** 135–140.

Alpert, E., Isselbacher, K. J., and Schur, P. H. (1971). *N. Engl. J. Med.* **285,** 185–189.

Andersen, P., and Andersen, H. K. (1975). *Clin. Exp. Immunol.* **22,** 22–29.

Arnstein, P., Levy, J. A., Oshiro, L. S., Price, P. J., Suk, W., and Lennette, E. H. (1974). *J. Natl. Cancer Inst.* **53,** 1787–1792.

Baldwin, R. W. (1973). *Adv. Cancer Res.* **18,** 1–75.

Baltimore, D. (1970). *Nature* (*London*) **226,** 1209–1211.

Barbieri, D., Belehradek, J., and Barski, G. (1971). *Int. J. Cancer* **7,** 364–371.

Benveniste, R. E., Lieber, M. M., and Todaro, G. J. (1974). *Proc. Natl. Acad. Sci. U.S.A.* **71,** 602–606.

Bernhard, W. (1960). *Cancer Res.* **20,** 712.

Bielschowsky, M., Helyer, B. J., and Howie, J. B. (1959). *Proc. Univ. Otago Med. Sch.* **37,** 9–11.

Bittner, J. J. (1936). *Science* **84,** 162.

Block, S. R., Winfield, J. B., Locksin, M. D., D'Angelo, W. A., and Christina, C. L. (1975). *Am. J. Med.* **59,** 533–552.

Braverman, I. M. (1968). *J. Invest. Dermatol.* **50,** 483–499.

Burch, G. E., and Colcolough, H. L. (1969). *Ann. Intern. Med.* **71,** 963–970.
Burnet, F. M., and Holmes, C. M. (1964). *J. Pathol. Bacteriol.* **88,** 229–241.
Chang, K. S. S., Law, L. W., and Aoki, T. (1974). *J. Natl. Cancer Inst.* **52,** 777–784.
Charman, H. P., Bladen, S., Gilden, R. V., and Coggins, S. (1976). *J. Virol.* **19,** 1073–1079.
Chase, D. G., and Piko, L. (1973). *J. Natl. Cancer Inst.* **51,** 1971–1975.
Chattopadhyay, S. K., Lowy, D. R., Teich, N. M., Levine, A. S., and Rowe, W. P. (1974). *Proc. Natl. Acad. Sci. U.S.A.* **71,** 167–171.
Chisari, F. V., and Edgington, T. S. (1975). *J. Exp. Med.* **142,** 1092–1107.
Chou, S. M. (1967). *Science* **158,** 1453–1455.
Claude, A., Porter, K. R., and Pickels, E. G. (1947). *Cancer Res.* **7,** 421.
Coovadia, H. M., and Soothill, J. F. (1976). *Clin. Exp. Immunol.* **23,** 562–567.
Cox, K. O., and Keast, D. (1973). *J. Natl. Cancer Inst.* **50,** 941–946.
Cremer, N. E. (1967). *J. Immunol.* **99,** 71–81.
Crocker, B. P., Del Villano, B. C., Jensen, F. C., Lerner, R. A., and Dixon, F. J. (1974). *J. Exp. Med.* **140,** 1028.
Dacie, J. V. (1955). *Am. J. Med.* **18,** 810–821.
Datta, S. K., and Schwartz, R. S. (1974). *N. Engl. J. Med.* **291,** 1304–1305.
Datta, S. K., and Schwartz, R. S. (1976). *Transplant. Rev.* **31,** 44–78.
De Horatius, R. J., and Messner, R. P. (1975). *J. Clin. Invest.* **55,** 1254–1258.
Del Villano, B. C., Nave, B., and Croker, B. P. (1975). *J. Exp. Med.* **141,** 172–187.
De Vries, M. J., and Hijmans, W. (1967). *Immunology* **12,** 179.
Dixon, F. J., Oldstone, M. B., and Tonietti, G. (1971). *J. Exp. Med.* **134,** 65–71.
Dixon, J. A., Sugai, S., and Talal, N. (1975). *Clin. Exp. Immunol.* **19,** 347–354.
Dubois, E. L., and Strain, L. (1973). *Biochem. Med.* **7,** 336–342.
Dunn, T. B., and Green, A. W. (1966). *J. Natl. Cancer Inst.* **36,** 987–1002.
East, J., de Sousa, M. A., and Parrott, D. M. V. (1965). *Transplantation* **3,** 711–729.
East, J., Prosser, P. R., Holborrow, E. J., Holborrow, E. J., and Jaquet, H. (1967). *Lancet* **1,** 755–757.
Ellerman, V., and Bang, O. (1908). *Zentralbl. Bakteriol., Parasitenkol., Infektionskr. Hyg., Abt. 1: Orig.* **46,** 595.
Feltkamp, T. E. W., van den Berg-Loonen, P. M., Nijenhuis, L. E., Engelfriet, C. P., van Rossum, A. L., Van Loghem, J. J., and Oosterhuis, H. J. G. H. (1974). *Brit. Med. J.* (Jan–Feb) 131–133.
Fernandes, G., Yunis, E. J., and Good, R. A. (1976). *Proc. Natl. Acad. Sci. U.S.A.* **73,** 1279–1283.
Fox, R. R., Meier, H., Crary, D. D., Norberg, R. F., and Myers, D. D. (1971). *Oncology* **25,** 372–382.
Fresco, R. (1970). *N. Engl. J. Med.* **26,** 1231–1232.
Furth, J., Seibold, H. R., and Rathbone, R. R. (1933). *Am. J. Cancer* **19,** 521–604.
Gabrielsen, A. E. (1974). *Lancet* (Oct–Dec), 1116–1118.
Gallagher, R. E., Todaro, G. J., Smith, R. G., Livingston, D. M., and Gallo, R. C. (1974). *Proc. Natl. Acad. Sci. U.S.A.* **71,** 1309–1313.

Gallo, R. C., Miller, N. R., Saxinger, W. C., and Gillespie, D. (1973). *Proc. Natl. Acad. Sci. U.S.A.* **70,** 3219–3224.

Gardner, M. B., Dubois, E. L., Ihle, J. N., Talal, N., and Levy, J. A. (1977). *Nature,* (In press).

Geering, G., Hardy, W. D., Old, L. J., de Harven, E., and Brodey, R. S. (1968). *Virology* **36,** 678–707.

Ghaffar, A., and Playfair, J. H. L. (1971). *Clin. Exp. Immunol.* **8,** 479–490.

Gilden, R. V., Oroszlan, S., and Huebner, R. J. (1971). *Nature* (*London*), *New Biol.* **231,** 107–108.

Gilliland, B. D., Leddy, J. P., and Vaughn, J. H. (1970). *J. Clin. Invest.* **49,** 898–906.

Gleichmann, E., Gleichmann, H., and Schwartz, R. S. (1972). *J. Natl. Cancer Inst.* **49,** 793–804.

Gocke, D. J., Morgan, C., Lockshin, M., Hsu, K., Bombardieri, S., and Christian, C. L. (1970). *Lancet* **2,** 1149–1153.

Goldberg, M. A., Arnett, F. C., Bias, W. B., and Shulman, L. (1976). *Arthritis Rheum.* **19,** 129–132.

Goldstein, J. L., and Brown, M. S. (1974). *J. Biol. Chem.* **249,** 5153.

Goodman, J. R., Sylvester, R. A., Talal, N., and Tuffanelli, D. L. (1973). *Ann. Intern. Med.* **79,** 396–402.

Goodpasture, E. W. (1919). *Am. J. Med. Sci.* **158,** 863–870.

Greenberger, J. S., and Aaronson, S. A. (1973). *J. Natl. Cancer Inst.* **51,** 1935–1938.

Greenspan, J. S., Gutman, G. A., Talal, N., Weissman, I. L., and Sugai, S. (1974). *Clin. Immunol. Immunopathol.* **3,** 32–51.

Greenwood, B M. (1968). *Lancet* **2,** 380.

Greenwood, B. M., Herrick, E. M., and Voller, A. (1970). *Nature* (*London*) **226,** 266–267.

Gregoriades, A., and Old, L. J. (1969). *Virology* **37,** 189–202.

Gross, L. (1951). *Proc. Soc. Exp. Biol. Med.* **76,** 27–32.

Gross, L. (1954). *Blood* **9,** 557.

Gross, L., (1974). *Proc. Natl. Acad. Sci. U.S.A.* **71,** 2013.

Gyorkey, F., Min, K. W., Sincovics, J. G. and Gyorkey, P. (1969). *N. Engl. J. Med.* **280,** 333.

Haran-Ghera, N., and Kotler, M. (1968). *Bibl. Haematol.* (*Basel*) **31,** 70–72.

Haran-Ghera, N., Ben-Yaakov, M., Peled, A., and Bentwich, Z. (1973). *J. Natl. Cancer Inst.* **50,** 1227–1235.

Hartley, J. W., and Rowe, W. P. (1976). *J. Virol.* **19,** 19–25.

Helyer, B. J., and Howie, J. B. (1963). *Br. J. Haematol.* **9,** 119.

Henson, J. B., and McGuire, T. C. (1971). *Am. J. Clin. Pathol.* **56,** 306–314.

Henson, J. B., and McGuire, T. C. (1974). *Prog. Med. Virol.* **18,** 143–159.

Henson, J. B., McGuire, T. C., and Gorham, J. R. (1971). *Arch. Gesamte Virusforsch.* **35,** 385–391.

Henson, J. B., McGuire, T. C., Crawford, T. B., and Gorham, J. R. (1973). *Proc. Int. Conf. Equine Infect. Dis., 3rd, 1972* pp. 228–241.

Hicks, J. D. (1966). *J. Pathol. Bacteriol.* **91,** 479–486.

Hirsch, M. S., Allison, A. C., and Harvey, J. J. (1969). *Nature* (*London*) **223,** 739–740.

Hirsch, M. S., Black, P. H., Tracy, G. S., Leibowitz, S., and Schwartz, R. S. (1970). *Proc. Natl. Acad. Sci. U.S.A.* **67,** 1914–1917.

Hirsch, M. S., Phillips, S. M., Solnik, C. Black, P. H., Schwartz, R. S., and Carpenter, C. B. (1972). *Proc. Natl. Acad. Sci. U.S.A.* **69,** 1069–1072.

Holmes, M. C., and Burnet, F. M. (1963). *Ann. Intern. Med.* **59,** 265–276.

Holmes, M. C., and Burnet, F. M. (1964). *Heredity* **19,** 419–434.

Huebner, R. J., and Igel, H. J. (1971). *Perspect. Virol.* **7,** 55–71.

Huebner, R. J., and Todaro, G. J. (1969). *Proc. Natl. Acad. Sci. U.S.A.* **64,** 1087–1095.

Ihle, J. N., Yurnonic, M., Jr., and Hanna, M. G., Jr. (1973). *J. Exp. Med.* **138,** 194–208.

Ikeda, H., Pincus, T., Yoshiki, T., Strand, M., August, J. T., Boyse, E. A., and Mellors, R. C. (1974). *J. Virol.* **14,** 1274–1280.

Imamura, M., Phillips, P. E., and Mellors, R. C. (1976). *Ann. J. Pathol.* **83**(2), 383–394.

Ishitani, R. (1970). *Natl. Inst. Anim. Health Q.* **10,** Suppl., 1–28.

James, D. G., Neville, E., and Walker, A. (1975). *Amer. J. Med.* **59,** 388–394.

Kalter, S. S., Helmke, R. J., Heberling, R. L., Panigel, P., Fowler, A. K., Strickland, J. E., and Hellman, A. (1973)*J. Natl. Cancer Inst.* **50,** 1081–1084.

Kawano, K., Miller, L., and Kimmelstiel, P. (1969). *N. Engl. J. Med.* **281,** 1228–1229.

Kennel, S. J., and Feldman, J. D. (1976). *Cancer Res.* **36,** 200–208.

Kobayashi, K., and Kono, Y. (1967). *Natl. Inst. Anim. Health Q.* **7,** 8–20.

Kono, Y. (1969). *Natl. Inst. Anim. Health Q.* **9,** 1–9.

Kono, Y. (1973). *Proc. Int. Conf. Equine Infect. Dis., 3rd, 1972,* pp. 242–254.

Kono, Y., and Kobayashi, K. (1966). *Natl. Inst. Anim. Health Q.* **6,** 204–207.

Kono, Y., and Kobayashi, K. (1967). *Natl. Inst. Anim. Health Q.* **7,** 138–144.

Kono, Y., and Yoshino, T. (1974). *Natl. Inst. Anim. Health Q.* **14,** 155–162.

Kono, Y., Kobayashi, K., and Fukunaga, Y. (1970). *Natl. Inst. Anim. Health Q.* **10,** 113–122.

Kono, Y., Kobayashi, K., and Fukunaga, Y. (1971). *Natl. Inst. Anim. Health Q.* **11,** 11–20.

Kono, Y., Kobayashi, K., and Fukunaga, Y. (1973). *Arch. Gesamte Virusforsch.* **4,** 1–10.

Kouttab, N. M., and Jutila, J. W. (1972). *J. Immunol.* **108,** 591–595.

Krontiris, T. G., Soeiro, R., and Fields, B. M. (1973). *Proc. Natl. Acad. Sci. U.S.A.* **70,** 2549–2553.

Kruger, G. (1971). *Verh. Dtsch. Ges. Pathol.* **55,** 200–204.

Lee, J. C., and Ihle, J. N. (1975). *J. Natl. Cancer Inst.* **55,** 831–838.

Lee, J. C., Hanna, M. G., Jr., Ihle, J. N., and Aaronson, S. A. (1974). *J. Virol.* **14,** 773–781.

Leong, J. C., Kane, J. P., Oleszko, O. and Levy, J. A. (1977) *Proc. Natl. Acad. Sci. U.S.A.* **74,** 276–280.

Lerner, R. A., Wilson, C. B., Del Villano, B. C., McCohahey, P. J., and Dixon, F. J. (1976). *J. Exp. Med.* **143,** 151–166.
Levy, J. A. (1973a). *Science* **182,** 1151–1153.
Levy, J. A. (1973b). *Abstr., Am. Soc. Microbiol.* p. 222.
Levy, J. A. (1974). *Am. J. Clin. Pathol.* **62,** 258–280.
Levy, J. A. (1975a). *Nature (London)* **253,** 140–142.
Levy, J. A. (1975b). *J. Rheumatol.* **2,** 135–148.
Levy, J. A. (1975c). *Proc. Am. Assoc. Cancer Res.* **16,** 190 (abstr.).
Levy, J. A. (1976a). *Biomedicine* **24,** 84–93.
Levy, J. A., (1977a). *Microbiology,* 559–563.
Levy, J. A. (1977b). *Virology* **77,** 797–810.
Levy, J. A., and Huebner, R. J. (1970). *Nature (London)* **222,** 949–950.
Levy, J. A., and Pincus, T. (1970). *Science* **170,** 326–327.
Levy, J. A., Ihle, J. N., Oleszko, O., and Barnes, R. D. (1975a). *Proc. Natl. Acad. Sci. U.S.A.* **72,** 5071–5075.
Levy, J. A., Kazan, P., Varnier, O., and Kleiman, H. (1975b). *J. Virol.* **16,** 844–853.
Levy, J. A., Datta, S., and Schwartz, R. S. (1977). *Clin. Immunol. Immunopathol.* **7,** 262–268.
Lewis, R. M., and Schwartz, R. S. (1971). *J. Exp. Med.* **134,** 417–438.
Lewis, R. M., Schwartz, R., and Henry, W. B. (1965). *Blood* **25,** 143–160.
Lewis, R. M., Andre-Schwartz, J., and Harris, G. S. (1973). *Clin. Invest.* **52,** 1893–1907.
Lewis, R. M., Tannenberg, W., Smith, C., and Schwartz, R. S. (1974). *Nature (London)* **252,** 78–79.
Lilly, F., and Pincus, T. (1973). *Adv. Cancer Res.* **17,** 231–277.
Lindenmann, J. (1974). *Biochim. Biophys. Acta* **49,** 355–375.
Lindenmann, J., and Klein, P. A. (1967). *J. Exp. Med.* **126,** 93–108.
McCoy, J. L., Fefer, A., Ting, R. C., and Glynn, J. P. (1972). *Cancer Res.* **32,** 1671–1678.
McDevitt, H. O., and Bodmer, W. F. (1974). *Lancet* **1,** 1269–1275.
McGuire, T. C., Henson, J. B., and Burger, D. (1969). *Immunology* **103,** 293–299.
McGuire, T. C., Van Hoosier, G. L., and Henson, J. B. (1971). *Immunology* **107,** 1738–1744.
Mellors, R. C. (1966). *Blood* **27,** 435–448.
Mellors, R. C., and Huang, C. Y. (1966). *J. Exp. Med.* **124,** 1031–1038.
Mellors, R. C., and Huang, C. Y. (1967). *J. Exp. Med.* **126,** 53–65.
Mellors, R. C., and Mellors, J. W. (1976). *Proc. Natl. Acad. Sci. U.S.A.* **73,** 223–237.
Mellors, R. C., Aoki, T., and Huebner, R. J. (1969). *J. Exp. Med.* **129,** 1045–1062.
Mellors, R. C., Shirai, T., Aoki, T., Huebner, R. J., and Krawczynski, K. (1971). *J. Exp. Med.* **133,** 113–132.
Metcalf, D. (1961). *Br. J. Cancer* **15,** 769–779.
Monier, J. C., Thivolet, J., and Sepetijian, M. (1969). *Ann. Inst. Pasteur, Paris* **116,** 646–656.
Monier, J. C., Thivolet, J., Beyvin, A. J., Czyba, J. C., Schmitt, D., and Salussola, D. (1971). *Pathol. Eur.* **6,** 357–383.

Moroni, C., Schumann, G., Robert-Guroff, M., Suter, E. R., and Martin, D. (1975). *Proc. Natl. Acad. Sci. U.S.A.* **72,** 535–538.

Myers, B. D., Griffel, B., Naveh, D., Jankielowitz, T. and Klajman, A. (1973). *Am. J. Clin. Pathol.* **59,** 222–228.

Nakajima, H. (1973). *Proc. Int. Conf. Equine Infect. Dis., 3rd, 1972* pp. 162–174.

Nakajima, H., Tajima, M., Tanaka, S., and Ushimi, C. (1969a). *Arch. Gesamte Virusforsch.* **28,** 348–360.

Nakajima, H., Tanaka, S., and Ushimi, C. (1969b). *Arch. Gesamte Virusforsch* **26,** 389–394.

Nakajima, H., Tanaka, S., and Ushimi, C. (1970). *Arch. Gesamte Virusforsch.* **31,** 273–280.

Nakajima, H., Kono, Y., and Ushimi, C. (1971). *J. Immunol.* **107,** 889–894.

Nakajima, H., Yoshino, T., and Ushimi, C. (1974). *Infect. Immunol.* **10,** 667–668.

Notkins, A. L. (1971). *J. Exp. Med.* **134,** 41–51.

Notkins, A. L., Mergenhagen, S. E., and Howard, R. J. (1970). *Annu. Rev. Microbiol.* **24,** 525–538.

Nowinski, R. C., and Klein, P. A. (1975). *J. Immunol.* **115,** 1261–1268.

Obara, J., and Nakajima, H. (1961). *Jpn. J. Vet. Sci.* **23,** 247–253.

Officer, J. E., Tecson, N., Estes, J. D., Fontanilla, E., Rongey, R. W., and Gardner, M. B. (1973). *Science* **181,** 945–947.

Oie, H. K., Russell, E. K., Dotson, J. H., Rhoads, J. M., and Gazdar, A. F. (1976). *J. Natl. Cancer Inst.* **56,** 423–425.

Oki, Y. (1961). *Tohoku J. Agric. Res.* **12,** 91–105.

Oldstone, M. B. A., and Dixon, F. J. (1969). *J. Exp. Med.* **129,** 483–499.

Oldstone, M. B. A., Aoki, T., and Dixon, F. J. (1972). *Proc. Natl. Acad. Sci. U.S.A.* **69,** 134–138.

Oshiro, L. S., Levy, J. A., Riggs, J. L., and Lennette, E. H. (1977). *J. Gen. Virol.* **35,** 317–323.

Panem, S., Prochownik, E. V., Reale, F. R., and Kirsten, W. H. (1975). *Science* **189,** 297–299.

Panem, S., Ordonez, N. G., Kirsten, W. H., Katz, A. I., and Spargo, B. H. (1976). *N. Engl. J. Med.* **295,** 470–475.

Papas, T. S., Dahlberg, J. E., and Sonstegard, R. A. (1976). *Nature (London)* **261,** 506–508.

Pascal, R. R., Koss, M. N., and Kassel, R. L. (1973). *Lab. Invest.* **29,** 159–165.

Perryman, D. E., McGuire, T. C., Banks, R. L., and Henson, J. B. (1971). *Immunology* **106,** 1074–1078.

Peterson, W. J., and Makinodan, T. (1972). *Clin. Exp. Immunol.* **12,** 273–290.

Phillips, P. E. (1975). *Ann. Intern. Med.* **83,** 709–715.

Phillips, P. E., and Christian, C. L. (1973). *Ann. Rheum. Dis.* **32,** 450–456.

Phillips, P. E., Hargrave, R., Stewart, E., and Sarkar, N. H. (1976). *Ann. Rheum. Dis.* **35,** 422–428.

Pincus, T., Schur, P. H., Rose, J. A., Decker, J. L., and Talal, N. (1969). *N. Engl. J. Med.* **281,** 701–705.

Pincus, T., Blacklow, N. R., Grimley, P. M., and Bellanti, J. A. (1970). *Lancet* **2,** 1058–1061.

Pisciotta, A. V., and Hinz, J. E. (1957). *Am. J. Pathol.* **27,** 619.

Plotz, P. H. (1975). *Med. Clin. North Am.* **59,** 869–876.

Popper, H., and Mackay, I. R. (1972). *Lancet* **1,** 1161–1164.

Porter, D. D., Larsen, A. E., and Porter, H. G. (1969). *J. Exp. Med.* **130,** 575–589.

Proffitt, M. R., Hirsch, M. S., and Black, P. H. (1973). *Science* **182,** 821–823.

Rasheed, S., Gardner, M. B., and Chan, E. (1976). *J. Virol.* **19,** 13–18.

Recher, L., Tanaka, T., Sykes, J. A., Yumoto, T., Seman, G., Young, L., and Dmuchowski, L. (1966). *Natl. Cancer Inst., Monogr.* **22,** 459–479.

Reilly, C. A., and Shloss, G. T. (1971). *Cancer Res.* **34,** 841–846.

Robinson, G. A., Butcher, R. W., and Sutherland, E. W. (1971). "Cyclic AMP." Academic Press, New York.

Rous, P. (1911). *J. Am. Med. Assoc.* **56,** 198.

Rowe, W. P. (1973). *Cancer Res.* **33,** 3061–3068.

Rowe, W. P., Pugh, W. E., and Hartley, J. W. (1970). *Virology* **42,** 1136–1139.

Russell, P. J., Hicks, J. D., Boston, L. E., and Abbott, A. (1970). *Clin. Exp. Immunol.* **6,** 227–239.

Schaap, O. L., de Groot, E. R., and Van Loghem, J. J. (1975). *Pathol. Microbiol.* **42,** 171–187.

Schrader, J. W., Cunningham, B. A., and Edelman, G. M. (1975). *Virus Immunol.* **72,** 5066–5070.

Schwartz, R. S. (1975). *N. Engl. J. Med.* **293,** 132–135.

Schwartz, R. S., and Beldotti, L. (1965). *Science* **149,** 1511–1514.

Sherr, C. J., and Todaro, G. J. (1974). *Proc. Natl. Acad. Sci. U.S.A.* **71,** 4703–4707.

Sherr, C. J., Lieber, M. M., and Todaro, G. J. (1974). *Cell* **1,** 55–58.

Shirai, T., and Mellors, R. C. (1971). *Proc. Natl. Acad. Sci. U.S.A.* **68,** 1412–1415.

Siegel, M., and Lee, S. L. (1973). *Semin. Arthritis Rheum.* **3,** 1–54.

Silagi, S., Beju, D., Wrathall, J., and de Harven, E. (1972). *Proc. Natl. Acad. Sci. U.S.A.* **69,** 3443–3447.

Simpson, R. W., and Iinuma, M. (1975). *Proc. Natl. Acad. Sci. U.S.A.* **72,** 3230–3234.

Squire, R. A. (1968). *Blood* **32,** 157–169.

Stanley, N. F., and Walters, N. I. M. (1966). *Lancet* **1,** 962–963.

Steeves, R. A., Strand, M., and August, J. T. (1974). *J. Virol.* **14,** 187–189.

Strand, M., and August, J. T. (1973). *J. Biol. Chem.* **214,** 5627–5633.

Strand, M., and August, J. T. (1974a). *J. Virol.* **13,** 171–180.

Strand, M., and August, J. T. (1974b). *J. Virol.* **14,** 1585–1596.

Sutherland, D. E. R., Archer, O. K., Peterson, R. D. A., Eckert, E., and Good, R. A. (1965). *Lancet* **1,** 130–133.

Sutherland, J. C., and Mardiney, M. R. (1973). *J. Natl. Cancer Inst.* **50,** 633–644.

Svet-Moldavsky, G. J., Mkheidze, D. M., Liozner, A. L., and Bykovsky, A. P. (1968). *Nature* (*London*) **217,** 102–104.

Tajima, M., Nakajima, H., and Ito, Y. (1969). *J. Virol.* **4,** 521–527.

Talal, N., and Steinberg, A. D. (1974). *Curr. Top. Microbiol. Immunol.* **64,** 79–103.

Talal, N., Steinberg, A. D., Jacobs, M. E., Chused, T. M., and Gazdar, A. F. (1971). *J. Exp. Med.* **134,** 52s–64s.

Tan, E. M., Schur, P. H., Carr, R. I., and Kunkel, G. (1966). *J. Clin. Invest.* **45,** 1732–1740.

Temin, H. M. (1971). *J. Natl. Cancer Inst.* **46,** III. (Feb.)

Temin, H. M., and Mizutani, S. (1970). *Nature* (*London*) **226,** 1211–1213.

Terasaki, P. I., Mottironi, V. D., and Barnett, E. V. (1970). *N. Engl. J. Med.* **283,** 724–728.

Thomas, L. (1964). *N. Engl. J. Med.* **270,** 1157–1159.

Tihon, C., and Green, M. (1973). *Nature* (*London*), *New Biol.* **244,** 227–231.

Todaro, G. J., and Gallo, R. C. (1973). *Nature* (*London*) **244,** 206–209.

Todaro, G. J., Arnstein, P., Parks, W. P., Lennette, E. H., and Huebner, R. J. (1973). *Proc. Natl. Acad. Sci. U.S.A.* **70,** 859–862.

Tonietti, G., Oldstone, M. B., and Dixon, F. J. (1970). *J. Exp. Med.* **132,** 89–109.

Vallée, H., and Carré, H. (1904). *C.R. Hebd. Seances Acad. Sci.* **139,** 331–333.

Van Loghem, J. J. (1965). *Ser. Haematol.* **9,** 1–16.

Vernon, M. L., Lane, W. T., and Huebner, R. J. (1973). *J. Natl. Cancer Inst.* **51,** 1171–1175.

Vernon, M. L., McMahon, M. J., and Hackett, J. J. (1974). *J. Natl. Cancer Inst.* **52,** 987–989.

Wanebo, H. J., Gallmeier, W. M., Boyse, E. A. *et al.* (1966). *Science* **154,** 901–903.

Weir, D. M. (1967). Lancet **2,** 1071–1073.

Wick, G., Sundick, R. S., and Albini, B. (1974). *Clin. Immunol. Immunopathol.* **3,** 272–300.

Williams, R. C., Kenyon, A. J., and Huntley, C. C. (1968). *Blood* **31,** 522–535.

Wilson, C. B., and Smith, R. C. (1972). *Ann. Intern. Med.* **76,** 91–94.

Witebsky, E., Kite, J. H., Jr., Wick, G., and Cole, R. K. (1969). *J. Immunol.* **103,** 708–715.

Wollmann, R. L., Pang, E. J., Evans, A. E., and Kirsten, W. H. (1970). *Cancer Res.* **30,** 1003–1010.

Yoshiki, T., Mellors, R. C., Strand, M., and August, J. T. (1974). *J. Exp. Med.* **140,** 1011–1027.

Yumoto, T., and Dmochowski, L. (1967). *Med. Rec. Annu.* **60,** 133–139.

Yunis, E. J., Teague, P. O., Stutman, O., and Good, R. A. (1969). *Lab. Invest.* **20,** 46–61.

Zavada, J. (1972). *J. Gen. Virol.* **15,** 183–191.

Zhdanov, V. M. (1975). *Nature* (*London*) **256,** 471–473.

Ziff, M. (1971). *Ann. Intern. Med.* **75,** 951–958.

Zinkernagel, R. M., and Doherty, P. C. (1974). *Nature* (*London*) **251,** 547–548.

Zuelzer, W. W., Stulberg, C. S., Page, R. H., Teruya, J., and Brough, A. J. (1966). *Transfusion* **6,** 438–461.

Part IV

CLINICAL ASPECTS

Chapter 15

Infection and Autoimmunity

RALPH C. WILLIAMS, JR.

I. INTRODUCTION

During the last two decades, it has become abundantly clear that various infectious processes may be associated with autoimmune reactions. Indeed, examples of autoantibodies produced during the course of clear-cut, well-defined bacterial or viral infections, provide support, although mostly by analogy, for the idea that certain diseases of unknown etiology may, indeed, be generated secondary to infectious agents as yet poorly defined. Examples of such diseases could be listed as disorders such as Hodgkin's disease (lymphocytotoxic antibody), systemic lupus erythematosus (anti-DNA antibody), or even rheumatoid arthritis (rheumatoid factor).

Several basic mechanisms may be operating whereby an infectious disease actually induces apparent autoimmune reactivity. During the course of an infection, tissues or normal body constituents may become damaged or altered secondary to release of bacterial or viral products or more often as a result of the general inflammatory reaction induced by the infectious agent itself. Thus, lysosomal enzymes released after polymorphonuclear leukocyte phagocytosis of bacterial products (Weissman, 1964; Weissman and Dukor, 1970) could alter autologous γ-globulins to such an extent that they might not be recognized as self and, thus, subsequently produce anti-γ-globulins or various rheumatoid factors. Antibodies with specificity for sites on γ-globulin revealed or exposed after proteolytic enzyme digestion have been extensively characterized and may occur in association with various infections (Osterland *et al.*, 1963; Waller, 1967; Lawrence and Williams, 1967; Mandy, 1967). In like manner, bacterial product-stimulated lysosomal enzyme release could alter other self-constituents, such as cell-surface antigens themselves, inducing apparent self-directed antibodies against granulocytes or various granulocyte precursors (Mahmoud *et al.*, 1974; Boxer and Stossel, 1974; Boxer *et al.*, 1972). The vast number of chronic infectious disease states known to be associated with rheumatoid factor production, for example, actually could be taken as evidence that production of antibodies to autologous γ-globulins may be a normal immune response engendered in the host during many reversible infectious diseases. Though not yet substantiated by clear experimental or clinical data, it seems possible that certain autoantibodies, such as rheumatoid factors or immunoconglutinin (Ingram, 1959a,b), may actually function in a helper or protective way, perhaps shifting the balance in favor of successful host responses.

Aside from the obvious idea of infection altering autologous self-markers on tissue or circulating proteins, several other possible mechanisms working towards autoimmunity during infection can be postulated. Recently, considerable attention has been directed at a detailed analysis of the importance of balance in the "immunostat" or regulatory setting governing various immune reactions. Thus, clear definition and understanding of the importance of both helper and suppressor T-cell populations has begun to emerge (Allison *et al.*, 1971; Allison, 1973). Evidence for defective suppressor cell function in NZB mouse disease (Chused *et al.*, 1973; Hardin *et al.*, 1973; Barthold *et al.*, 1974) and the concomitant amplification of autoreactive mechanisms might be explained by direct infection and, thus, functional impairment of suppressor T cells. In like manner, the striking elevations of immunoglobulins, anti-self-directed antibodies, and immune derangement recorded in lepromatous leprosy might be a result of direct infection, intracellular replication, and consequent damage to suppressor T cells in this disorder. A similar situation may obtain in the case of infectious mononucleosis where lymphoid cell increases in the face of an acute or subacute intracellular viral infection are often associated with a host of autoantibodies. Thus, intracellular parasitism by the EB virus of suppressor T cells could be involved. At present, however, there is no direct evidence to support such a hypothesis. In the case of lepromatous leprosy, there is already a considerable body of evidence suggesting that T cell functions are depressed in the face of a variety of autoantibodies possibly representing unbridled B cell hyperactivity. In similar fashion preferential intracellular specificity for either suppressor or helper cell populations may be an important feature in facilitating autoantibody reactions among a host of other infections characterized by intracellular replication, particularly with respect to chronic or subacute viral infections.

Finally, there are several features peculiar to a number of bacterial infections which may predispose to accentuating detectable autoimmune reactions. In particular, certain bacterial polysaccharides or cell wall products such as endotoxin, C polysaccharide, or myobacterial fractions are well known for their clear adjuvant effects (Freund and McDermott, 1942; Raffel and Forney, 1948; Johnson *et al.*, 1956; Neter, 1969). Thus, a normal or relatively low level of autoimmune reactivity may be amplified by adjuvants intrinsic to the particular infectious agent itself. Endotoxin, known to be a B cell mitogen in mice, can stimulate the formation of anti-DNA antibodies in a wide variety of mouse strains (Fournie *et al.*, 1974). Many other mechanisms may be operating in the way of an adjuvant effect to facilitate autoantibody formation. Thus, infection with lymphocytic choriomeningitis has been shown to accelerate DNA–anti-DNA immune complex disease in NZB mice (Tonietti *et al.*, 1970). Whether or not such superimposed viral infection acts in the true sense as an adjuvant or whether it functions to further depress intrinsic immunoregulatory control by further depleting suppressor cell function is not yet clear.

Finally, another possible mechanism involved in autoimmunity and infections may be classified under the category of bacterial mimicry. Several convincing lines of evidence have already been developed to support the idea that certain infectious agents may be preferentially capable of infecting a particular host since they share structures which are extremely similar in antigenic composition and immunologic constitution to those possessed by the host (Springer and Horton, 1964; Drach, 1973). Some evidence has now accumulated implicating this type of mechanism in the genesis of isoagglutinins (Springer and Horton, 1969), some urinary tract infections (Drach *et al.*, 1971), pneumococcal pneumonia (Reed *et al.*, 1974), and possibly in some parasitic infections such as schistosomiasis (Dean, 1974). A variation on this theme might, therefore, include the concept that slight antigenic differences between infecting bacteria or viruses and host cell surface markers, for instance, could set the stage for harmful cross-reactions capable of inducing substantial host damage. Of particular importance with regard to this concept is the incorporation of virally induced antigens into cell-surface markers during certain viral infections. Such a mechanism might be utilized to explain the occurrence of lymphocytotoxic antibodies after viral infections such as measles, varicella, or infectious mononucleosis (Mottironi and

TABLE I

Mechanisms by Which Autoimmune Reactions Are Induced by Various Infections

Basic Mechanism	Resulting autoantibody or autoimmune response	Possible example
I. Lysosomal enzyme release during phagocytosis or tissue damage produces alteration or denaturation of cell constituents or circulating protein.	Immunoconglutinin, pepsin agglutinators, rheumatoid factors	Subacute bacterial endocarditis
	Anti-lymphocyte antibody	Measles, varicella infection. Infectious mononucleosis
II. Infecting agent actually resides in suppressor T cells and/or activates helper T cells producing accentuation of normal background low-level autoimmune response	Anti-smooth muscle antibody	Cytomegalovirus infection
	Rheumatoid factor; anti-nuclear antibody	Lepromatous leprosy; infectious mononucleosis
III. Infecting agent bypasses ordinary immunologic control through production of adjuvant substances	Rheumatoid factors	Subacute bacterial endocarditis; pulmonary tuberculosis; long-standing brucellosis
IV. Infecting agent actually gains access to host by sharing of antigenic determinants on host cells; when immune response occurs to antigens close to, but not identical, tissue damage follows	Antibody to cardiac myocardial membranes or heart valve glycoprotein	Acute rheumatic fever

Terasaki, 1970; Kreisler *et al.*, 1971). This general concept and variations upon it have also evolved in the demonstration of cross-reactions between streptococcal antigens and cardiac muscle, heart valves, or myocardial cell membranes (Kaplan and Svec, 1964; Zabriskie, 1967; Goldstein *et al.*, 1968). Such bacterial mimicry cannot, by strict standards, be judged as true autoimmunity. However, the importance and prevalence of this type of mechanism remain to be completely identified and documented. Several of these possible categories of autoimmune reactions occurring in response to infections are outlined in Table I.

With these possible mechanisms in way of introduction, several types of autoantibody occurring in specific infectious disease states provide examples of well-documented autoimmune reactions.

II. RHEUMATOID FACTORS

Many chronic or subacute human infectious diseases are associated with the production of rheumatoid factors or anti-γ-globulin antibodies of diverse specificity. Representative infections accompanied by rheumatoid factor are listed in Table II. One of the most interesting of these is subacute bacterial endocarditis (SBE), where moderate to high titers of rheumatoid

TABLE II

Infections Known to Be Associated with Production of Rheumatoid Factors

Infection or disease state	Reference
Syphilis	Peltier and Christian, 1959
Lepromatous leprosy	Cathcart *et al.*, 1961
Tuberculosis	Singer *et al.*, 1962
Subacute bacterial endocarditis	Williams and Kunkel, 1962
Aleutian mink disease	Williams *et al.*, 1966
Malaria	Houba and Allison, 1966
Schistosomiasis	R. C. Williams, Jr. and J. D. Emmons, unpublished observations, 1975
Infectious mononucleosis	Kaplan, 1968
Kala-azar	Kunkel *et al.*, 1958
Visceral larva migrans	Huntley *et al.*, 1966
Infectious hepatitis, hepatitis (B)	Hoofnagle *et al.*, 1973
Influenza A	Svec and Dingle, 1965
Cytomegalovirus	Langenhuysen, 1971
Rubella	Johnson and Hall, 1958
Herpes zoster	Dresner and Trombly, 1959

factors have been documented in approximately half of the patients studied (Williams and Kunkel, 1962; Gutman *et al.*, 1972). Of note is the fact that no particular organism seems to be preferentially involved, and rheumatoid factor production has been noted in association with infections caused by *Staphylococcus aureus, Staphylococcus albus,* pneumococci, *Streptococcus viridans*, as well as numerous anerobic streptococci or fecal streptococci. Currently, it is felt that the disorder of subacute bacterial endocarditis represents a situation where the lesion engrafted as it is on heart valves and endocardium constantly bathed by the circulating blood is in an ideal site to provide rather constant infusion of bacterial products, whole bacteria, and their antigenic consitituents into the circulation. Clear documentation of the relatively low order of magnitude of the bacteremia associated with SBE has been provided by previous studies (Werner *et al.*, 1967). That an indolent rather than a rapidly overwhelming bacteremia exists may be an important feature in bacterial endocarditis, since it allows the host sufficient time to generate a broad spectrum of antibodies to various antigenic determinants related to the infecting organism.

Of particular interest is the finding that disappearance of rheumatoid factor frequently follows the successful antimicrobial treatment of the disease (Henney and Ishizaka, 1968). In general, rheumatoid factors associated with disorders other than rheumatoid arthritis show primary specificity for human rather than other species of γ-globulins. Thus, latex fixation tests may be strongly positive, whereas sensitized sheep cell tests using rabbit hemolysin coating indicator erythrocytes may be negative or weakly positive.

Of interest is the concomitant striking improvement of immune complex-mediated renal disease after successful therapy and transient maintenance dialysis in such patients (Perez *et al.*, 1976). Examples of striking interval decrements in rheumatoid factor after completion of antibiotic treatment for SBE are shown in Fig. 1. Of particular interest was the virtual disappearance of rheumatoid factor in a culture-negative individual studied by us and later shown at autopsy to have healed bacterial endocarditis (Williams and Kunkel, 1962). Similar findings have also been reported in studies by Gutman *et al.* (1972).

Most rheumatoid factors can be shown to have a spectrum of immunologic specificities towards different determinants present either on apparently native or unaltered autologous IgG or against minor modifications or alterations presumably produced by structural or conformational changes in IgG molecules engendered by their actual combination with their respective antigens. The principal antigenic site for reactivity of most rheumatoid factors appears to be located on the Fc portions of IgG. However, specificities for sites on L chains (Williams, 1964), $F(ab')_2$,

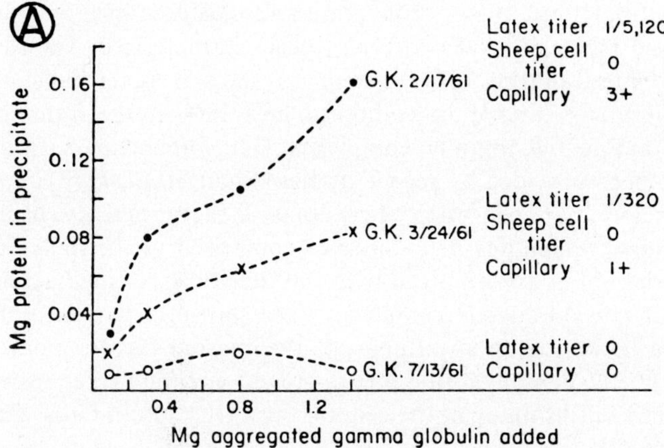

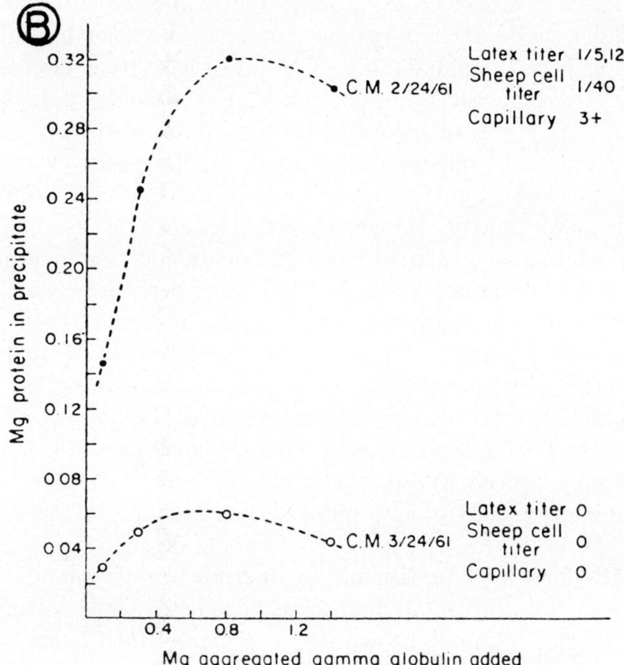

Fig. 1. (A) Change in precipitin curves and other measurement of rheumatoid factors in patient G. K. after treatment of the subacute bacterial endocarditis. (B) Change in precipitin curves and other measurement of rheumatoid factors in patient C. M. after treatment of the subacute bacterial endocarditis. [Reproduced with permission of *J. Clin. Invest.* **41,** 666 (1962).]

(Waller and Blaylock, 1966), or determinants clustered in aggregates of IgG (Henney and Ishizaka, 1968) have also been characterized. The rheumatoid factors produced during SBE appear to show a remarkable degree of autospecificity for altered or combined host IgG as the immunoglobulin portion of autologous immune complexes. Data supporting such autospecificity have been provided by recent studies (Phair *et al.*, 1972) appearing to indicate preferential absorption of rheumatoid factor activity, using autologous immune precipitates or complexes comprised of the individual's own anti-bacterial antibody combined with the specific infecting bacteria. Other similar, but not autologous complexes were shown in parallel not to be as effective in inhibiting or absorbing out rheumatoid factors from the same serum. Thus, the demonstration of a degree of apparent true autospecificity in this regard fulfills many of the criteria for a true autoimmune reaction.

Other possibilities must be considered when the whole question of rheumatoid factors and bacterial endocarditis is considered. Data from the work of Bokisch *et al.* (1973) using sera from rabbits hyperimmunized with various cellular products of A-variant streptococci appear to indicate that rather homogeneous populations of 7 S IgG rheumatoid factors may be induced secondary to such immunizations. Experimental data have been produced by this group to indicate that absorption or direct reactivity of isolated rheumatoid factors from such rabbit sera with purified peptidoglycans from immunizing A-variant antigen effectively reduces rheumatoid factor activity (Johnson and Hall, 1958). Such data may provide an alternative explanation for production of rheumatoid factors essentially as cross-reacting antibodies—directed perhaps primarily toward bacterial cell wall peptidoglycans—but reacting also with cross-specific or very similar determinants on Fc portions of Ig molecules. More direct testing of this latter hypothesis needs to be undertaken before either explanation—(1) reactivity for conformational changes in autologous IgG as produced by the combined antibody in immune complexes or (2) cross-reaction between peptidoglycan determinants and similar chemical immunodominant groups of IgC molecules—can stand as the most likely resolution.

Several attempts have been made to interpret the physiological significance of rheumatoid factors in diseases such as SBE. Under certain experimental conditions, it can be shown that rheumatoid factors are capable of actually blocking polymorphonuclear leukocyte phagocytosis of test bacteria by combining with Fc portions of opsonic antibodies and, thus, preventing their effective combination with phagocytic cell receptors (Messner *et al.*, 1968; Quie *et al.*, 1968). An example of rheumatoid factor inhibition of phagocytosis mediated by IgG antibody is shown in Fig. 2. On the other hand, other studies utilizing complement in addition to rheumatoid factors

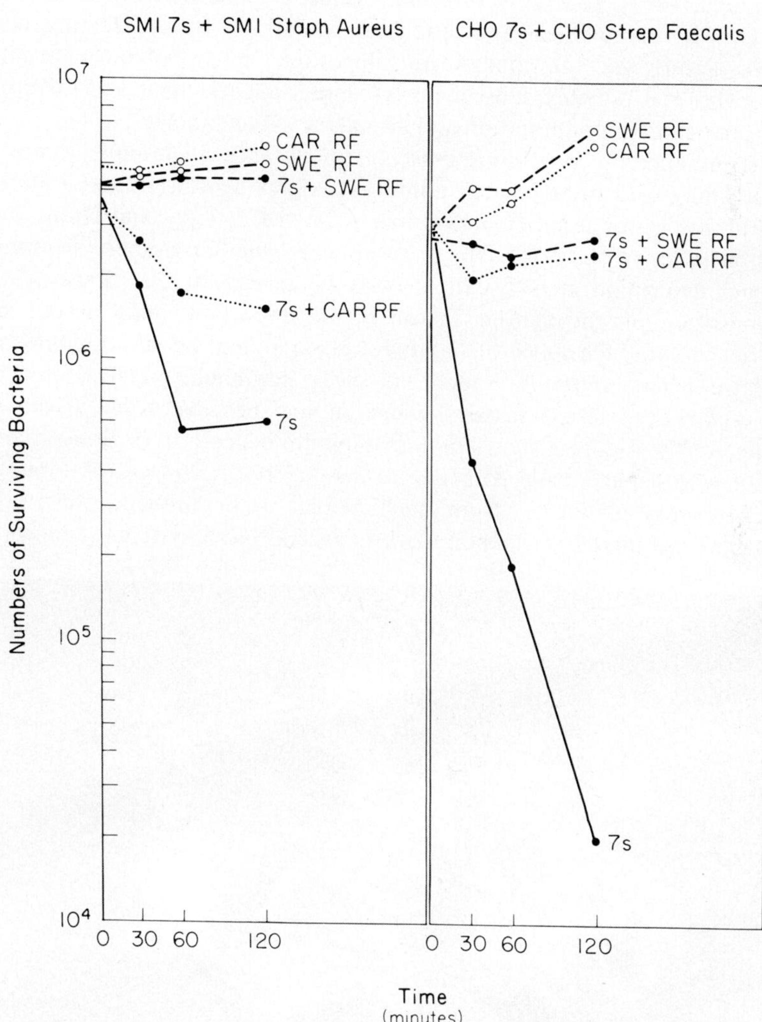

Fig. 2. Inhibition of phagocytosis following addition of isolated 19 S rheumatoid factors to 7 S IgC opsonin and bacteria. [Reproduced with permission of *J. Clin. Invest.* **47**, 1109 (1968).]

have shown that, under proper conditions, rheumatoid factors may actually facilitate complement-dependent phagocytic mechanisms (McDuffie and Brumfield, 1972). It is easy to visualize how rheumatoid factors acting in concert with complement and opsonized bacteria or other infecting agents might accelerate the phagocytic ingestion into polymorphonuclear leukocytes and possibly subsequent lysosomal engorgement and disruption with surrounding inflammation and attendant tissue damage.

The presence of chronic intravascular persistence of immune complexes in SBE may lead to associated immune complex deposition and a glomerulonephritis in some patients (Gutman *et al.*, 1972; Levy and Hong, 1973; Boulton-Jones *et al.*, 1974). The question as to whether glomerular immune complex deposition in such patients may be accentuated or aggravated by the presence of rheumatoid factor is an important one. In our own experience, although subepithelial and mesangial deposits of IgG, IgM, and C3 have been commonly found, no clear immunohistological proof of glomerular rheumatoid factor deposition has been recorded (Svec and Dingle, 1965). Figure 3 shows immunoglobulin deposition in glomeruli of a patient with nephritis and SBE due to *Streptococcus viridans*. Attempts to elute rheumatoid factor from such tissues were unsuccessful in this particular instance. Exerimental work in several other systems supports the

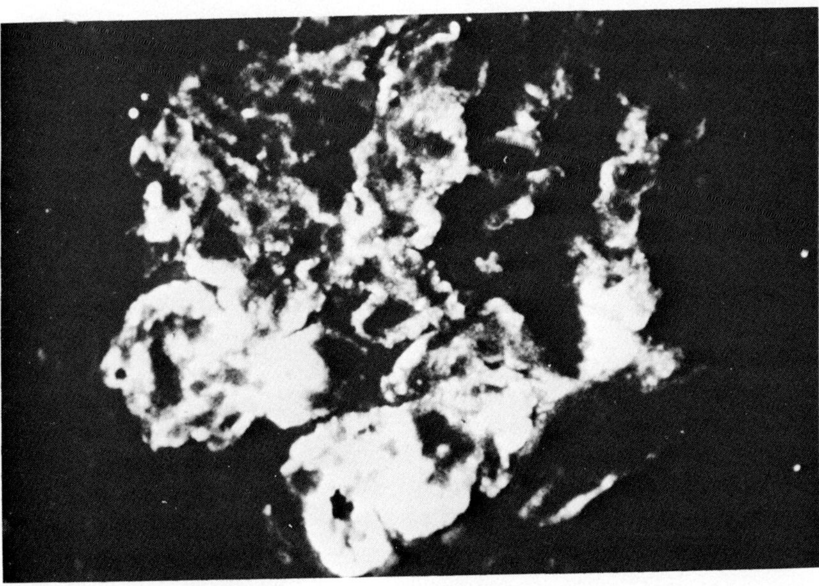

Fig. 3. Immunofluorescent studies of glomeruli from a patient with subacute bacterial endocarditis. Staining for IgM is shown. No rheumatoid factor activity could be demonstrated in glomerular eluates (× 350).

concept that aggravation or accentuation of the inflammatory process related to immune complex deposition may indeed be produced by rheumatoid factor (McCormick *et al.*, 1969; De Horatius and Williams, 1972). In addition, recent studies of tissues obtained from a broad spectrum of patients with various forms of glomerular injury appear to indicate an association between the presence of apparent tissue-bound anti-γ-globulin activity and the degree of glomerular damage (Rossen *et al.*, 1975). However, considerably more experimental data must be developed before the exact mechanisms involved are entirely clear.

In subacute bacterial endocarditis, one other lesion occurs which is highly reminiscent of a vasculitis possibly mediated by immune complexes. This is the Osler's node or Janeway lesion occurring as it does in small capillaries associated with the glomus tuft of fingers. Although as yet immunofluorescent studies have not been accomplished, microscopic examination of such lesions suggests a picture very similar to an acute or subacute Arthus reaction. In such an anatomic setting with bacterial antigen and antibody participating directly in an acute inflammatory reaction within the capillary tufts, it is again easy to visualize how rheumatoid factors possibly activating or facilitating the complement cascade might participate directly in the basic lesion. In our own experience, the association between Osler's nodes and the occurence of rheumatoid factor has been striking. Unfortunately, direct immunocytological proof of tissue deposition of rheumatoid factor in such instances is still lacking.

As shown in Table II, many other infectious disease states besides subacute bacterial endocarditis have been associated with the presence of rheumatoid factors. Among these are syphilis, lepromatous leprosy, tuberculosis, malaria, shistosomiasis, visceral larva migrans, and leishmaniasis of kala-azar (Peltier and Christian, 1959; Cathcart *et al.*, 1961; Singer *et al.*, 1962; Honba and Allison, 1966; R. C. W. Williams, Jr. and J. D. Emmons, unpublished observations, 1975; Huntley *et al.*, 1966; Kunkel *et al.*, 1958); In addition, the transient appearance of anti-γ-globulins has also repeatedly been recorded with hepatitis B infection or even following prophylactic or booster immunizations in normal adults. In many of the above infectious diseases, a situation obtains where the ground is ripe for intense prolonged exposure to a huge load of bacterial or parasitic antigenic material. Certainly such would be the case in malaria, leprosy, shistosomiasis, or kala-azar. Many of these disorders, like SBE, are chronic and allow sufficient time for a global and profound immune response within the infected host. Generation of a wide spectrum of humoral antibodies to antigenic determinants of the invading agent or parasite may be an important feature in the mechanisms leading to production of rheumatoid factors. Thus, bacterial- or parasite-directed hypergammaglobulinemia may be essential to provide sufficient altered γ-globulin—either in the form of autologous immune complexes or partially degraded Ig—to allow an adequate stimulus for rheumatoid factor production. In this regard, the situation encountered in lepromatous leprosy is particularly interesting, since studies of heavily involved lepromatous tissues show extensive tissue-bound immunoglobulins. Apparently, uninvolved skin from such patients has been shown to contain extensive deposits of fixed immunoglobulins (Bullock *et al.*, 1974; Quismorio *et al.*, 1975) (Fig. 4). Whether or not such Ig deposits all represent specific anti-leprosy antibody, anti-tissue antibody, or whether

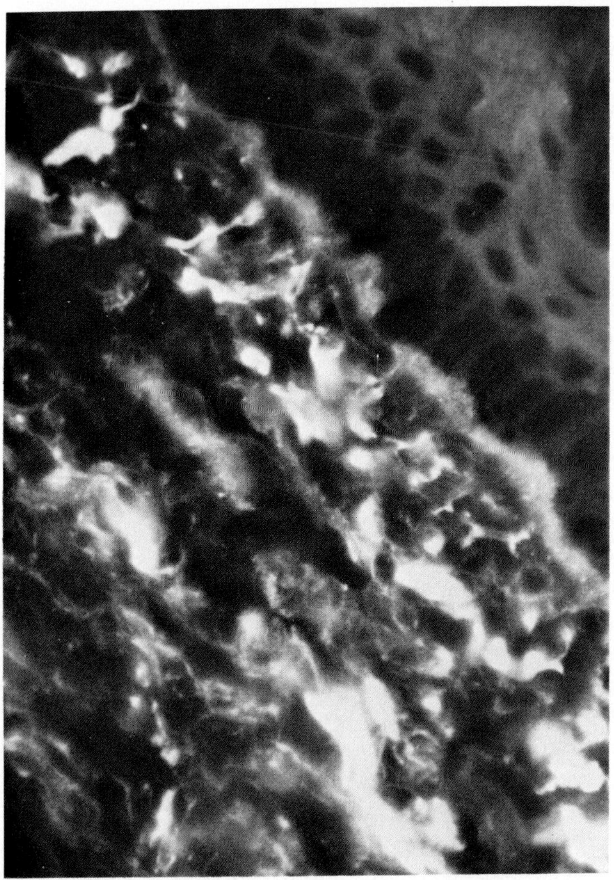

Fig. 4. Section of clinically normal skin from patient with lepromatous leprosy showing deposition of IgM along fibers in dermis. Small amounts of IgM are also present at dermoepidermal junction (× 560). [Published by permission of Drs. Quismorio *et al.* and *Arch. Dermatol.* **111,** 331 (1975).]

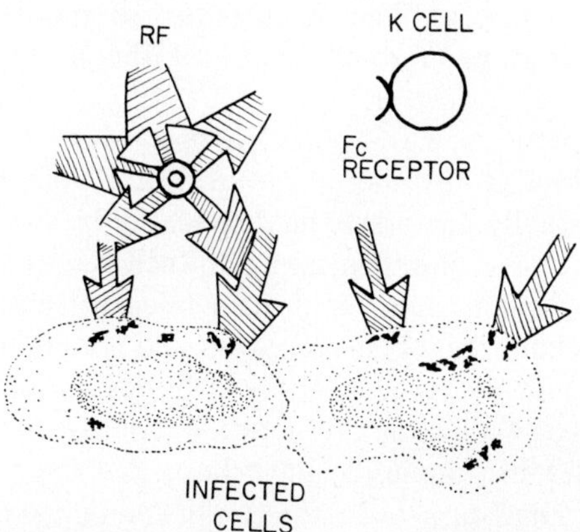

Fig. 5. 7 S IgC molecules bound to infected cells containing parasitizing bacteria are shown reacting with 19 S rheumatoid factor through Fc structures. Thus rheumatoid factors occupy Fc areas on tissue reacting IgC antibodies and could conceivably protect such cells from antibody dependent cytotoxicity by preventing attachment of Fc receptors on killer cell (K cells) in area.

they may be, in large part, IgG or IgM rheumatoid factors has not been settled. It is conceivable that in disorders such as schistosomiasis, leprosy, or malaria where tissues may, indeed, contain large amounts of tissue-fixed specific antibody along with absorbed rheutmatoid factors, a protective role for the latter could be operative. Thus, autologous cells coated with antibody might be unduly susceptible to inadvertent killing through mechanisms similar to that of antibody mediated cytotoxicity (Gale *et al.*, 1975; Calder *et al.*, 1974; Perlmann *et al.*, 1975). In this way, innocent bystander killer cells possessing Fc receptors might be prevented from affixing to autologous infected tissues and killing them by having rheumatoid factors absorbed to their Fc portions and, thus, tying up vital receptors necessary for killer cell attachment. Such a potential mechanism is diagrammed in Fig. 5. Evidence has recently been accumulated substantiating that rheumatoid factors can indeed block or modulate antibody-dependent lymphocytotoxicity *in vitro* (Diaz-Jouanen *et al.*, 1976). Whether or not similar mechanisms obtain *in vivo* remains to be established.

Several of the infectious disease conditions associated with rheumatoid factor production have also been noted to be accompanied by cryoglobulins. These include subacute bacterial endocarditis (Hurwitz *et al.*, 1975; Dreyfuss and Librach, 1952), and infectious mononucleosis (Kaplan, 1968). Extensive characterization of autoantibody content as well as relative concentration of anti-γ-globulin or rheumatoid factor activity indicates that many such cryoprecipitates contain anti-γ-globulins as part of the cryoprecipitating complex. The occurrence of cryoglobulins in such disorders may indeed be a rough index of the presence of circulating immune complexes.

Integrity of structures within the Fc portion of IgG appears to be important for efficient catabolic removal and turnover as antibody molecules are eventually degraded and disposed of by the body. Tissue-fixed rheumatoid factors, therefore, depending on their relative avidity or level of binding constants actually deter or protect infected cells from overzealous normal body mechanisms of Ig removal and catabolism. This sort of mechanism would not be expected to alter Ig desorption or elimination in the case of IgM or IgA rheumatoid factors where association constants of a relatively low order of magnitude have been described (Abraham *et al.*, 1972; Normansell and Stanworth, 1968). On the contrary, with respect to IgG rheumatoid factors such as those recently described by Pope *et al.* (1974) where much higher association costants have been described, a significant physiological effect on antibody catabolism and removal could be envisaged.

Under appropriate conditions as previously noted, rheumatoid factors can be shown to activate the complement cascade (Schmid *et al.*, 1970; Tesar and Schmid, 1973; Tanimoto *et al.*, 1975). Thus, it has been postulated that they may be important in helping or giving an assist to normal body mechanisms of inactivation of infecting organisms. Evidence supporting this concept has recently been presented by several groups (Gipson *et al.*, 1974; Gipson and Daniels, 1975). Diagrammatic expression of how such an adjuvant effect of rheumatoid factor might operate is shown in Fig. 6. As in previous work, it was recently shown, using solid phase radioimmunoassay, that rheumatoid factors reacting with hepatitis B–antigen–anti-

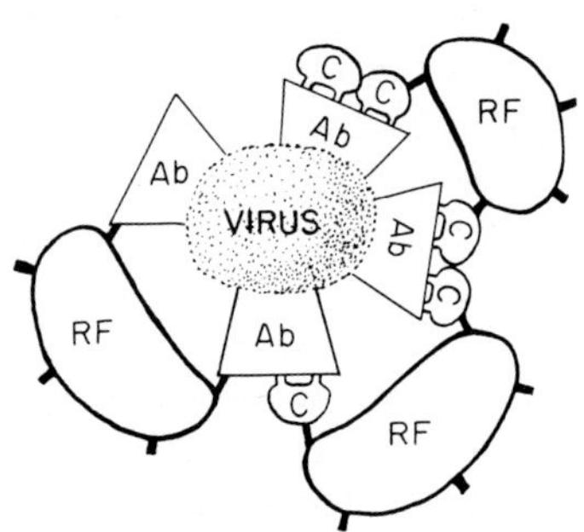

Fig. 6. Virus particle diagrammatically shown reacting with anti-viral antibody (Ab) and complement (C) being fixed to the latter. Possible additional contribution of rheumatoid factor (RF) is shown. The mass of immunoreactants, thus, could conceivably effectively interfere with the ability of the virus subsequently to bind to and infect cells.

TABLE III

Infections in Which Anti-Nuclear Antibodies Have Been Described

Infection	Reference
Tuberculosis	Seligmann *et al.*, 1965
Leprosy	Petchelai *et al.*, 1973
Infectious mononucleosis	Kaplan, 1968
Lymphocytic choriomeningitis (mice)	Tonietti *et al.*, 1970
Rauscher and Graffi viruses	Cannat and Varet, 1972
Cytomegalovirus	Andersen and Andersen, 1975

body complexes showed specificity for the complexes and not for either antigen or antibody alone (Markenson *et al.*, 1975). Presumably, infection with hepatitis B virus first induces antigenemia, followed by formation of antibodies and, finally, some degree of immune complexes. No direct correlation has been noted, however, between presence of rheumatoid factor and detectable hepatitis B antigen in a large series of patients with hepatitis (Hoofnagle *et al.*, 1974). Further studies are clearly needed to settle the question as to whether rheumatoid factors actually aid or assist the host in effectively dealing with infecting organisms.

Many of the infectious disease states associated with production of anti-γ-globulins are characterized by relative hypergammaglobulinemia. Several possible models for rheumatoid factor production have been established in animals, which involve long-term immunizations with coliform or other bacteria (Abruzzo and Christian, 1961), or immunizations with autologous γ-globulins or immune complexes (Williams and Kunkel, 1963; Milgrom and Witebsky, 1960; McCluskey *et al.*, 1962). It is still not clear whether anti-γ-globulin antibodies formed during hyperimmunization may indeed be merely an accentuation of a normal process. Their widespread occurrence in association with many forms of infection or hyperimmunization suggests that this may be the case.

III. ANTI-NUCLEAR ANTIBODIES

Clear or broad knowledge of the extent to which numerous infectious diseases may be associated with other autoantibodies is not yet available. However, certain diseases of infectious nature have from time to time been associated with the production of antibodies to nuclear components. A summary of positive reactions for anti-nuclear antibodies associated with some infections is given in Table III. Exactly how this comes about is open to a great deal of question, since it is conceivable that various drugs used in the treatment of some of these disorders actually may be involved in ANA induction (Seligmann *et al.*, 1965; Cannat and Seligmann, 1966). The other simplistic explanation which has been offered revolves around the idea that diseases associated with extensive tissue damage and, therefore, alteration of autologous nuclear material may be the natural reservoir of antigenic stimulation as a normal consequence of the inflammatory process itself. Interesting in this regard is the relative absence of clear-cut positive reactions for anti-native DNA in diseases such as tuberculosis or leprosy. This latter specificity seems to be considerably more limited to individuals with systemic lupus, although occasionally seen in association with other conditions (Bell *et al.*, 1975).

The mechanisms underlying acceleration or increments in anti-nuclear antibody following viral infections appear to be more complex. Whether or not viral replication acts as a nonspecific adjuvant or complexes with endogenous nucleic acids to form haptenic immunostimulatory antigens is not clear.

IV. SMOOTH MUSCLE ANTIBODIES

In the past, a great deal of interest has centered around the genesis of smooth muscle antibodies (SMA). Although most frequently related to diseases of unknown etiology, such as chronic active hepatitis or plasma cell hepatitis, SMA have also been described in association with viral hepatitis and infectious mononucleosis (Farrow *et al.*, 1970; Holborrow *et al.*, 1973). Considerable insight into the different possible specificities of smooth muscle antibody has been afforded by the studies of Trenchev *et al.* (1974) which have divided the antigens involved into several distinct groups. Smooth muscle antibodies have also been recently described among patients with cytomegalovirus infections (Andersen and Andersen, 1975). Recent studies by Fagraeus *et al.* (1974, 1975) have suggested that contractile elements on lymphocytes and other mononuclear cells may be related to the same general antigenic specificities as those classically described for contractile proteins of ordinary smooth muscle substrates. In our laboratory, absorption studies showing smooth muscle antibody from a group of heroin addicts (Husby *et al.*, 1975) suggest cross-reactions between smooth muscle and lymphocytotoxic antibodies. The frequent association of smooth muscle antibodies with intracellular infections such as infectious mononucleosis, viral hepatitis, or cytomegalovirus infection suggests that alterations in cell-surface membranes and, perhaps, thereby contractile surface projections may play a role in the induction of SMA in these instances.

V. LYMPHOCYTOTOXIC ANTIBODY

The occurrence of lymphocyte directed lymphocytotoxic antibodies appears to be a reaction common to a large number of human disease states (Messner, 1975; Strickland *et al.*, 1975), including conditions as divergent as regional ileitis, Hodgkin's disease, or systemic lupus erythematosus. However, it is clear that many viral infections are followed by the occurrence of lymphocytotoxic antibodies (Mottironi and Tersaki, 1970; Kreisler *et al.*, 1971; Huang *et al.*, 1973). In comparison to what is known concerning anti-nuclear antibodies or rheumatoid factors, very little is understood of the true specificity of such lymphocyte-directed antibodies. Molecular and immunoglobulin class characterizations now available largely from studies of cold-reactive lymphocytotoxins in sera of patients with systemic lupus (Winfield *et al.*, 1975) or regional ileitis (R. G. Strickland, C. A. Henderson, and R. C. Williams, Jr., unpublished observations 1975) indicate that they fall into the IgM class and are most active at 4°C. Attempts to uncover uniform auto- or hetero- specificity among this group of anti-lymphocyte antibodies have not produced a clearcut definition or system of reactivity (Messner, 1975; Terasaki; *et al.*, 1970).

In the case of lymphocytotoxins associated with infectious mononucleosis, there is some evidence that such antibodies are heterogeneous and may in some instances show reactivity for lymphocyte cell-surface determinants somehow peculiar to or exposed on dividing or immature cells (Thomas and Phillips, 1973a,b). Whether this type of buried specificity may be a general feature of anti-lymphocyte antibodies associated with many other viral infections has not been established. If anti-lymphocyte antibodies are indeed directed at virally induced antigens or alterations on lymphocyte membrances, it is difficult to understand why they appear to show such broad reactivity with a large panel of normal test lymphocytes (Messner, 1975). The possibility remains of course that many normal lymphocytes retain cell-surface antigens encoded by previous infection as vestiges of previous viral exposure.

Very little is known concerning the possible physiological importance of naturally occurring anti-lymphocyte or lymphocytotoxic antibodies. Arising as they do in such infections as infectious mononucleosis, cytomegalovirus infections, or infectious hepatitis—where the occurrence of other autoantibodies also seems to be increased—the possibility arises that they may somehow be directed at suppressor T cells or the basic immunostat mechanism. If this were the case, suppressor cells, muted or somehow covered up by antilymphocyte antibody, might be unable to contain autoreactive clones, thereby favoring the production of various autoantibodies. As yet, no clear evidence for suppressor T-cell specificity of lymphocytotoxic antibodies has been found particularly in the case of the several infectious diseases where they occur. We have recently accumulated some evidence, on the other hand, that lymphocytotoxic antibodies associated with conditions such as systemic lupus erythematosus or regional ileitis may actually be directed not against suppressor cells, but against nonsuppressor lymphocyte populations (Korsmeyer *et al.*, 1976). This general area provides an avenue where considerable progress must await definitive methods whereby suppressor and helper T cells can be separated and studied directly with respect to the effect of such lymphocyte-directed naturally occurring autoantibodies. The frequent occurrence of similar apparently T-specific lymphocytotoxins in the sera of NZB mice (Shirai *et al.*, 1972, 1973) in association with decline in apparent suppressor T cell functions makes the above hypothesis an attractive one.

VI. MISCELLANEOUS AUTOANTIBODIES ASSOCIATED WITH INFECTIONS

Perhaps the first autoantibody clearly linked to infection was the Wasserman or anti-cardiolipin reaction (Hanis *et al.*, 1948; Wallace and Norrins, 1969). Although, from a practical point, extremely useful in the serological diagnosis of syphilis, the reagin producing positive reactions in the RPR or conventional flocculation tests used for the serological diagnosis of syphilis may actually be an autoantibody directed against altered self-constituents. The occasional occurrence of positive tests for reaginlike antibodies in association with other diseases such as malaria is well known (Mayer and Heidelberger, 1946; Kitchen *et al.*, 1939). The use of a test for apparent autoantibody in the practical diagnosis of syphilis seems paradoxical and enigmatic, but has stood the test of time in its proven usefulness (Jaffe, 1975).

Several infections have frequently been associated with the occurrence of antibodies showing specificity for erythrocyte antigens. The most well defined of these is the association between mycoplasmal pneumonia and cold agglutinins. In many of the cases where cold agglutinins are produced in response to mycoplasmal infection, the rises in titer and clear anti-I specificity are not as well defined as is the case in so-called cold agglutinin disease (Schubothe, 1965; Roelcke, 1974). Of interest in this regard are the cold agglutinins with apparent anti-I specificity, which have been described in the sera of patients with infectious mononucleosis (Goldberg and Barnett, 1967; Roelcke, 1974). Mechanisms operative in the production of anti-i or anti-I cold agglutinins might well fall under category II or III shown previously in Table I.

Several heterogeneous syndromes involving unusual autoantibody profiles have been reported in association with various infections. Shaper *et al.* (1968) described an immunologic syndrome of high titer of malarial antibody in conjunction with high levels of IgM and circulating antibody to heart, thyroid, and gastric parietal cells among certain populations in Uganda. The direct relationship to malaria or to other possible indigenous variables, however, was not clear-cut.

Many autoimmune reactions and examples of autoantibody formation can be listed as various infections are studied. Some of them can be judged as potentially harmful, however, considerably more information is needed before the physiological role of such reactions can be finally understood and defined.

REFERENCES

Abraham, G. N., Clarke, R. A., and Vaughan, J. H. (1972). *Immunochemistry* **9,** 301–315.

Abruzzo, J. L., and Christian, C. L. (1961). *J. Exp. Med.* **114,** 791–806.

Allison, A. C. (1973). *Ann. Rheum. Dis.* **32,** 283–293.

Allison, A. C., Denman, A. M., and Barnes, R. D. (1971). *Lancet* **2,** 135–140.

Andersen, P., and Anderson, H. K. (1975). *Clin. Exp. Immunol.* **22,** 22–29.

Barthold, D. R., Kysela, S., and Steinberg, A. D. (1974). *J. Immunol.* **112,** 9–16.

Bell, C., Talal, N., and Schur, P. H. (1975). *Arthritis Rheum.* **18,** 535–540.

Bokisch, V. A., Chiao, J. W., Bernstein, D., and Krause, R. M. (1973). *J. Exp. Med.* **138,** 1184–1193.

Boulton-Jones, J. M., Sissons, J. G. P., Evans, D. J., and Peters, D. K. (1974). *Br. Med. J.* **2,** 11–14.

Boxer, A. L., and Stossel, T. P. (1974). *J. Clin. Invest.* **53,** 1534–1545.

Boxer, A. L., Yokoyama, M., and Wiebe, R. A. (1972). *Am. J. Med.* **52,** 279–282.

Bullock, W. E., Callerame, M. L., and Panner, B. J. (1974). *Am. J. Trop. Med. Hyg.* **23,** 78–83.

Calder, E. A., Urbaniak, S. J., and Penhale, W. J. (1974). *Clin. Exp. Immunol.* **18,** 579–593.

Cannat, A., and Seligmann, M. (1966). *Lancet* **1,** 185–187.

Cannat, A., and Varet, B. (1972). *Proc. Soc. Exp. Biol. Med.* **141,** 1077–1080.

Cathcart, E. S., Williams, R. C., Jr., and Ross, H. (1961). *Am. J. Med.* **31,** 758–765.

Chused, T. M., Steinberg, A. D., and Parker, L. M. (1973). *J. Immunol.* **111,** 52–57.

Dean, D. A. (1974). *J. Parasitol.* **60,** 260–263.

De Horatius, R. J., and Williams, R. C., Jr. (1972). *Arthritis Rheum.* **15,** 293–301.

Diaz-Jouanen, E., Bankhurst, A. D., and Williams, R. C., Jr. (1976). *Arthritis Rheum.* **19,** 133–141.

Drach, G. W. (1973). *Surg. Forum* **24,** 35–37.

Drach, G. W., Reed, W. P., and Williams, R. C., Jr. (1971). *J. Lab. Clin. Med.* **78,** 725–735.

Dresner, E., and Trombly, P. (1959). *N. Engl. J. Med.* **261,** 981–988.

Dreyfuss, F., and Librach, G. (1952). *J. Lab. Clin. Med.* **40,** 489–497.

Fagraeus, A., Lidman, K., and Biberfeld, G. (1974). *Nature* (*London*) **252,** 246–247.

Fagraeus, A., Lidman, K., and Norberg, R. (1975). *Clin. Exp. Immunol.* **20,** 469–477.

Farrow, L. J., Holborrow, E. J., Johnson, G. D., Lamb, S. G., Stewart, J. S., Taylor, P. E., and Zuckerman, A. J. (1970). *Br. Med. J.* **2,** 693–695.

Fournie, G. J., Lambert, P. H., and Miescher, P. A. (1974). *J. Exp. Med.* **140,** 1189–1206.

Freund, J., and McDermott, K. (1942). *Proc. Soc. Exp. Biol. Med.* **49,** 548–553.

Gale, R. P., Zighelboim, J., and Ossorio, R. C. (1975). *Clin. Immunol. Immunopathol.* **3,** 377–384.

Gipson, T. G., and Daniels, C. A. (1975). *Clin. Immunol. Immunopathol.* **4,** 16–23.

Gipson, T. G., Daniels, C. A., and Nofkins, A. L. (1974). *J. Immunol.* **112,** 2087–2093.

Goldberg, L. S., and Barnett, E. V. (1967). *J. Immunol.* **99,** 803–809.

Goldstein, I., Rebeyrotta, P., Parlebas, J., and Halpern, B. (1968). *Nature* (*London*) **219,** 866–868.

Gutman, R. A., Striker, G. E., Gilliland, B. C., and Cutler, R. E. (1972). *Medicine* (*Baltimore*) **51,** 1–25.

Hanis, A., Rosenberg, A. A., and Del Vecchio, E. R. (1948). *J. Vener. Dis. Inf.* **29,** 313–316.

Hardin, J. A., Chused, T. M., and Steinberg, A. D. (1973). *J. Immunol.* **111,** 650–651.

Henney, C. S., and Ishizaka, K. (1968). *J. Immunol.* **100,** 718–725.

Holborrow, E. J., Hemsted, E. H., and Mead, S. V. (1973). *Br. Med. J.* **3,** 323–325.

Hoofnagle, J. H., Markenson, J. A., Gerety, R. J., Daniels, C. A., and Barker, L. F. (1973). *Bacteriol. Proc.* **73,** 198 (V20 Abstract).

Hoofnagle, J. H., Markenson, J. A., Daniels, C. A., Gerety, R. J., Notkins, A. L., and Barker, L. F. (1974). *Am. J. Med. Sci.* **268,** 23–29.

Houba, V., and Allison, A. C. (1966). *Lancet* **1,** 848–852.

Huang, S. W., Lattos, D. B., Nelson, D. B., Reeb, K., and Hong, R. (1973). *J. Clin. Invest.* **52,** 1033–1040.

Huntley, C. G., Costas, M. C., Williams, R. C., Jr., Lyerly, A. D., and Watson, R. G. (1966). *J. Am. Med. Assoc.* **197,** 552–556.

Hurwitz, D., Quismorio, F. P., and Friou, G. J. (1975). *Clin. Exp. Immunol.* **19,** 131–141.

Husby, G., Pierce, P. E., and Williams, R. C., Jr., (1975). *Ann. Intern. Med.* **83,** 801–805.

Ingram, D. G. (1959a). *Immunology* **2,** 322–333.

Ingram, D. G. (1959b). *Immunology* **4,** 334–345.

Jaffe, H. W. (1975). *Ann. Intern. Med.* **83,** 846–850.

Johnson, A. G., Gaines, S., and Landy, M. (1956). *J. Exp. Med.* **103,** 225–246.

Johnson, R. E., and Hall, A. P. (1958). *N. Engl. J. Med.* **258,** 743–745.

Kaplan, M. E. (1968). *J. Lab. Clin. Med.* **71,** 754–765.

Kaplan, M. H., and Svec, K. H. (1964). *J. Exp. Med.* **119,** 651–666.
Kitchen, S. F., Webb, E. L., and Kupper, W. H. (1939). *J. Am. Med. Assoc.* **112,** 1143–1449.
Korsmeyer, S. J., Strickland, R. G., Amman, A. J., Waldmann, T. A., and Williams, Jr., R. C. (1976). *Clin. Immunol. Immunopathol.* **5,** 67–73.
Kreisler, M. J., Naito, S., and Terasaki, P. I. (1971). *Transplant. Proc.* **3,** 112–114.
Kunkel, H. G., Simon, H. J., and Fudenberg, H. (1958). *Arthritis Rheum.* **1,** 289–296.
Langenhuysen, M. M. A. C. (1971). *Clin. Exp. Immunol.* **9,** 393–398.
Lawrence, T. G., Jr., and Williams, R. C., Jr. (1967). *J. Exp. Med.* **125,** 233–248.
Levy, R. L., and Hong, R. (1973). *Am. J. Med.* **54,** 645–652.
McClusky, R. T., Miller, F., and Benacerraf, B. (1962). *J. Exp. Med.* **115,** 253–273.
McCormick, J. N., Day, J., and Morris, C. J. (1969). *Clin. Exp. Immunol.* **4,** 17–28.
McDuffie, F. C., and Brumfield, H. W. (1972). *J. Clin. Invest.* **51,** 3007–3014.
Mahmoud, A. F., Kellermeyer, R. W., and Warren, K. S. (1974). *Lancet* **2,** 1163–1166.
Mandy, W. J. (1967). *J. Immunol.* **99,** 815–824.
Markenson, J. A., Daniels, C. A., Notkins, A. L., Hoofnagle, J. H., Gerety, J., and Barker, L. F. (1975). *Clin. Exp. Immunol.* **19,** 209–217.
Mayer, M. M., and Heidelberger, M. (1946). *J. Immunol.* **54,** 89–102.
Messner, R. P. (1975). *In* "Lymohocytes and Their Interactions" (R. C. Williams, Jr., ed.), pp. 169–181. Raven, New York.
Messner, R. P., Laxdal, T., Quie, P. G., and Williams, Jr., R. C. (1968). *J. Clin. Invest.* **47,** 1109–1120.
Milgrom, F., and Witebsky, E. (1960). *J. Am. Med. Assoc.* **174,** 56–63.
Mottironi, V. D., and Terasaki, P. I. (1970). *In* "Histocompatibility Testing" (P. I. Teresaki, ed.), p. 301–308. Williams & Wilkins, Baltimore, Maryland.
Neter, E. (1969). *Curr. Top. Microbiol. Immunol.* **47,** 92–96.
Normansell, D. E., and Stanworth, D. R. (1968). *Immunology* **15,** 549–560.
Osterland, C. K., Harboe, M., and Kunkel, H. G. (1963). *Vox Sang.* **8,** 133–152.
Peltier, A., and Christian, C. L. (1959). *Arthritis Rheum.* **2,** 1–7.
Perez, G. O., Rothfield, N., and Williams, R. C., Jr. (1976). *Arch. Intern. Med.* **136,** 334–336.
Perlmann, P., Perlmann, H., and Müller-Eberhard, H. J. (1975). *J. Exp. Med.* **141,** 287–296.
Petchelai, B., Chuthanondh, Rungruong, S., and Ramasoota, T. (1973). *Lancet* **1,** 1481–1482.
Phair, J. P., Klippel, J., and MacKenzie, M. R. (1972). *Infect. Immun.* **5,** 24–26.
Pope, R. M., Teller, D. C., and Mannik, M. (1974). *Proc. Natl. Acad. Sci. U.S.A.* **71,** 517–521.
Quie, P. G., Messner, R. P., and Williams, R. C., Jr. (1968). *J. Clin. Invest.* **47,** 1109–1120.
Quismorio, F. P., Rea, T. H., Levan, N. E., and Friou, G. J. (1975). *Arch. Dermatol.* **111,** 331–334.
Raffel, S., and Forney, J. E. (1948). *J. Exp. Med.* **88,** 485–501.
Reed, W. P., Drach, G. W., and Williams, R. C., Jr. (1974). *J. Lab. Clin. Med.* **78,** 725–735.

Roelcke, E. (1974). *Clin. Immunol. Immunopathol.* **2,** 266–280.

Rossen, R. D., Reisberg, M. A., Sharp, J. T., Suki, W. N., Schloeder, F. X., Hill, L. L., and Eknoyan, G. (1975). *J. Clin. Invest.* **56,** 427–437.

Schmid, F. R., Roitt, I. M., and Rocha, M. J. (1970). *J. Exp. Med.* **132,** 673–683.

Schubothe, H. (1965). *Ann. N.Y. Acad. Sci.* **124,** 484–490.

Seligmann, M., Cannat, A., and Hamard, M. (1965). *Ann. N.Y. Acad. Sci.* **124,** 816–832.

Shaper, A. G., Kaplan, M. H., Mody, N. J., and McIntyre, P. A. (1968). *Lancet* **1,** 1342–1347.

Shirai, T., Yoshiki, T., and Mellors, R. C. (1972). *Clin. Exp. Immunol.* **12,** 455–465.

Shirai, T., Yoshiki, T., and Mellors, R. C. (1973). *J. Immunol.* **110,** 517–523.

Singer, J. M., Plotz, C. M., Peralta, F. M., and Lyons, H. C. (1962). *Ann. Intern. Med.* **56,** 545–552.

Springer, G. F. (1971). *Prog. Allergy* **15,** 9–77.

Springer, G. F., and Horton, R. E. (1964). *J. Gen. Physiol.* **47,** 1229–1250.

Springer, G. F., and Horton, R. E. (1969). *J. Clin. Invest.* **48,** 1280–1291.

Strickland, R. G., Friedler, E. M., Henderson, C. A., Wilson, I. D., and Williams, Jr., R. C. (1975). *Clin. Exp. Immunol.* **21,** 384–393.

Svec, K. H., and Dingle, J. H. (1965). *Arthritis Rheum.* **8,** 524–529.

Tanimoto, K., Cooper, N. R., Johnson, J. S., and Vaughan, J. H. (1975). *J. Clin. Invest.* **55,** 437–445.

Terasaki, P. I., Mottironi, V. D., and Barnett, E. V. (1970). *N. Engl. J. Med.* **283,** 724–728.

Tesar, J. T., and Schmid, F. R. (1973). *J. Immunol.* **110,** 993–1002.

Thomas, D. B., and Phillips, B. (1973a). *Clin. Exp. Immunol.* **14,** 91–96.

Thomas, D. B., and Phillips, B. (1973b). *J. Exp. Med.* **138,** 64–70.

Tonietti, G., Oldstone, M. B. A., and Dixon, F. J. (1970). *J. Exp. Med.* **132,** 89–109.

Trenchev, P., Snyd, P., and Holborrow, E. J. (1974). *Clin. Exp. Immunol.* **16,** 125–136.

Wallace, A. L., and Norrins, L. C. (1969). *Prog. Clin. Pathol.* **2,** 198–215.

Waller, M., and Blaylock, K. (1966). *J. Immunol.* **97,** 438–443.

Weissman, G. (1964). *Lancet* **2,** 1373–1375.

Weissman, G., and Dukor, P. (1970). *Adv. Immunol.* **12,** 283–331.

Werner, A. S., Cobbs, C. G., Kaye, D., Hook, E. W., and Werner, A. S. (1967). *J. Am. Med. Assoc.* **202,** 199–203.

Williams, R. C., Jr. (1964). *Proc. Natl. Acad. Sci. U.S.A.* **52,** 60–64.

Williams, R. C., Jr., and Kunkel, H. G. (1962). *J. Clin. Invest.* **41,** 666–675.

Williams, R. C., Jr., and Kunkel, H. G. (1963). *Proc. Soc. Exp. Biol. Med.* **112,** 554–561.

Williams, R. C., Jr., Russell, J., and Kenyon, A. J. (1966). *Am. J. Vet. Res.* **27,** 1447–1454.

Winfield, J. B., Winchester, R. J., Wernet, P., Fu, S. M., and Kunkel, H. G. (1975). *Arthritis Rheum.* **18,** 1–8.

Zabriskie, J. B. (1967). *Adv. Immunol.* **7,** 147–188.

Chapter 16

Immunodeficiency Disorders and Autoimmunity

ARTHUR J. AMMANN

I. INTRODUCTION

Various theories have been proposed to explain the loss of tolerance to self and the subsequent development of autoimmune disease. Virtually all of these theories invoke some alteration in the immune system, the consequence of which is the development of autoimmunity. One of the earliest theories, proposed by Burnet (1959), suggested that cells capable of synthesizing autoantibodies are destroyed in the embryonic state or in the thymus as "forbidden clones." The appearance of autoantibodies would be a result of somatic mutations of cells that would not be destroyed and that could produce antibody. In a somewhat "opposite" theory, Fudenberg (1971b) proposed that autoimmunity was a result of immunodeficiency, which could allow the survival of mutant cells capable of producing autoantibody and/or autoimmune destruction of normal tissue.

The first clinical association of immunodeficiency and autoimmunity was reported by Bruton (1952) in a report of a patient with hypogammaglobulinemia. The patient had a clinical history of recurrent infection and intermittent arthritis. Subsequently, there were numerous reports of autoimmune disease occurring in patients with both congenital and acquired hypogammaglobulinemia (Table I). In 1955, Collins described the occurrence of autoimmune hemolytic anemia in a patient with hypogammaglobulinemia (Collins and Dudley, 1955). Autoimmune phenomenon and autoimmune disease were subsequently described in other immunodeficiency disorders including "dysgammaglobulinemia," selective IgA deficiency, selective IgM deficiency, chronic mucocutaneous candidiasis, ataxia-telangiectasia, Wiskott–Aldrich syndrome, chronic granulomatous disease, and complement deficiencies. In this chapter, the association of autoimmunity and abnormalities of antibody-mediated immunity, cell-mediated immunity, and phagocytosis will be discussed in detail.

TABLE I

"Rheumatoid Arthritis" Associated with Hypogammaglobulinemia

Congential		No.
Bruton	1952	1
Hayles *et al.*	1954	2
Fisher	1955	1
von Kulneff *et al.*	1955	1
Janeway *et al.*	1956	5
Good *et al.*	1960	6
Fudenberg *et al.*	1962	3
Acquired		**No.**
Grant and Wallace	1954	1
Lang *et al.*	1954	1
Collins and Dudley	1955	1
Good *et al.*	1960	2
Kushner *et al.*	1960	1
Barnett *et al.*	1970	1

II. DISORDERS OF ANTIBODY-MEDIATED IMMUNITY ASSOCIATED WITH AUTOIMMUNITY

A. Hypogammaglobulinemia

Two major forms of hypogammaglobulinemia exist: congenital hypogammaglobulinemia and acquired hypogammaglobulinemia. Congenital hypogammaglobulinemia is a sex-linked recessive disorder which becomes symptomatic beyond 6 months of age and coincides with the loss of passively transferred maternal immunoglobulin. In this form of hypogammaglobulinemia, cell-mediated immunity is intact, and there is absence of all five immunoglobulin classes (IgG, IgM, IgA, IgD, and IgE). Recent studies of peripheral blood lymphocytes indicate that patients with congenital hypogammaglobulinemia lack circulating B cells (cells which have immunoglobulin or immunoglobulinlike receptors on their surface (Grey *et al.*, 1971). These patients also lack plasma cells containing immunoglobulin in their tissue. As patients with congenital hypogammaglobulinemia become older, they may "acquire" some degree of immunodeficiency. The majority of patients, however, survive for prolonged periods of time with only antibody deficiency.

The common variable onset form of hypogammaglobulinemia (acquired hypogammaglobulinemia) is usually detected as a result of clinical symptomatology consisting of recurrent infections and/or malabsorption. The disorder may appear at any age and is usually unassociated with any predisposing cause. Rarely, a thymoma may be found before the onset of hypogammaglobulinemia or is detected years after the onset of hypogammaglobulinemia. Although thymoma and acquired hypogammaglobulinemia appear to be definitely related, the reason for this association is not clear.

Patients with acquired hypogammaglobulinemia lack all five immunoglobulin classes but, in contrast to patients with congenital hypogammaglobulinemia, may also have defective cell-mediated immunity. Recent studies indicate that the majority of patients with acquired hypogammaglobulinemia have circulating peripheral blood lymphocytes which bear B lymphocyte markers (Grey *et al.*, 1971), indicating that these patients have B lymphocytes but are unable to synthesize and/or release immunoglobulins. Studies by Waldmann *et al.* (1974) have added a new dimension to an understanding of the etiology of acquired hypogammaglobulinemia. These investigators demonstrated the presence of suppressor cells which are capable of suppressing the immunoglobin production of normal cells in the blood of some patients with acquired hypogammaglobulinemia. Some forms of acquired hypogammaglobulinemia may, therefore, result from an excessive number of suppressor cells, rather than a diminished number of immunoglobulin producing cells.

TABLE II

Autoimmune Disease and Hypogammaglobulinemia

Pernicious anemia		No.
Larsson	1962	1
Conn *et al.*	1968	2
Twomey *et al.*	1969	10
Gelfand *et al.*	1972	1
Autoimmune hemolytic anemia		**No.**
Collins and Dudley	1955	1
Fudenberg and Soloman	1961	2
Thyroiditis		**No.**
Hilton and Doyle	1974	1
Dermatomyositis		**No.**
Janeway *et al.*	1956	1
Good *et al.*	1957	1
Gotoff *et al.*	1972	1
Scleroderma		**No.**
Good *et al.*	1957	1
Polymyositis		**No.**
Giuliano	1974	1

The first clear association of immunodeficiency and autoimmune disease was made by Janeway *et al.* (1956) in 12 patients with congenital hypogammaglobulinemia (Table I). The association was based on the clinical observation that 5 out of 12 patients with hypogammaglobulinemia had symptons which could not be distinguished from juvenile rheumatoid arthritis. One patient had a syndrome identical to dermatomyositis. The arthritis appeared in these patients 1½–7½ years after the onset of recurrent infections. Large joints were involved preferentially over smaller joints. Janeway *et al.* (1956) observed that pain was severe initially but became minimal with time. Little tenderness, heat, or limitation of movement was recorded. Aspiration of the joint fluid usually revealed a thick turbid fluid with a total white blood cell count ranging from 1,730/ml^3 to 24,000/ml^3 with a predominance of polymorphonuclear cells. No organisms were cultured. On biopsy, there was thickening of the synovial membrane without any apparent injury to cartilage, proliferation of mesothelial lining, and deposition of fibrin.

In 1957, Good *et al.* reported three patients who had hypogammaglobulinemia and arthritis, one who had scleroderma, and one who had dermatomyositis (Table I,II). Good *et al.* (1960) observed that in the original case of congenital hypogammaglobulinemia described by Bruton (1952), two attacks of arthritis occurred unassociated with infection. In their review of the literature prior to 1957, they uncovered a total of five patients with congenital hypogammaglobulinemia and three patients with acquired hypogammaglobulinemia who had arthritic episodes. Good *et al.* (1957) felt that the arthritic symptoms were indistinguishable from rheumatoid arthritis (in two instances, the illness was initially diagnosed as rheumatoid arthritis). In contrast to the report of Janeway *et al.* (1956), they observed involvement of metacarpal–phalangeal and interphalangeal joints, as well as large joints, and the association of heat and tenderness with active joint involvement. Some of the patients had stiffness of the joints, which was more troublesome early in the morning and gradually diminished during the day. In patients who had long-standing symptoms, X-rays of the joints revealed destructive changes and osteoporosis. One patient developed arthritis, anemia, leukopenia, and splenomegaly resulting in a diagnosis of Felty's syndrome. In another patient, the arthritis subsided following an episode of acute infectious hepatitis. This is similar to the report of Kornreich *et al.* (1971) who observed that patients with juvenile rheumatoid arthritis may have a remission of symptoms during an episode of infectious hepatitis.

Good *et al.* (1960) in reviewing 28 patients with hypogammaglobulinemia found a total of 9 with "collagen–vascular" disease. Subcutaneous nodules were found in three out of eight with rheumatoid arthritis, and the presence of fibrin deposits in biopsied tissues was described. One important difference between patients with classical rheumatoid arthritis and arthritis associated with hypogammaglobulinemia was the lack of plasma cells in synovial biopsies. Two of the eight patients with arthritis had spontaneous remissions, while the others went on to chronic disease. No description of a relationship between the arthritis and γ-globulin therapy was given.

Barnett *et al.* (1970) described a 4-year-old child with congenital hypogammaglobulinemia. In detailed immunologic studies, they found an absence of immunoglobulin in the serum, with the presence of immunoglobulins in the synovial fluid of involved joints. Following the institution of γ-

globulin therapy, the polyarthritis and subcutaneous nodules receded completely.

Collins and Dudley (1955) and Fudenberg and Solomon (1961) described the association of acquired hypogammaglobulinemia and autoimmune hemolytic anemia (Table II). One of the patients had a long-standing history of hypogammaglobulinemia prior to the development of autoimmune hemolytic anemia. Studies revealed a positive direct Coombs' test with an autoantibody that was active at 37°C. The anemia and an associated thrombocytopenia responded to steroid therapy. A splenectomy was performed in the patient who expired shortly thereafter. At autopsy, the patient was found to have a lymphoma of the spleen. A second patient also had acquired hypogammaglobulinemia, autoimmune hemolytic anemia, and a positive direct Coombs' test, which was active at 37°C and responded to steroid therapy.

The association of hypogammaglobulinemia and pernicious anemia was first described by Larsson (1962) (Table II). Subsequently, a series of 10 patients were evaluated by Twomey *et al.* (1969), who compared their 10 patients with hypogammaglobulinemia and pernicious anemia to 25 patients with pernicious anemia and normal immunoglobulins. The patients with hypogammaglobulinemia had a significantly earlier onset of pernicious anemia than patients with classical pernicious anemia. Eight of the ten patients had episodic diarrhea and *Giardia lamblia* was found in four of five patients in whom studies were performed. One of the patients had ulcerative colitis in association with pernicious anemia and a second patient had rheumatoid arthritis associated with subcutaneous nodules. None of the ten patients with pernicious anemia and hypogammaglobulinemia had antibodies against parietal cell, intrinsic factor, or antibody binding with vitamin B_{12}. Biopsy of the gastric mucosa in seven patients revealed infiltration with lymphocytes, but a lack of plasma cells. One patient developed a gastric adenocarcinoma. Nine of the patients had achlorhydria with severe vitamin B_{12} malabsorption. The vitamin B_{12} malabsorption was not corrected with exogenous instrinsic factor in four of the patients. Assays showed an absence of intrinsic factor. Conn *et al.* (1968) confirmed the early onset of pernicious anemia in patients with hypogammaglobulinemia. They also found an increased incidence of *Giardia lamblia* which was present in 50% of their patients. As in previous reports, none of their patients had antibody against parietal cell or intrinsic factor.

A single case of acquired hypogammaglobulinemia and autoimmune thyroiditis has been described (Hilton and Doyle, 1974). Detailed investigation for autoantibody did not reveal any antibodies against thyroid nuclear material. A biopsy of the thyroid demonstrated extensive infiltration by lymphocytes but absence of plasma cells.

B. Selective IgA Deficiency

Selective IgA deficiency has been defined as a disorder associated with a serum IgA value of less than 5 mg/dl, no deficiency of other immunoglobulins, normal antibody-mediated immunity, and normal cell-mediated immunity (Ammann and Hong, 1971c). This definition was devised to exclude other disorders associated with selective IgA deficiency which have in addition, moderate or severe defects in cell-mediated immunity, e.g., ataxia-telangiectasia (Peterson *et al.*, 1966). The original intent of a restrictive definition was to ascertain the specific clinical and laboratory disorders associated with a single abnormality of the immune system. However, with the use of more sophisticated studies of cell-mediated immunity, it was apparent that some patients who were previously thought to have selective IgA deficiency alone also have additional, more subtle, defects in cell-mediated immunity. Epstein and Amman (1974) described an inability of some patients with selective IgA deficiency to form T cell interferon following stimulation by phytohemagglutinin. Recently, we have found that some patients with selective IgA deficiency have depressed numbers of T cell rosettes. When these patients are followed sequentially, the T cell rosettes frequently return to normal. Thus, some of the cellular immunodeficiencies that are observed in patients with selective IgA deficiency are of a mild and transient nature. It is possible that they represent a form of secondary immunodeficiency as a consequence of the recurrent viral illnesses which these patients experience. In contrast, deficiency of IgA is a permanent abnormality and, in only one instance, has the serum IgA returned to normal (Petty *et al.*, 1973).

IgA is distinct from other immunoglobulins in that it exists in two separate forms. In the serum, IgA circulates in a monomeric (7 S) form, while in the secretions, IgA exists in a dimeric (11 S) form. Secretory IgA is composed of two molecules of IgA linked together by a separately synthesized and secreted protein termed "secretory component." Over 98% of patients with selective IgA deficiency lack both secretory and serum IgA. However, they have normal levels of secretory component (Ammann and Hong, 1971c). A few patients have absent serum IgA with normal levels of secretory IgA and normal numbers of IgA containing plasma cells along the gastrointestinal tract. There is a single report of a patient with normal levels of serum IgA and absent secretory IgA, as well as secretory component (Strober *et al.*, 1976).

Selective IgA deficiency is the most common immunodeficiency disorder in man. The incidence in the normal population varies from 1 in 600 to 1 to 900 (Bachmann, 1965; Hobbs, 1968; Johansson *et al.*, 1968). It is found more frequently in individuals with allergic disorders. Buckley and Dees

(1969) found an incidence of 1 in 200 in the population of individuals attending an allergy clinic.

Initially, selective IgA deficiency was felt to be an incidental finding in normal individuals (Rockey *et al.*, 1964; Bachmann, 1965; Goldberg *et al.*, 1968). Subsequently, numerous cases were reported in which selective IgA deficiency was associated with a variety of clinical disorders. The majority of patients with selective IgA deficiency suffered from recurrent sinopulmonary tract infections. An increased incidence of allergic phenomenon has also been found in patients with selective IgA deficiency (Buckley and Dees, 1969). This may be a result of the lack of formation of blocking or competing antibodies of the IgA class.

West *et al.* (1962) first recognized the association of selective IgA deficiency and autoimmune disease. In 1971, Ammann and Hong (1971) presented a detailed clinical and laboratory evaluation of 30 patients with selective IgA deficiency and suggested that there was a clear association between selective IgA deficiency, autoimmune disease, and autoimmune phenomenon. It is not known if there is a direct link between IgA deficiency and each autoimmune disease reported in association with this deficiency (Table III). However, in certain disorders there are a sufficient number of cases for a statistical analysis. Utilizing the data of Cassidy *et al.* (1968) on the incidence of selective IgA deficiency in systemic lupus erythematosus and rheumatoid arthritis, the probability of the chance simultaneous occur-

TABLE III

Autoimmune Disorders Associated with Selective IgA Deficiency

Systemic lupus erythematosus
Rheumatoid arthritis
Dermatomyositis
Pernicious anemia
Thyroiditis
Celiac disease
Addison's disease
Idiopathic thrombocytopenic purpura
Coombs'-positive hemolytic anemia
Transfusion reaction
Regional enteritis
Ulcerative colitis
Lupoid hepatitis
Sjögren's syndrome
Cerebral vasculitis

rence of either rheumatoid arthritis or systemic lupus erythematosus and selective IgA deficiency is $p < 0.0001$.

Several series have reported an increased incidence of selective IgA deficiency among patients with systemic lupus erythematosus (Cassidy *et al.*, 1968; Claman *et al.*, 1966; Stobo and Tomasi, 1967). The onset and severity of disease in patients with systemic lupus erythematosus and selective IgA deficiency does not differ from that found in patients with systemic lupus erythematosus and normal or elevated immunoglobulins. Patients with selective IgA deficiency and systemic lupus erythematosus have not been followed long enough to determine if the prognosis is different from that of patients with sytemic lupus erythematosus and normal or elevated immunoglobulins. One might expect that patients with IgA deficiency would have frequent exacerbations of systemic lupus secondary to recurrent viral illness, but this has not been documented in the literature, nor is there evidence that they respond differently to immunosuppressive therapy. As patients with systemic lupus and selective IgA deficiency lack normal levels of serum IgA, they are unable to form antibodies against nuclear material in the IgA class. The lack of serum IgA might, from a theoretical point, result in greater deposition of immune complexes in the kidney, since greater amounts of antigenic material would be available to bind with IgG and IgM, both of which, in contrast to IgA, fix complement well. However, a greater severity of renal disease has not been observed in patients with systemic lupus erythematosus and selective IgA deficiency.

Stobo and Tomasi (1967) studied a series of patients with systemic lupus, some of whom had selective IgA deficiency. When the saliva of these individuals was analyzed and compared to that of normals, they found an increased secretion of a low molecular weight (7 S) IgM. Increased secretion of 7 S IgM may provide a compensatory mechanism for protection against foreign antigens in those patients who lack secretory IgA.

The association of selective IgA deficiency and rheumatoid arthritis was first described by Cassidy *et al.* (1966). This was confirmed by Huntley *et al.* (1967) and Bluestone *et al.* (1970). In these series, the incidence of selective IgA deficiency varied from 2 in 100 to 8 in 100. The clinical symptomatology, course, and response to treatment of patients with selective IgA deficiency and rheumatoid arthritis did not appear to differ significantly from patients with rheumatoid arthritis and normal or elevated levels of serum IgA.

Impaired cell-mediated immunity, as measured by lymphocyte responsiveness to phytohemagglutinin, has been described in patients with selective IgA deficiency and rheumatoid disease. However, Panush *et al.* (1972) also described impaired cell-mediated immunity, but found that it was associated with activity and chronicity of disease and was independent of IgA deficiency.

An interesting patient with juvenile rheumatoid arthritis and selective IgA deficiency was reported by Petty *et al.* (1973). A 10-year-old female patient had a 3-year history of polyarthritis involving peripheral joints and cervical spine and recurrent sinopulmonary infection. The patient was diagnosed as having juvenile rheumatoid arthritis and was treated with infusions of fresh frozen plasma. She subsequently had marked clinical improvement of arthritis and recurrent infection that was concomitant with the return of the serum IgA to normal. No other instances of a nonpermanent form of selective IgA deficiency have been reported.

In a recent study, we investigated 14 patients with selective IgA deficiency for the presence of a variety of autoantibodies. Anti-nuclear antibodies were detected using the indirect immunofluorescence technique. Antibodies against DNA and single and double-stranded RNA [poly(A) and poly(A:U), respectively] were determined, utilizing a radioimmunoassay technique. Table IV summarizes the results found in patients with selective IgA deficiency, compared to patients with other immunodeficiency disorders. Out of 14 patients tested, only 1 had a positive antinuclear antibody. This patient had systemic lupus erythematosus. Two patients were positive for antibodies against DNA. One of these had systemic lupus erythematosus. Eight out of 14 patients were positive for antibodies against double-stranded RNA, while none had antibodies against single-stranded RNA.

Patients with selective IgA deficiency have an increased incidence of various types of rheumatoid factor. Ammann and Hong (1971c) reported

TABLE IV

Autoantibodies Associated with Immunodeficiency Disorders

	Autoantibody (No. positive/total No.)				
Disorder	Total studied	Rheumatoid factor	Anti-DNA	Anti-poly(A:U)[a]	Anti-poly(A)[b]
Selective IgA deficiency	14	3/14	2/14	8/14	0/14
Wiskott–Aldrich syndrome	8	1/8	0/8	1/8	1/8
Ataxia-telangiectasia	4	1/4	1/4	3/4	0/4
Chronic granulomatous disease	11	1/11	1/11	6/11	1/11
Female carriers of chronic granulomatous disease	8	2/8	3/8	3/8	1/8

[a] Anti-Poly(A:U), anti-double-stranded RNA.
[b] Anti-poly(A), anti-single-stranded RNA.

that anti-IgG antibodies were found in 37% of the individuals studied, while anti-IgA antibodies were found in 40%. There has been some debate as to whether anti-IgA antibodies are true "autoantibodies" or represent sensitization to exogenous IgA. As patients with selective IgA deficiency lack IgA (none have been shown to be totally lacking IgA by radioimmunoassay), it is postulated that they will recognize exogenous IgA as foreign and form antibodies against it. The majority of patients with selective IgA deficiency who have antibodies directed against IgA lack a history of administration of exogenous IgA. Possible sources of sensitization that have been suggested include blood transfusion, γ-globulin administration, breast feeding, and cross-reactivity with bovine IgA in the diet.

The presence of high titers of antibody directed against IgA has correlated with anaphylactic transfusion reactions (Vyas *et al.*, 1968). Initially, it was felt that patients with selective IgA deficiency, with and without antibody against IgA might be distinguished on the basis of the presence or absence of IgA-bearing B cells. To date, however, all patients with selective IgA deficiency, whether or not they have antibodies against IgA, have normal numbers of circulating IgA-bearing B cells (Grey *et al.*, 1971). This strongly suggests that the antibodies formed against IgA in IgA-deficient individuals represent "autoantibodies."

"Reverse rheumatoid factors" have been described in the sera of patients with selective IgA deficiency by several investigators. Wells *et al.* (1972) found that 30% of patients with selective IgA deficiency had IgG antibodies directed against human IgM. They were unable to correlate the presence of antibodies with any particular clinical abnormality.

The various rheumatoid factors observed in patients with selective IgA deficiency may be a result of sensitization that follows exposure to immunoglobulin in the diet. Lopez and Hyslop (1968) observed an increased incidence of antibody against goat, sheep, and cow sera in patients with IgA deficiency. They suggested that this was related to an abnormal mucosa with absorption of animal protein. These results were further investigated by Ammann and Hong (1971a), who demonstrated that the antibody in the patients was in the IgG class and directed against the IgM of the bovine immunoglobulins. In addition, the antibody only reacted with immunoglobulins of the bovidae species and did not cross-react with other animal species.

Many forms of gastrointestinal tract disease have been described in patients with selective IgA deficiency with celiac disease as the most common (Crabbé and Heremans, 1967). A deficiency of serum IgA is found in approximately 2 out of 100 patients with celiac disease (Booth, 1970). The remainder have normal or elevated levels of serum IgA. Within the group of patients who have IgA and celiac disease, some are found who have a loss

TABLE V

Clinical Disorders Associated with Anti-Basement Membrane Antibodies

Disorder	No. tested	No. positive
Celiac disease without IgA deficiency	8	2
Celiac disease with selective IgA deficiency	3	3
Selective IgA deficiency without celiac disease	40	1
Hypogammaglobulinemia	12	0
Thymic hypoplasia	6	0
Systemic lupus	10	0
Chronic active hepatitis	5	0
Normals (2–40 years)	40	0

of IgA containing plasma cells on intestinal biopsy. In celiac patients deficient in serum and secretory IgA, the IgA plasma cells are replaced by IgM-containing plasma cells (Crabbé and Heremans, 1967). Of additional interest are the observations of Beale *et al.* (1971) that the response of celiac patients to oral polio vaccine is quantitatively deficient in the IgA class.

Unique autoantibodies have been demonstrated in patients with celiac disease with and without IgA deficiency (Ammann and Hong, 1971b). The incidence of some of these autoantibodies (anti-basement membrane) is greater in IgA-deficient celiac patients (Table V). This autoantibody is distinct from that found in Goodpasture's syndrome. Its activity is directed primarily against the basement membrane of Bowman's capsule and renal tubules, bile canaliculi, and sarcolemma sheath of muscle (Table VI). The antibody does not react with the basement membrane of the skin and is

TABLE VI

Tissue Reactivity of Anti-Basement Membrane Activity

Structure	Anti-IgG fluorescent antibody reactivity
Bowman's capsule	+
Glomerular basement membrane	−
Kidney tubule basement membrane	+
Bile canaliculi	+
Sarcolemma sheath	+
Epithelial portion of ileum	+
Esophagus basement membrane	−
Salivary duct	+
Cornea basement membrane	−

therefore, distinct from anti-basement antibody found in pemphigoid. There is some reactivity of the antibody with collagen as well as basement membrane (Figs. 1–3). A similar autoantibody, termed anti-reticulin antibody, has been described by Seah *et al.* (1971) in celiac patients. It appears that autoimmunity, celiac disease, and selective IgA deficiency are related in some as yet unexplained manner.

Numerous reports of autoimmune hemolytic anemia and selective IgA deficiency have appeared. Patients range in age from young children to adults. The anemia may be mild to moderate and is usually associated with a positive Coombs' test. In one study, the antibody eluted from the red cells was found to be of the IgG class (Gosh and Harris-Jones, 1974). The majority of patients reported with autoimmune hemolytic anemia and selective IgA deficiency did not have other autoantibodies or other autoimmune disease (Heinz and Boyer, 1963; Bergström *et al.*, 1973; Gosh and Harris-Jones, 1974; Hobbs, 1968).

The mild and transient nature of the autoimmune hemolytic anemia found in patients with selective IgA deficiency suggests that the etiology of these episodes may be related to increased susceptibility to infection and subsequent adsorption of bacterial and/or viral products onto erythrocyte membranes. Although the majority of patients reported in the literature have responded well to treatment, certain cases have had chronic relapses and an

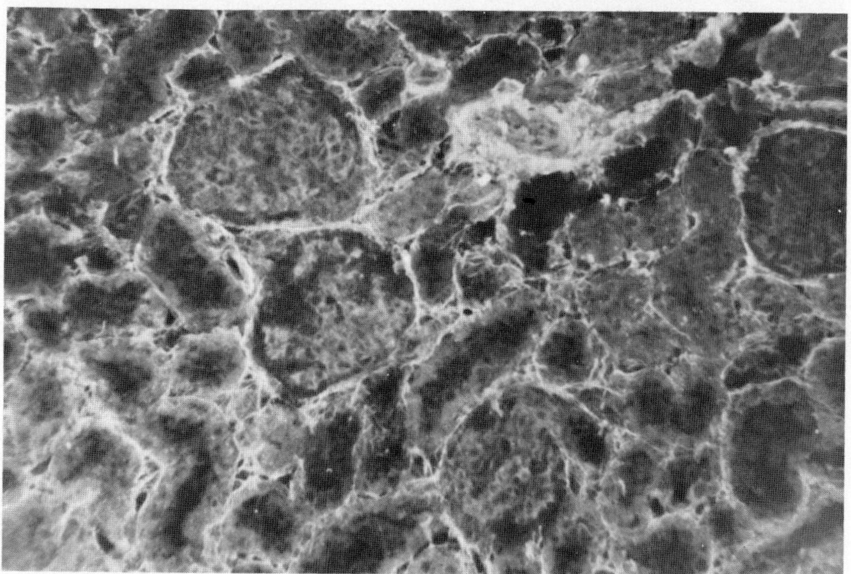

Fig. 1. Fluorescent photomicrography of isolated IgG on rat kidney section. Positive staining of basement membrane of Bowman's capsule and tubules is seen (IgG obtained from patient with IgA deficiency).

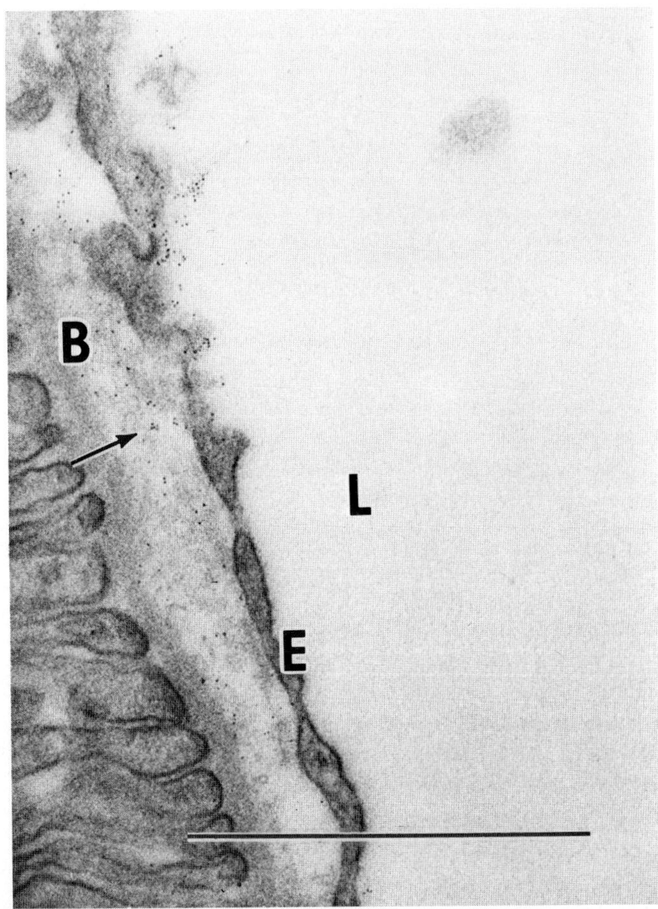

Fig. 2. Electron micrographs of ferritin molecules within the basement membrane (B) of this tubular cell can be seen (arrow). There is also some ferritin in the endothelial cell (E) lining the capillary lumen (L). The scale is μm. Isolated IgG from patient with IgA deficiency was placed on kidney tissue. Subsequently ferritin labeled anti-IgG was placed on the tissue.

unfavorable prognosis (Gosh and Harris-Jones, 1974). This would be anticipated in view of the life-long susceptibility to infection found in these patients.

Idiopathic thrombocytopenic purpura has been described as an isolated finding in at least three patients with selective IgA deficiency (Claman *et al.*, 1966; Lang *et al.*, 1973). In one instance, a child responded completely and permanently to the administration of steroids. In an adult with idiopathic thrombocytopenic purpura and selective IgA deficiency, reported by Lang *et al.* (1973), steroid therapy was unsuccessful, but the patient responded completely to splenectomy.

At least 24 individuals with selective IgA deficiency and pernicious anemia and/or thyroiditis have been reported (Ammann and Hong, 1971c). An even greater number of patients with selective IgA deficiency, who have antibodies against thyroglobulin and/or parietal cells also have been reported. The relationship of antibodies to the pathogenesis of pernicious anemia is uncertain, however, as it is known that patients with hypogam-

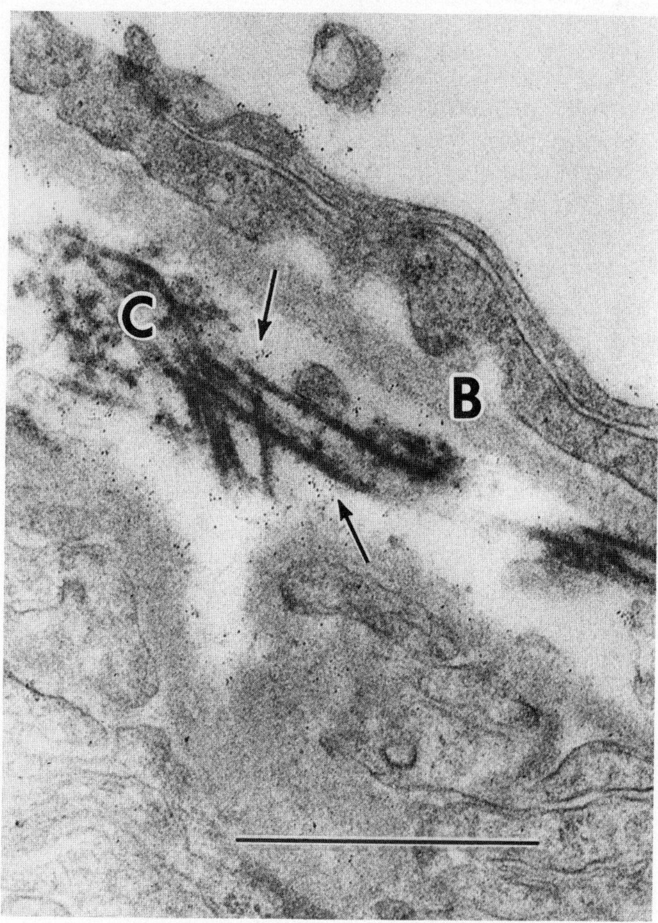

Fig. 3. Electron micrograph of a small cluster of collagen fiber (C) which have a scatter of ferritin molecules (arrows) on and near their surface. There is also some ferritin in the basement membrane (B) of this tubule cell. The scale is μm. Isolated IgG from a patient with IgA deficiency was placed on kidney tissue. Subsequently ferritin labeled anti-IgG was placed on the tissue.

maglobulinemia (and, therefore, absent antibodies) may also develop pernicious anemia (see Section II,A).

Several patients with selective IgA deficiency and pernicious anemia have developed malignancies (Fraser, 1969). A patient reported by Ginsberg and Mullinax (1970) had a monoclonal gammopathy. In this patient, the isolated M protein did not have antibody activity against parietal cells or intrinsic factor. A patient with selective IgA deficiency and a 22-year history of pernicious anemia and hypothyroidism developed rheumatoid arthritis and pulmonary failure during the last year of life. At autopsy, he was shown to have rheumatoid arthritis, chronic thyroiditis, pernicious anemia, atrophic gastritis, adenocarcinoma of the stomach, and pulmonary interstitial fibrosis (Case Records of the Massachusetts General Hospital, 1975).

Other autoimmune diseases have been reported in association with IgA deficiency, e.g., Sjögrens syndrome (Hobbs, 1968; Claman *et al.*, 1966), "lupoid" hepatitis (Claman *et al.*, 1966), and ulcerative colitis (Ammann and Hong, 1971c). The number of these patients is too small to indicate a clear association with IgA deficiency.

The large number of autoimmune diseases associated with selective IgA deficiency (Table III) could be interpreted as either showing a significant association between autoimmune disease and selective IgA deficiency or merely the fortuitous association of autoimmune disease with a common immunodeficiency disorder. Where complete data is available for statistical analysis, a significant association of certain of these disorders and selective IgA deficiency can be documented, e.g., systemic lupus erythematosus and rheumatoid arthritis. The multiplicity of autoimmune diseases found in association with IgA deficiency may be related to chronic antigenic stimulation, which results in the development of autoantibody and/or autoimmune disease. Patients with selective IgA deficiency are distinct from other immunodeficiency disorders in that they possess the "mildest" form of immunodeficiency. Although they lack IgA, they are capable of making normal or even increased amounts of antibodies in the other immunoglobulin classes. In addition, they possess T cell immunity in the majority of instances. Thus, the selective nature of the immunodeficiency permits long-term survivial. Concomitantly, this increases the number of infections experienced and the possibility that these infections might result in the development of autoantibody or autoimmune disease. The multiplicity of autoimmune diseases that have been reported in association with selective IgA deficiency could be, therefore, a result of more prolonged exposure to a variety of agents capable of triggering autoimmune diseases.

Autoimmunity may also be brought about by exposure to foreign antigens that cannot be excluded from the gastrointestinal tract. The high incidence of antibody against bovine protein argues strongly for such an association. Of interest is a report by Butler and Oskvig (1974) presenting data on the occurence of antibodies against bovine-associated mucroprotein. Antibody against this protein was demonstrated in patients with selective IgA deficiency, systemic lupus erythematosus, rheumatoid arthritis, and malignancies of the epithelial surfaces. The bovine protein was also found in human cancer tissue, as well as human embryonic tissue. These studies point to an association between the development of autoimmune disease, malignancy, and the occurrence of antibodies against bovine-associated mucoprotein.

An abnormality of the immunoregulation of antibody production is another means by which an increased incidence of autoimmunity could result. The majority of patients with selective IgA deficiency have abnormal levels (usually elevated) of IgG as well as IgM. Abnormal κ/λ ratios have been found in 37% of the patients. 7 S IgM has been found in the serum of 10% of the patients and may be found in the secretions as well (Stobo and Tomasi, 1967; Ammann and Hong, 1971c). These studies indicate that patients with selective IgA deficiency are unable to control the normal level of immunoglobulin, the ratio of immunoglobulin subgroups, and the production of normal molecular forms of immunoglobulins. This would offer an additional explanation for the increased incidence of autoantibody formation observed in these patients. Whether the defect is primarily in the B cells or in the cooperative or suppressive effects of T cells has not been demonstrated at this time. The lack of normal T cell interferon production observed in some patients (Epstein and Ammann, 1974) suggests that defective T cell regulatory mechanisms may also play a role in recurrent and/or chronic viral infection and subsequent susceptibility to autoimmune disease. The increased incidence of antibody directed against single and double-stranded RNA, immunoglobulin, and other native antigens (Table V), even in the absence of overt autoimmune disease, suggests that the immunologic aberrations described in patients with selective IgA deficiency, result in a significant abnormality of immunoregulation and predisposition to autoimmune disease.

C. Other Antibody Deficiency Disorders Associated with Autoimmune Phenomonen

Several immunodeficiency disorders are associated with various combinations of a deficiency or increase of one or more immunoglobulin classes. Previously, the term "dysgammaglobulinemia" was applied to these disorders. However, as studies of cell-mediated immunity became available, it was apparent that many of these diseases were primarily a defect in cell-mediated immunity with secondary deficiencies in antibody function. From a historical point of view, these disorders are discussed in this section. A variety of autoimmune disorders have been described in association with dysgammaglobulinemia (Table VII).

Heinz and Boyer (1963) described a 62-year-old female patient who presented with pallor, jauntice, and a palpable liver and spleen. The patient was found to have a positive direct and indirect Coombs' with the use of "non-γ" antiglobulin antisera. The patient improved markedly following transfusions and steroid therapy. The patient's antibody had activity against M red blood cells and cross-reactivity against the N antigen. Activity was present at both 25° and 1°C. Specific immunoglobulin quantitation was not peformed in this patient; however, crude separation of proteins indicated that the patient had a deficiency of 7 S immunoglobulin with an elevation of 19 S. An additional patient with decreased levels of IgG and IgA and increased levels of IgM and autoimmune disease was reported by Smith *et al.* (1970). The patient had both systemic lupus erythematosus and lymphoma. Anti-nuclear antibody was present but was found only in the IgM class. A cryoglobulin of the IgM class was also demonstrated.

The association of a Coombs'-positive hemolytic anemia in an unusual form of immunodeficiency consisting of decreased IgG, normal IgM, and increased IgA was reported by Goldman *et al.* (1967). The patient was lymphopenic and sick from birth until the time of death at 2½ years of age. At autopsy, the thymus was hypoplastic, and generalized lymphoid hypoplasia was found. Of interest was the presence of a generalized erythematous rash which first appeared at age 3 months and continued until the

TABLE VII

Autoimmune Disease Associated with "Dysgammaglobulinemia"

Autoimmune hemolytic anemia		No.
Stoelinga *et al.*	1969	1
Heinz	1963	1
Schaller *et al.*	1966	1
Goldman *et al.*	1967	1
Systemic lupus erythematosus		**No.**
Smith *et al.*	1970	1
Idiopathic thrombocytopenic purpura		**No.**
Rosen *et al.*	1961	1

death of the patient. The rash was noted to exacerbate intermittently and, on one occasion, became quite severe following typhoid immunization. A description of the rash and subsequent course of the patient suggests that the patient might have had a graft versus host reaction. On several occasions, we have observed the presence of a Coombs'-positive hemolytic anemia following a graft versus host reaction. In these instances, it is assumed that the Coombs' test is a result of antibody formed by the graft cells against host cells.

Selective IgM deficiency is an antibody deficiency disorder associated with intact cell-mediated immunity and normal levels of immunoglobulins, except for IgM. This is a rare antibody deficiency with an extremely poor prognosis. Patients behave in a manner similar to that of a young splenectomized patient, with susceptibility to overwhelming infection by polysaccharide-containing organisms. Stoelinga *et al.* (1969) reported a 13-year-old boy with a history of recurrent bacterial infection since birth. The patient was unable to make normal amounts of antibody against substances presumed to be in the IgM class, e.g., antibody directed against polysaccharide antigen, while the antibody response to immunization with polio and tetanus was normal. At age 13, the patient developed an autoimmune hemolytic anemia, and the direct Coombs' test was positive with an anti-IgG serum. The patients red cells agglutinated with an anti-complement serum. No red cell antigen specificity of the autoantibody could be demonstrated.

Schaller *et al.* (1966) reported a patient with elevated levels of IgG and IgA and depressed levels of IgM. The patient was intermittently lymphopenic and, prior to death, developed nephritis and an autoimmune hemolytic anemia. In this patient, the Coombs' test was positive, and the antibody was found to be in the IgG class with activity against blood group A. Prednisone therapy stabilized the anemia, but the patient subsequently died of *Pneumocystis carinii* pneumonia. At autopsy, atrophy of the thymus and hypoplasia of the lymph nodes was found.

Although patients with "dysgammaglobulinemia" have a variety of immunoglobulin abnormalities, they have in common an inability to form normal amounts of antibody and varying degrees of cellular immunodeficiency. It is clear that these patients have an increased incidence of autoimmune hemolytic anemia. Even if one carefully sorts out those patients who might have experienced a graft versus host reaction, there remains a significant number with autoimmune hemolytic anemia. These patients, therefore, represent another form of immune imbalance that predisposes to the development of autoimmune phenomenon. Their limited ability to form antibody probably accounts for the restricted manifestations of autoimmune phenomenon and autoimmune disease.

III. DISORDERS OF CELL-MEDIATED IMMUNITY ASSOCIATED WITH AUTOIMMUNITY

A. Chronic Mucocutaneous Candidiasis

Chronic mucocutaneous candidiasis is characterized by persistent candida infection involving the mucous membranes, various areas of the skin, and the nails. The candida infection is most commonly present in the oral cavity, but certain patients may develop candida granuloma which results in extensive skin involvement. Rarely, patients may have only chronic nail infection. Various forms of treatment have been devised to eradicate the candida, which is resistant to local antifungal treatment. Unmatched lymphocytes were utilized by Chilgren *et al.* (1969). Intravenous amphotericin has been found to be partially successful by a number of investigators (Heremans *et al.*, 1969; Kirkpatrick *et al.*, 1971). More recently, approximately one-half of the patients have been found to respond to a combination of treatment with transfer factor and amphotericin (Kirkpatrick *et al.*, 1971). A single patient was successfully treated utilizing a fetal thymus transplant (Levy *et al.*, 1971).

Approximately one-half of the patients with chronic mucocutaneous candidiasis have idiopathic endocrinopathy. All forms of endocrinopathy have been described, but Addison's disease and hypoparathyroidism are the most frequent. Other patients have been reported to have pernicious anemia, diabetes, hypothyroidism, and hypopituitarism (Kirkpatrick *et al.*, 1971). Separation of chronic mucocutaneous candidiasis into two disorders, one with and one without endocrinopathy, has been proposed, but family studies indicate that some patients have the onset of the disorder with chronic candida, while others have the onset with endocrinopathy. The complete syndrome may not be manifest until 15–20 years after the initial symptoms. In the majority of instances, however, the time interval between the development of the two major features of this disorder is less than 10 years.

Typically, patients with chronic candidiasis have elevated levels of antibody directed against candida antigens (Chilgren *et al.*, 1969). Studies of cell-mediated immunity may be abnormal. Some patients lack only a positive delayed hypersensitivity skin test to candida. These patients are able to produce migration inhibition factor (MIF), and the lymphocytes respond to stimulation with candida antigen. Other patients have a more severe defect in cell-mediated immunity, including absent delayed hypersensitivity skin tests to candida, absent MIF production, and absent *in vitro* lymphocyte blastogenesis to candida antigen (Kirkpatrick *et al.*, 1971).

Autoantibody directed against endocrine organs is frequently positive in patients with chronic mucocutaneous candidiasis with or without endocrinopathy. Studies by Blizzard and Gibbs (1968) indicate that a wide variety of autoantibodies are found, including antibody against kidney, parietal cells, adrenal, thyroid, and ovary. The studies of Wuepper and Fudenberg (1967) indicate that autoantibody may be present only transiently and absent when specific endocrine organ involvement occurs. Studies have not been performed in patients with chronic mucocutaneous candidiasis and liver disease to determine if the liver disease is associated with autoantibody, such as is found in chronic active hepatitis, e.g., anti-mitochondrial and anti-smooth muscle. Rheumatoid factor has been found in an increased incidence (Kirkpatrick *et al.*, 1971).

Several theories have been presented to explain the association of chronic candida and idiopathic endocrinopathy. Initially, it was suggested that the chronic candida infection was a result of chronic hypoparathyroidism. The improvement in the candida infection following correction of the hypoparathyroidism was cited as evidence in favor of this theory. However, well over 50% of patients with chronic mucocutaneous candidiasis and endocrinopathy have the onset of candida several years prior to any evidence of hypoparathyroidism.

It is possible to propose a theory that the entire syndrome of chronic mucocutaneous candidiasis and idiopathic endocrinopathy is related to a basic endocrine disturbance. The thymus is known to elaborate several humoral substances that will partially or completely replace the cellular function of the intact gland. Several thymic "hormones" have been studied *in vitro* and *in vivo* in animals (see Chapter 8). One of these, thymosin, has also been utilized for *in vitro* and *in vivo* therapy in man (Wara *et al.*, 1975a). The effect of this substance in providing *in vitro* and *in vivo* immunologic reconstitution suggests that the thymus gland, indeed, elaborates a thymic "hormone" or multiple hormones. If one considers the thymus to be an endocrine organ, then the syndrome of chronic mucocutaneous candidiasis with endocrinopathy could be a primary endocrine organ disease. The variable presentation in the syndrome would be dependent upon which endocrine organ was first involved. This theory does not explain the "trigger" which initiates the endocrinopathy, although it is possible that an autoimmune process could involve destruction of the thymus, as well as other endocrine organs.

Regardless of the basic etiology of chronic mucocutaneous candidiasis with and without endocrinopathy, there is a clear association between a basic defect in cell-mediated immunity to candida and the progressive development of autoimmune endocrine disease.

B. Wiskott–Aldrich Syndrome

The Wiskott–Aldrich syndrome is a sex-linked recessive immunodeficiency disorder characterized by eczema, thrombocytopenia, and recurrent infections. Patients with this disorder have variable life expectancies. Early in infancy, bleeding, secondary to thrombocytopenia, is the primary cause of death. If the patients survive the bleeding episodes, they may experience repeated infections with polysaccharide-containing organisms (*Pneumococcus, Hemophilus influenzae, Escherichia coli*. Immunologically, the patients are characterized as having normal levels of IgG, depressed levels of IgM, and elevated levels of IgA and IgE. Characteristically, the patients are unable to form antibodies when immunized with purified polysaccharide, although they may form antibodies when immunized with protein antigens (Cooper *et al.*, 1968). Early in life, the patients have primarily a defect in antibody-mediated immunity, and, as they become older, defective cell-mediated immunity (Blaese *et al.*, 1968).

A basic defect linking the inability to form antibody to polysaccharide organisms, the eczema, and the thrombocytopenia is not available. Two of the earliest immunolic abnormalities found in the Wiskott–Aldrich syndrome are the inability to form antibody to polysaccharide and hypercatabolism of immunoglobulins. The thrombocytopenia is always present at the time of birth.

The occurrence of autoimmunity in patients with Wiskott–Aldrich syndrome was not appreciated until recent years. Autoimmune hemolytic anemia in a patient with Wiskott–Aldrich syndrome following treatment with transfer factor was described by Ballow *et al.* (1973). They described a 3-year-old patient who previously had a negative Coombs' test. Following treatment with transfer factor, he developed a weakly positive direct Coombs' test. Additional transfer factor therapy resulted in a strongly positive direct and indirect Coombs' test, associated with severe hemolysis and ultimate death. During the episode of hemolytic anemia, coxsackie B-5 was isolated from the stool associated with a rise in serum antibody. Evaluation of the autoantibody in the patient revealed a warm IgG panagglutinin. IgA, IgM, C3, C4, and C5 were not found on the surface of the red blood cells.

Three additional cases of a Coombs'-positive hemolytic anemia have been described in 100 patients with the Wiskott–Aldrich syndrome (Cummins *et al.*, 1959; Wolff, 1967; Douglas and Fudenberg, 1969). In one of these cases (Douglas and Fudenberg, 1969), the hemolytic anemia was associated with a graft versus host reaction. It is likely that this was not an autoimmune hemolytic anemia but, rather, represented the formation of graft antibodies against host cells. Ballow *et al.* (1973) uncovered an additional seven cases of Coombs'-positive hemolytic anemia in a survey of immunologists. In our own experience, we have seen four patients with Coombs'-positive hemolytic anemia. These studies suggest that a Coombs'-positive hemolytic anemia is a more frequent finding in the Wiskott–Aldrich syndrome than previously appreciated.

Ballow *et al.* (1973) suggested that the hemolytic anemia seen in their patient was associated with partial reconstitution of cellular immunity by transfer factor and that the hemolytic anemia developed as a result of reconstitution of helper T cell function. The hemolytic anemia observed in two of our four patients was also associated with transfer factor therapy. However, the majority of patients reported in the literature developed hemolytic anemia prior to the use of transfer factor. In addition, many of the patients with Wiskott–Aldrich syndrome are treated with multiple drugs that have the potential of causing autoimmune hemolytic anemia. One of our patients developed hemolytic anemia in association with cephalothin therapy.

In a study of autoantibodies in patients with various immunodeficiency disorders, we were unable to detect an increased incidence of other autoantibodies in patients with the Wiskott–Aldrich syndrome (Table IV). Therefore, these patients appear to be uniquely susceptible to the development of autoimmune hemolytic anemia. The basic immunologic defect in these patients, that of an inability to form antibody directed against polysaccharide antigen, is also unique to immunodeficiency disorders, but an etiologic relationship between this defect and autoimmune hemolytic anemia has not been uncovered.

C. Ataxia-Telangiectasia

Ataxia-telangiectasia is an immunodeficiency disorder with a characteristic triad of progressive ataxia, recurrent sinopulmonary infection, and telangiectasis. The disorder is inherited in an autosomal recessive manner. The ataxia, which is of a cerebellar type, usually makes its appearance shortly after 1 year of age. In certain patients, the ataxia may be delayed for as long as 4–6 years. Telangiectasis involves the bulbar conjunctivae, the ear lobe, the bridge of the nose, and the antecubital fossa. The characteristic telangiectatic blood vessels may not appear until several years of age or may be delayed as long as 8 years. Sinopulmonary tract infection may also have a variable onset and severity. Only when the primary clinical symptomatologies are present simultaneously and can a diagnosis be made with certainty.

The first immunologic deficiency described was that of an absence of serum IgA (Thieffry *et al.*, 1961). Peterson *et al.* (1966) presented evidence for defective cell-mediated immunity. Deficiency of IgE was first described by Ammann *et al.* (1969a).

As more detailed studies of ataxia-telangiectasia become available, it was apparent that the disorder had more widespread involvement of various organs than previously appreciated. Ovarian dysgenesis was described by Boder and Sedgwick (1957), testicular atrophy and involvement of the anterior pituitary cells were described by Strich (1966), abnormalities of growth hormone response by Ammann *et al.* (1969b), an unusual form of diabetes by Schalch *et al.* (1970), and increased urinary excretion of FSH by Ammann *et al.* (1969b).

Various theories have been proposed to explain the varied clinical and laboratory abnormalities observed in ataxia-telangiectasia. Any single theory must explain the variable onset of the disorder, the progression of the disease, and the multisystem involvement (central and peripheral nervous system, endocrine organ, vascular, and immunologic). Peterson *et al.* (1966) described telangiectatic blood vessels in the lung and skin and suggested that the telangiectasis, gonadal abnormalities, and thymic defect were related to defective embryogenesis of mesenchyme. These studies have not been confirmed by other investigators, nor have abnormalities of the blood vessels in the central nervous system been described. An alternate theory, proposed by Ammann and Hong (1971d) following the observations of an increased incidence of autoantibodies in patients with ataxia-telangiectasia, suggested that the recurrent and chronic viral infections observed in these patients resulted in gradual and progressive destruction of various organs, with autoantibodies as the indicators of this destructive process. Another interpretation suggested that a basic thymic deficiency resulted directly in autoimmune phenomenon and gradual destruction of various organs.

A variety of autoantibodies have been described in patients with ataxia-telangiectasia (Ammann and Hong, 1971d). Of 18 patients studied, a total of 8 had one or more autoantibodies directed against IgG, IgA, thyroglobulin, parietal cell, smooth muscle, mitochondria, striated muscle, bile canaliculi, nuclear material, or basement membrane. Antibodies against IgA were found in the majority of the patients, and, in this respect, these patients are similar to patients with IgA deficiency. Six of the nine patients who had antibody against IgA lacked serum IgA. Patients with ataxia-telangiectasia and IgA deficiency had a greater frequency of autoantibodies, when compared to patients with selective IgA deficiency alone. Significantly, 12 out of 18 patients with ataxia-telangiectasia had other immunologic abnormalities in addition to IgA deficiency. This would suggest that the greater degree of immunodeficiency found in these patients enhanced their susceptibility to autoantibody formation when compared to patients with IgA deficiency alone.

Recent studies performed by us (Table IV) in a smaller number of patients with ataxia-telangiectasia indicate that the majority have antibodies against double-stranded RNA. Four patients were tested for antibody directed against DNA, double-stranded RNA, and single-stranded RNA. The results are similar to those found in patients with selective IgA deficiency who have an increased incidence of antibodies directed against double-stranded RNA (Table IV). Of interest is the fact that all three ataxia-telangiectasia patients with antibodies against double stranded RNA had an IgA deficiency.

Studies have not been performed in patients with ataxia-telangiectasia to determine if the autoantibodies are cytotoxic to cells against which they are directed, nor have studies been performed to determine if cellular sensitivity might be present in these patients. It would also be of interest to determine if patients with ataxia-telangiectasia had autoantibodies directed against central nervous system antigens. Such studies might provide a unifying hypothesis for the multisystem involvement, which is a characteristic feature of the disease, as the thymus, brain, and gonads are known to share antigenic determinants (Leiken and Oppenheim 1971; Lamelin *et al.*, 1972).

IV. ABNORMALITIES OF PHAGOCYTOSIS ASSOCIATED WITH AUTOIMMUNITY: CHRONIC GRANULOMATOUS DISEASE

Normal phagocytosis is dependent upon a number of extracellular and intracellular events. Prior to phagocytosis, most bacteria require the interaction of specific antibodies and complement. Phagocytic cells have membrane receptors for both the Fc portion of immunoglobulin molecules and various complement components. These receptors enhance the adherence of opsonized bacteria and subsequent ingestion. The process of ingestion is active, requiring ATP, glycolysis, glycogenolysis, and oxidative phosphorylation. Ingestion is followed by the formation of a phagosome within the phagocytic cell. Degranulation occurs with the release of enzymes that act in conjunction with other metabolic products to destroy bacteria. The process of ingestion is also associated with an increase in oxygen consumption, hydrogen peroxide production, oxidation of glucose, and an increase in the hexose monophosphate shunt. The oxidative burst within the neutrophil has been associated with two enzymes: NADH oxidase and NADPH oxidase, which reduce oxygen to a superoxide anion (Curnutte *et al.*, 1974). Another enzyme, myeloperoxidase, found within phagocytic cells, acts upon hydrogen peroxide plus halogen anions to generate potent bactericidal halogen (Fridovich, 1974). The hydrogen peroxide–myeloperoxide–halide system is extremely important in bacterial killing within phagocytic cells.

Phagocytic disorders are associated with both extrinsic and intrinsic abnormalities. Deficiency of both complement components and immunoglobulin will result in abnormal phagocytosis. Several disorders have been described, which are felt to be associated with intracellular defects: myeloperoxidase deficiency (Lehrer and Cline, 1969), glucose-6-phosphate dehydrogenase deficiency (Cooper *et al.*, 1972), Chediak-Higashi syndrome (Blume *et al.*, 1968), and chronic granulomatous disease (Holmes *et al.*, 1970). Of these disorders, only the complement deficiencies and chronic granulomatous disease have been associated with significant autoimmune disease. The complement disorders are discussed in another chapter.

Chronic granulomatous disease is a sex-linked inherited disorder of bacterial killing. The disease is a result of an enzymatic defect (NADP oxidase or NADPH oxidase) which results in the failure to produce free hydrogen radicals, decreased oxygen consumption, and diminished hydrogen peroxide production. Superoxide production is also abnormal in these patients, and there is a lack of iodination of bacterial cell walls. The net effect is a failure to kill certain bacteria. A female variant of the disease has been described. Children with this disease have a susceptibility to certain microbial agents. These are generally of low virulence in normal individuals and include *Staphylococcus epidermidis, Serratia marcescens, Candida, Aspergillus*, and certain species of *Pseudomonas*. The onset of symptoms occurs by 2 years of age in most instances. Chronic diarrhea, perianal abscess, ulcerative stomatitis, osteomyelitis, and hepatosplenomegaly are frequent findings. One of the most characteristic features of the disorder is chronic draining lymphadenopathy. Patients with this disorder rarely live beyond 16 years of age (Good *et al.*, 1968).

The association of autoimmune disease and chronic granulomatous disease was first made in the female carriers, some of whom were observed to have discoid lupus erythematosus (McFarlane *et al.*, 1967; Quie and Davis, 1973; Thompson and Soothill, 1970; Schaller, 1972). As a result of these observations, we evaluated a population of female carriers of chronic granulomatous disease and patients with chronic granulomatous disease for clinical and laboratory evidence for autoimmune disease (Table IV).

Of eight female carriers of chronic granulomatous disease, three had clinical evidence of discoid lupus, and one had clinical evidence of systemic lupus erythematosus. One female carrier grandmother of a patient with chronic granulomatous disease expired with systemic lupus erythematosus prior to our evaluation. Eleven males with chronic granulomatous disease were studied. None of these had evidence of autoimmune disease.

Laboratory studies consisted of anti-nuclear antibody and antibody against DNA and single- and double-stranded RNA [poly(A) and poly(A:U), respectively]. Table IV lists the abnormalities found in patients with chronic granulomatous disease and female carriers. Six out of 11 patients with chronic granulomatous disease had antibodies to poly(A:U) and 1 out of the 11 to poly(A) and DNA. None had anti-nuclear antibodies. In the study of the female carriers, three out of eight had antibodies to DNA, on out of eight to poly(A), three out of eight to poly(A:U), and two out of eight had anti-nuclear antibody. It is apparent that both the female carriers of chronic granulomatous disease and patients with chronic granulomatous disease are significantly positive for autoantibodies associated with autoimmune disease.

Tubular reticular structures have been described in chronic granulomatous disease (Wara *et al.*, 1975b) and provide further evidence for an association of features common to autoimmune disorders and immunodeficiency. The first description of tubular reticular structures by Fresco (1968) and, subsequently, by Grausz *et al.* (1970) and Gyorkey *et al.* (1972) resulted in the suggestion that they might be viral particles. Originally, they were found in renal biopsies of patients with systemic lupus erythematosus, but were subsequently described in patients with scleroderma, Goodpasture's syndrome, and Sjögren's syndrome (Grausz *et al.*, 1970). They were described in the peripheral blood lymphocytes of patients with discoid and systemic lupus erythematosus by Goodman *et al.* (1973). The occurence of tubular reticular structures in normal individuals has been reported (Huhn, 1968), but the structures are frequently confused with parallel tubular arrays, which are found in normals (Goodman *et al.*, 1973). Fresco (1968) considered that tubular reticular structures morphologically resembled paramyxoviruses and presented evidence that the structures may contain RNA. However, studies performed on EB virus-infected lymphoid cells suggested that tubular reticular structures consisted primarily of phospholipid and acetic glycoprotein (Schaff *et al.*, 1973).

There is a distinct difference between the autoantibodies found in patients with chronic granulomatous disease and female carriers. Patients have a high incidence of antibodies to poly(A:U), but a low incidence of antibodies to poly(A) and DNA. Female carriers have a high incidence to both DNA and poly(A:U). There are several possibilities to explain this difference. The antibody in patients with chronic granulomatous disease may reflect chronic infection. This is felt to be unlikely, since patients with chronic granulomatous disease do not have an increased incidence of other antibodies found in patients with chronic infection, e.g., the patients lacked an increased incidence of rheumatoid factor, such as is seen in patients with subacute bacterial endocarditis. The autoantibody in female carriers is not felt to be a result of chronic infection, as the majority of these patients are free of infection of the types encountered in patients with chronic granulomatous disease. Another possibility is that the autoantibodies in patients represent a pre-lupus state and that clinical lupus would develop if these patients survived longer. The oldest patient in our series was 18 years of age, and the youngest female carrier was 26 at the time of onset of discoid lupus. Of interest is one female carrier who developed autoantibodies and tubular reticular structures 1 year prior to the onset of clinical discoid lupus erythematosus.

Studies have been performed in patients with systemic lupus erythematosus to determine if they have laboratory abnormalities similar to those found in patients with chronic granulomatous disease or female carriers of the disease. Douwes (1972) found normal nitroblue tetrazolium dye reduction in patients with systemic lupus erythematosus. Besana *et al.* (1975) demonstrated an impairment of nitroblue tetrazolium (NBT) reduction in patients with systemic lupus erythematosus. They utilized endotoxin and latex stimulation in the nitroblue tetrazolium assay and reported their results as the percentage of NBT-reducing cells. This method of assay is not diagnostic of chronic granulomatous disease, however, and similar results may be found in other disorders unassociated with autoimmune disease.

Currently, there is no well-defined theory linking the etiology of chronic granulomatous disease and autoimmune disease. It is apparent from the studies performed that both the disease and the carrier state have antibodies and tubular reticular structures in common. It can be postulated that the basic defect in chronic granulomatous disease, which is partially shared by female carriers, predisposes to the development of autoimmune disease.

V. CONCLUSIONS

An increased incidence of autoimmune phenomenon and autoimmune disease has been described in immunodeficiency disorders involving each of the major immune systems: antibody-mediated immunity, cell-mediated immunity, phagocytosis, and complement. It is not necessary to invoke a unifying hypothesis to explain the increased incidence of autoimmunity in these disorders based on a single etiology. It is apparent from recent studies that the immune system is not merely a unidirectionally responsive system, but one in which numerous control mechanisms regulate the degree of immunologic responsiveness. Within the antibody-mediated immune system, antibodies are formed which may either enhance or suppress a variety of biologic responses. Enhancing antibody, blocking antibody, and cytotoxic antibody are all terms utilized to describe various biologic observations, but which also indicate that antibody may have multiple functions. Within the cell-mediated immune system, there are also controlling mechanisms that determine the degree of immunologic responsiveness. T cells must cooperate with B cells for a normal antibody response to occur. However, suppressor T cells exist which regulate the degree of responsiveness. Excess suppressor cell activity may result in diminished antibody production (Waldmann *et al.*, 1974), while diminished suppressor cell activity results in enhanced antibody formation (Morse *et al.*, 1976). Interaction of T cells, B cells, and macrophages is required for normal antibody synthesis, but little information is currently available to determine the role of this three-cell cooperative effect on the regulation of antibody formation in man.

The increased incidence of autoimmune disease found in patients with hypogammaglobulinemia in the absence of antibody strongly suggests that certain autoimmune disorders are initiated and perpetuated by sensitized lymphocytes alone. Conclusive proof and the demonstration of specific lymphocyte sensitization is lacking in the majority of instances. Selective immunoglobulin deficiencies also predispose to autoimmunity as observed in patients with selective IgA deficiency and selective IgM deficiency. In selective IgA deficiency, a broad spectrum of autoantibodies and autoimmune disorders are observed.

Cellular immunodeficiency disorders are also associated with an increased incidence of autoantibody and autoimmune disease. However, in contrast to antibody deficiency disorders, where the autoimmune disorders take the form of arthritis, systemic lupus, hemolytic anemia, and pernicious anemia, cellular immunodeficiency disorders are more frequently associated with endocrinopathy. An exact interpretation of this segregation of disorders is difficult, however, because some overlap occurs.

The association of defective phagocytosis and autoimmunity is difficult to explain. In chronic granulomatous disease, there is a susceptibility to infection by certain bacteria. Although female carriers have a partial defect, as measured by laboratory studies, they do not have an increased incidence of infection. In both the patients and the carriers, increased autoantibody formation is found. In the carriers, systemic lupus and discoid lupus are observed with an increased frequency.

Many theories can be proposed to explain the increased incidence of autoimmunity in immunodeficiency disorders. Complete or partial deficiency of antibodies may result in an increased susceptibility to infection with an increased risk of "neoantigens" or in an inability to dispose of antigens altered by the consequences of microbial infection. The lack of antibody might also result in a greater access of antigens to the systemic circulation and induction of autoimmunity. Antibody may be necessary for the elimination of "antigen-positive cells" which have the potential of producing autoimmunity (Fudenberg, 1971a,b). Complete or partial deficiency of cell-mediated immunity could be postulated to predispose to autoimmunity in a manner similar to that of antibody deficiency.

The most intriguing association of autoimmunity and immunodeficiency is that of chronic granulomatous disease. The theory of autoimmunity proposed by Grabar (1975) provides a clue to a possible mechanism. Grabar postulated that autoantibodies are "natural" mechanisms for disposing of debris and that autoantibody increases when there is a diminished disposal by nonimmunologic means or an increased "load" due to increased tissue or cell destruction. It is possible that, in chronic granulomatous disease and the carrier state, decreased phagocytosis results in an increased antigenic load and subsequent autoimmunity.

There are many areas of immunodeficiency and autoimmunity yet to be explored. Little is known concerning the relationship of a deficiency of suppressor cells or enhanced numbers of suppressor cells and the development of autoimmunity. As new methods of assay for selective deficiencies of T cells become available, greater insight into the pathogenesis of autoimmune disease will be made.

REFERENCES

Ammann, A. J., and Hong, R. (1971a). *J. Immunol.* **106,** 567–569.

Ammann, A. J., and Hong, R. (1971b). *Lancet* (*Baltimore*) **,** 1264–1266.

Ammann, A. J., and Hong, R. (1971c). *Medicine* (*Baltimore*) **50,** 223–236.

Ammann, A. J., and Hong, R. (1971d). *J. Pediatr.* **78,** 821–826.

Ammann, A. J., Cain, W. A., Iskizaka, K., Hong, R., and Good, R. A. (1969a). *N. Engl. J. Med.* **281,** 469–472.

Ammann, A. J., DuQuesnoy, R. J., and Good, R. A. (1969b). *Clin. Exp. Immunol.* **6,** 587–595.

Bachmann, R. (1965). *Scand. J. Clin. Lab. Invest.* **17,** 316–320.

Ballow, M., Dupont, B., and Good, R. A. (1973). *J. Pediatr.* **83,** 772–780.

Barnett, E. V., Winkelstein, A., and Weinberg, H. J. (1970). *Am. J. Med.* **48,** 40–47.

Beale, A. J., Parish, W. E., Douglas, A. P., and Hobbs, J. R. (1971). *Lancet* **1,** 1198–1202.

Bergström, K., Britton, M., Hanson, L. A., Holm, G., Kardos, M., and Webster, P. O. (1973). *Scand. J. Haematol.* **11,** 87–91.

Besana, C., Lazzarin, A., Capsoni, F., Carredda, F., and Moroni, M. (1975). *Lancet* **2,** 918.

Blaese, R. M., Strober, W., Brown, R. S., and Waldmann, T. A. (1968). *Lancet* **1,** 1056–1061.

Blizzard, R. M., and Gibbs, J. H. (1968). *Pediatrics* **42,** 321–327.
Bluestone, R., Goldberg, L. S., Katz, R. M., Marchesano, J. M., and Colabro, J. J. (1970). *J. Pediatr.* **77,** 98–102.
Blume, R. S., Bennett, J. M., Yantee, R. A., and Wolf, S. M. (1968). *N. Engl. J. Med.* **279,** 1009–1015.
Boder, E., and Sedgwick, R. P. (1957). *Univ. South Calif. Med. Bull.* **9,** 15–27.
Booth, C. C. (1970). *Br. Med. J.* **3,** 725–726.
Bruton, O. C. (1952). *Pediatrics* **9,** 722–728.
Buckley, R. H., and Dees, S. C. (1969). *N. Engl. J. Med.* **281,** 465–469.
Burnet, F. H. (1959). "The Clonal Selection Theory of Acquired Immunity." Vanderbilt Univ. Press, Nashville, Tennessee.
Butler, J. E., and Oskvig, R. (1974). *Nature* (*London*) **249,** 830–833.
Case Records of the Massachusetts General Hospital. (1975). *N. Engl. J. Med.* **292,** 95–102.
Cassidy, J. T., Burt, A., Sullivan, D. B., and Dickinson, D. G. (1966). *Arthritis Rheum.* **9,** 851.
Cassidy, J. T., Burt, A., Petty, R., and Sullivan, D. (1968). *N. Engl. J. Med.* **280,** 275.
Chilgren, R. A., Quie, P. G., Meuwissen, H. J., Good, R. A., and Hong, R. (1969). *Lancet* **1,** 1286–1288.
Claman, H. N., Harley, T. F., and Merrill, D. (1966). *J. Allergy* **38,** 215–225.
Collins, H. D., and Dudley, H. R. (1955). *N. Engl. J. Med.* **252,** 255–259.
Conn, H. O., Binder, H., and Burns, B. (1968). *Ann. Intern. Med.* **681,** 603–612.
Cooper, M. D., Chase, H. P., Lowman, J. T., Krivit, W., and Good, R. A. (1968). *Am. J. Med.* **44,** 499–513.
Cooper, M. R., DeChatelet, L. R., LaVia, M. F., McCall, C. E., Spurr, C. L., and Baehner, R. L. (1972). *J. Clin. Invest.* **51,** 769–778.
Crabbé, P. A., and Heremans, J. F. (1967). *Am. J. Med.* **42,** 319–326.
Cummins, L., Spearer, W., and Levenson, S. (1959). *Am. J. Dis. Child.* **98,** 579–580.
Curnutte, J. T., Whitten, D. M., and Babior, B. M. (1974). *N. Engl. J. Med.* **290,** 583–597.
Douglas, S. D., and Fudenberg, H. H. (1969). *Vox Sang.* **16,** 172–178.
Douwes, F. R. (1972). *N. Engl. J. Med.* **287,** 822.
Epstein, L., and Ammann, A. J. (1974). *J. Immunol.* **112,** 617–626.
Fisher, C. C. (1955). *Postgrad. Med.* **17,** 406–409.
Fraser, K. J. (1969). *Med. J. Aust.* **1,** 298–299.
Fresco, R. (1968). *Fed. Proc., Fed. Am. Soc. Exp. Biol.* **27,** 246.
Fridovich, I. (1974). *N. Engl. J. Med.* **290,** 624–625.
Fudenberg, H. H. (1971a). *Am. J. Med.* **51,** 295–298.
Fudenberg, H. H. (1971b). *In* "Immunobiology" (R. Good and D. W. Fisher, eds.), pp. 175–183. Sinauer Assoc., Stamford, Connecticut.
Fudenberg, H. H., and Soloman, A. (1961). *Vox Sang.* **6,** 68–79.
Fudenberg, H. H., Gorman, S. L., and Kunkel, H. G. (1962). *Arthritis Rheum.* **5,** 565–588.

Gelfand, E. W., Berkel, A. L., Godwin, H. A., Rocklin, R. E., David, J. R., and Rosen, F. S. (1972). *Clin. Exp. Immunol.* **11,** 187–199.

Ginsberg, A., and Mullinax, F. (1970). *Am. J. Med.* **48,** 787–791.

Goldberg, L. S., Burnet, E. V., and Fudenberg, H. H. (1968). *J. Lab. Clin. Med.* **72,** 204–212.

Goldman, A. S., Haggard, M. E., McFadden, J., Ritzman, S. E., Houston E. W., Bratcher, R. L., Weiss, K. G., Box, E. M., and Szrekrenyes, J. W. (1967). *Pediatrics* **39,** 348–362.

Good, R. A., Rotstein, J., and Mazzitello, W. F. (1957). *J. Lab. Clin. Med.* **49,** 342–357.

Good, R. A., Zak, S. J., Cordie, R. M., and Bridges, R. A. (1960). *Pediatr. Clin. North Am.* **7,** 397–433.

Good, R. A., Quie, P. G., Windhorst, D. B., Page, A. R., Rodeym, G. E., White, J., Wolfson, J. J., and Holmes, B. H. (1968). *Sem. in Haematol.* **5,** 215–254.

Goodman, J. R., Sylvester, R. A., Talal, N., and Tuffanelli, D. L. (1973). *Ann. Intern. Med.* **79,** 396–402.

Gosh, M. L., and Harris-Jones, J. N. (1974). *Am. J. Clin. Pathol* **62,** 40–46.

Gotoff, S. P., Smith, R. D., and Sugar, O. (1972). *Am. J. Dis. Child.* **123,** 53–56.

Grabar, P. (1975). *Clin. Immunok Im unopathol.* **4,** 453–466.

Grant, G. H., and Wallace, W. D. (1954). *Lancet* **2,** 671–673.

Grausz, H., Laurence, L. E., Stephens, B. G., Lee, J. C., and Hooper, J. (1970). *N. Engl. J. Med.* **283,** 506–511.

Grey, H. M., Rabellino, E., and Pirofsky, B. (1971). *J. Clin. Invest.* **50,** 2368–2375.

Gyorkey, F., Sinkovics, J. G., MIn, K. W., and Gyorkey, P. (1972). *Am. J. Med.* **53,** 148–157.

Hayles, A. B., Stickler, G. B., and McKenzie, B. E. (1954). *Pediatrics* **14,** 449–454.

Heinz, C. F., and Boyer, J. T. (1963). *N. Engl. J. Med.* **269,** 1329–1335.

Heremans, P. E., Ulrich, J. A., and Markowitz, H. (1969). *Am. J. Med.* **47,** 503–519.

Hilton, A. M., and Doyle, L. (1974). *Postgrad. Med.* **50,** 303–305.

Hobbs, J. R. (1968). *Lancet* **1,** 110–114.

Holmes, B., Park, B. H., Malawista, S. E., Quie, P. G., Nelson, D. L., and Good, R. A. (1970). *N. Engl. J. Med.* **283,** 217–231.

Huhn, D. (1968). *Dtsch. Med. Wochenschr.* **93,** 2099–2100.

Huntley, C. C., Thorpe, D. P., Lyerly, A. D., and Kelsey, W. M. (1967). *Am. J. Dis. Child.* **113,** 411–418.

Janeway, C. A., Gitlin, P., Craig, J. M., and Grice, D. S. (1956). *Trans. Assoc. Am. Physicians* **69,** 93–97.

Johansson, S. G. O., Hogman, C. F., and Killander, J. (1968). *Acta Pathol. Microbiol. Scand.* **74,** 519–530.

Kirkpatrick, C. H., Rich, R. R., and Bennett, J. E. (1971). *Ann. Intern. Med.* **74,** 955–978.

Kornreich, H., Molouf, N. N., and Hanson, V. (1971). *J. Pediatr.* **79,** 27–35.

Kushner, D. S., Dubin, A., Donlon, W. P., and Bransky, D. (1960). *Ann. Intern. Med.* **29,** 33–42.

Lamelin, J. P., Lisowska-Bernstein, B., Matter, A., Ryser, J. E., and Vassalli, P. (1972). *J. Exp. Med.* **136,** 984–1007.

Lang, N., Schettler, G., and Wildhack, R. (1954). *Klin. Wochenschr.* **32,** 856–863.

Larsson, S. O. (1962). *Acta Med. Scand.* **172,** 195–199.

Lehrer, R., and Cline, M. J. (1969). *J. Clin. Invest.* **48,** 1478–1488.

Leiken, S., and Oppenheim, J. J. (1971). *Lancet* **2,** 876–877.

Levy, R. L., Bach, M. L., Hunag, S., Bach, F. H., Hong, R., Ammann, A. J., Bortin, M., and Kay, H. E. M. (1971). *Lancet* **2,** 898–900.

Lopez, M., and Hyslop, E. (1968). *Fed Proc., Fed. Am. Soc. Exp. Biol.* **27,** 684.

McFarlane, P. S., Speirs, A. L., and Sommerville, R. G. (1967). *Lancet* **1,** 408–410.

Morse, H. C., Prescott, B., Cross, S. S., Stashak, P. W., and Baker, P. J. (1976). *J. Immunol.* **116,** 279–287.

Odgers, R. J., and Wangel, A. G. (1968). *Lancet* **2,** 846–849.

Panush, R. S., Bianco, N. E., Cheer, P. H., Rocklin, R. E., David, J. R., and Sillman, J. S. (1972). *Clin. Exp. Immunol.* **10,** 103–115.

Peterson, R. D. A., Cooper, M. D., and Good, R. A. (1966). *Am. J. Med.* **41,** 342–359.

Petty, R. E., Cassidy, J. T., and Sullivan, D. B. (1973). *Pediatrics* **51,** 44–48.

Quie, P. G., and Davis, T. (1973). *In* "Immunologic Disorders in Infants and Children" (E. R. Stiehm and V. Fulginiti, eds.), pp. 273–288. Saunders, J. Philadelphia, Pennsylvania.

Rockey, J. H., Hanson, L. A., Heremans, J. F., and Kunkel, H. G. (1964). *Lab. Clin. Med.* **63,** 205–212.

Rosen, F. S., Kevy, S. V., Merler, E., Janeway, C. A., and Gitlin, D. A. (1961). *Pediatrics* **28,** 182–195.

Schaff, Q., Barry, D. W., and Grimley, P. M. (1973). *Lab. Invest.* **29,** 577–586.

Schalach, D. S., McFarlin, D. E., and Barlow, M. H. (1970). *N. Engl. J. Med.* **282,** 1396–1402.

Schaller, J. (1972). *Ann. Intern. Med.* **76,** 746–749.

Schaller, J., Davis, S. D., Ching, Y., Lugunoff, D., Williams, C. P. S., and Wedgwood, R. J. (1966). *Lancet* **2,** 825–829.

Seah, P. P., Fry, L., Hoffbrand, A. V., and Holborow, E. J. (1971). *Lancet* **1,** 834–836.

Smith, C. K., Cassidy, J. T., and Bole, G. G. (1970). *Am. J. Med.* **48,** 113–119.

Spitler, L. E., Levin, A. S., Stites, D. P., Fudenberg, H. H., and Huber, H. (1975). *Cell. Immunol.* **19,** 201–218.

Stobo, J. D., and Tomasi, T. B. (1967). *J. Clin. Invest.* **46,** 1329–1337.

Stoelinga, G. B. A., vanMunster, P. J. J. J., and Sloof, J. P. (1969). *Acta Paediatr. Scand.* **58,** 352–362.

Strich, S. J. (1966). *Neurol., J. Neurosurg. Psychiatry* **29,** 489–499.

Strober, W., Krakauer, R., Klaverman, H. L., Reynolds, H. Y., and Nelson, D. L. (1976). *N. Engl. J. Med.* **294,** 351–356.

Thieffry, S., Arthuris, M., Aicardi, J., and Lyon, G. (1961). *Rev. Neurol.* **105,** 390–405.

Thompson, E. N., and Soothill, J. F. (1970). *Arch. Dis. Childh.* **45,** 24–32.

Twomey, J. J., Jordan, P. H., Jarrold, T., Trubowitz, S., Ritz, N. D., and Conn, H. O. (1969). *Am. J. Med.* **47,** 340–349.

von Kulneff, N., Pederson, K. O., and Waldenstrom, J. (1955). *Schweiz. Med. Wochenschr.* **85,** 363–368.

Vyas, G. N., Perkins, H. A., and Fudenberg, H. H. (1968). *Lancet* **2,** 312–315.

Waldmann, R. A., Broder, S., Durm, M., Blackman, M., Blaese, R. M., and Strober, W. (1974). *Lancet* **2,** 609–613.

Wara, D. W., Goldstein, A. L., Doyle, N. E., and Ammann, A. J. (1975a). *N. Engl. J. Med.* **292,** 70–74.

Wara, D. W., Goodman, J. R., Ochs, H., Doyle, N. E., and Ammann, A. J. (1975b). *Clin. Exp. Immunol.* **21,** 54–58.

Wells, J. V., Bleumers, J. F., and Fudenberg, H. H. (1972). *Clin. Exp. Immunol.* **12,** 305–313.

West, C. A., Hong, R., and Holland, N. H. (1962). *J. Clin. Invest.* **41,** 2054–2064.

Wolff, J. A. (1967). *J. Pediatr.* **70,** 221–232.

Wuepper, K. D., and Fudenberg, H. H. (1967). *Clin. Exp. Immunol.* **2,** 71–82.

Chapter 17

Autoimmunity and Aging

F. M. BURNET

Clinical experience indicates that a number of manifestations of autoimmunity are commonly seen in old age and provides a *prima facie* case for discussing the relationship. However, there is as yet no clear delineation or accepted physiopathological interpretation of either autoimmunity or the process of senescence. Any discussion of relationships will be, therefore, considerably influenced by the general attitude of the author to those two soft-edged fields. In the context of a work on all aspects of autoimmunity, it seems important that the present contribution should open with a brief account of those aspects of aging that seem to be relevant to the topic.

I. CURRENT VIEWS OF THE AGING PROCESS

Aging in mammals is all that needs to be considered in the present context. Even within those limits there is certainly no uniformity as to how the aging process should be interpreted. There is, however, a fairly general appreciation of the importance of accumulating genetic error and its secondary effects in somatic cells, and I feel justified in outlining the variation of that point of view, which I have written about extensively in the last 2 years (Burnet, 1973, 1974a,b). It is essentially a genetic approach, based on three generalizations.

1. Each species of mammal that has been adequately studied under sheltered conditions has an average life span (Comfort, 1964), which must be regarded as a genetically determined characteristic subject to evolutionary control.
2. Bodily changes in aging are evidenced by a diffuse reduction of efficiency in virtually all measurable functions of the body (Shock, 1960) associated with an increasing vulnerability to all types of potentially lethal impacts of the environment. Such changes are interpreted as resulting from the accumulation of genetic errors in somatic cells (Orgel, 1963; Medvedev, 1964).
3. In addition to diffuse changes, there are a number of age-associated diseases apart from those arising from simple increase in vulnerability. They include neoplastic and autoimmune diseases and a variety of degenerative diseases of the central nervous system. All of these can be regarded as being derived predominantly from somatic mutational changes.

On that basis, the essence of any theory of aging is to devise a means whereby the information in the genome that codes for the quality life span (1) can be expressed in a definable rate of somatic genetic error responsible for the bodily changes of age (2 and 3). In some way, a connection must be found; it may be relatively direct or it may function through a very complex web of interacting structural and regulatory genes. If there is some central genetic control of the rate of somatic mutation, the necessary first hypothesis is that the control is concerned with the structure of certain enzymes or other structural proteins. After all, it is a dogma of modern biology that every macromolecule of nucleic acid or protein is directly, and every other organic molecule produced by the body indirectly, coded for in every molecular detail by the genome (Watson, 1970). In a healthy body, at least 99.9% of its macromolecules are certifiably correct according to genetic specification. Any process leading to a progressive accumulation of genetic errors in the somatic cells of the body will result eventually in malfunction of cells, overall inefficiency, and, in the limit, death. Genetic error is especially important when it primarily involves DNA. If the cell concerned undergoes clonal proliferation, all descendant cells will manifest any mutant quality resulting from the primary genetic error. This would not be the case if the primary error involved some other type of informational macromolecule. The error, whatever physical form it takes, must be located somewhere in the nucleotide sequence of DNA if it is to be transmitted clonally.

In seeking an enzyme or complex of enzymatic functions that might control somatic mutation rates, and having in mind what is known of mutator and anti-mutator mutants of bacteria and bacterial viruses, the obvious candidate was the complex of enzymes and auxiliary proteins responsible for the functions of DNA replication and repair and originally spoken of as DNA polymerase (DP). This led to the development of a general concept of intrinsic mutagenesis. In brief, this is that the rate of genetic error, i.e., mutation in somatic cells, could be regulated by the degree of error proneness of DNA polymerase complexes concerned with replication and, more particularly, with repair of DNA damaged by physical or chemical mutagens. There is a certain amount of direct evidence in favor of this view, e.g., Hart and Setlow's (1974) demonstration that efficiency in DNA repair increases in the same linear order as life span from shrewmouse to man. From the present point of view, however, all that is relevant is that, with aging, there is a progressive increase in errors involving effector and receptor proteins of lymphocytes and other immunologically significant cells (Burnet, 1974c). This makes it inevitable that inefficiency must develop in the highly organized homeostatic and self-monitoring system that is responsible for immune function.

II. THE SELF-MONITORING FUNCTION OF THE IMMUNE SYSTEM IN RELATION TO AGING

An aspect of autoimmunity, which is of special relevance in its relation to aging, is the probability that, in many instances, the appearance of autoimmune disease represents a breakdown in the self-monitoring function of the immune system. Aspects of this concept are touched on in several other chapters, but it seems desirable to expand it here in its relevance to aging.

Jerne's network theory (1974) of the functional structure of the immune system is now well known. Basically, it depends on the fact that an immunoglobulin present as antibody or as Ig receptor on an immunocyte presents only one set of antigenic determinants that can be recognized as nonself by its own immune system. These are the specifically modified areas of the V segments that make up the antigen-combining site of the immunoglobulin. Such antigenic potentiality is referred to as the idiotype of the antibody or Ig receptor. Since the idiotypic antigen can react with appropriate immunoglobulin molecules that possess complementary binding sites, we have, in principle, the possibility of specific control by the immune system over any clone of antibody-producing cells and—though it is not yet possible to define the situation precisely—each specific population of T cells.

Although Jerne confines his discussion to B cells and immunoglobulins in their functions both as antibody and antigen, the same principles can be elaborated in other directions. It seems to be self-evident that, in addition to its immune specificity, any immunocyte, T or B, which has some other distinctively individual activity, whether physiological or pathological, will differ in regard to some surface component from the common qualities of normal lymphocytes. Such distinctive components are likely to be immunologically recognizable and, therefore, in principle, can come under the control of the self-monitoring activities of the immune system. Malignant lymphoid cells and forbidden clones of B or T cells associated with autoimmune conditions are specially important in this regard. Others have expressed similar ideas. The H-2 system in mice, and presumably the corresponding genetic region in man, according to Shreffler and David (1975), is a complex of many genes with diverse functions, most or all of which seem to control cell membrane functions. Some of these concern cell–cell interactions, including almost certainly many of the interactions among lymphocytes and of lymphocytes with other cells that are responsible for the organization and control of the immune system.

The best interpretation of the finding that lymphoreticular tumors are especially conspicuous in persons who are immunodeficient, whether from drugs (Starzl *et al.*, 1971; Hoover and Fraumeni, 1973) or from some subacute immunodeficiency disease (Good, 1970), is that malignant change is common within the cells of the immune system, but equally that the normal monitoring system is particularly effective in recognizing and eliminating initiated clones of malignant lymphocytes. On a number of occasions, I have referred to the "forbidden clones" of autoimmune diseases essentially as examples of conditioned malignancy (Burnet, 1959, 1965), and, in a slightly different sense, this seems to hold for all types of lymphoid cell malignancies. Both malignant transformation and change to autoimmune capacity in lymphocytes are, as it were, commonly occurring anomalies against which there are effective counter measures. In the case of autoimmune disease, they can be regarded as part of a set of fail-safe mechanisms.

The implications of such a self-monitoring system are clearly important for aging. Any homeostatic and self-monitoring system, whether industrial or biologic, is necessarily dependent on arrays of sensors and effectors linked by a variety of positive and negative feedbacks. In the biologic situation, special requirements are for proteins of defined configuration to be embedded in the double phospholipid layer of cell membranes (Singer and

Nicolson, 1972; Singer, 1974) and capable of recognizing and being recognized by whatever other molecular pattern has a complementary structure. It is obvious that both complementary patterns must have a genetically accurate structure if effective recognition and signal generation is to occur. Any considerable amount of genetic error will interfere seriously with function, particularly since most corrective moves in the immune system will demand the clonal expansion of appropriate cell types. If the cell from which a new clone is developed has changed by somatic genetic error, all the descendants will have a similar fault, so that the error may have a magnified effect in making the normally adequate response to some threatening situation quite ineffective. If the interpretation of aging that I have adopted is correct, the accumulation of genetic error in the stem cells, lymphocytes, and ancillary cells of the immune system will make it inevitable that there will be a progressive and universal increase in minor inefficiencies and another progressive but rarer and later increase in major life-threatening conditions, such as lymphoreticular cell malignancies or gross autoimmune disease.

In old age one finds that chronic lymphocytic leukemia, multiple myeloma, and a variety of solid lymphomatous tumors, including late-onset Hodgkin's disease, show a typical age-associated character. Autoantibodies are more frequently found, though overt autoimmune disease is not commonly initiated in old age. Amyloid deposition, however, increases strikingly with age.

In Walford's (1969) view, most of the characteristics of aging can be ascribed to increasing inefficiency of the immune system, particularly of T cell functions. At one stage, I (Burnet, 1970) was interested in the possibility that the early atrophy of the thymus could mean that, in a sense, the thymus was the clock that set the pace for senescence. There is no doubt that the immune system plays a very important part in aging, but its progressive loss of efficiency with age must itself be accounted for. In line with the approach which has already been outlined, I prefer, therefore, to look for genetic errors in the controlling mechanisms of the immune system as the primary source of immune dysfunction and to regard it as only one, though possibly the most important, of the body systems whose weaknesses produce the clinical phenomena of aging.

III. THE AGE-SPECIFIC INCIDENCE OF AUTOIMMUNE DISEASE

In looking at the age-specific incidence of autoimmune disease, it is important to consider briefly the possibility espoused by Burch (1963,

1968), that such data can be handled mathematically to provide a stochastic interpretation in terms of the distribution in time of the sequential genetic errors that were involved. Where, for instance, a disease shows an age-specific incidence, which when plotted on a double logarithmic scale falls on a straight line sloping upward with a slope X, one interpretation would be that any unit in the system must suffer a series of $X + 1$ random events whose rate of occurrence is stochastically uniform over the whole period being considered. This type of curve is characteristic of most human cancers, with a slope of 5–6, and among a rather wide range of possible interpretations that have been given are (1) that the initiating cell of the cancer must undergo a series of six to seven mutations with cumulative effect, only the last one being effective in initiating malignant growth; or (2) at least two somatic mutations are required, one or more of the earlier ones inducing an accelerated rate of proliferation in the mutant and its descendant clone without the other aspects of malignancy.

Burch has published extensively in this area and has considerably influenced my outlook on the nature of autoimmune disease and its relation to age. Like other critics of Burch's methods, e.g., Maynard Smith (1962), I feel that he has insufficient appreciation of the flexibility of biologic phenomena and has tried to include too wide a range of clinical conditions within his autoaggressive diseases. The most significant aspect of Burch's work is his need to postulate changes in somatic cells that persist in descendants and on which other random changes can have an additive and equally persisting effect. Somatic mutation, informational error in DNA, is the only biologic episode that fits the requirement. Possibly even more important is the necessity for workers concerned with cellular processes, immunologists and oncologists in particular, to think stochastically whenever the conventional method of explaining disease as the determinative effect of some environmental agent, toxin, antigen, mutagen, or virus is being obviously unsuccessful.

Autoimmune disease is, at first glance, by no means a characteristic disease of old age. The most conspicuous autoimmune conditions are probably thyrotoxicosis, systemic lupus, myasthenia gravis, and autoimmune hemolytic anemia, none of which is commonly associated with old age. Following Burch, and bearing in mind the correlation of most of the conditions with a particular HLA group, one can feel confident that in all of them there is an important genetic component in the absence of which the disease cannot appear. It is obvious that any genetic factor is only part of the etiology; environmental influences and accumulating genetic errors in lymphocyte lines must also be thought of.

Disease in old age in general tends to be slow moving, and this holds quite strikingly for autoimmune conditions. They give the impression of conditions arising by age-associated accumulations of genetic error without any specifically active genetic factor. Arthritic conditions are almost universal in the very old. Some represent residual activity or the "burnt-out" manifestations of rheumatoid arthritis, but most will be classified as osteoarthroses and spoken of as degenerative. Their more detailed etiology is unknown, but many or all may contain an autoimmune component.

The most characteristic feature of autoimmune conditions in old age is their common occurrence, but generally inconspicuous character. Many investigators testing sera from old people with the standard battery of tests for autoantibodies have found a fairly steady increase in the number of positive findings (Hooper *et al.*, 1972), with, as a rule, no significant relationship to any corresponding clinical finding. It is also common to find some degree of hyperglobulinemia quite apart from the monoclonal paraproteinemias to be mentioned later. A curious feature to be seen in several graphic representations of both the proportion of people with autoantibodies and the mean concentration of immunoglobulins (Kipshidze, 1968; Acheson and Jessop, 1962) at different ages is a dip after 70 or 75, followed by a new rise in the 80's. It is conceivable that this may point to the existence of two subpopulations with a genetic difference in life span.

Thyroid glands examined at autopsy in elderly women contain a proportion showing atrophy with mononuclear cellular infiltration, probably lymphocytic (Bastenie, 1967). These may be representative of other low grade cellular infiltrations and represent some partial breakdown of homeostasis to an autoimmune condition, most likely involving an autoantibody-based cytotoxic attack by nonspecific T cells and monocytes.

IV. ASSOCIATION OF AUTOIMMUNE DISEASE WITH CERTAIN HLA TYPES

Although it is only indirectly related to aging, brief mention should be made of recent work on HLA groups in relation to disease, which has shown a clear indication that only diseases that are either generally accepted as autoimmune in character or have some other immunopathological quality show significant correlations with a given histocompatibility antigen. Among whites, but not necessarily in other races, the relevant antigens are HLA-8, W-27, and HLA-7 (McDevitt and Bodmer, 1974; Svejgaard *et al.*, 1975). This finding seems now to be sufficiently well established for an excess of one of these three types among patients with a disease of doubtful etiology to provide a *prima facie* case for regarding the disease as one with an important autoimmune component. This has both theoretical and practical implications.

In view of the fact that most discussions of the etiology of autoimmune disease make no more than cursory mention of genetic or somatic genetic factors, it is worth pointing out that the findings summarized in Tables I and II indicate quite definitely the presence of a genetic association linked to the locus concerned with major histocompatibility antigens, presumably the human equivalents of the Ir genes, and, therefore, closely concerned with the control of the immune system. Although not included in Table I, it should be added that da Costa *et al.* (1974) have also found a positive association of HLA-8 with autoimmune hemolytic anemia.

The finding in almost every type of autoimmune disease in which it is practicable to make the test, including NZB mice hybrids (Warner, 1974) of monoclonal B cell populations, indicates equally strongly that genetic error in a single somatic cell has played a significant part in initiating the condition. Overall, this seems to strengthen the view central to this article that genetic errors, usually involving both germ-line and somatic genomes and interfering with the self-monitoring function of the immune system, are the principal cause of autoimmune disease. It supports equally strongly the contention that genetic errors accumulating with age in the various cell lines that make up the immune system are responsible for the increasing inci-

TABLE I

Positive Associations of HLA and Disease[a]

SD2 type HLA	Disease	Relative risk associated with HLA type[b]
HLA-27	Ankylosing spondylitis	121++
(W-27)	Reiter's syndrome	40++
	Reactive arthritis (yersinia)	++
	Psoriatic arthritis	4.7++
	Juvenile rheumatoid arthritis	11.5++
	Acute anterior uveitis	31++
HLA-8	Dermatitis herpetiformis	4.3++
	Celiac disease (gluten-sensitive enteropathy)	9.5++
	Chronic active hepatitis	3.6++
	Myasthenia gravis	4.5++
	Insulin-dependent diabetes	2.1+
	Addison's disease	6.4+
	Graves' disease	3.6+
HLA-7	Multiple sclerosis	1.49+

[a] Abbreviated from Svejgaard *et al.* (1975).

[b] ++ = highly significant. + = moderately significant.

TABLE II

Positive Associations of Alleles of LD1 Loci and Disease[a]

LD1 type	Disease	Relative risk in comparison with corresponding HLA	
8A	Myasthenia gravis (F)[b]	Lower	
	Celiac disease	Higher	
	Addison's disease	Higher	10.5/6.4
	Graves' disease	Equivalent	
	Juvenile diabetes	Higher	4.5/2.1
7A	Multiple sclerosis	Higher	5.0/1.49

[a] Data from Svejgaard *et al.* (1975) and Möller *et al.* (1976).
[b] F, females only.

dence of low-grade autoimmune disease in old people. This does not refute the possibility that, for autoimmune disease to be initiated, other factors may be needed. It is obvious that the autoantigen involved must be accessible in adequate amount, and, if circumstances not yet established for any condition result in modification of the structure of the autoantigen so that it becomes analogous to the corresponding antigen of another species, this may have an additional effect (Weigle, 1965). The part played by a variety of bacterial or viral infections as initiating agents is also to be kept in mind, though it is unlikely to be much concerned with the autoimmune conditions of old age. Recent work from Finland (Aho *et al.*, 1974, 1975) that yersinia infections can induce noninfectious arthritis and spondylitis, but only in persons with HLA W-27, is illuminating in this regard.

As in all genetic approaches to disease, we are concerned essentially with the reasons why, in normal people, infections, drugs, and other possible initiating agents of autoimmune disease have no effect. The clue offered by one of the "marker" HLA antigens gives positive evidence of the importance of the genetic factor, which otherwise could be claimed only on logical grounds by exclusion of other possibilities.

If the full significance of autoimmune processes for aging is to be gauged, much more work in this field will be needed. There is already a suggestion from the epidemiologic survey of an Australian community (Mackay, 1972) that the presence of autoantibodies—of the types conventionally tested for—in people over 70 is of bad prognostic import. Among 97 people in the study group dying during the test period, there was a significantly higher proportion with autoantibodies than in a group of survivors matched for age and sex. This could be an important lead to further research, but, even if it fails to be confirmed, it is to be hoped that, in the near future, HLA typing and parallel work on the LD1 system, making use of mixed lymphocyte reactions (Jersild *et al.*, 1973, 1975), will be used extensively in gerontological research. It would be most enlightening to determine whether there is any characteristic change in the distribution of SD2 and LD types in the population as it becomes progressively reduced by death.

In this connection, it may be noted that a recent paper by Mathews (1975) shows a significant correlation of the incidence by countries of death from ischemic heart disease and the prevalence of HLA-8 in the population. It will obviously be of interest to establish whether the significance of this finding is supported by an excess of HLA-8 among diagnosed cases of coronary disease. At present, the evidence does not justify including it as a possible autoimmune condition, but it is an index of what might happen in the future. Another possibility that may emerge is that there is a specific correlation of an autoimmune disease with a certain HLA group only within a certain kinship (Sever, 1975) or racial group (Whittingham *et al.*, 1973). In other assemblages, the association is with a different HLA type. There are many combinations of degenerative changes in old age where it would not be surprising to find an indication of autoimmune processes at work. Possible examples in addition to ischemic heart disease are osteoarthrosis and senile psychosis.

V. LYMPHOPROLIFERATIVE PROCESSES

Reasons have already been given for regarding autoimmune disease as a conditioned malignancy, and there are some interesting associations among lymphoid cell malignancies, autoimmune diseases, and aging.

A good practical criterion for deciding whether a proliferative condition has sprung from a change in a single cell, i.e., by somatic mutation, is to demonstrate that the cell population has a monoclonal character. Where an immunoglobulin-producing cell is concerned, monoclonality can be shown by demonstrating the single antigenic nature of the light chain κ (I, II, and III) or λ, or by showing that the immunoglobulin in question is uniform in quality by tests for specificity for idiotype or for amino acid sequence. If other types of cell are concerned, the only procedure that is commonly available is to test for a character coded for by a gene in the X chromosome in women who are heterozygous for two distinguishable alleles. As is well known, only one X chromosome is active in any somatic cell, the distribution being essentially a random one. Almost invariably, the enzyme glucose 6-phosphate dehydrogenase (G6PD) is used in women of African origin heterozygous for A and B types of the enzyme (Fialkow, 1972).

It is very difficult in most cases to establish whether an autoimmune disease is a monoclonal condition or not, except in the case of the autoimmune hemolytic anemias. The great majority of warm, cold, and Donath–Landsteiner varieties that have been tested appear to be monoclonal. The general method of investigation is to elute the autoantibody attached to the circulating red cells or taken up by them on cooling, and determine the antigenic type (κ or λ) of the light chain. Leddy and Bakemeier (1965) were the first to find that, with only a small proportion of exceptions showing both κ and λ, all eluted immunoglobulins were pure κ or pure λ, and, as would be expected, about twice as many κ as λ.

Cold autoimmune hemolytic anemia is often associated with a monoclonal hyperglobulinemia and has a considerable resemblance to the paraproteinemias (Cooper, 1968). These proteins are, for some unknown reason, all κ, but their monoclonal character is established by examining for the different κI, κII, and κIII types (Capra *et al.*, 1972). Each is one or the other, and κIII is the one most frequently found as the cold agglutinin. It is obvious that some nonrandom factors are at work here, but the monoclonal origin is undoubted.

Cold autoimmune hemolytic anemia, like some of the purely lymphoproliferative conditions considered below, is a typical age-associated disease in the sense that age-specific incidence of the condition rises steadily with age. In this, it differs from warm type autoimmune hemolytic anemia which can affect any age from infancy onward.

Chronic lymphocytic leukemia is a typical age-associated disease and, in most cases, represents a monoclonal proliferation of B cells (Aisenberg and Bloch, 1972). A considerable proportion produce detectable amounts of monoclonal immunoglobulin in the serum (Seligmann and Preud'homme, 1973). I am not aware of studies to determine whether any of these immunoglobulins are reactive as antibody with a known antigen or hapten. It is well known that terminal symptoms of hemolytic anemia or thrombocytopenia may occur, but it is not likely that the initial clone was responsible for the autoimmune acitivity. Much more probably, the appearance of a terminal autoimmune condition is a manifestation of the progressive inefficiency of self-moitoring function in the immune system, with the uncontrolled appearance of a pathogenic clone which is wholly distinct from the clone responsible for the chronic lymphocytic leukemia as such.

Multiple myelomatosis is generally interpreted as representing the activity of a malignant plasma cell clone, apparently derived from genetic error occurring in a cell that had already taken on plasma cell quality. A considerable number of myeloma proteins and of the IgM paraproteins from Waldenström's macroglobulinemia patients are reactive as antibodies with some of the antigens that have been used to test them (Gajdusek and Mackay, 1958; Metzger, 1967). Among them are some that react like rheumatoid factor or other autoantigen. A proportion of macroglobulinemia patients may, in fact, be suffering from an autoimmune condition in which the aberrant clone is being stimulated to proliferate by an autoantigen. Both myeloma and nonmalignant paraproteinemias are strongly age-associated diseases, the latter being much more common. About 3% of males over 75 show a monoclonal increase in immunoglobulin (Kohn and Srivastava, 1973). Isobe and Osserman (1971) found a highly significant correlation of malignancy in prostate and rectum with paraproteinemia in males. Tumor in these cases was often infiltrated with plasma cells, but no reason for the association was found.

VI. AMYLOIDOSIS

Amyloid disease, in its classical form, was associated with chronic sepsis or tuberculosis. These have virtually disappeared, and most amyloidosis today is associated with Hodgkin's disease, rheumatoid arthritis, paraproteinemia, and old age. Although only one autoimmune disease is included in that list, recent work on amyloidosis points to its resulting from an immunologic process occurring in an immune system under stress and inadequately controlled (Franklin and Zucker-Franklin, 1972). Amyloid as deposited in spleen or kidney can be recognized by staining with Congo red and by the typical fibrillar structures seen in electron micrographs. It is characteristically associated with cellular debris in which occasional plasma cells can often be recognized.

Two different types of fibrillar protein, A and B (Benditt and Eriksen, 1973), and a nonfibrillar P component have been described, of which the B form is best understood (Hobbs, 1973). It is made up of fragments of κ or λ light chains, modified in some respect, that makes them resistant to proteolysis (Glenner *et al.*, 1970). Similar material has been prepared by *in vitro* action of proteolytic or kidney lysosomal enzymes on Bence Jones protein (Glenner *et al.*, 1971; Epstein *et al.*, 1974). Amyloid protein B is mainly seen in cases associated with the presence of a monoclonal immunoglobulin in the blood. Fibrillar protein AS (or AA) is not an immunoglobulin product and has a molecular weight (MW) of 7000–8000. It has a specific antigenicity, and material reactive with anti-A is found in serum from amyloid patients (Husby *et al.*, 1973). A nonfibrillar minor component, P, has been defined and shown to be present in the serum of both amyloid patients and some normal individuals in the form of an α-

globulin (Cathcart *et al.*, 1967). The immunologic significance of A and P components is uncertain, but it seems likely that they also represent accumulation at the site of deposition of material concerned with inflammatory or immune responses.

Any interpretation of the amyloid lesion must be tentative, but in the light of its pathology in man, and of experimental results, such as those of Cathcart *et al.* (1970), with casein-induced amyloidosis in the guinea pig, there is justification for regarding autoimmune processes associated with hyperglobulinemia and circulating antigen–antibody complexes as playing a major role. Deposition of immune complex, with tissue damage and local accumulation of circulating cells, including T and B lymphocytes and plasma cells, could initiate a focus whose extension would result if a low-grade autoimmune process leads to more deposition of the autoantigen with accumulation of T and B cells carrying autoantibody specificity and their destruction by high antigen concentration, presumably accentuated by the local action of lymphokines liberated from stimulated and damaged cells.

One of the characteristic pathological features of old age, especially seen in senile psychosis, is the presence of "senile plaques" in the brain (Wolstenholme and O'Connor, 1970). These are composed of amyloid associated with cellular debris from nerve cells and, presumably, also from lymphocytes or plasma cells. Plaques are regular in Alzheimer's disease and in senile psychosis, and tend to be correlated with the degree of fallout of neurons. There is a suggestion here that autoimmune processes play an unsuspected part in the central nervous system degenerations of old age, but the converse possibility that any autoimmune reaction is secondary to a primary degenerative process seems at least as likely.

VII. AGE AND AUTOIMMUNITY IN ANIMAL MODELS

Virtually the only animal models in which the "spontaneous" appearance of autoimmune conditions can be related to age are among the mouse strains of the laboratory. Occasional instances of disease with autoimmune features are seen in dogs, mink, and other animals, but, in the present context, only murine conditions warrant consideration.

During the 1950's, a group of pure-line mouse strains were developed in New Zealand by the Bielschowskys, as described by Bielschowsky and Goodall (1970). The strain NZB and its F_1 hybrid, with another of their strains, NZW, are now the standard examples of autoimmune disease in mice. Both show the appearance of autoimmune hemolytic anemia and antigen–antibody complex-induced glomerulonephritis, the former being more conspicuous in NZB and the latter in F_1 NZB/NZW, where it almost invariably causes death around 300–400 days of age. In NZB, the appearance of Coombs-type antibody begins around 4 or 5 months of age and shows an age-associated rise until the whole population is positive. When tests for cells capable of producing plaques on mouse cells were developed by Wilson *et al.* (1971), only very small numbers of plaque-forming cells were present in spleens of young mice, with a sharp increase in animals over 9 months of age. Similar findings were reported by Hildemann and Walford (1966) for an F_1 hybrid strain unrelated to the NZ strains.

A relatively large number of mouse strains and at least two outbred populations devleop anti-nuclear factor in the serum as they age; a brief review will be found in an earlier paper (Burnet, 1974c).

Other immunopathological conditions in mice not strictly autoimmune in quality are also age associated. Lymphoreticular tumors become common with age in many, probably all, strains of mice, notably so in NZB. A typically age-associated incidence of such tumors has also been shown for wild mice kept under laboratory conditions (Gardner *et al.*, 1973). Finally, the strain SJL/J is reported to develop paraproteinemia in a proportion of older mice, usually with subsequent appearance of reticulum cell tumors of the spleen. An interesting postscript to this finding is the recent observation that SJL/J mice are susceptible to paralysis when injected with "basic protein" from brain tissue. This susceptibility to experimental autoallergic encephalomyelitis differentiates it from the other mouse strains that have been studied in this regard.

The nature of the immunological changes in NZB and its hybrids and their etiology is extensively discussed by others in this volume. Here I am only justified in outlining the part played by genetic and somatic genetic factors in accounting for the characteristic age incidence of the autoimmune signs. The NZB strain breeds true to type, and part of the etiology of the hemolytic disease must be gene based. Warner (1973) reported that two genes are concerned, one being also carried by the strain NZC. In part, these genetic factors may be expressed in the exceptional resistance of NZB mice to tolerization by a number of antigens, including deaggregated bovine γ-globulin (Staples and Talal, 1969). I should consider it likely that the characteristic age incidence of the appearance of Coombs antibody can best be ascribed to somatic mutation in B cells or their precursors. Evidence for this is provided in Warner's (1974) finding that, where circumstances allow the test to be made, the autoantibody in NZB F_1 hybrids is monoclonal in character. Sugai *et al.* (1973) also observed a monolonal IgM in NZB mice, but this was not identified as a Coombs-type antibody and may be an unrelated paraprotein.

Another factor which may be relevant to the age incidence is the loss with age of some of the self-monitoring capacity associated with suppressor T cells. According to Barthold *et al.* (1974), the antibody response to a pneumococcal polysaccharide is highest in old NZB mice and can be reduced by injection of cells (presumably suppressor T cells) from young NZB mice.

My summary following a more extensive discussion in 1974 (Burnet, 1974c, pp. 31–32) still holds. The relationship of age to the development of signs of disease in NZB mice depends initially on the balance between the buildup of appropriate somatic mutations in cells already genetically susceptible and the controlling influence of suppressor cells forming part of the self-monitoring mechanism of the immune system. As monitoring acitivity diminishes with age, the effect of autoantibodies on red cells and via Ag–Ab complexes in the kidney becomes progressively more apparent.

VIII. CONCLUSION

Autoimmune disease is by no means a conspicuous disability of old age, but, at the same time, a rather large proportion of elderly people show evidence of low-grade autoimmune conditions, as well as of other anomalies or deficiencies of the immune system.

Neither autoimmunity nor aging is well understood at the molecular level, and there are widely discrepant theoretical approaches to each. It would be a legitimate criticism of this contribution to say that its chief concern has been to show how the genetic and somatic genetic approaches to aging and to autoimmune disease that I have favored in the past allow the association of autoimmunity with aging to take a logically consistent form. Both are manifestations of cumulative genetic error in somatic cells on a genetic background controlled by the germ-line genome. In both, there is a large random element at genetic levels and the possibility of significant, essentially accidental influence by a wide variety of environmental impacts.

Autoimmune disease on this view requires, first, the appearance, often against a genetic background anomaly, of a mutant cell sufficiently resistant to avoid early elimination. The potentially pathogenic cells of the developing clone find themselves part of an immune system, which for one reason or another lacks a normally adequate self-monitoring capacity, and where the potentially pathogenic cells find adequate opportunity for specific stimulation by accessible autoantigen. On such a view it is inevitable, when somatic genetic error in old age has diminished the efficiency of control within the immune system, that many clones of relatively trivial degrees of pathogenicity should be able to persist producing irregularly, detectable autoanitbody, minor symptoms, and focal deposition of amyloid.

REFERENCES

Acheson, M., and Jessop, W. J. E. (1962). *Gerontologia* **6,** 195.

Aho, K., Ahvonen, P., Lassus, A., Sievers, K., and Tiilikainen, A. (1974). *Arthritis Rheum.* **17,** 521–526.

Aho, K., Ahvonen, P., Alkio, P., Lassus, A., Sairanen, E., Sievers, K., and Tiilikainen, A. (1975). *Ann. Rheum. Dis. Suppl.* **34,** 29–30.

Aisenberg, A. C., and Bloch, K. J. (1972). *N. Engl. J. Med.* **287,** 272–276.

Barthold, D. R., Kysela, S., and Steinberg, A. D. (1974). *J. Immunol.* **112,** 9–16.

Bastenie, P. A., Neve, P., Bonnyns, M., Vanhaelst, L., and Chailly, M. (1967). *Lancet* **1,** 915–918.

Benditt, E. P., and Eriksen, N. (1973). *Protides Biol. Fluids, Proc. Colloq.* **20,** 81–85.

Bielschowsky, M., and Goodall, C. M. (1970). *Cancer Res.* **30,** 834–836.

Burch, P. R. J. (1963). *Lancet* **1,** 1253–1257.

Burch, P. R. J. (1968). "An Inquiry Concerning Growth, Disease and Ageing." Oliver & Boyd, Edinburgh.

Burnet, F. M. (1970). *Lancet* **2,** 358–360.

Burnet, F. M. (1973). *Lancet* **2,** 480–483.

Burnet, F. M. (1974a). *Pathology* **6,** 1–11.

Burnet, F. M. (1974b). "Intrinsic Mutagenesis." MTP (Medical and Technical Publishing), Lancaster.

Burnet, F. M. (1974c). *Prog. Immunol., Int. Congr. Immunol., 2nd, 1974.* Vol. 5, pp. 27–36.

Burnet, M. (1959). *Br. Med. J.* **2,** 720–725.

Burnet, M. (1965). *Br. Med. J.* **1,** 338–342.

Capra, J. D., Kehoe, J. M., Williams, R. C., Feizi, T., and Kunkel, H. G. (1972). *Proc. Natl. Acad. Sci. U.S.A.* **69,** 40–43.

Cathcart, E. S., Shirahama, T., and Cohen, A. S. (1967). *Biochim. Biophys. Acta* **147,** 392–393.

Cathcart, E. S., Mullarkey, M., and Cohen, A. S. (1970). *Lancet* **2,** 639–640.

Comfort, A. (1964). "Ageing—The Biology of Senescence." Routledge & Kegan Paul, London.

Cooper, A. G. (1968). *Clin. Exp. Immunol.* **3,** 691–702.

da Costa, J. A. G., White, A. G., Parker, A. C., and Grigor, G. B. (1974). *J. Clin. Pathol.* **27,** 353–355.

Epstein, W. V., Tan, M., and Wood, I. S. (1974). *J. Lab. Clin. Med.* **84,** 107–110.

Fialkow, P. J. (1972). *Adv. Cancer. Res.* **15,** 191–226.

Franklin, E. G., and Zucker-Franklin, D. (1972). *Adv. Immunol.* **15,** 249–304.

Gajdusek, D. C., and Mackay, I. R. (1958). *Arch. Intern. Med.* **101,** 30–46.

Gardner, M. B., Henderson, B. E., Estes, J. D., Menck, H., Parker, J. C., and Huebner, R. J. (1973). *J. Natl. Cancer Inst.* **50,** 1571–1579.

Glenner, G. G., Harbaugh, J., Ohms, J. I., Harada, M., and Cuatrecasas, P. (1970). *Biochem. Biophys. Res. Commun.* **41,** 1287–1289.

Glenner, G. G., Ein, D., Eanes, E. D., Bladen, H. A., Terry, W., and Page, D. L. (1971). *Science* **174,** 712–714.

Good, R. A. (1970). *In* "Immune Surveillance" (R. T. Smith and M. Landy, eds.), pp. 442–444. Academic Press, New York.

Hart, R. W., and Setlow, R. B. (1974). *Proc. Natl. Acad. Sci. U.S.A.* **71,** 2169–2173.

Hildemann, W. H., and Walford, R. L. (1966). *Proc. Soc. Exp. Biol. Med.* **123,** 417–421.

Hobbs, J. R. (1973). *Proc. R. Soc. Med.* **66,** 705–710.

Hooper, B., Whittingham, S., Mathews, J. D., Mackay, I. R., and Curnow, D. H. (1972). *Clin. Exp. Immunol.* **12,** 79–87.

Hoover, R., and Fraumeni, J. F. (1973). *Lancet* **2,** 55–57.

Husby, G., Sletten, K., Michaelsen, T. E., and Natvig, J. B. (1973). *Scand. J. Immunol.* **2,** 395–404.

Isobe, T., and Osserman, E. F. (1971). *Ann. N.Y. Acad. Sci.* **190,** 507–517.

Jerne, N. K. (1974). *Ann. Immunol.* (*Paris*) **125c,** 373–389.

Jersild, C., Fog., T., Hansen, G. S., Thomsen, M., Svejgaard, A., and Dupont, B. (1973). *Lancet* **2,** 1221–1225.

Jersild, C., Dupont, B., Fog, T., Platz, P. J., and Svejgaard, A. (1975). *Transplant. Rev.* **22,** 148–163.

Kipshidze, N. N. (1968). *Cancer Aging, Thule Int. Symp., 2nd, 1967.* pp. 49–57.

Kohn, J., and Srivastava, P. C. (1973). *Protides Biol. Fluids, Proc. Colloq.* **20,** 257–261.

Leddy, J. P., and Bakemeier, R. F. (1965). *J. Exp. Med.* **121,** 1–17.

McDevitt, H. O., and Bodmer, W. F. (1974). *Lancet* **1,** 1269–1275.

Mackay, I. R. (1972). *Gerontologia* **18,** 285–304.

Mathews, J. D. (1975). *Lancet* **2,** 681–682.

Maynard Smith, J. (1962). *Proc. R. Soc. London, Ser. B* **157,** 115–127.

Medvedev, Z. A. (1964). *Adv. Gerontol. Res.* **1,** 181–206.

Metzger, H. (1967). *Proc. Natl. Acad. Sci. U.S.A.* **57,** 1490–1497.

Möller, E., Link, H., Matell, G., Olhagen, B., and Stendahl, L. (1976). *Histocompat. Test.* (in press).

Orgel, L. E. (1963). *Proc. Natl. Acad. Sci. U.S.A.* **49,** 517–521.

Seligmann, M., and Preud'homme, J. L. (1973). *Protides Biol. Fluids, Proc. Colloq.* **20,** 211–213.

Sever, J. L. (1975). *Neurology* **25,** 486–488.

Shock, N. W. (1960). *In* "Aging—Some Social and Biological Aspects" (N. W. Shock, ed.), Publ. No. 65, pp. 241–260. Am. Assoc. Adv. Sci., Washington, D.C.

Shreffler, D. C., and David, C. S. (1975). *Adv. Immunol.* **20,** 125–195.

Singer, S. J. (1974). *Adv. Immunol.* **19,** 1–66.

Singer, S. J., and Nicolson, G. L. (1972). *Science* **175,** 729–731.

Staples, P. J., and Talal, N. (1969). *J. Exp. Med.* **129,** 123–139.

Starzl, T. E., Penn, I., Putnam, C. W., Groth, C. G., and Halgrimson, C. G. (1971). *Transplant. Rev.* **7,** 112–145.

Sugai, S., Pillarisetty, R., and Talal, N. (1973). *J. Exp. Med.* **138,** 989–1002.

Svejgaard, A., Platz, P., Ryder, L. P., Staub Nielsen, L., and Thomsen, M. (1975). *Transplant. Rev.* **22,** 3–43.

Walford, R. L. (1969). "The Immunologic Theory of Aging." Munksgaard, Copenhagen.

Warner, N. L. (1973). *Clin. Immunol. Immunopathol.* **1,** 353–363.

Warner, N. L. (1974). *Clin. Immunol. Immunopathol.* **2,** 556–562.

Watson, J. D. (1970). "Molecular Biology of the Gene," 2nd ed. Benjamin, New York.

Weigle, W. O. (1965). *J. Exp. Med.* **121,** 289–307.

Whittingham, S., Mackay, I. R., Thanabalasundrum, R. S., Chuttani, H. K., Manjuran, R., Seah, C. S., Yu, M., and Viranuvatti, V. (1973). *Br. Med. J.* **4,** 517–519.

Wilson, J. D., Warner, N., and Holmes, M. C. (1971). *Nature (London), New. Biol.* **233,** 80–82.

Wolstenholme, G. E. W., and O'Connor, M., eds. (1970). "Alzheimer's Disease and Related Conditions," Ciba Found. Symp. Churchill, London.

Chapter 18

Autoimmunity and Systemic Lupus Erythematosus

DAVID GLASS AND PETER H. SCHUR

I. INTRODUCTION

Systemic lupus erythematosus (SLE) is one of a group of diseases of unknown etiology associated with evidence for abnormal humoral and cellular immune responses. Most studies indicate that the immune response is directed primarily to a range of constituents of normal human cells. These findings have warranted the inclusion of SLE among those diseases which have been labeled "autoimmune." This involvement of the immunologic system may lead to anergy or to immune complex formation with subsequent tissue deposition and injury. SLE has also been considered as a prototype for "immune complex" disease.

In mice, there is an association between the major histocompatibility complex (MHC) and immune responses. In certain strains, immune complex deposition has been associated with MHC markers. These observations have prompted examination in man for possible association between the MHC and diseases in which immune response genes may be of relevance. The availability of tissue typing methods has, therefore, provided an opportunity to reevaluate the genetic background of these diseases, including SLE, in which immune system appears to be important. The association between HLA types and SLE is not as complete as in other diseases. Sufficient data is available though to reinforce the earlier population studies, suggesting some degree of genetically determined predisposition for the disease.

While the primary cause of the disease remains an enigma, it is possible to draw up a hypothesis that includes infection or invasion with a microorganism in a genetically susceptible individual. This may cause the release of "hidden" cellular autoantigens or the development of new antigens which are then associated with an (abnormal) immune response by the host. The evidence of this hypothesis will be reviewed in this chapter.

II. SLE: GENETIC PREDISPOSITION

A. Epidemiology of the Disease

The methods used for the initial studies relating to predisposition to the disease were those available to the epidemiologist studying particular racial groups, families, and when possible, twins. The disease occurs in females more commonly than males. Siegel and Lee (1973) established that the female to male preponderance was most marked among black Americans, compared to their white counterparts, there being an approximately threefold increase in incidence in the black population. This racial difference was found in urban and rural communities; both groups had a higher incidence (130/100,000) in an urban environment (New York), compared to the rural area (63/100,000) (Alabama). This finding of susceptibility of black American females to the disease has been confirmed by the Kaiser Permanente Medical Group (Fessel, 1975). The increased incidence in urban areas is presumed to represent an environmental influence, as yet undefined, in addition to any genetic predisposition that might exist.

Family studies have shown an increased incidence, although there are conflicting reports. Estimates of overall incidence of disease range between 1 per 100,000 (Block and Christian, 1975) and 2.5 per 1000 (Arthritis Foundation booklet). First-degree relatives have been reported to have an incidence approaching 15 per 1000 (Masi, 1968). Block *et al.* (1975) noted Raynaud's phenomenon and polyarteritis nodosa frequently among the first-degree relative of their patients. Anti-nuclear antibodies (ANA) were found in 4–33% of first degree relatives, compared with 0–1.3% in normal controls (Block *et al.*, 1975). ANA were found in 4–14% of nonconsanguineous relatives of probands. This suggestion of an environmental effect is reinforced by the study of De Horatius and Messner (1975) who noted antilymphocyte antibodies in 57% of 124 relatives of 28 SLE patients, compared with 4% of 76 control individuals. However, a higher incidence of antibodies was found in consanguineous than in nonconsanguineous household contacts (73% versus 50%) and a higher incidence in consanguineous household contacts than nonhousehold consanguineous contacts (73% versus 23%). We have not been able to confirm these findings (Raum *et al.*, 1977).

Anti-RNA antibodies were found in only 16% of SLE family members, in 21% of household contacts, in 27% of consanguineous household contacts, but not in nonconsanguineous household or nonhousehold contacts (De Horatius *et al.*, 1975). A significant correlation was noted between anti-RNA antibodies and lymphocytotoxic antibodies in household contacts (De Horatius *et al.*, 1975). These findings can be interpreted, as can the rural versus urban studies, as evidence of the interaction of genetic and environmental factors, since the overall incidence in relatives not sharing a household with the propositus with SLE was still higher than in control families.

Analysis of twins, both monozygous and dizygous, has demonstrated a 57% concordance rate for SLE in monozygous pairs, and concordance ratio of 71% for ANA, and 87% for hypergammaglobulinemia (Block *et al.*, 1975). Similarities of age of onset and clinical presentation seem to have been a feature of these twin studies. In one pair of monozygotic twins, separated in infancy and concordant for SLE, the disease was found at a similar age in both individuals. The rate for concordance in dizygous twins appears to be substantially lower, although one of three pairs had marked serological abnormalities.

B. Predisposition to SLE Associated with Genetically Determined Deficiencies in Immune Response-Related Proteins

1. *Immunoglobulins*

Global deficiencies of immunoglobulins are associated with connective tissue disorders, including rheumatoid arthritis and dermatomyositis, but not with SLE. However, isolated deficiencies of IgA has been noted in 4.1% (4 out of 87) patients with SLE, compared with 0.14% for controls (Cassidy *et al.*, 1969). The comparable figure for juvenile rheumatoid arthritis (JRA) in this study was 10 out of 294 (4%) of affected individuals. That the IgA deficiency is inherited, rather than acquired, was not established. Supporting evidence for the role of IgA deficiency as a predisposing factor in SLE is provided by the recent report of an increased frequency of ANA among IgA-deficient individuals (11 of 37) (Gershwin *et al.*, 1975).

2. *Complement Components*

Components of the classic complement pathway have been found to be deficient in the sera of several family groups, inheritance of the deficiency in those identified thus far being autosomal codominant. Some of the members of these families have rheumatic diseases, including SLE, which has been reported to be associated with a range of deficiencies including C1r, C1s, C1 INH, C4, C5, C8, and, most commonly, with C2 (Moncado *et al.*, 1972; Day *et al.*, 1972, 1973; Pondman *et al.*, 1968; Kohler *et al.*, 1974; Hauptmann *et al.*, 1974; Cooper *et al.*, 1968; Agnello *et al.*, 1972; Stern *et al.*, 1976; Wild *et al.*, 1976; Jasin, 1976; Glass *et al.*, 1976). The syndromes resembling SLE in these patients have not been entirely typical, warranting the description SLE-like in some instances. A feature common to some of these patients has been the relative lack of antinuclear antibodies (Table I). The manner, or even the extent in which complement deficiencies predispose to disease, if at all, is not clear. Asymptomatic familes with complement deficiencies, particularly of C2, are described. An incidence of hypocomplementemia of 14 out of 41,083 and 1 out of 10,000 "normal" individuals has been reported (von Hassig *et al.*, 1964; F. Stratton, quoted in Lachmann, 1974). These studies probably relate to homozygous deficiency. In the later study, the one hypocomplementemic individual was C2 deficient. Therefore, the predicted incidence of C2 heterozygous deficiency will be 1:50. In our laboratory we have noted 6 presumed heterozygous deficient individuals amongst 509 blood bank donors (Glass *et al.*, 1976).

In these and related studies the identity of C2 deficient individuals was assisted by analysis of HLA antigens, since the majority of C2 deficient individuals carry either antigen A10 or B18, or the combination A10, B18 (Fu *et al.*, 1974; Gibson *et al.*, 1975, Schur, 1977). Using HLA antigens in addition to complement measurements, we were able to identify C2 deficient individuals amongst 137 patients with SLE (Glass *et al.*, 1976). These

TABLE I

Complement Component Deficiencies Associated with SLE or Variants

Component deficiency	Study	Comments
C1r	Pickering *et al.* (1970), Mancado *et al.* (1972), Day *et al.* (1972)	ANA/LE cells absent
C1s	Pondman *et al.* (1968)	ANA developed late in the course of the disease
C1 INH	Kohler *et al.* (1974), Donaldson *et al.* (1977)	Angioedema and SLE
C4	Hauptman *et al.* (1974), Gilliland *et al.* (1975)	ANA, immunoglobulin in skin absent
C2	Agnello *et al.* (1972), Day *et al.* (1973), Fu *et al.* (1974), Osterland *et al.* (1975), Friend *et al.* (1975), Gibson *et al.* (1975), Glass *et al.* (1976), Stein, *et al.* (1976), Wild *et al.* (1976)	"Lupus-like" syndrome atypical skin changes late development of ANA Discoid LE and SLE
C5	Rosenfeld and Leddy (1974)	
C8	Jasin (1976)	

findings would suggest that complement component deficiencies, even in the heterozygous form, can predispose to SLE and in the instance of C2, do so to an extent similar to that of IgA deficiency.

C. Histocompatibility Loci Markers in SLE

Evidence is accumulating in man to suggest that the histocompatibility loci are on the sixth autosomal chromosome. In an analogous situation to that existing in experimental animals, notably the H-2 locus on the seventeenth mouse chromosome, specific immune response genes are probably situated on this chromosome, although the data in man is as yet limited. The histocompatibility antigens in man, closest to the suggested site for the immune response genes are those of the HLA-B, or second series antigens, and those of the D or MLC/MLR series. The demonstration of an association between disease and histocompatibility (HLA) antigens could, therefore, provide evidence both for the existence of genetic control and, by inference, suggest an immune basis for disease, assuming Ir genes and HLA antigens are as closely related in man as is currently believed. The lack of antisera for use in the definition of the MLC loci, as are available for the HLA antigens, is a limiting factor at present in the application of some of these techniques to clinical investigation. The studies of HLA antigens in patients with SLE (Table II) do not show as clear associations as, for example, that between B27 and spondylitis in which the strong family history suggests a greater genetic component in etiology. Perhaps the major point of significance in the SLE studies is the presence of some association, even if of small degree, between HLA-B series antigens and SLE. Although different antigens have been reported in these studies, it is of interest that the antigens B5 reported by Stastny (1972), Nies (1974), and BW35 reported by Bitter (1974) are cross-reacting as part of the 4c locus, antigens that have also been associated with lymphoma, particularly Hodgkin's disease. In our own studies, an increased frequency of B18 have been noted (Glass) (Table II). The negative findings by Kissmeyer-Nielsen *et al.* (1975) in a group of Danish patients in one of the largest series published, presumably drawn from a homogeneous population, emphasizes the problems involved in drawing conclusions from the data thus far available.

The value of haplotype or at least of first and second series antigen pair analysis, has recently been emphasized; additional evidence can result for HLA linkages not obtained by single antigen analysis (Terasaki and Mickey, 1975). The finding of the A1, B8 haplotype in increased frequency in two series of SLE patients is of interest (Goldberg *et al.*, 1973; Glass *et al.*, 1976). This combination, the commonest in white populations, has been associated with a range of diseases including chronic active hepatitis and celiac disease, in which immunologic mechanisms and viruses (in the former)

TABLE II

SLE-HLA Antigens

	Antigens	Patients[a]	Controls[a]	Race	Study
Single antigens	BW15			Black	Waters *et al.*, 1971
	B8	36 (25)	16 (82)	White	Grumet *et al.*, 1971
	BW15 (LND)	36 (25)	10 (82)	White	Grumet *et al.*, 1971
	B13	15 (40)	0 (40)	Black	Arnett *et al.*, 1972
	AW33	21 (40)	3 (40)	Black	Stastny, 1972
	B5	Twice as frequent as controls		Black	Stastny, 1972
	B7	54 (28)	10 (280)	Black	Bitter, 1974; Bitter *et al.*, 1972
	BW35	82 (28)	23 (280)	Black	Bitter, 1974; Bitter *et al.*, 1972
	A1	14 (71)		Black	Goldberg *et al.*, 1973
	B8	35 (49)	12	White	Goldberg *et al.*, 1973
	B5	24 (42)	11 (886)	White	Nies *et al.*, 1974
	B5	23 (40)	5 (120)	Black	Nies *et al.*, 1974
	No diff.	— (65)	— (502)	White	Kissmeyer-Nielson *et al.*, 1975
	B18	20 (44)	5 (346)	White	Glass and Schur (unpublished observations)
Haplotypes	A1, B8	12 (120)	5 (120)	Mixed	Goldberg *et al.*, 1973
	A1, B8	34 (44)	15 (346)	White	Glass and Schur (unpublished observations)
	A2, B12[b]	0	5.9	White	Terasaki and Mickey, 1975
	B7, BW35	50 (28)	10%	Black	Bitter *et al.*, 1972

[a] Percent positive (numbers in parens indicate total number of people typed).
[b] A "significant" absence of this haplotype.

may contribute toward pathogenesis (Svejgaard *et al.*, 1975). Bitter *et al.* (1972) noted a marked increase in the second series antigens B7 and BW35, especially when found together in black patients with SLE (Table II). We have not noted this combination in our white lupus patients. Terasaki and Mickey (1975) noted an absence of A2,B12 in their white lupus patients. We have noted A2,B12 in 9% of our 44 SLE patients and 10% of controls. Differences in HLA types between races, diversity of predisposing factors, as in C2 and IgA deficiency, may contribute toward the varying HLA results reported. Further elucidation of histocompatibility loci in SLE may have to await the availability of I-a and/or MLC-typed cells or antisera.

III. IMMUNE STATUS OF SLE PATIENTS

The extent to which recognizable genetically determined defects may predispose to SLE has been reviewed in the preceding section. The numbers accounted for by IgA and C2 deficiency represent a minority of patients only. Other genetically determined defects of the immune system, as yet unrecognized, may govern susecptibility to the disease. Studies of general immune responsiveness in SLE are, therefore, of interest.

Predisposition to infection has been reported, as have defects in neutrophil function, including diminished bone marrow reserves and defective *in vitro* chemotaxis (Ropes, 1964; Staples *et al.*, 1974; Kimball *et al.*, 1973; Clark *et al.*, 1974). Similarly macrophage function, as evaluated by monocyte ingestion of yeast, has been found to be impaired in patients with SLE (Svensson and Hedberg, 1973). Problems of interpretation are presented in these studies in the differentation between preexisting defects and the acquired effects of the disease. Both immunosuppressive drugs and chronic renal failure may increase susceptibility to infection.

Similarly, the incidence of neoplasia in SLE may be increased due to a defect in immune surveillance and/or suppression. Eight of 70 patients with SLE developed malignancies over nearly 7 years of follow-up (Canoso and Cohen, 1974). More extensive studies are required for fuller elucidation. In complimentary studies, the general ability of SLE patients to develop humoral and cellular immune responses to a range of common antigens has been evaluated.

A. The Capacity for Antibody Responses in SLE

There is no indication from a number of studies that the wide range of B cell activity directed toward cells and some macromolecules seen in active SLE is a general hyperresponsiveness to all antigens.

1. Antibodies to Microorganisms

Phillips and Christian (1970) reported on a higher titer of anti-myxovirus antibodies in SLE patients than in controls. Subsequently, when antibodies to other viruses were examined it was noted that high titers were found to many viruses, especially measles, rubella, parainfluenza, reovirus, and not to only one in particular (Hollinger *et al.*, 1971; Phillips, 1975; Hurd *et al.*, 1972; Rothfield *et al.*, 1973). These antibody levels were higher than in normal controls, but not greater than in patients with tuberculosis (Hurd *et al.*, 1972; Phillips and Christian, 1972). Titers of antibodies to Epstein-Barr virus may be higher among SLE patients than controls (Evans *et al.*, 1971), although other investigators could not confirm this (Phillips and Hirshaut, 1973). Titers of antibodies to the following viruses were usually normal:

influenza, Newcastle disease, respiratory syncytial, OC43 coronavirus, adenovirus, *Herpes simplex*, cytomegalovirus, papovavirus, and hepatitis B (Phillips, 1975). In contrast to elevated anti-viral antibody titer, a specific immune hyporesponsiveness, using migration inhibition, to measles (but not to rubella or parainfluenza) virus has been noted in SLE patients (Untermohlen *et al.*, 1974).

Titers of *Proteus* OX-2 agglutinins and antistreptolysin O were the same in SLE patients and normals (Muschel, 1961), while antibody titers (particularly 19 S antibodies) to *Shigella* and *Escherichia coli* were lower in SLE patients than controls (Baum, 1967).

The response of SLE patients to immunization has yielded variable results. High antibody titers were noted in response to immunization with Vi antigens (Stevens *et al.*, 1967); however, hyporesponsiveness to immunization was noted with *Brucella* antigens by Baum (1967) but not by others (Meiselas *et al.*, 1961). Lupus patients respond normally to immunization with tetanus toxoid (Abe and Homma, 1971). Patients with SLE have antibodies to bovine proteins in the same frequency as do normals, but the titers are higher in SLE patients (Carr *et al.*, 1972). Interferon produced by the viral stimulation of lymphocytes drawn from SLE patients has been found to be similar to that of lymphocytes from a control population (Alarcón-Segovia *et al.*, 1974).

B. The Capacity for "Delayed Hypersensitivity" Type Responses in SLE

To evaluate cellular immune function, skin tests and *in vitro* assays with a range of antigens have been investigated. The reports have been conflicting, some demonstrating depression of the skin response to a number of common antigens, including those from tuberculin, trichophyton, candida, and streptokinase (Bitter *et al.*, 1971; Abe and Homma, 1971; Horwitz, 1972; Rosenthal and Franklin, 1975; Hahn *et al.*, 1973). Others have found more selective hyporesponsiveness. Block *et al.* (1968) found a reduced reaction to tuberculin alone with normal responses to histoplasmin and candida. There are also reports of normal responses to all bacterial or fungal antigens tested (Goldman *et al.*, 1972; Senyk *et al.*, 1974). The correlation between skin testing with *in vitro* responses has not been consistent. The reduced skin response to tuberculin, observed by Hahn and colleagues, was not paralleled by a reduction in the *in vitro* responses of lymphocytes to the same antigen (Hahn *et al.*, 1973). Dinitrochlorobenze, which is not normally encountered in the human environment, has been used to assess cellular immunity in SLE. Hyporesponsiveness was demonstrated (Abe and Homma, 1971). *In vitro* lymphocyte responsiveness to concanavalin A and pokeweed mitogens were found to be depressed in a study of 21 patients;

controls included patients with RA and inflammatory diseases (Locksin *et al.*, 1975). The conclusion was reached that a specific cellular immunodeficiency exists in the disease. Others (Suciu-Foca *et al.*, 1974) have also noted lymphocyte hyporeactivity to PHA and allogenic cells among SLE patients. Patients were not tested in remission and, therefore, conclusions as to the relevance of those defects to predisposition to the disease cannot be evaluated. The findings of Rosenthal and Franklin (1975) give some indication that the *in vitro* defects are reversible in that some patients initially giving negative tests were positive after treatment with corticosteroids.

C. Characteristics of Circulating Lymphocytes in SLE

An alternative approach to the evaluation of the patients' immune status has been the enumeration of T and B cell markers of lymphocytes. The percentage of T lymphocytes, enumerated either by formation of rosettes with sheep red cells or by the use of T cell-specific antibody, were reduced, as were the absolute numbers of T cells (Messner *et al.*, 1973; Scheinberg and Cathcart, 1973). B cell lymphocytes assessed by surface immunoglobulin and/or formation of EAC rosettes were normal, decreased or elevated (Williams *et al.*, 1973a; Messner *et al.*, 1973; Tannenbaum and Schur, 1974; Scheinberg and Cathcart, 1973). More recently, Winchester and colleagues (1974) have demonstrated that cold-reactive lymphocytotoxic antibodies and immune complexes can cause overestimation of the number of B lymphocytes, using surface immunoglobulin as a criterion. The "acquired" antibody can be washed off cells by overnight incubation. Their data that resulted from this methodological change is at variance with that reported previously in that the percentage of B cells was reduced and that of T cells increased (Winchester *et al.*, 1974). The increase in T cells was not marked, the values being just above the normal levels. Estimates of B cells previously recorded, based on an Ig marker, may well have been too high. The difference between cells with the Ig marker and EAC rosette cells reported by Messner and colleagues (1973) may be a reflection of this.

More recently Schneider *et al.* (1975) have noted decreased antibody-dependent lymphocyte-mediated cytotoxicity among SLE patients, especially during active disease.

IV. IMMUNE RESPONSE TO NUCLEAR SUBSTANCES

A. The LE Cell

The first autoantibody discovered in patients with LE were those to nucleohistone, i.e., the complex formed between DNA and histone (Holman and Deicher, 1959; Holman *et al.*, 1959). This antibody or LE cell factor reacts and complexes with nuclei from disrupted leukocytes; the immune complex is subsequently phagocytosed by viable leukocytes to form the LE cell. LE cells are detected at some time in the course of the disease in over 75% of patients with SLE, usually during active disease (Dubois, 1971). The correlation with disease activity is not necessarily good, and the phenomenon is seen in other diseases and may be absent in SLE. LE cells have been noted in 0.6–24% of patients with rheumatoid arthritis (Goldfine *et al.*, 1965; Sigler *et al.*, 1958), 10% of patients with Sjögren's syndrome (Bloch *et al.*, 1965), 4–14% of patients with scleroderma (Dubois, 1971), patients with liver disease (namely, by definition in patients with lupoid hepatitis), and occasionally in patients with drug hypersensitivity (e.g., procainamide, hydralazine, anticonvulsants). As the LE cell is difficult and tedious to perform and lacks specificity, it has been generally replaced by other assays for the detection of anti-nuclear antibodies.

B. Anti-Nuclear Antibodies Detected by Immunofluorescence (ANA, ANF, FANA)

By far the most commonly utilized method for recognizing antibodies to nuclei is the immunofluorescent technique. This method detects ANA in 86–100% of patients with SLE (Gonzalez and Rothfield, 1966; Mandema *et al.*, 1961). The absence of ANA has been said to negate a diagnosis of SLE.

TABLE III

Autoantibodies in LE

Cells	Cytoplasm
Lymphocytes	Ribosomes
Red Blood Cells	Mitochondria
Platelets	Lysosomes
Neutrophils	Ro
	La
Nuclei	Nucleic Acids
Nucleoprotein (NP, SNP)	DNA-ds, ss
DNA	RNA-ds, ss
Histones	DNA/RNA
Sm	Other
RNP-Mo	Rheumatoid factors
RNA-nucleoli	Circulating anticoagulants
	Biologic false-positive test for syphilis

Negative tests have been noted in patients with circulating DNA (Koffler *et al.*, 1967), those receiving excessive amounts of corticosteroids and/or immunosuppressives, those in remission, and in association with inherited deficiencies of complement components. The presence of ANA is not specific for SLE, being found in approximately 33% of patients with RA, 31% with JRA (Schur *et al.*, 1974), 40% with scleroderma (Rothfield and Rodnan, 1968), 48–68% with Sjögren's syndrome (Alspaugh and Tan, 1975), 25% with liver disease, and frequently in association with leprosy, pulmonary disease, and other chronic inflammatory disorders. The administration of certain drugs will also induce ANA (reviewed by Alarcón-Segovia, 1969). This lack of specificity for LE has prompted investigations to improve specificity. High titers of complement-fixing ANA are seen frequently in patients with SLE, especially those with active nephritis, while non-complement-fixing ANA are seen in SLE patients without nephritis and in those with other diseases (Tojo *et al.*, 1970).

The ANA test can also help differentiate the presence of antibodies to different nuclear antigens. This is accomplished by the recognition of different patterns of fluorescence-peripheral (also called rim or shaggy), diffuse (or homogeneous), speckled, and nucleolar. The peripheral pattern recognizes primarily anti-DNA antibodies, the diffuse or homogeneous pattern anti-nucleoprotein (NP) antibodies, the speckled pattern anti-Sm and RNP antibodies, and the nucleolar pattern anti-RNA antibodies. The peripheral pattern, by virtue of its relative anti-DNA antibody specificity is found primarily in patients with SLE; other patterns of fluorescence, particularly the diffuse form, may also be found.

ANA in patients with SLE, RA, and other connective tissue disorders have been found in IgG, IgM, IgA, IgD, and IgE classes (Gonzalez and Rothfield, 1966; Jackson *et al.*, 1973). Although there was no association between disease activity and IgG, IgA, or IgM class ANA, IgD and IgE ANA were more likely to be present in patients with active disease (Jackson *et al.*, 1973), although this may reflect an increase in the total antibody present.

C. Antibodies to "Specific" Nuclear Antigens

Antibodies to nucleoprotein (NP) can be recognized in the ANA test as a diffuse or homogeneous pattern (Lachmann and Kunkel, 1961). Antibodies to NP can also be detected by precipitation in gel or by radioimmunoassays (Notman *et al.*, 1975). Using immunofluorescence, the anti-NP antibodies are not specific for SLE, but, when detected by radioimmunoassay, they are said to be relatively specific for SLE (Notman *et al.*, 1975). The biologic role of these antibodies in patients with LE or other diseases is unclear. In patients with SLE, their presence correlates to a certain extent with nephritis (Townes, 1963). Furthermore, antibodies to NP have been eluted from the kidneys of SLE patients with dying nephritis (Koffler *et al.*, 1967). These observations suggest that, at least in some SLE patients, complexes of NP and anti-NP may cause nephritis.

Anti-nuclear antibodies giving a speckled pattern in the ANA test have been found frequently among patients with SLE and related diseases. These represent antibodies to a group of nuclear extracts that contain protein and nucleic acids, but not DNA. Their terminology is confusing. The most heterogeneous nuclear extracts have been called CTN or ENA (Schur and Sandson, 1968; Sharp *et al.*, 1972). These consist of two or more substances: one a glycoprotein called Sm, and, another, a ribonucleoprotein (RNP or MO) (Tan and Kunkel, 1966b; Notman *et al.*, 1975; Reichlin and Mattioli, 1973–1974). Antibodies to CTN have been found in 23% of patients with SLE, 2% with RA, 1% with JRA (Schur *et al.*, 1974); high titers of antibodies to ENA have been used to distinguish a group of patients with some features of SLE and scleroderma, a steroid responsive disorder, which has been called mixed connective tissue disease (Sharp *et al.*, 1972). Others have noted antibodies to ENA in patients with SLE and other diseases (Notman *et al.*, 1975; Reichlin and Mattioli, 1973–1974). Antibodies to ENA have been thought to protect against SLE nephritis (Sharp *et al.*, 1972), perhaps by formation of complexes with DNA, retarding the formation of anti-DNA–DNA complexes (Hamburger *et al.*, 1974). However, antibodies to CTN (and Sm) were found in equal frequency among LE patients with and without nephritis (Notman *et al.*, 1975; Reichlin and Mattioli, 1973–1974; Schur and Sandson, 1968) and antibodies to CTN were eluted from kidneys of SLE patients dying with nephritis (Koffler *et al.*, 1967). The presence of antibodies to Sm is highly suggestive of SLE (Notman *et al.*, 1975) but is found in only 28% of patients. Antibodies to RNP are found in 26% of patients with SLE, in 10% with RA, 22% with scleroderma, and by definition, in all patients with mixed connective tissue disease (Notman *et al.*, 1975). Reichlin and Mattioli (1973–1974) noted that patients with SLE and antibodies to "MO" (i.e., the same as RNP) had a low incidence of nephritis and anti-DNA antibodies.

1. *Antibodies to DNA*

Shortly after the discovery of antibodies to NP in patients with LE, it became apparent that some of these antibodies were directed to the DNA portion of NP. These antibodies have been detected by immunodiffusion, complement fixation, immunofluorescence, spot test, and hemagglutination (Kunkel and Tan, 1964; Koffler *et al.*, 1971; Schur *et al.*, 1974; Levine and

Stollar, 1968). By immunofluorescence, a peripheral pattern ANA may indicate anti-DNA activity (Casals *et al.*, 1963), as can immunofluorescence using hemoflagellates containing mitochondrial double-stranded DNA (dsDNA), as a substrate (Aarden *et al.*, 1975). The development of radioimmunoassays (Wold *et al.*, 1968; Pincus *et al.*, 1969) has resulted in a greater ease and sensitivity of assay. Most earlier papers felt that these antibodies were found only in patients with SLE and probably not in patients with other disorders (Levine and Stollar, 1968). More recently, the more sensitive radioimmunoassays have suggested that these antibodies are found in normal individuals and in some patients with other connective tissue disorders (Hasselbacher and LeRoy, 1974; Notman *et al.*, 1975; Schur *et al.*, 1974). Although not absolutely diagnostic, high titers of anti-DNA antibodies are not only highly suggestive of SLE, but are also probably of biologic significance in SLE patients.

There are three types of anti-DNA antibodies; the most prevalent are those that react with sites on both native or double-stranded DNA (dsDNa), as well as on the denatured or single-stranded form (ssDNA); some that react with only dsDNA; and some that react with only ssDNA. The presence of high titers of anti-dsDNA antibodies correlates well with active nephritis in SLE patients (Schur and Sandson, 1968). The class antibodies to dsDNA appears to be both IgG and IgM. There is some evidence that patients with IgM antibodies do not develop nephritis (Talal and Pillarisetty, 1975); similarly, patients with both precipitating and DNA-binding antibodies have a high incidence of nephritis while those patients' sera which precipitate with, but do not form soluable complexes in a redioimmunoassay have nephritis infrequently (Holgate *et al.*, 1976; Johnson *et al.*, 1973). The IgG antibodies are primarily IgG1 and IgG3 globulins (Schur *et al.*, 1972), i.e., those IgG subclasses that fix complement well (Ishizaka *et al.*, 1967). Differences in avidity of anti-DNA antibodies has been described in sera from patients with nephritis and without lupus nephritis (Steward *et al.*, 1974; Gershwin and Steinberg, 1974). These observations point to the importance of both qualitative and quantitative differences between anti-DNA antibodies with respect to lupus nephritis. Persistently high titers of anti-dsDNA antibodies have also been associated with lupus vasculitis (Johnson *et al.*, 1973). Antibodies to dsDNA have been eluted off the kidneys of SLE patients (Koffler *et al.*, 1967) and have been found in the CSF of SLE patients with CNS involvement (Carr *et al.*, 1975). Antibodies to dsDNA are thought to mediate inflammation when complexed with DNA as immune complexes (Cochrane and Koffler, 1973). The origin of the DNA remains unknown but is probably endogenous (Harbeck *et al.*, 1975). Free serum DNA has been detected in SLE sera, especially in patients with acute, active disease (Tan *et al.*, 1966; Hughes *et al.*, 1971), but is not diagnostic of SLE having been found in sera other conditions associated with tissue breakdown (Tan *et al.*, 1966; Davis and Davis, 1973) and in normal sera (Davis and Davis, 1973).

While antibodies to dsDNA appear to be directed to the carbohydrate phosphate backbone on one strand, antibodies to ssDNA are directed to the purine and pyrimidine bases (Stollar, 1975). Antibodies to ssDNA are found in up to 87% of patients with SLE, but also in up to 60% of patients with rheumatoid arthritis, 58% of patients with chronic hepatitis, and up to 55% of patients with procainamide-induced lupus (Koffler *et al.*, 1971). Antibodies to ssDNA are found in higher titers in SLE patients with nephritis than in those without (Schur and Sandson, 1968).

The separation of antibody specificities to DNA has been complicated by the problems involved establishing antigenic purity. Native DNA may not be entirely free of breaks in one or other of the strands. The methods used to circumvent these technological difficulties include separation of the two DNA types by chromatography (Epstein, 1975; Tan and Natali, 1970; Samaha and Irvin, 1975), by enzymatic digestion of ssDNA (Harbeck *et al.*, 1975), by assay for ssDNA (Schur *et al.*, 1974), and by removal of ssDNA by binding to cellulose nitrate filters (Ginsberg and Keiser, 1973). Two preparations of DNA that should not contain denatured contaminants include an nDNA, poly(dAT) (Ginsberg and Keiser, 1973), and a include synthetic poly(dAT) (Steinman *et al.*, 1975), and a hemoflagellate, *Crithidia luciliae*, containing mitochondrial dsDNA (Aarden *et al.*, 1975).

D. Antibodies to Other Nucleic Acids

In addition to antibodies to DNA, antibodies to RNA and RNA/DNA hybrids have been recognized in SLE patients. While more readily detected using synthetic polyribonucleotides, they can also be detected using viral RNA. Antibodies to ds or ssRNA are not diagnostic for SLE, but are found more frequently and in higher titer in SLE patients than in patients with other diseases (Koffler *et al.*, 1971; Schur *et al.*, 1971; Schur and Monroe, 1969). As dsRNA appears to occur in only trace amounts, if at all, in normal tissue, but in higher amounts in (RNA) virally infected tissue, antibodies thereto may represent part of an immune response to a virus (Schur and Monroe, 1969). Anti-dsRNA antibodies are both 7 S and 19 S immunoglobulins (Talal and Pillarisetty, 1975).

Antibodies to RNA/DNA hybrids have also been described (Talal and Gallo, 1972). Antibodies to a nuclear 7 S RNA are thought to represent antibodies to nucleoli (Miyawaki and Ritchie, 1973; Pinnas *et al.*, 1972). These antibodies were found in 26% of patients with SLE, 9% RA, 8% JRA, and 54% scleroderma. The presence of antibodies to nucleoli correlated with Raynaud's phenomenon (Ritchie, 1970).

E. Cell-Mediated Immunity to Nucleic Acids

As evidence for antibody responses to nucleic acids accumulated, studies reflecting cellular responsiveness to nuclear antigens have also been carried out. These studies were initially of skin tests using leukocytes and various nuclear extracts, including calf thymus nucleoprotein, DNA, and histone (Friedman *et al.*, 1960; Azoury *et al.*, 1966). Positive responses were recorded in lupus patients and not in healthy or in ill controls. The positive tests were observed initially within 10–18 hours of the intradermal injection. However, others (Hahn *et al.*, 1973; Block *et al.*, 1968) have noted no difference in skin reactions to DNA between patients with SLE or RA and normals. Subsequently *in vitro* lymphocyte responsiveness was studied, and conflicting reports resulted. Patrucco and colleagues (1967) noted lymphocyte blast transformation to DNA in 11 of 12 SLE patients and a much lower degree of response in cells from normal individuals and from RA patients. Evidence of lymphocyte responsiveness, as assessed by lymphocyte transformation and increased uptake of radiolabeled thymidine has been obtained with nuclear antigens, including native and denatured DNA (Goldman *et al.*, 1972; Senyk *et al.*, 1974). Migration inhibition was tested with positive results, both directly by inhibition of cell migration from capillaries with the nuclear antigens and indirectly using MIF generated by a reaction of DNA with lymphocytes (Abe *et al.*, 1973; Galanud *et al.*, 1971). Others have not been able to confirm these results by *in vitro* stimulation (Rosenthal and Franklin, 1975). Lack of correlation of these presumed tests of thymic-dependent lymphocyte function and circulating anti-nuclear antibody has been reported (Senyk *et al.*, 1974) in addition to the more evident dissociation, as suggested by the negative lymphocyte studies previously discussed. Senyk and colleagues (1974) found lymphocyte responsiveness to DNA/nucleohistone in 2 of 16 individuals and in 5 of 16 with synthetic RNA. The conflicting reports are probably inevitable in a field of investigation where standardization of methodology has not been evident.

F. Anti-Cytoplasmic Antibodies

Antibodies to a number of cytoplasmic fractions have been found in some LE patients and appear to be as heterogeneous as the anti-nuclear antibodies. The presence of these antibodies has never been considered to be diagnostic of LE. They are, however, of interest in analyzing the immune status of SLE patients. Thus, while some LE patients have antibodies to mitochondria, they are found more frequently among patients with primary biliary cirrhosis (Deicher *et al.*, 1960; Asherson, 1959; Doniach *et al.*, 1966). Antibodies to ribosomes and lysosomes, while found in some SLE patients

(41% and 62%, respectively), have been noted infrequently in other rheumatic conditions (Schur *et al.*, 1967; Lamon and Bennett, 1970; Wiedermann and Miescher, 1965; Bell *et al.*, 1975). Antibodies to ribosomes appear to be directed to either RNA, proteins or both (Schur *et al.*, 1967; Bianchi *et al.*, 1974; Lamon and Bennett, 1970). Antibodies to a cytoplasmic, periodate-sensitive, glycoprotein (Ro) are found in 30% of SLE patients and infrequently in patients with connective tissue disorders other than Sjögren's syndrome (25%) (Reichlin and Mattioli, 1973–1974). Antibodies to Ro are usually found in association with antibodies to a soluble cytoplasmic RNA protein called La, but rarely in conjunction with antibodies to Sm (Reichlin and Mattioli, 1973–1974). Three of the patients studied (with anti-La and anti-Ro antibodies) had features suggestive of SLE but were ANA-negative (Mattioli and Reichlin, 1974). Antibodies reactive with the cytoplasm of neurons were found in 41% of SLE patients with active neurological disease, 9% in those without a history of neurological involvement, and in 0.9% of non-SLE controls (Quismorio and Friou, 1972).

G. Antibodies to Cellular Elements

Antibodies to red blood cells, white blood cells, and platelets have been noted frequently in patients with SLE. Antibodies to red blood cells are usually detected by the γ and non-γ-Coombs' test. Many SLE patients have both γ-globulin and complement on red blood cells, some have only complement, but few, if any, have γ-globulin alone (Mongan *et al.*, 1967; Gilliland *et al.*, 1970). Overt hemolytic anemia is uncommon and even a positive Coombs' test does not necessarily indicate accelerated hemolysis (Mongan *et al.*, 1967). Patients with SLE were found to have normal levels of isohemagglutinins (Muschel, 1961), but SLE patients, after transfusion, may develop antibodies to rare Rh determinants; patients with SLE have higher titers of antibodies in response to isologous blood group substances than do controls (Zingale *et al.*, 1963).

Antibodies to platelets are common (Karpatkin and Siskind, 1969). These antibodies involve all four IgG subclasses, in contrast to the IgG3 subclass anti-platelet antibodies found in patients with ATP (Karpatkin *et al.*, 1973). While 25–50% of patients with SLE have thrombocytopenia, about 8% of patients have thrombocytopenia and bleeding (reviewed in Lee and Miotti, 1975).

Antibodies to white blood cells in SLE patients have become the object of recent intensive investigation. Antibodies that are cytotoxic *in vitro* to lymphocytes have been noted in over 80% of SLE patients (Terasaki *et al.*, 1970; Mittal *et al.*, 1970). Their presence correlates with lymphopenia

(Butler *et al.*, 1972), hypocomplementemia (Nies *et al.*, 1974; Butler *et al.*, 1972), and the presence of fever and dermatologic manifestations (Butler *et al.*, 1972). They are directed primarily to T lymphocytes (Lies *et al.*, 1973), but separate B cell specificity has been noted as well (Winfield *et al.*, 1975b). These antibodies are primarily IgM, bind to lymphocyte maximally at 4°C, but are maximally cytotoxic at 15° (Winfield *et al.*, 1975b). These antibodies appear to interfere with HLA typing in SLE (Winfield *et al.*, 1975b).

Anti-lymphocyte antibodies in SLE sera have also been known to suppress (Wernet and Kunkel, 1973; Williams *et al.*, 1973b; Suciu-Foca *et al.*, 1974) or enhance (Suciu-Foca *et al.*, 1974) mixed lymphocyte cultures (MLC) rections. This suppression of MLC could have identified a specific surface antigen on T cells (Wernet and Kunkel, 1973). By allowing lymphocytes to shed antibodies, normal MLC reactivity was restored (Wernet *et al.*, 1973). SLE sera also suppressed mitogen-induced proliferation of lymphocytes (Cousar and Horwitz, 1973; Rosenthal and Franklin, 1973). The antibodies that suppress lymphocyte function are IgG (Wernet *et al* 1973; Williams *et al.*, 1973b; Cousar and Horwitz, 1973; Rosenthal and Franklin, 1973), in contrast to the IgM lymphocytotoxic antibodies.

V. OTHER AUTOIMMUNE ANTIBODIES

Positive serological tests for syphilis have been noted in 0–44% of SLE patients (Harvey and Schulman, 1974). While some of these individuals have syphilis, most have "biologic false-positive" (BFP) tests confirmed by doing more specific tests, e.g., the TPI. Seven percent of patients with chronic BFP have SLE. Even the highly specific test for syphilis, the FTA-ABS test, has been noted to be positive with SLE sera, however, the beaded pattern of fluorescence distinguishes it from the homogeneous pattern of treponemal antibodies (Kraus *et al.*, 1970).

Anti-γ-globulins, inlcuding rheumatoid factors, have been noted in up to 30% of patients with SLE (Miescher *et al.*, 1973). In contrast to RA, they fluctuate with clinical activity but do not correlate with the presence of arthritis. They have also been detected in the kidneys of patients with lupus nephritis (Agnello *et al.*, 1971).

Circulating anticoagulants are found in about 10% of SLE patients (Lee and Miotti, 1975). Most of these antibodies inhibit the coagulation system in the region of the prothrombin converter. The anticoagulant is usually IgG antibody, but IgM has also been occasionally noted. Where studied, they were primarily IgG4 (Robboy *et al.*, 1970). Curiously, the presence of anticoagulants in SLE sera is often (64%) associated with positive serological tests for syphilis (Lee and Miotti, 1975).

VI. DRUG-INDUCED LUPUS

A number of drugs, used to treat individuals for certain non-SLE diseases, are occasionally associated with the development of anti-nuclear antibodies (Alarcón-Segovia, 1969). This may even be associated with a lupuslike syndrome. This is especially so with the use of procainamide and hydralazine and, less frequently, with the use of anticonvulsants, isoniazid, and methyldopa. Sporadic associations with other drugs have also been cited. Individuals with drug-induced ANA or "lupus" rarely, if ever, develop renal disease, anti-dsDNA antibodies, or hypocomplementemia. The mechanism for the induction of ANA and "lupus" remains unknown, but hypotheses include activation of a latent virus (Blomgren *et al*., 1972), activation of a genetically determined diathesis (Alarcón-Segovia, 1969), or alteration of cell constituents, making them antigenic (Blomgren *et al*., 1972). Support for the latter hypothesis has been gained from the observations of reactions between these drugs and nucleic acids inducing immunogenicity (Blomgren *et al*., 1972; Tan, 1968).

VII. SLE AS AN IMMUNE COMPLEX-MEDIATED DISEASE

Investigation of some of the mechanisms of tissue injury suggests that SLE is at least in part an immune complex deposition disease. The skin and kidneys are the tissues in SLE patients in which there is most evidence for immune complex deposition; by inference from animal models, such deposition could result in tissue injury. The extent to which these concepts have been documented for formation, detection, and characterization of these complexes in serum, and the evidence that the γ-globulin in tissue represents part of an immune complex will be reviewed in this section.

A. Blood and CSF

1. Complement Levels in Serum and Other Fluid Compartments

Disorders of the complement system in patients with SLE reflect, to a large extent, activation and fixation by circulating immune complexes. However, blood levels may be affected by varying rates of synthesis and catabolism of complement components, as well as by genetic control of complement levels. This subject has recently been reviewed (Schur, 1975) and will be only briefly discussed here; the genetics of the complement system have been discussed above.

Serum complement levels are decreased in most patients with SLE at some time during their illness, especially when disease activity is present. Complement levels are infrequently depressed in patients with discoid LE or serositis; somewhat depressed in association with severe skin lesions, arthritis, and hemolytic anemia; and often severely depressed in patients with active lupus nephritis. Patients without nephritis tended not to have so severe a degree of hypocomplementemia as those with this complication. Serum complement levels often decreased (usually 50%) in association with an increase in levels of antibodies to DNA prior to clinical or laboratory features of an exacerbation of nephritis, suggesting the formation of DNA–anti-DNA immune complexes. These decreases usually occurred gradually over weeks, but they can occur suddenly in response to an acute stress (e.g., infections, surgery). Analysis of complement components in those with low total hemolytic (CH50) levels, reveals primarily low levels of the classical complement system, that is, C1 (including C1q, C1r, C1s), C4, and C3. This pattern suggests activation by circulating immune complexes—sera with this pattern are usually anti-complementary (*in vitro*) and contain high molecular weight IgG, presumably in the form of immune complexes. C2 (protein) levels are rarely depressed, except in association with genetic defects. When the C3 levels are moderately or markedly depressed, there is usually associated depression of properdin components (e.g., Factors P and B). Low levels of C5 and other later-acting components are infrequently encountered but may occur during exacerbations of nephritis.

Serial determinations of complement levels are often useful in following and managing patients with SLE. While serum C4 protein levels are the first to fall in the majority of patients in association with or prior to an exacerbation, in others, CH50, C1q, or C3 levels can fall before C4. In the majority of instances, a fall in C4 protein levels is followed by fall in serum C3, CH50, and C1q; C2 protein levels are rarely depressed. Exacerbation of nephritis was also occasionally associated with activation of the properdin system. Patients with persistently very low levels (i.e., less than 25% of the normal mean) of either CH50, C1q, C4, or C3 are either ill at the time or will shortly become so and usually have nephritis. Very low levels of C1q tended to be associated with high morbidity and mortality, and very low levels of C3 were invariably accompanied by active and severe nephritis. Complement levels have varied in patients with nephrotic syndrome. Levels tended to be low, particularly CH50, C1q, C4, and C3 when proteinuria was associated with a telescopic urine; complement levels tended to be normal, however, when there was a fixed proteinuria without cellular elements in the urine, reflecting preexisting renal disease rather than active inflammation. Patients with complement levels at, or somewhat below the lower limit of normal, are usually well. These relatively minor depressions could represent synthetic defects of complement or low-grade utilization.

Soter *et al.* (1974) has analyzed complement levels in patients with SLE and necrotizing angiitis. The patients tend to have low levels of CH50, C1, C4, C2, C3, C9, factor B, and especially very low C1q levels at the time they had active disease. A few studies have noted low complement levels in pleural, synovial, and pericardial fluid from patients with SLE. C4 levels in the cerebrospinal fluid tend to be low normal in patients with active CNS involvement.

2. *Cryoglobulins in SLE*

Cryoprecipitable material in serum has been found in patients with SLE and associated with both disease activity and hypocomplementemia. That the cryoglobulins are complement-fixing immune complexes formed in the circulation and do not merely represent an *in vitro* phenomenon has been harder to establish. Initial studies in SLE concerned the demonstration of complement proteins in addition to immunoglobulins in the cryoglobulins. Christian *et al.* (1963) demonstrated the presence of C1q in the cryoglobulins of SLE patients, and, in a later study, Hanauer and Christian (1967) found C4 and C3 proteins in addition to IgG and IgM. The IgM possessed anti-IgG activity. Cryoglobulins were associated in these studies with active disease being found in 18 of 33 SLE sera, 15 of these 18 patients having "significant" renal disease. Similarly, Stastny and Ziff (1969) noted an association between cryoglobulins and renal lupus. Sera of 11 out of 31 patients had cryoglobulins, and 8 of these 11 had renal disease. Ten of the 11 patients with cryoglobulins and 3 of the 25 patients without cryoglobulins had low C3 protein levels. The isolated cryoproteins were capable of fixing complement *in vitro*. Druet *et al.* (1973) also observed the association between renal disease and cryoglobulins; the latter were found in 12 of 13 patients with lupus nephritis, compared with 2 of the 12 patients without renal involvement. The renal disease was biopsy proven, IgG and IgM were found in both cryoglobulins and in the renal glomeruli.

If cryoprecipitates do represent circulating immune complexes of possible pathogenic significance, then they ought to contain antigen and specific antibody. Recent studies support this concept, both anti-lymphocyte and anti-nuclear antibodies having been found in cryoprecipitates to a greater degree than anticipated from their concentration in serum. The lymphocyte antibodies were of IgM class, and, although specificity for lymphocytes was demonstrated, the possibility that these antibodies have additional specificities remains (Winfield *et al*., 1975c). Winfield *et al*. (1975a) were able to demonstrate an increased concentration of anti-nuclear antibodies and the presence of nucleic acids in the cryoprecipitates. The antibodies found were those to native DNA, single-strand DNA, and ribonucleoprotein. Although antibodies to double-stranded RNA were present in serum, these were not found in the cryoprecipitates. Antibodies to tetanus toxoid were similarly found in serum, but not in the cryoprecipitates. A major proportion of the γ-globulin in some cryoproteins was antibody with anti-nuclear specificity.

3. *C1q Binding in Sera*

As an alternative to detection of immune complexes by cryoprecipitation, binding of C1q has been used either in gel or fluid phase systems. Agnello *et al*. (1971) found C1q precipitins in 23 of 30 hypocomplemtemic SLE patients and in none of 53 normocomplementemic SLE patients. Both high and low molecular weight reactants were found; in those sera with low molecular weight reactants, C1q serum levels were lower than in those with high molecular weight reactants.

In a fluid-phase system with ^{125}I-C1q, Nydegger *et al*. (1974) found in C1q binding in 22 of 52 sera drawn from 22 patients. The greatest degrees of binding were found in those with most active disease. The isotope-labeled system should have advantages of sensitivity over the gel precipitation method, but the possibility of binding to substances other than immune complexs exists. Bacterial polysaccharides and DNA have been demonstrated to bind C1q.

4. *Release of DNA Antibody by Enzymes*

One approach used to infer the presence of circulating immune complexes in SLE has been the treatment of serum with the enzyme DNase, the assumption being that any resulting increase in DNA binding represents release of hitherto bound antibody in immune complexes. Harbeck *et al*. (1973) reported an increase in DNA binding in 11 of 15 patients with SLE and renal involvement. Maximum effect of the enzyme was found during exacerbations of renal disease. The specificity for DNA–anti-DNA immune complexes is suggested by the absence of an effect by RNase. Those patients whose sera do not contain DNA antibodies cannot be evaluated in this system for the presence or absence of immune complexes. This DNase digestion has been applied to CSF, one patient with lupus cerebritis having increased binding of DNA in both serum and CSF after enzyme digestion (Keeffe *et al*., 1974). Because of clinical problems in the diagnosis of CNS involvement in lupus and the uncertain state of complement assays in CSF, this approach could have a useful diagnostic role.

5. *Cell Receptor Assays for Immune Complexes*

Immune complexes can be detected by their binding to receptors on human lymphoblastoid cell lines (Theofilopoulos *et al.*, 1974). Sera from 13 patients bound these to receptors. The amount bound correlated merely to some degree with the CH50 levels, the presence of DNA antibody, and clinical exacerbation. The validation of this, as with other recently described methods, is less complete than that of cryoglobulin detection.

B. Skin

Evidence for immune complex deposition in the form of electron microscopy, immunofluorescent studies for immunoglobulin, and complement proteins, has been sought in tissues including the skin. Where feasible, elution studies have also been carried out. Using electron microscopy, Grishman and Churg (1970) found electron-dense deposits at the dermal–epidermal junction in the skin of six patients with SLE. That these deposits might represent immune complexes is reinforced by the findings from immunofluorescent studies. γ-Globulins and complement have demonstrated in the skin of lupus patients. The area of deposition is consistently the dermal–epidermal junction, and both complement and immunoglobulins have been found in association by numerous investigations (Tan *et al.*, 1966a; Percy and Smith, 1969; Tuffanelli *et al.*, 1969; Burnham and Fine, 1971). Tuffanelli *et al.* (1969) found positive biopsies in 34 of 37 biopsies of clinically involved areas and in 27 of 45 biopsies from noninflamed skin areas. "Positive" biopsies in these instances included IgG, IgM, IgA, and C3 proteins. Patients with discoid lupus have positive biopsies in affected areas only. Circulating anti-basement antibodies were not found. Burnham and Fine (1971) noted positive dermal–epidermal fluorescence in 16 of 44 SLE patients. These patients with positive biopsies had more severe disease with more fever and renal disease than those not so affected. This collected evidence for immune complex deposition is reinforced by the findings of antinuclear antibodies in elution studies from skin (Landry and Sams, 1973).

C. Kidneys

The kidneys are perhaps the tissues most extensively studied for evidence of immune complex deposition. The indirect evidence previously discussed for skin damage mediated by immune complexes includes association with hypocomplementemia, cryoglobulinemia, and the deposition of γ-globulin and complement. Immune complexes with complement are thought to be deposited initially in the mesangial area [which may represent part of the host's defense reticuloendothelial system; the cells appear to have some phagocytic function (Cochrane and Koffler, 1973)]. If the mesangial area is the only site involved, it is accompanied by mild nephritis with minimal proteinuria, hematuria, and pyuria and with little histological damage. If, however, this system becomes overloaded, it is postulated that these immune complexes then deposit along the glomerular basement membrane, first in a fine granular fashion and then, subsequently, in a more intense lumpy, bumpy fashion (Comerford and Cohen, 1967). Studies in rabbits strongly suggest that an IgE-mediated mechanism, resulting in the release of vasoactive amines from platelets, appears to potentiate this deposition along the glomerular basement membrane (Cochrane and Koffler, 1973). Furthermore, receptors for C3 in the glomeruli may enhance immune complex deposition (Gelfand *et al.*, 1975). The antigen–antibody complexes, through activation of C3 in particular, are thought to generate chemotactic factors, resulting in the attraction of macrophages, phagocytosis of immune complexes, and release of lysosomal enzymes perpetuating the renal inflammation (Cochrane and Koffler, 1973; Koffler *et al.*, 1969). Although immune complexes per se have not been demonstrated in the glomeruli, complement components have been noted to be deposited in the same location as immunoglobulins and DNA in kidneys of patients with lupus nephritis (Koffler *et al.*, 1967; Andres *et al.*, 1970). In addition, γ-globulin, eluted from some of these kidneys, has been demonstrated to be antibody, particularly anti-nuclear antibody, with specificities for nucleoprotein and for DNA—antibodies to cytoplasmic antigens were also eluted (Koffler *et al.*, 1967). Control eluates did not contain ANA. The ANA activity of eluted γ-globulin was greater than that of γ-globulin from serum. The ANA was capable of fixing complement. Krishnan and Kaplan (1967) reported similar findings, and, in a later study, Koffler *et al.* (1974) established further that the increased concentration of ANA in the glomeruli did not involve all specificities of ANA found in serum. Studying eluates for nine kidneys, antibodies to native (6/9) and single-stranded DNA (8/9), and antibodies to RNA protein (3/9) were found in concentrations above that found in serum, whereas antibodies to double-stranded RNA, found in serum from four of the six patients were not present in the eluates. The evidence then for immune complex deposition in kidneys is reinforced by this demonstration of selectivity in antibody specificities involved.

Study of complement components in renal tissues has given evidence, as in serum, of classic complement pathway activation, a subject reviewed recently by Schur (1975). Thus, C1q, C4, and particularly, C3 have been noted in lupus nephritis biopsies. In addition to these early classical complement components, deposition of properdin, but not of factor B, has also been noted. This contrasts to the more frequent observations of low serum levels of factor B than of properdin. Observations on a few specimens by Verroust *et al.* (1974) have shown deposition of late complement components in addition.

In this laboratory, we have had occasion to study biopsies from 53 SLE patients. As noted by others (reviewed in Schur, 1975), the majority of specimens examined had IgG; somewhat more than half had IgM; less than one-third had IgA. IgD and IgE were usually only weakly present and were detected infrequently. Deposition of complement-fixing IgG3 and non-complementing-fixing IgG2 were observed to a greater extent than of IgG1 and 4. C1q and C3 were detected in over half but C4 infrequently. Examination for late components was generally performed only when C3 was present, and C5, C6, and C9 were usually detected in these instances. Similarly, properdin was seen often in biopsies with C3, but factor B only rarely. There were no apparent differences in the deposition of immunoglobulins or complement components in SLE or non-SLE patients who had membranous or proliferative glomerulonephritis.

The presence of early and late complement components in renal lesions, as well as their depletion in patients with active nephritis, argues the evidence of an immune complex-mediated nephritis with activation of the classical complement pathway. Whether the activation and deposition of components of the properdin patheway is a result of direct activation by immunoglobulins or other factors or indirect by recruitment secondary to classical pathway activation is unknown.

D. Blood Vessels

1. Small Vessel Inflammation

Necrotizing angiitis (vasculitis), a rare complication of SLE associated in some instances with immunoglobulin and complement deposition in the small blood vessels, the arterioles and venules being generally involved. Tan and Kunkel (1966a), while studying skin biopsies, observed immunoglobulin by immunofluorescence in the arterioles of three of the nine skin biopsies. The entire blood vessel wall was involved, but particularly the intima. These changes were not found in patients with dermatomyositis or polymyositis.

2. Large and Medium-Sized Vessels

Inflammatory lesions suggestive of immune complex deposition, have been found in larger blood vessels. Grishman and Churg (1970) have found electron-dense deposits similar to those found in the dermal–epidermal junction. Immunoglobulins and complement have been found by immunofluorescent methods in blood vessel walls (Lachmann *et al.*, 1962; Koffler *et al.*, 1967). Paronetto and Koffler (1965) demonstrated immunoglobulin, complement, and fibrinogen in the vessels of kidneys, spleen, heart, and liver. Elution studies were carried out by Svec and Allen (1970) who obtained anti-nuclear antibodies from the blood vessels of the spleen of a patient dying from SLE. The anti-nuclear antibody was of IgG, IgM, and IgA classes and had, in part, specificity for DNA.

E. Brain

The evidence for deposition of immune complexes in central nervous system is much less well defined than in the tissues previously discussed, in contrast to the frequency with which lupus is clinically associated with neurological abnormalities. In studies of the choroid plexus of two patients dying of SLE with cerebral involvement, IgG and IgG with IgM were found by immunofluorescence, but not C3 complement protein. In one patient, electron-dense deposits were seen in the choroid plexus basement membrane, the possibility being raised that there were immune complexes, although the blood vessels were noted to be free of vasculitic changes (Atkins *et al.*, 1972).

VIII. DISCUSSION

Early reviewers have generally considered SLE as an autoimmune disease. To the limited extent that autoantibodies can be demonstrated *in vitro*, that immune complexes consisting in part of these antibodies are associated with nephritis, and that anti-RBC and platelet antibodies may contribute to accelerated clearance, SLE can indeed by regarded as an autoimmune disease (Stiller *et al.*, 1975). Neither this concept nor that of T and B lymphocyte imbalance will suffice to explain the type of primary events currently envisaged as initiating the disease. Failure of suppressor T cell function has been proposed as an initiating event in autoimmune disease (Talal, 1975). The absence of data on T cell function before the onset of disease, as well as the rise and fall in antibody titers and periodic nature of cellular immune defects, makes it difficult at this time to give T cell malfunction a primary role in etiology, although it may play a secondary role.

An immune response, in some way genetically controlled to environmental agents, seems to provide the hypothesis that best lends itself to the evidence at hand and to further investigation. Evidence is now available from other diseases, e.g., subacute bacterial endocarditis, infectious hepatitis, and diabetes, in which autoimmune phenomenon have been documented to suggest that this type of concept can be of relevance to SLE.

Most individuals with chronic active hepatitis, a disease of probable viral etiology, associated with hepatitis B antigenemia, immune complexes, and autoantibodies, have the A1,B8 HLA haplotype and also a common HLA-D cell type (Page *et al.*, 1975). Juvenile onset diabetes mellitus, a disease in which autoimmune phenomena (Nerup *et al.*, 1971; Moore and Neison, 1963; Maclaren *et al.*, 1975) can be found, and in which lymphocytes infiltrate the pancreas, suggests a chronic immune response, and is also associated with particular HLA antigens B8, BW15, and LD-8a (Thomsen *et al.*, 1975). Recent epidemiology studies strongly support the concept of a viral etiology in this disease, mumps and coxsackievirus being implicated (Maugh, 1975). The example of Reiter's syndrome may be relevant, since this disease can be triggered by shigella, yersinia, salmonella, and presumably other as yet not identified microorganisms in the HLA-BW27 susceptible individual (Aho *et al.*, 1975). While a similar series of events seems to be involved in these diseases, a multiplicity of infectious agents can be implicated.

Does evidence exist for such a mechanism in SLE? The primary events in the etiology of SLE are, as emphasized previously, unknown. There are two statements, however, concerning pathogenesis that can be made with some certainty at this time. The first of these is that there is evidence for a genetic predisposition to the disease, which would seem to exist as some kind of immunodeficiency, of which C2 and IgA are the best documented to date. The precise nature of the genetic predisposition to the disease should be defined more exactly, since other markers, in addition to C2, C4, C6, and properdin factor B are localized on the sixth human chromosome, close to or as part of the HLA complex. The recently described B lymphocyte specific antisera may be particularly relevant (Fu *et al.*, 1975). These antisera may detect products of HLA loci which are closer to the proposed site for IR genes than those currently available. The levels at which such genetic background may be operative can be multiple and include a direct role for IR genes or genetically determined deficiency leading to infection. The documentation of deficiencies in the complement system in SLE patients may be of relevance here since the early components of the classical pathway are particularly involved in viral neutralization (Daniels *et al.*, 1970). The control of the nature of the antibody response may be equally important, antibody levels of the IgM class having been demonstrated to be higher in females than males (Allansmith *et al.*, 1968; Rowley and Mackay, 1969; Bartfeld, 1969). The greater prevalence of the disease among females may be due in part to a malfunctioning of IgM regulation. The antibody responsiveness to DNA, a particular feature of SLE, may represent the extreme degree of ANA formation seen in the disease or could represent a genetically determined unique immune responsiveness. However, the ubiquitous nature of DNA antibody (Hasselbacher and LeRoy, 1974) and (specifically) sensitized responsive lymphocytes in normals (Bankhurst and Williams, 1975) makes this seem unlikely. Genetically determined deficiencies of the receptors on cell surfaces, which seem to be critical both in immune recognition and immune elimination, are possibilities as yet unexplored.

The second point concerns tissue injury, particularly the nephritis of lupus, which regardless of initiating events, probably results from immune complex deposition. These immune complexes contain both nucleic acids and their antibodies. The pathogenesis of tissue injury can probably be adequately explained for renal involvement, but not necessarily for other sites of injury. The reasons for differences in patterns of disease between individuals, or why some get certain organ involvement and others do not, is not understood. This applies particularly to the observation that only about one-half of SLE patients develop nephritis; why do not the other half? Better understanding of the role of immune complexes in healthy individuals and the factors involved in their clearance by the reticuloendothelial system will be required before mechanisms of tissue injury in SLE are further defined. The function of lymphocyte subpopulations, particularly those with Fc and complement receptors, may also be relevant.

The third facet of disease, namely, the specific triggering event, is the least comprehended at this time, in spite of extensive investigation. While a viral etiology is currently favored, the evidence at this time is far from being decisive. Patients with SLE do not appear to have had any particular type of unique infection. Some of the evidence for viral etiology is indirect, being dependent on the nature and distribution of autoantibodies in patients and their families, particularly lymphocytotoxic and anti-RNA antibodies. As viruses alter cell-surface antigenicity and since lymphocytotoxic antibodies have been associated with viral infection, a viral etiology for these antibodies and/or SLE represents an attractive hypothesis (De Horatius *et al.*, 1975). The presence of lymphocytotoxic antibodies more frequently in (related or unrelated) household contacts of SLE patients than in nonhousehold relatives, further supports the concept that these may relate to environmental agents. The fact that these antibodies were also present more frequently among nonhousehold relatives than controls suggest that this represents part of the genetic contribution to the disease. Similarly, the presence of anti-RNA antibodies may also reflect genetic and viral factors, since they were found only among related household blood relatives and not other household contacts or nonhousehold relatives (De Horatius *et al.*, 1975). The presence of anti-dsRNA antibodies may also reflect exposure to

RNA viral infection (Schur and Monroe, 1969). The observation that (synthetic) dsRNA can act as an adjuvant on T and B cells (in mice) (Cone and Wilson, 1972) can lead to the speculation that (viral) dsRNA released from (viral) damaged cells might not only be immunogeneic but might also boost the titers of other antibodies in SLE patients. Similarly as lymphocytes shed cell-surface antigens, these may combine with lymphocytotoxic antibodies to form circulating immune complexes (Winfield *et al.*, 1975a). In that regard, lymphocytotoxic antibodies have been noted among cryoglobulins (Winfield *et al.*, 1975a). The observations of Fournie *et al.* (1974) are of interest in that injections of bacterial lipopolysaccharides into mice resulted in the release of DNA into the circulation and subsequent formation of anti-DNA antibodies.

The likely viral agents have been much less clearly defined than those drugs that are associated with the onset of SLE. A role for C-type viruses in SLE has been suggested by the observation of Lewis *et al.* and Strand and August of antigens in some SLE patients' cells and tissues (Lewis *et al.*, 1974; Strand and August, 1974). The role of these viruses found in mice with and without immune complex disease is presently the subject of much speculation. Their role in SLE is unlikely to be clarified until there is greater understanding of their biology in man (see Chapter 14). The fact that there is evidence of high titers of antibodies to a multiplicity of the viruses commonly encountered in the human environment would suggest that many events, including uv light and drugs, will trigger the syndrome we now recognize as SLE.

IX. SUMMARY

Current hypotheses regarding the etiology of SLE are depicted in Fig. 1. Possible sites of genetic influence on the pathogenesis of SLE are indicated by //. Susceptible individuals, when exposed to microorganisms and/or drugs, can have triggered in themselves the events depicted in Fig. 1. The ability of the individual to respond to these exogenous agents is influenced by inherited deficiencies of the host's immune defense mechanisms. Microorganisms may then infect and/or effect mononuclear cells, with persistence, or may be acitivated by environmental factors including uv light or various infections. If cell lysis results, antibodies can then be made to cell products (ANA, etc.). The antibodies to lymphocyte membranes may interfere with lymphocyte function in a number of ways including immunosuppression and could also cause reactivation of this cycle (Fig. 1). The antibodies may combine with antigens to form immune complexes that can be efficiently cleared by the reticuloendothelial system (RES), have a

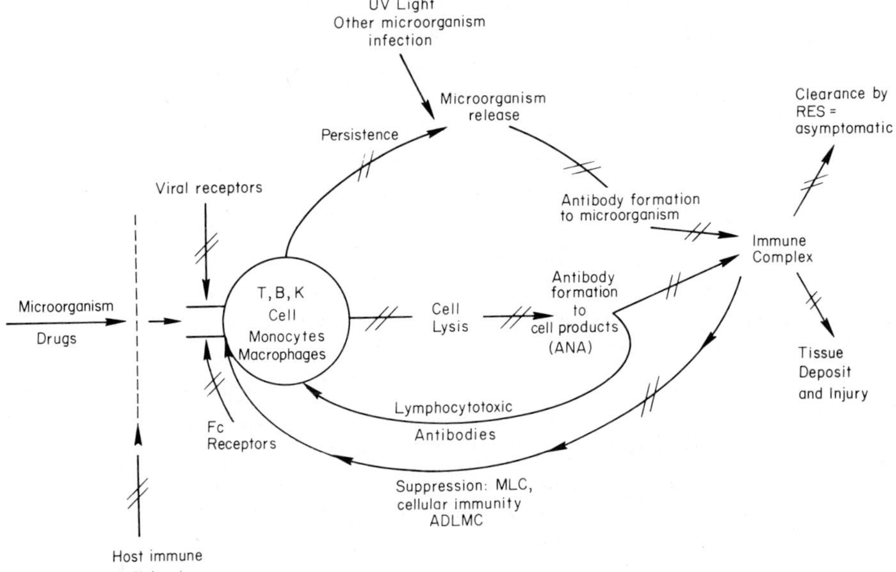

Fig. 1. Current hypothoses regarding the etiology of SLE. Possible sites of genetic influence on the pathogenesis of SLE are indicated by //.

feedback role in lymphocyte regulation, or in susceptible individuals deposit in tissue, with subsequent inflammation.

ACKNOWLEDGMENT

Supported by USPHS Grants AM11414, AM05577, AM05076, and AI00366. Dr. Glass is a Fellow of the Arthritis Rheumatism Council, United Kingdom.

REFERENCES

Aarden, L. A., deGroot, E. R., and Feltkamp, T. E. W. (1975). *Ann. N.Y. Acad. Sci.* **254,** 505–514.

Abe, T., and Homma, M. (1971). *Acta Rheum. Scand.* **17,** 35–46.

Abe, T., Hara, M., Yamasaki, K., and Homma, M. (1973). *Arthritis Rheum.* **16,** 688–694.

Agnello, V., Koffler, D., Eisenberg, J. W., Winchester, R. J., and Kunkel, H. G. (1971). *J. Exp. Med.* **134,** 228s-241s.

Agnello, V., deBracco, M. M. E., and Kunkel, H. G. (1972). *J. Immunol.* **108,** 837–840.

Aho, K., Ahvonen, P., Alkio, P., Lassus, A., Saivanen, E., Sievens, K., and Tiilikainen, T. (1975). *Ann. Rheum. Dis.* **34,** Suppl. 1, 29–32.

Alarcón-Segovia, D. (1969). *Mayo Clin. Proc.* **44,** 664–681.

Alarcón-Segovia, D., Ruiz-Gomez, J., Fishbein, E., and Bustamante, M. E. (1974). *Arthritis Rheum.* **17,** 590–597.

Allansmith, M., McClennan, B. H., Butterworth, M., and Maloney, J. R. (1968). *J. Pediatr.* **72,** 276–290.

Alspaugh, M. A., and Tan, E. M. (1975). *J. Clin. Invest.* **55,** 1067–1073.

Andres, G. A., Accinni, L., Beiser, S. M., Christian, C. L., Cinotti, G. A., Erlanger, B. F., Hsu, K. C., and Seegal, B. C. (1970). *J. Clin. Invest.* **49,** 2106–2118.

Arnett, F. C., Bias, W. B., and Shulman, L. E. (1972). *Arthritis Rheum.* **15,** 428.

Arthritis Foundation Booklet on SLE.

Asherson, G. L. (1959). *Br. J. Exp. Pathol.* **40,** 209–215.

Atkins, C. J., Kandon, J. J., Quismorio, F. P., and Frious, G. J. (1972). *Ann. Intern. Med.* **76,** 65–72.

Azoury, F. J., Jones, H. E., Derbes, V. J., and Gum, O. B. (1966). *Ann. Intern. Med.* **65,** 1221–1228.

Bankhurst, A. D., and Williams, R. C., Jr. (1975). *J. Clin. Invest.* **56,** 1378–1385.

Bartfeld, H. (1969). *Ann. N.Y. Acad. Sci.* **168,** 30–38.

Baum, J. (1967). *Arthritis Rheum.* **10,** 265.

Beighlie, D. J., and Teplitz, R. L. (1975). *J. Rheumatol.* **2,** 149–160.

Bell, D. A., Thiem, P. A., Vaughan, J. H., and Leddy, J. P. (1975). *J. Clin. Invest.* **55,** 256–268.

Bianchi, F. B., Rizzetto, M., Penfold, P., Swana, G. T., and Doniach, D. (1974). *Clin. Exp. Immunol.* **17,** 629–636.

Bitter, T. (1974). *Rheumatology* **5,** 49–243.

Bitter, T., Bitter, F., Silberschmidt, R., and Dubois, E. L. (1971). *Arthritis Rheum.* **14,** 152–153.

Bitter, T., Mottironi, W. D., and Terasaki, P. T. (1972). *N. Engl. J. Med.* **286,** 435–436.

Bloch, K. J., Buchanan, W. W., Wohl, M. J., and Bunim, J. J. (1965). *Medicine* (*Baltimore*) **44,** 187–231.

Block, S. R., and Christian, C. L. (1975). *Am. J. Med.* **59,** 453–456.

Block, S. R., Gibbs, C. B., Stevens, M. B., and Shulman, L. E. (1968). *Ann. Rheum. Dis.* **27,** 311–317.

Block, S. R., Winfield, J. B., Lockshin, M. D., D'Angelo, W. A., and Christian, C. L. (1975). *Am. J. Med.* **59,** 533–552.

Blomgren, S. E., Condemi, J. J., and Vaughan, J. H. (1972). *Am. J. Med.* **52,** 338–348.

Burnham, T. K., and Fine, G. (1971). *Arch. Dermatol.* **103,** 24–32.

Butler, W. T., Sharp, J. T., Rossen, R. D., Liddy, M. D., Mittal, K. K., and Gard, D. A. (1972). *Arthritis Rheum.* **15,** 231–238.

Canoso, J. J., and Cohen, A. S. (1974). *Arthritis Rheum.* **17,** 383–390.

Carr, R. I., Wold, R. T., and Farr, R. S. (1972). *J. Allergy Clin. Immunol.* **50,** 18–30.

Carr, R. I., Harbeck, R. J., Hoffman, A. A., Pirofsky, B., and Bardana, E. J. (1975). *J. Rheumatol. 2, 184–193.*

Casals, S. P., Friou, G. J., and Teague, P. O. (1963). *J. Lab. Clin. Med.* **62,** 625–631.

Cassidy, J. T., Burt, A., Petty, R., and Sullivan, D. (1969). *N. Engl. J. Med.* **280,** 275.

Christian, C. L., Hatfield, W. B., and Chase, P. H. (1963). *J. Clin. Invest.* **42,** 823–829.

Clark, R. A., Kimball, H. R., and Decker, J. L. (1974). *Ann. Rheum. Dis.* **33,** 167–172.

Cochrane, C. G., and Koffler, D. (1973). *Adv. Immunol.* **16,** 185–264.

Comerford, F. R., and Cohen, A. S. (1967). *Medicine* (*Baltimore*) **46,** 425–473.

Cone, R. E., and Wilson, J. D. (1972). *Int. Arch. Allergy Appl. Immunol.* **43,** 123–130.

Cooper, N. R., Ten Bensel, R., and Kohler, P. F. (1968). *J. Immunol.* **101,** 1176–1182.

Cousar, J. B., and Horwitz, D. A. (1973). *Arthritis Rheum.* **16,** 539.

Daniels, C. A., Borsos, T., Rapp, H. J., Snyderman, R., and Notkins, H. L. (1970). *Proc. Natl. Acad. Sci. U.S.A.* **65,** 528–535.

Davis, G. L., and Davis, J. S. (1973). *Arthritis Rheum.* **16,** 52–58.

Day, N. K., Geiger, H., Stroud, R., deBracco, M., Moncado, B., Windhorst, D., and Good, R. A. (1972). *J. Clin. Invest.* **51,** 1102–1108.

Day, N. K., Geiger, H., McLean, R., Michael, A., and Good, R. A. (1973). *J. Clin. Invest.* **52,** 1601–1607.

De Horatius, R. J., and Messner, R. P. (1975). *J. Clin. Invest.* **55,** 1254–1258.

De Horatius, R. J., Pillarisetty, R., Messner, R. P., and Talal, N. (1975). *J. Clin. Invest.* **56,** 1149–1154.

Deicher, H. R. G., Holman, F. R., and Kunkel, H. G. (1960). *Arthritis Rheum.* **3,** 1–15.

Doniach, D., Roitt, I. M., Walker, J. G., and Sherlock, S. (1966). *Clin. Exp. Immunol.* **1,** 237–262.

Druet, P., Letontuiner, P., Contet, A., and Mandet, C. (1973). *Clin. Exp. Immunol.* **15,** 483–496.

Dubois, E. L. (1971). *Semin. Arthritis Rheum.* **1,** 97–115.

Epstein, W. V. (1975). *J. Rheumatol.* **2,** 215–220.

Evans, A. S., Rothfield, N. F., and Niederman, J. C. (1971). *Lancet* **1,** 167–168.

Federlin, K., and Helme, U. (1972). *Lancet* **1,** 596–597.

Fessel, W. J. (1975). *Arch. Intern. Med.* **134,** 1027–1035.

Fournie, G. J., Lambert, P. H., and Miescher, P. A. (1974). *J. Exp. Med.* **140,** 1189–1200.

Friedman, E. A., Bardawil, W. A., Merrill, J. P., and Chim, C. H. (1960). *N. Engl. J. Med.* **262,** 486–491.

Fu, S. M., Kunkel, H. G., Brusman, H. P., Allen, F. H., Jr., and Fotino, M. (1974). *J. Exp. Med.* **140,** 1108–1111.

Fu, S. M., Winchester, R. J., and Kunkel, H. G. (1975). *J. Exp. Med.* **142,** 1334–1338.

Galanud, P., Dorman, T. J., Crosnier, J., and Mery, J. P. H. (1971). *Lancet* **2,** 923.

Gelfand, M. C., Frank, M. M., and Green, I. (1975). *J. Exp. Med.* **142,** 1029–1034.

Gershwin, M. E., and Steinberg, A. D. (1974). *Arthritis Rheum.* **17,** 947–954.

Gershwin, M. W., Blaese, R. M., Wistar, R., and Steinberg, A. D. (1975). *Arthritis Rheum.* **18,** 400.

Gibson, D., Glass, D., Carpenter, C. B., and Schur, P. H. (1975). *Arthritis Rheum.* **18,** 401.

Gilliland, B. C., Leddy, J. P., and Vaughan, J. H. (1970). *J. Clin. Invest.* **49,** 898–906.

Ginsberg, B., and Keiser, H. (1973). *Arthritis Rheum.* **16,** 199–207.

Glass, D., Raum, Gibson, D., Stillman, J. S., and Schur, P. H. (1976). *J. Clin. Invest.* **58,** 853–861.

Goldberg, M. A., Arnett, F. C., and Shulman, L. E. (1973). *Arthritis Rheum.* **16,** 546.

Goldfine, L. J., Stevens, M. B., Masi, A. T., and Shulman, L. E. (1965). *Ann. Rheum. Dis.* **24,** 153–160.

Goldman, J. A., Litwin, A., Adams, L. E., Krueger, R. C., and Hess, E. V. (1972). *J. Clin. Invest.* **51,** 2669–2677.

Gonzalez, E. N., and Rothfield, N. F. (1966). *N. Engl. J. Med.* **274,** 1333–1338.

Grishman, E., and Churg, J. (1970). *Lab. Invest.* **22,** 189–197.

Grumet, F. C., Coukell, A., Bodmer, J. G., Bodmer, W. F., and McDevitt, H. O. (1971). *N. Engl. J. Med.* **285,** 193–196.

Hahn, B. H., Bagby, M. K., and Osterland, C. K. (1973). *Am. J. Med.* **55,** 25–31.

Hamburger, M., Friedlander, L., and Barland, P. (1974). *Arthritis Rheum.* **17,** 469–475.

Hanauer, L. B., and Christian, C. L. (1967). *J. Clin. Invest.* **46,** 400–408.

Harbeck, R. J., Bandana, E. J., Kohler, P. T., and Carr, R. I. (1973). *J. Clin. Invest.* **52,** 789–795.

Harbeck, R. J., Hoffman, A. A., and Carr, R. I. (1975). *J. Rheumatol.* **2,** 194–203.

Harvey, A. M., and Shulman, L. E. (1974). *In* "Lupus Erythematosus" (E. L. Dubois, ed.), 2nd ed. pp. 196–205.

Hasselbacher, P., and LeRoy, E. C. (1974). *Arthritis Rheum.* **17,** 63–71.

Hauptmann, G., Grosshans, E., and Reid, E. (1974). *Ann. Dermatol. Syphiligr.* **101,** 479–496.

Holgate, S., Glass, D., Haslam, P., Maini, T., Turner-Warwick, M. (1976). *Clin. Exp. Immunol.* **24,** 385–395.

Hollinger, F. B., Sharp, J. T., Lidsky, M. D., and Rawls, W. E. (1971). *Arthritis Rheum.* **14,** 1–11.

Holman, H., and Deicher, H. (1959). *J. Clin. Invest.* **38,** 2059–2072.

Holman, H., Deicher, H., and Kunkel, H. G. (1959). *Bull. N.Y. Acad. Med. [2]* **35,** 409–418.

Horwitz, D. A. (1972). *Arthritis Rheum.* **15,** 353–359.

Hughes, G. R. V., Cohen, S. A., Lightfoot, R. W., Meltzer, J. I., and Christian, C. L. (1971). *Arthritis Rheum.* **14,** 259–266.

Hurd, E. R., Dowdle, W., Casey, H., and Ziff, M. (1972). *Arthritis Rheum.* **15,** 267–274.

Ishizaka, T., Ishizaka, K., Salmon, S., and Fudenberg, H. (1967). *J. Immunol.* **99,** 82–91.

Jackson, J., DeAngelis, D., and Schur, P. H. (1973). *Clin. Res.* **21,** 581.

Jasin, H. (1976). *Arthritis Rheum.* **19,** 803–804.

Johnson, G. D., Edmonds, J. P., and Holborow, E. J. (1973). *Lancet* **2,** 883–885.

Karpatkin, S., and Siskind, G. W. (1969). *Blood* **33,** 795–812.

Karpatkin, S., Schur, P. H., Strick, N., and Siskind, G. W. (1973). *Clin. Immunol. Immunopathol.* **2,** 1–8.

Keeffe, E. B., Bardana, E. J., Harbeck, R. J., Pirofsky, B., and Carr, R. I. (1974). *Ann. Intern. Med.* **80,** 58–60.

Kimball, H. R., Wolff, S. M., Talal, N., Plotz, P. H., and Decker, J. L. (1973). *Arthritis Rheum.* **16,** 345–352.

Kissmeyer-Neilsen, F., Kjerbye, K. E., Andersen, E., and Halberg, P. (1975). *Transplant. Rev.* **22,** 164–167.

Koffler, D., Schur, P. H., and Kunkel, H. G. (1967). *J. Exp. Med.* **126,** 607–623.

Koffler, D., Agnello, V., Carr, R. I., and Kunkel, H. G. (1969). *Am. J. Pathol.* **56,** 305–316.

Koffler, D., Carr, R. I., Angello, V., Thoburn, R., and Kunkel, H. G. (1971). *J. Exp. Med.* **134,** 294–312.

Koffler, D., Agnello, V., and Kunkel, H. G. (1974). *Ann. J. Pathol.* **74,** 109–122.

Kohler, P. F., Percy, J., Campion, W. M., and Smyth, C. J. (1974). *Ann. J. Med.* **56,** 406–411.

Kraus, S. J., Haserick, J. R., and Lantz, M. A. (1970). *J. Am. Med. Assoc.* **211,** 2140–2141.

Krishnan, C., and Kaplan, M. H. (1967). *J. Clin. Invest.* **46,** 569–579.

Kunkel, H. G., and Tan, H. G. (1964). *Adv. Immunol.* **4,** 351–395.

Lachmann, P. J. (1974). *Boll. Ist. Sieroter. Milan.* **53,** 195–207.

Lachmann, P. J., and Kunkel, H. G. (1961). *Lancet* **2,** 436–437.

Lachmann, P. J., Müller-Eberhard, H. J., Kunkel, H. G., and Panoretto, F. (1962). *J. Exp. Med.* **115,** 63–82.

Lamon, E. W., and Bennett, J. C. (1970). *Immunology* **19,** 439–442.

Landry, M., and Sams, W. M., Jr. (1973). *J. Clin. Invest.* **52,** 1871–1880.

Lee, S. L., and Miotti, A. B. (1975). *Semin. Arthritis Rheum.* **4,** 241–252.

Levine, L., and Stollar, B. D. (1968). *Prog. Allergy* **12,** 161–191.

Lewis, R. M., Tannenberg, W., Smith, C., and Schwartz, R. S. (1974). *Nature (London)* **252,** 78–79.

Lies, R. B., Messner, R. P., and Williams, R. C., Jr. (1973). *Arthritis Rheum.* **16,** 369–375.

Lockshin, M. D., Eisenhauer, A. C., Kohn, R., Weksler, M., Block, S., and Mushlin, S. B. (1975). *Arthritis Rheum.* **18,** 245–250.

Maclaren, N. K., Huang, S., and Fogh, J. (1975). *Lancet* **1,** 997–1000.

Mandema, E., Pollak, V. E., Kark, R. M., and Rezaian, J. (1961). *J. Lab. Clin. Med.* **58,** 337–352.

Masi, A. T. (1968). *In* "Proceedings of the Third International Symposium" (P. H. Bennett and P. H. N. Wood, eds.), Int. Congr. Ser. No. 148, p. 267. Excerpta Med. Found., Amsterdam.

Mattioli, M., and Reichlin, M. (1974). *Arthritis Rheum.* **17,** 421–429.

Maugh, T. H. (1975). *Science* **188,** 347–351.
Meiselas, L. E., Zimgale, S. B., Lee, S. L., Richman, S., and Siegel, M. (1961). *J. Clin. Invest.* **40,** 1872–1881.
Messner, R. P., Lindstrom, F. D., and Williams, R. C., Jr. (1973). *J. Clin. Invest.* **52,** 3046–3056.
Miescher, P. A., Rothfield, N., and Miescher, A. (1973). *In* "Lupus Erythematosus" (E. L. Dubois, ed.), 2nd ed. pp. 153–163.
Mittal, K. K., Rossen, R. D., Sharp, J. T., Lidsky, M. D., and Butler, W. T. (1970). *Nature* (*London*) **225,** 1255–1256.
Miyawaki, S., and Ritchie, R. R. (1973). *Arthritis Rheum.* **16,** 726–736.
Moncado, B., Day, N. K. B., Good, R. A., and Windhorst, D. B. (1972). *N. Engl. J. Med.* **286,** 689–693.
Mongan, E. S., Leddy, J. P., Atwater, E. C., and Barnett, E. V. (1967). *Arthritis Rheum.* **10,** 502–508.
Moore, J. M., and Neison, J. M. E. (1963). *Lancet* **2,** 645.
Muschel, L. H. (1961). *Proc. Soc. Exp. Biol. Med.* **106,** 622–625.
Nerup, J., Ortred, A. O., Bendixen, G., Egebjerg, J., and Paulsen, J. E. (1971). *Diabetes* **20,** 424.
Nies, K. M., Brown, J. C., Dubois, E. L., Quismorio, F. P., Friou, G. J., and Terasaki, P. I. (1974). *Arthritis Rheum.* **17,** 397–402.
Notman, D. D., Kurato, N., and Tan, E. M. (1975). *Ann. Intern. Med.* **83,** 464–469.
Nydegger, M. E., Lambert, P. H., Gerber, H., and Miescher, P. A. (1974). *J. Clin. Invest.* **54,** 297–309.
Osterland, C. K., Espinoza, L., Parker, L. P., and Schur, P. H. (1975). *Ann. Intern. Med.* **82,** 323–328.
Page, A. R., Sharp, H. L., Greenberg, L. S., and Yunis, E. J. (1975). *J. Clin. Invest.* **56,** 661–667.
Paronetto, F., and Koffler, D. (1965). *J. Clin. Invest.* **44,** 1657–1664.
Panush, R. S., Bianco, N. E., Schur, P. H., Rocklin, R. E., David, J. R., and Stillman, J. S. (1972). *Clin. Exp. Immunol.* **10,** 103–115.
Patrucco, A., Rothfield, N. F., and Hirschorn, K. (1967). *Arthritis Rheum.* **10,** 32–37.
Percy, J. S., and Smyth, C. J. (1969). *J. Am. Med. Assoc.* **208,** 485.
Phillips, P. E. (1975). *Ann. Intern. Med.* **83,** 709–715.
Phillips, P. E., and Christian, C. L. (1970). *Science* **168,** 982–984.
Phillips, P. E., and Christian, C. L. (1972). *Proc. Soc. Exp. Biol. Med.* **140,** 1340.
Phillips, P. E., and Hirshaut, Y. (1973). *Arthritis Rheum.* **16,** 97–101.
Pickering, R. J., Natt, G. B., Stroud, R. M., Good, R. A., Gewurz, H. (1970). *J. Exptl. Med.* **131,** 803–815.
Pincus, T., Schur, P. H., Rose, J. A., Decker, J. L., and Talal, N. (1969). *N. Engl. J. Med.* **281,** 701–705.
Pinnas, J. L., Northway, J. D., and Tan, E. M. (1972). *Arthritis Rheum.* **15,** 450.
Pondman, K. W., Stoop, J. W., Cormane, R. H., and Hannema, A. J. (1968). *J. Immunol.* **101,** 811.
Quismorio, F. P., and Friou, G. J. (1972). *Int. Arch. Allergy Appl. Immunol.* **43,** 740–748.

Raum, D., Glass, D., Soter, N. A., Stillman, J. S., Carpenter, C. B., and Schur, P. H. (1977). *Arthritis Rheum.* (in press).
Reichlin, M., and Mattioli, M. (1973–1974). *Bull. Rheum. Dis.* **24,** 756–760.
Ritchie, R. F. (1970). *N. Engl. J. Med.* **282,** 1174–1178.
Robboy, S. J., Lewis, E. J., Schur, P. H., and Colman, R. W. (1970). *Am. J. Med.* **49,** 742–752.
Ropes, M. W. (1964). *Medicine (Baltimore)* **43,** 387–391.
Rosenfeld, S. I. and Leddy, J. P. (1974). *J. Clin. Invest.* **53,** 67a.
Rosenthal, C. J., and Franklin, E. C. (1973). *Arthritis Rheum.* **10,** 565.
Rosenthal, C. J., and Franklin, E. C. (1975). *Arthritis Rheum.* **18,** 207–217.
Rothfield, N. F., and Rodnan, G. P. (1968). *Arthritis Rheum.* **11,** 607–617.
Rothfield, N. F., Evans, A. S., and Niederman, J. C. (1973). *Ann. Rheum. Dis.* **32,** 238–246.
Rowley, M. J., and Mackay, I. R. (1969). *Clin. Exp. Immunol.* **5,** 407–418.
Samaha, R. J., and Irvin, W. S. (1975). *J. Clin. Invest.* **56,** 446–457.
Scheinberg, M. A., and Cathcart, E. S. (1973). *Arthritis Rheum.* **16,** 566.
Schneider, J., Chin, W., Friou, G. J., Cooper, S. M., Harding, B., Hill, R. L., and Quismorio, F. P. (1975). *Clin. Exp. Immunol.* **20,** 187–192.
Schur, P. H. (1975). *Clin. Rheum. dis.* **1,** 519–544.
Schur, P. H. (1977). *Arthritis Rheum.* (in press).
Schur, P. H, and Monroe, M. (1969). *Proc. Natl. Acad. Sci. U.S.A.* **63,** 1108–1112.
Schur, P. H., and Sandson, J. (1968). *N. Engl. J. Med.* **278,** 533–538.
Schur, P. H., Moroz, L. A., and Kunkel, H. G. (1967). *Immunochemistry* **4,** 447–453.
Schur, P. H., Stollar, B. D., Steinberg, A. D., and Talal, N. (1971). *Arthritis Rheum.* **14,** 342–347.
Schur, P. H., Monroe, M., and Rothfield, N. (1972). *Arthritis* **15,** 174–182.
Schur, P. H., DeAngelis, D., and Jackson, J. (1974). *Clin. Exp. Immunol.* **17,** 209–218.
Senyk, G., Hadley, W. K., Attias, M. R., and Talal, N. (1974). *Arthritis Rheum.* **17,** 553–562.
Sharp, G. C., Irvin, W. S., Tan, E. M., Gould, R. G., and Holman, H. (1972). *Am. J. Med.* **52,** 148–159.
Siegel, M., and Lee, S. L. (1973). *Semin. Arthritis Rheum.* **3,** 1–54.
Sigler, J. W., Monto, R. W., Ensign, D. C., Wilson, G. M., Jr., Rebuch, J. W., and Loveth, J. D. (1958). *Arthritis Rheum.* **1,** 115–121.
Soloway, R. D., Summerskill, W. H. J., Baggenstoss, A. H., and Schoenfield, L. J. (1972). *Gastroenterology* **63,** 458–465.
Soter, N., Austen, K. F., and Gigli, I. (1974). *J. Invest. Dermatol.* **63,** 219–226.
Staples, P. J., Gerding, D. N., Decker, J. L., and Gordon, R. S., Jr. (1974). *Arthritis Rheum.* **17,** 1–10.
Statsny, P. (1972). *Arthritis Rheum.* **15,** 455–456.
Statsny, P., and Ziff, M. (1969). *N. Engl. J. Med.* **280,** 1376–1381.
Steinman, C. R., Deesomchok, U., and Spiera, H. (1975). *Arthritis Rheum.* **18,** 429.
Stern, R., Fu, S. M., Agnello, V. *et al.* (1976). *Arthritis Rheum.* **19,** 517–522.

Stevens, M. B., Urowitz, M. B., Mulhern, L. M., and Shulman, L. E. (1967).*Arthritis Rheum.* **10,** 317.
Steward, M. W., Glass, D. N., Maini, R. N., and Scott, J. T. (1974). *J. Rheum.* **1,** 41.
Stiller, C. R., Russell, A. S., and Dossetor, J. B. (1975). *Ann. Intern. Med.* **82,** 405–410.
Stollar, B. D. (1975). *Crit. Rev. Biochem.* **3,** 45–69.
Strand, M., and August, J. T. (1974). *J. Virol.* **14,** 1584–1596.
Suciu-Foca, N., Buda, J. A., Thiem, T., and Reemtsma, K. (1974). *Clin. Exp. Immunol.* **18,** 295–301.
Svec, K. H., and Allen, S. T. (1970). *Science* **170,** 550–551.
Svejgaard, A., Platz, Rev., Ryder, P., Nielsen, L. S., and Thomson, M. (1975). *Transplant. Rev.* **22,** 4–43.
Svensson, B., and Hedberg, H. (1973). *Scand. J. Rheumatol.* **2,** 78–80.
Talal, N. (1970). *Arthritis Rheum.* **13,** 887–894.
Talal, N. (1975). *Clin. Rheum. Dis.* **1,** 82, 405–410, and 485–496.
Talal, N., and Gallo, R. C. (1972). *Nature* (*London*) **240,** 240–242.
Talal, N., and Pillarisetty, R. (1975). *Clin. Immunol. Immunopathol.* **4,** 24–31.
Tan, E. M. (1968). *Arthritis Rheum.* **11,** 515.
Tan, E. M., and Kunkel, H. G. (1966a). *Arthritis Rheum.* **9,** 37–46.
Tan, E. M., and Kunkel, H. G. (1966b). *J. Immunol.* **96,** 464–471.
Tan, E. M., and Natali, P. G. (1970). *J. Immunol.* **104,** 902–906.
Tan, E. M., Schur, P. H., Carr, R. T., and Kunkel, H. G. (1966). *J. Clin. Invest.* **45,** 1732–1740.
Tannenbaum, H., and Schur, P. H. (1974). *J. Rheumatol.* **14,** 392.
Terasaki, P., and Mickey, M. R. (1975). *Transplant. Rev.* **22,** 105–119.
Terasaki, P. I., Mottironi, V. D., and Barnett, E. V. (1970). *N. Engl. J. Med.* **283,** 724–728.
Theofilopoulos, A. N., Wilson, C. B., Bokisch, V. A., and Dixon, F. J. (1974). *J. Exp. Med.* **140,** 1230–1244.
Thomsen, M., Platz, P., Andersen, O. O., Christy, M., Lyngsxe, J., Nerup, J., Rasmussen, K., Ryder, L. P., Nielsen, L. S., and Svejgaard, A. (1975). *Transplant. Rev.* **22,** 125–147.
Tojo, T., Friou, G. J., and Spiegelberg, H. L. (1970). *Clin. Exp. Immunol.* **6,** 145–151.
Townes, A. S. (1963). *Bull. Johns. Hopkins Hosp.* **112,** 183–202.
Tuffanelli, D. L., Kay, D., and Fukuyama, K. (1969). *Arch. Dermatol.* **99,** 652–662.
Utermohlen, V., Winfield, J. B., and Kunkel, H. G. (1974). *J. Exp. Med.* **139,** 1019.
Verroust, P. J., Wilson, C. B., Cooper, N. R., Edgington, T. S., and Dixon, F. J. (1974). *J. Clin. Invest.* **53,** 77–84.
von Hassig, A., Borel, J. F., Ammann, P., Thorii, M., and Bütler, R. (1964). *Pathol. Microbiol.* **27,** 542–547.
Waters, Konrad, P., and Walford, R. L. (1971). *Tissue Antigens* **1,** 68–73.
Wernet, P., and Kunkel, H. G. (1973). *J. Exp. Med.* **138,** 1021.
Wernet, P., Fotino, M., Thoburn, R., Moore, A., and Kunkel, H. G. (1973). *Arthritis Rheum.* **16,** 137.

Wiedermann, G., and Miescher, P. A. (1965). *Ann. N.Y. Acad. Sci.* **124,** 807–815.

Wild, J. H., Zvaifler, N. J., Muller-Eberhard, H. J. *et al.* (1976). *Clin. Exp. Immunol.* **24,** 238–248.

Williams, R. C., Jr., DeBoard, J. R., Mellbye, O. J., Messner, R. P., and Lindstrom, F. D. (1973a). *J. Clin. Invest.* **52,** 283–295.

Williams, R. C., Jr., Lies, R. B., and Messner, R. P. (1973b). *Arthritis Rheum.* **16,** 597–605.

Winchester, R. J., Winfield, J. B., Siegal, F., Wernet, P., Bentwich, Z., and Kunkel, H. G. (1974). *J. Clin. Invest.* **54,** 1082–1092.

Winfield, J. B., Koffler, D., and Kunkel, H. G.(1975a). *J. Clin. Invest.* **56,** 563–570.

Winfield, J. B., Winchester, R. J., Wernet, P., Fu, S. M., and Kunkel, H. G. (1975b). *Arthritis Rheum.* **18,** 1–8.

Winfield, J. B., Winchester, R. J., Wernet, P., and Kunkel, H. G. (1975c). *Clin. Exp. Immunol.* **19,** 399–406.

Wold, R. T., Young, F. E., Tan, E. M., and Farr, R. S. (1968). *Science* **161,** 806–807.

Zingale, S. B., Avalos, J. C. S., Anrada, J. A., Stringa, S. G., and Manni, J. A. (1963). *Arthritis Rheum.* **6,** 581–598.

Chapter 19

Rheumatoid Arthritis

NATHAN J. ZVAIFLER

I. CLINICAL FEATURES OF RHEUMATOID ARTHRITIS

Rheumatoid arthritis is a chronic inflammatory disorder of unknown etiology which is systemic in nature and characterized by the manner in which it involves joints (Short *et al.*, 1957). In general, articular involvement is remitting; episodes of joint inflammation usually occur against a backdrop of progressive articular destruction and deformity, leading ultimately to a highly variable degree of incapacitation. Extraarticular features, such as rheumatoid nodules, arteritis, neuropathy, scleritis, pericarditis, lymphadenopathy, and splenomegaly occur with considerable frequency. Once considered to be complications of rheumatoid arthritis, these manifestations are now recognized as integral parts of the disease process and serve to emphasize the truly systemic nature of this disorder.

The disease occurs at all ages, with a generally increasing incidence through the sixth decade. Women are affected two or three times more commonly than men. The onset of rheumatoid arthritis is frequently heralded by prodromal symptoms, such as fatigue, anorexia, weakness, and generalized aching and stiffness that is not clearly localized to articular structures. Some patients provide a history of one or more disturbing events in the weeks or months preceding the onset of arthritis, most commonly infection, surgery, trauma, childbirth, or emotional stress. The significance of these observations is questionable. Joint symptoms usually appear gradually and insidiously over a period of weeks to months. Occasionally, there are brief remittent episodes of articular involvement prior to the development of more persistent arthritis; approximately 20% of patients have an abrupt onset with the rapid development of polyarthritis, often accompanied by fever, prostration, and severe constitutional symptoms. The mode of onset is not clearly related to the subsequent course or prognosis of the disease.

Articular involvement is manifested clinically by pain, stiffness, limitation of motion, and the signs of inflammation, i.e., swelling, warmth, erythema, and tenderness. Pain need not be proportional to the degree of inflammation, and is usually most pronounced on movement of the afflicted joint. Morning stiffness lasting more than 30 minutes (and frequently several hours) is highly characteristic of rheumatoid arthritis and is thought to be due to an accentuation of the congestion and edema in the synovium, joint capsule, and periarticular tissues resulting from inactivity. This "gelling" phenomenon often recurs after periods of inactivity later in the day, typically after sitting in a movie theater or watching television. Joint swelling results from synovial hypertrophy, thickening of the joint capsule, and, frequently, from an increase in the volume of synovial fluid (effusion). Early in the disease, limitation of motion is usually due to pain, but later may be caused by capsular fibrosis, bony or fibrous ankylosis, muscle contracture and/or rupture, and laxity or shortening of tendons and ligaments.

Any of the diarthrodial joints of the body can be affected; initially, those most commonly involved are the small joints of the hands, the wrists, knees, and feet. At the outset, there may be any pattern of joint disease. Usually it is bilateral and polyarticular, but in a small percentage of patients, the arthritis remains unilateral or monarticular (usually the knees) for periods of months to years, and considerable diagnostic confusion may result. As the disease becomes established, the arthritis spreads to the elbows, shoulders, hips, ankles, subtalar, and sternoclavicular joints. Less commonly, the temporomandibular and cricoarytenoid joints are affected. Spinal involvement is usually limited to the upper cervical articulations. Radiographic evidence of sacroiliac disease is not uncommon, but this assumes little clinical importance.

Subcutaneous nodules, perhaps the most commonest extraarticular feature of rheumatoid arthritis, appear at some time in approximately 20–25% of patients. They are almost invariably associated with seropositive (rheumatoid factor) disease and, hence, a more severe and destructive arthritis (see below). The nodules characteristically are firm, nontender, rounded or oval masses in the subcutaneous or deeper connective tissues, varying in size from less than 0.5 cm to several centimeters in diameter. Areas subjected to mechanical pressure are common sites—especially the olecranon and extensor surface of the forearms and the Achilles tendon—as are articular and periarticular structures. Visceral involvement by rheumatoid nodules will be discussed in more detail later. Except for cosmetic complaints, subcutaneous nodules seldom cause symptoms, but occasionally they break down or become infected. Typically, they develop insidiously and, once present, either persist indefinitely or regress at any time. Histologically, the rheumatoid nodule is composed of an irregular central zone of fibrinoid necrosis surrounded by a palisade of elongated connective tissue cells arranged radially in a corona about the necrotic zone; this core is enveloped by an outer zone of granulation tissue containing chronic inflammatory cells, chiefly lymphocytes and plasma cells.

A number of laboratory abnormalities appear regularly in rheumatoid arthritis. A moderate degree of anemia, usually associated with low serum iron and normal or decreased iron-binding capacity is a common feature. The erythrocyte sedimentation rate is elevated to a variable degree in most patients and roughly parallels disease activity. Serum proteins are often normal, but electrophoretic analysis may reveal mild to moderate decreases in albumin, elevation of the α_2-globulins and a polyclonal increase in γ-globulin. But no component of serum has attracted so much attention as the rheumatoid factors. These antibodies to the patient's own γ-globulin are the hallmark of rheumatoid arthritis and have fascinated investigators since their initial description in the early 1930's. Research in each subsequent decade defined, first, their diagnostic and prognostic significance, then their autoreactive (autoimmune) nature, and , finally, their probable role in the pathogenesis of rheumatoid arthritis (Franklin *et al.*, 1957; Kunkel and Tan, 1964; Stage and Mannik, 1973; Williams, 1974).

II. RHEUMATOID FACTORS

Rheumatoid factor(s) are antibodies with specificity for antigenic determinants on the Fc fragment of human or animal IgG. The usual clinical tests for rheumatoid factor are agglutination procedures that employ sheep red blood cells, sensitized with rabbit anti-sheep cell antibodies or inert particles (latex or bentonite) with human IgG adsorbed onto their surface. The sensitized sheep cell test is more specific for rheumatoid arthritis, but is infrequently used in clinical practice because it is more laborious than the latex agglutination or bentonite flocculation tests. All of these systems detect primarily 19 S IgM rheumatoid factors because these molecules are very potent agglutinators, as compared to other classes of immunoglobulins with similar specificities. More recently developed methods can demonstrate anti-γ-globulins (rheumatoid factor) in IgG and IgA immunoglobulins in a large percentage of rheumatoid sera (Torrigiani and Roitt, 1967). The latter, in fact, are occasionally detected in the absence of IgM rheumatoid factor.

Using the latex agglutination or bentonite flocculation tests, IgM rheumatoid factors can be detected in approximately 70% of adult patients with rheumatoid arthritis. A positive test is by no means diagnostic of this disorder, since rheumatoid factors are also found in 1–5% of normal subjects, the incidence increasing with advancing age, and in a variety of disease states. Conversely, its absence does not exclude rheumatoid arthritis. Rheumatoid patients usually have more rheumatoid factor than normals or those with other diseases. High titers of rheumatoid factor are associated with more severe and active joint disease, the presence of nodules, greater frequency of systemic complications of rheumatoid arthritis, and a poorer outcome (Epstein and Engleman, 1959; Mongan *et al.*, 1969).

The antibody nature of rheumatoid factors is demonstrated by specificity for both genetic (e.g., Gm)* and nongenetic (structural) determinants on the IgG molecule, most commonly located in the amino terminal portion of the Fc fragments from IgG_1, IgG_2, and IgG_4 molecules. This reactivity may be to autologous (patient's own), isologous (other human), or heterologous (other species) IgG, in either the native or denatured state. Individual sera, in general, contain an array of anti-γ-globulins with differing specificities. The majority lack specificity for genetic determinants and react preferentially with aggregated IgG or antigen–antibody complexes. Reactivity with native and autologous IgG can be demonstrated for some rheumatoid factors; this presumably accounts for the occurrence of circulating 22 S complexes made of IgM rheumatoid factor and IgG in the serum of some patients with rheumatoid arthritis. "Intermediate complexes" containing only 7 S IgG, part having rheumatoid factor activity, can also be detected in some sera. Some rheumatoid factors react with both heterologous and isologous IgG, reflecting shared antigenic determinants, and a minority with heterologous IgG only (Williams, 1974). Anti-γ-globulin antibodies have also been described, with reactivity limited to anti-

* Gm determinants are genetically determined antigenic specificities that reside on the heavy chain of certain human IgG molecules.

genic determinants on immunoglobulins uncovered by digestion with pepsin or other proteolytic enzymes; others are specific for sites on L chains. Rheumatoid factors in nonrheumatoid sera do not usually combine with the heterologous (e.g., rabbit) IgG, and this fact explains the negative sensitized sheep cell test in the majority of these patients (Stage and Mannik, 1973). Currently, the most popular notion is that rheumatoid factors arise as antibodies to "altered" autologous IgG. Alteration is thought to occur when a native IgG antibody molecule combines with its specific antigen. This antigen–antibody interaction changes the configuration of the IgG molecule revealing new or previously buried antigenic determinants, thereby rendering it an autoimmunogen. Support for this hypothesis comes from animal experiments in which chronic intense immunization with bacteria or bacterial cell wall antigens results in the production of anti-γ-globulin factors and from the finding of rheumatoid factors in bacterial endocarditis and other human diseases that have chronic antigenic stimulation as a common denominator (Abruzzo and Christian, 1961; Bokisch *et al.*, 1973; Williams and Kunkel, 1962).

The exact biologic role of rheumatoid factors is unknown. Anti-viral properties have been ascribed to them, and, under certain circumstances, they can augment the inflammatory response by enhancing complement fixation, by altering the properties (e.g., size or solubility) of immune complexes, or by rendering them more susceptible to ingestion by phagocytic cells. It should be appreciated, however, that these effects are only operative under very restricted *in vitro* conditions, and many experiments show opposing reactions as the conditions are altered. Indeed, it is possible that rheumatoid factors act differently in the circulation, in synovial tissues and in synovial fluids. The complex literature on this subject has been reviewed elsewhere (Zvaifler and Greenberg, 1977).

III. PATHOGENESIS OF RHEUMATOID JOINT DISEASE

Although rheumatoid arthritis remains a disease of unknown etiology, an increasing number of observations suggest that both cellular and humoral immunologic events mediate its pathogenesis. Thus,the detection of large numbers of lymphocytes identifiable as T cells in synovial tissues and the presence of lymphokines (soluble mediators of T cell origin) in synovial fluid imply a role for cell-mediated immunity. In addition, the capacity of rheumatoid synovium in culture to produce antibody, the demonstration of immunoglobulin and complement in phagocytic synovial cells and in blood vessels at sites of extraarticular lesions, as well as the identification of immune complexes and associated complement consumption in synovial fluid assert the importance of humoral immune mechanisms. Furthermore, features consistent with a disturbance of immune regulation, such as hypergammaglobulinemia and antibodies to "self-proteins" (i.e., autoantibodies to IgG and nucleoprotein) are regular findings in rheumatoid arthritis. Finally, the clinical observations of a close association of rheumatoid arthritis with other "autoimmune" diseases and the therapeutic efficacy of cytotoxic (immunosuppressive) drugs and lymphocyte depletion by thoracic duct drainage also support an immune pathogenesis of this disease (Pearson *et al.*, 1975).

The earliest clues came from the demonstration of anti-γ-globulins in the circulation. Subsequently, attention was directed to the articular cavity as evidence appeared for complement fixation and rheumatoid factor containing immune complexes in rheumatoid synovial effusions. Based on these observations, and others to be detailed below, the following working hypothesis has been constructed. An undefined inciting antigen establishes itself in the articular cavity and stimulates the local production of antibody. The interaction of antigen and antibody (and probably later anti-γ-globulins) in synovial tissues and fluid initiates the complement sequence, generating a number of biologically active products. Some of these cause increased vascular permeability, allowing an influx of serum proteins and cellular blood elements into the site where the complexes reside. Polymorphonuclear leukocytes are attracted by complement-derived chemotactic factors, and the complexes are attached to their cell surfaces by receptors for IgG and C3. Engulfment follows, with a concomitant release of large quantities of hydrolytic enzymes. These lysosomal enzymes are thought to directly mediate much of the inflammation and some of the tissue damage (Weissman, 1972; Zvaifler, 1973). According to this scheme, rheumatoid arthritis is "an extravascular immune complex disease" whose focus is in the synovium and articular cavity (Zvaifler, 1974).

But immune complexes alone cannot explain all the joint changes in rheumatoid arthritis. Indeed, many investigators are of the opinion that cell-mediated immune injury and the development of granulation tissue are more responsible for the proliferative and destructive elements of rheumatoid joint disease. Viewed from this perspective, the changes in the synovial fluid are only reflections of the primary pathogenetic events. Undoubtedly, each of these mechanisms is important and intimately interrelated, but for the sake of clarity they will be described separately in the sections to follow.

A. Synovial Membrane

Most studies of the joint lining have been made in chronic and well-established disease. Observations on the earlier stages of rheumatoid arthritis are limited because of difficulties in documenting the disorder at this time. Synovial biopsy taken in the first 2 months of disease demonstrate evidence of microvascular injury; it is manifested by gaps between endothelial cells, extravasation of erythrocytes, small vessel thrombosis, and endothelial cell injury. Polymorphonuclear cells predominate, infiltrating the superficial synovium and perivascular locations. Mononuclear cells are observed in the synovial effusions, which is in direct contrast to the findings later in the disease (Kulka *et al.*, 1955; Schumacher and Kitridou, 1974).

As time passes, the rheumatoid synovitis becomes more characteristic, demonstrating hypertrophied, edematous, and inflamed synovial lining surface, protruding into the joint space as slender villous projections. Normally few in number, the lining cells become multilayered, occasionally reaching a depth of 10–20 cells with multinucleated giant cells interspersed among them. Most typical, however, is the intense infiltration of the synovium by mononuclear cells, largely lymphocytes and plasma cells. These are frequently collected into aggregates or follicles, particularly around the small blood vessels, but true germinal centers are rarely seen (Gardner, 1965; Hamerman *et al.*, 1969). The predominant cell in these nodules is a lymphocyte, but about the periphery are typical plasma cells that by immunofluorescent analysis contain deposits of immunoglobulins (Fish *et al.*, 1966).

What kind of lymphocytes infiltrate rheumatoid synovial membranes? Electron micrographs of areas rich in lymphocytes reveal predominantly small lymphocytes, less than 5% transformed blastlike cells, and variable numbers of plasma cells (Kobayashi and Ziff, 1973). Fluoresceinated rabbit anti-human T cell antiserum applied to frozen sections of human rheumatoid synovium stains the majority of the cells within the lymphoid infiltrates, suggesting that the predominant cell is a T lymphocyte (Williams, 1974, p. 130). The technique of cytoadherence applied to the study of rheumatoid synovial membranes, has yielded conflicting data. When suspensions of sheep erythrocytes (E) or erythrocytes coated with antibody and the third component of complement (EAC) are layered over frozen serial sections of rheumatoid synovium, these respective T and B lymphocyte markers adhere to areas corresponding to those of lymphoid infiltration. Van Boxel and Paget (1975) claim the major lymphocyte is a T cell, whereas Sheldon and Holborow (1975) concluded that B lymphocytes predominate. There is a general agreement, however, that the majority of viable lymphocytes extracted from rheumatoid synovial membranes are T cells, and the proportion of B lymphocytes identified by membrane-bound immunoglobulin or C3 receptors are usually below levels normally found in the blood (Abrahamsen *et al.*, 1975; Van Boxel and Paget, 1975; Wangel and Klockars, 1977).

There is ample evidence that the rheumatoid synovium contains large amounts of immunoglobulin, much of it locally synthesized (Sliwinski and Zvaifler, 1970; Smiley *et al.*, 1968). IgG and IgM, singly or in combination, are regularly demonstrated by immunofluorescence in synovial lining cells, in blood vessels, and in the interstitial connective tissue of the synovial membrane. The IgG, generally found in abundance, is in areas that also stain for complement components (C3 and C4), whereas the IgM is in lesser amounts and not identified with complement. IgG is frequently present in early rheumatoid lesions, in children with rheumatoid arthritis, and in adults with seronegative rheumatoid arthritis, when little or no IgM is detectable (Zvaifler, 1973).

Immunofluorescent examination of the plasma cells present in the deeper layers of the membrane shows IgG to be the predominant immunoglobulin, both in seropositive and seronegative patients. Munthe and Natvig (1972a) demonstrated that the IgG within many of these plasma cells had anti-γ-globulin (rheumatoid factor) activity. Theoretically, IgG rheumatoid factor is difficult to detect, because it complexes with itself. This problem was circumvented by pepsin digestion of the tissue sections, which removes the antigenic (Fc) portion of the IgG molecule but leaves the reactive $F(ab)_2$ fragments intact. Before pepsin treatment, there was no binding of fluorescein-labeled aggregated IgG to the plasma cells, but afterward binding to a large proportion of the IgG containing cells was observed. Native IgG blocked the reaction, but it was not abolished by reduction and alkylation of the aggregated IgG, implying that these were true anti-IgG reactions. The results were similar in tissues from either seronegative or seropositive patients, namely, 20–60% of the IgG plasma cells showed anti-γ-globulin activity (Munthe and Natvig, 1972a). The absence of direct staining with anti-C1q or anti-C3 of fresh tissues suggested little *in vivo* complement fixation, but strong immunofluorescence was observed after C1q or a fresh serum source of C3 was applied to the tissues (Munthe and Natvig, 1972b). The authors (Natvig and Munthe, 1975) interpret their findings to indicate that many of the plasma cells in the rheumatoid synovium make an IgG rheumatoid factor that combines with similar IgG molecules ("self-associating IgG") within the cell. Although these complexes do not appear to activate or bind complement within the plasma cell cytoplasm, they might have important complement-fixing activities after secretion from the cells. It is somewhat surprising to note, however, that the results obtained are similar in patients with seronegative and seropositive joint disease, since the latter are generally accepted to have more aggressive and destructive arthritis and more profound intraarticular complement consumption. Perhaps a better understanding of the antibodies from the remaining 40–

50% of IgG-producing plasma cells or the role of IgM rheumatoid factors will shed light on these differences.

B. Synovial Fluid

Normal synovial fluid has been characterized as a dialysate of plasma to which hyaluronate has been added (Sandson and Hamerman, 1964). In the normal joint, the amount and type of protein is carefully regulated. Plasma proteins with a high molecular weight or asymmetrical shape, such as fibrinogen, are not detected in normal synovial fluid. However, synovial inflammation permits introduction of increased amounts of both large and small molecular weight proteins to the synovial fluid.

1. The Complement System

As a rule, the total hemolytic complement activity in the serum of rheumatoid arthritis patients is normal. Since the proteins of synovial fluid are derived from the blood, complement proteins should be present in synovial fluid in an equivalent concentration to proteins of similar size. But complement levels in rheumatoid arthritis effusions are significantly lower than in companion serum samples or synovial fluids from other forms of inflammatory joint disease (Hedberg, 1964; Pekin and Zvaifler, 1964). These early observations prompted a number of studies to determine if only a few critical complement components were lacking or whether the individual components were depleted in an orderly manner.

According to current understanding, the complement system is comprised of a group of serum proteins whose sequential interaction generates a number of biologically important factors. Most of these are derived from the terminal components (C5–C9). Activation of the terminal portion of the sequence can be accomplished by two discrete mechanisms. The first, known as the "classical pathway," is initiated by the binding of C1 through its C1q subunit to a site on the Fc portion of IgM or most IgG molecules. Binding of C1 results in its conversion to an enzyme whose two natural substrates are the fourth (C4) and second (C2) complement components. Their interaction causes the formation of a new bimolecular complex of fragments of C2 and C4 ($\overline{\text{C4b, 2a}}$), which becomes membrane bound and is capable of cleaving the third component (C3), and subsequently activates the terminal components (Müller-Eberhard, 1972).

Another pathway has recently been recognized that can bypass the early components and leads directly to the cleavage of C3. This "alternate pathway" (or properdin system) is readily activated by complex polysaccharides, such as inulin or zymosan, bacterial lipopolysaccharides or endotoxin, some immune complexes, aggregates of IgA, and a "nephritic factor" isolated from serum of patients with chronic membranoproliferative glomerulonephritis. The known components of this pathway include a recently described initiating factor (related to nephritic factor), properdin, factor D or C3 proactivator convertase (C3PAse), factor A which is probably native C3, and factor B or C3 proactivator (C3PA) (Medicus *et al.*, 1976). The precise mechanisms involved in the alternate pathway are still being defined, but it appears to include an activating substance and the assembly of a C3 converting enzyme from the interaction of initiating factor, factor B, factor D, native C3, and magnesium. The C3 converting enzyme deposits C3b on the surface of the activating substance where it combines with factor B to form an exceedingly labile enzyme ($\overline{\mathrm{C3b, B}}$) with C3 and C5 convertase activity. Properdin appears to act by stabilizing this enzyme (Medicus *et al.*, 1976).

In the majority of rheumatoid arthritis joint fluids, the C1 hemolytic activity is not significantly reduced (Ruddy and Austen, 1966), but inferential evidence for the activation of C1 comes from the observation of a parallel reduction in the intraarticular activity of its two natural substrates, C4 and C2. Ruddy and Austen found that the mean C4 hemolytic activity per gram of synovial fluid protein of seropositive rheumatoid arthritis patients was 700 $\pm$ 200 units, as compared to 4300 $\pm$ 500 units in fluids from seronegative patients and 7800 $\pm$ 1100 units in fluids from patients with degenerative arthritis. Measurement of synovial fluid C2 activity yielded analogous results (Ruddy and Austen, 1970). C3 levels in synovial fluids are generally decreased proportional to total hemolytic complement (Hedberg *et al.*, 1970; Ruddy and Austen, 1970; Zvaifler, 1969). The reduction of these early complement components is what would be expected if there was activation of the classical pathway by aggregated γ-globulin or immune complexes.

There is also evidence of activation of the alternate complement pathway in rheumatoid synovial fluids. The average C3PA (factor B) concentration in the effusions of seropositive rheumatoid arthritis patients is significantly less than in fluids from patients with infectious arthritis or nonrheumatoid inflammatory joint disease (Zvaifler, 1974). Ruddy *et al.* (1975) found a similar reduction of factor B concentration and properdin levels in seropositive rheumatoid arthritis joint fluids. Immunoelectrophoretic evidence of C3A (the alternate pathway convertase) was found in three of nine rheumatoid arthritis effusions and in three of six joint fluids from infectious arthritis, but was absent from nine other fluids of inflammatory nonrheumatoid arthritis and in the osteoarthritis group. Addition of inulin to rheumatoid fluids to test for residual alternate pathway activity caused no conversion of C3PA to C3A, while it did in fluids from other joint diseases (Zvaifler, 1974).

Reaction products from C3 and the terminal components of the complement sequence have been identified in rheumatoid synovial fluids. Cleavage of C3 (by either pathway) produces two biologically active substances—C3a, an anaphylatoxin, and C3b, responsible for the immune adherence phenomenon and enhanced phagocytosis of immune complexes. C3b is split by an enzyme (C3b inactivator) into two additional small molecular weight fragments (3c and 3d). These cleavage products of C3b have been detected by immunoelectrophoresis in synovial fluids from patients with a variety of joint diseases, but a significant correlation exists between their presence and the diagnosis of rheumatoid arthritis, particularly seropositive rheumatoid arthritis (Hedberg *et al.*, 1970; Zvaifler, 1969). Approximately two-thirds of rheumatoid synovial fluids contain substances that are chemotactic for granulocytes; a macromolecular complex (C567) and a low molecuar weight cleavage products of C5 (C5a) (Ward and Zvaifler, 1971). Finally, the suggestion that the complement sequence goes to completion is supported by the finding of a relative depletion of C9. Serum levels of C9 are increased almost twice normal in patients with both seropositive and seronegative rheumatoid arthritis; however, the synovial fluid C9 levels of seronegative patients are significantly higher than those from seropositive patients (Ruddy *et al.*, 1971).

2. *Immune Complexes*

Almost coincident with the finding of complement depletion in rheumatoid joint fluids, Hollander and his associates (1965) reported that these effusions contained white blood cells whose cytoplasm was filled with numerous dense particles. Immunofluorescent staining disclosed that they were composed, at least in part, of immunoglobulins and complement components. IgG and C3 were present in phagocytic cells from both seronegative and seropositive effusions, whereas IgM and anti-γ-globulin inclusions were limited to cells from the joints of seropositive rheumatoid arthritis patients. Generally, the representation of a single complement component within the inclusion is inversely proportional to its concentration in the accompanying fluid (Britton and Schur, 1971).

Synovial fluids also contain an ill-defined material called rheumatoid biologically active factor (RBAF) that releases histamine from perfused guinea pig lungs, a recognized property of immune complexes. RBAF positive fluids have a lower mean complement level (35.7 ± 3.9 units) than the RBAF negative ones (57.7 ± 7.3); this finding is consistent with the observation that RBAF in synovial fluid is associated with complement-fixing activity (Russell *et al.*, 1974).

Immune complexes are directly demonstrable in joint fluids by a number of techniques including analytical ultracentrifugation (Winchester *et al.*, 1970), sodium sulfate fractionation (Winchester, 1975), cryoprecipitation (Cracchiolo *et al.*, 1971; Marcus and Townes, 1971; Zvaifler, 1973), and precipitation with C1q (Agnello *et al.*, 1970) and polyclonal or monoclonal rheumatoid factors (Luthra *et al.*, 1975; Winchester, 1975; Winchester, *et al.*, 1970). Hannestad (1967) observed the formation of a precipitate when certain rheumatoid synovial fluids were reacted in gel with sera containing high titers of IgM rheumatoid factor and suggested that the reactant material behaved like aggregated IgG. Winchester and his associates (1970; Winchester, 1975) found similar complexes to be composed of IgG rheumatoid factor and autologous IgG. They noted a direct relationship between the amount of IgG–anti-IgG complexes in the joint fluid and the decrease in total hemolytic complement. Precipitation of these complexes with C1q did not require participation of IgM rheumatoid factor, since treatment of the joint fluid with 2-mercaptoethanol sufficient to destroy the IgM antiglobulin activity did not alter the amount of precipitate. On the other hand, addition of serum from patients with seropositive rheumatoid arthritis to joint fluids containing IgG complexes enhanced the anticomplementary effect of the joint fluid, suggesting that the serum IgM rheumatoid factor increased complement consumption.

Deoxyribonucleic acid and soluble nucleoprotein are regularly found in exudates from all inflamed joints. This prompted speculation that nuclear antigens, derived from disintegrating granulocytes, might complex with anti-nuclear antibodies to aggravate or perpetuate the articular inflammation (Zvaifler, 1965). Support for this idea comes from the observation that 8 of 31 (26%) rheumatoid synovial fluids contained antibody to soluble nucleoprotein and/or native DNA antigens, as compared to only 1 of 23 inflammatory nonrheumatoid effusions (Robitaille *et al.*, 1973). The fact that these antigens are rarely found in rheumatoid serum implies their local production.

Proteins that spontaneously precipitate upon standing at 4°C are found in rheumatoid arthritis synovial fluids, but not in other inflammatory joint effusions. These cryoprecipitates consist, in the main, of immunoglobulins—predominantly IgG and IgM—and fibrinogen or fibrin degradation products. Deoxyribonucleic acid has been detected in the majority by both the diphenylamine reaction and immunologic techniques (Cracchiolo *et al.*, 1971; Marcus and Townes, 1971). Cryoprecipitates contain anti-γ-globulin antibody, predominantly of the IgM class, and anti-nuclear activity (Cracchiolo *et al.*, 1971; Zvaifler, 1973). Marcus and Townes (1971) found anticomplementary activity of solubilized cryoprecipitates in density gradient fractions greater than 19 S. These same fractions contained variable amounts of DNA and rheumatoid factor, but the complement fixation appeared distinct from the anti-γ-globulin activity.

A number of other antibodies of potential pathogenetic significance have been recognized in inflammatory joint effusions. They are of interest because their antigens are constituents of articular tissues or by-products of the inflammatory process. These include antibodies to collagen, cartilage, fibrinogen, and fibrin degradation production and partially digested IgG (pepsin agglutinators) (Zvaifler, 1973). Evidence that they are present more often in rheumatoid arthritis effusions is lacking.

Immunoglobulins and complement components have been demonstrated in hyaline articular cartilage and menisci from 90% of patients with classical seropositive rheumatoid arthritis and 67% of seronegative patients (Cooke *et al.*, 1975). The authors have proposed that such immune complexes are sequestered in a location where their gradual release acts as a chronic inflammatory stimulus. These observations are of interest in light of the findings that neutrophils encountering immune complexes along a non-phagocytosable surface discharge their lysosomal enzymes although they cannot ingest the complexes. Only minute amounts of antibody are required (Henson, 1971). Thus, neutrophils could be continually discharging their enzymes in proximity to articular cartilage in response to minute doses of sequestered complexes that cannot be removed by conventional phagocytic mechanisms. It remains to be determined whether this mechanism is peculiar to rheumatoid arthritis or is a generalized phenomenon contributing to all chronic synovitis.

3. *Lymphokines*

Since the synovial membrane in rheumatoid arthritis is heavily populated by lymphocytes, plasma cells, and mononuclear cells, it is not surprising that substances produced by sensitized lymphocytes are present in rheumatoid synovial effusions. These include factors that lead to the accumulation and stimulation of macrophages and factors that act on lymphocytes to cause them to proliferate and differentiate (Maini *et al.*, 1975; Stastny *et al.*, 1975b). Addition of synovial fluids or supernatants from cultures of rheumatoid synovial tissues cause human peripheral blood lymphocytes to synthesize immunoglobulins (Stastny *et al.*, 1975a). It is not clear that this B cell stimulating factor is derived exclusively from T cells, because it is known that antigen–antibody complexes can induce blastic transformation. The significance of these observations, therefore, awaits further characterization of the factors with reference to known lymphokines generated *in vitro*, and the demonstration that these by-products of lymphocyte activation are limited to rheumatoid joint fluids. Of interest, however, is the observation that an experimental arthritis of rabbits can be produced by the intraarticular injection of lymphokines (Andreis *et al.*, 1974).

C. Rheumatoid Granulation Tissue

While there is a consensus that the acute inflammatory phase of rheumatoid arthritis results from immune reactions, there is less agreement about the mechanisms responsible for the chronic proliferative lesions leading to the destruction of cartilage, bone, and periarticular structures. An appreciation of the characteristics of the tissues involved is helpful in understanding this process.

Cartilage and other articular connective tissues are comprised primarily of a ground substance (proteoglycans) and collagen. The former is composed of repeating disaccharide subunits linked covalently to a protein core. Initial evidence of injury to cartilage is a loss of metachromatic staining due to a leaching out of the proteoglycans (Hamerman *et al.*, 1967). Cartilage that has lost ground substance has a diminished capacity to resist deformation and is at risk for permanent damage through mechanical disruption. Proteoglycan loss is reversible, however, and complete recovery is possible. But once collagen, which forms the structural skeleton, is lost, cartilage disintegration becomes irreversible (Harris *et al.*, 1972).

In rheumatoid arthritis the cartilage appears to be injured by a dual process, from without by enzymes in the synovial fluid and from above and below by granulation tissue. A number of potentially damaging enzymes released from phagocytic synoviocytes and polymorphonuclear leukocytes are in the fluid that continually bathes the cartilage surfaces. These include acid and neutral proteases, that can split proteoglycan from its protein matrix, and collagenases (Dingle, 1971; Harris *et al.*, 1969; Oronsky *et al.*, 1973). Collagen, when in its triple helical conformation, resists degradation by nonspecific proteases. However, specific collagenases derived from polymorphonuclear leukocytes and rheumatoid synovial cells can cleave the collagen polypeptide chains into two fragments, exposing them to further degradation by proteolytic enzymes (Krane, 1974). Both the collagenolytic and proteolytic enzymes are active at neutral pH and body temperature. The observation of proteoglycan depletion and cartilage injury at sites distant from the advancing margin of the proliferating synovial membrane (see below) is additional confirmation of the importance of enzymes derived from white blood cells (Hamerman *et al.*, 1967).

Another feature of the pathology of rheumatoid arthritis is the formation of pannus, a vascular granulation tissue composed of proliferating fibroblasts, numerous small blood vessels, and variable numbers of inflammatory cells (Gardner, 1965; Hamerman *et al.*, 1969). This aggressive material seems to be responsible for the ultimate destruction of joints in rheumatoid arthritis. Studies of early rheumatoid arthritis lesions show proliferation of synovial lining cells beginning at the joint margin where periosteum, perichondrium, and synovium attach (Hammerman *et al.*, 1969; Kulka *et al.*, 1955). As the disease progresses, pannus spreads and begins to adhere to the cartilage surface. Three types have been described (Kobayashi and Ziff, 1975). The first, a cellular pannus, has the appearance of synovium and infiltrates the cartilage with proliferating blood vessels and perivascular mononuclear cells. Collagen and proteoglycans seem to be dissolved in the region immediately surrounding the nests of cells. A second type of pannus resembles a granulation tissue composed of monocytic cells and fibroblasts. Multiple filopodia extend from these cells into the cartilage matrix and degradation proceeds around them. Another variety of pannus is composed of a dense avascular, acellular, fibrous tissue tightly adherent to cartilage.

It seems likely that the first type of pannus, which has the appearance of an "activated" synovial membrane, produces cartilage destruction by enzymatic degradation (Kobayashi and Ziff, 1975; Krane, 1974). The second "cellular" form of pannus may operate the same way, but its similarity to granulation tissue seen at other sites of injury suggests the alternate possibility that this cellular and fibrous infiltrate is the result of cartilage injury, rather than the cause. The third type of pannus probably acts as a mantle interfering with cartilage nutrition (Hamerman *et al.*, 1969). Although three types of pannus can be found simultaneously in the same joint, it is not clear that they represent sequential phenomenon or that each develops independently.

IV. EXTRAARTICULAR MANIFESTATIONS OF RHEUMATOID ARTHRITIS

Although characteristically a joint disease, rheumatoid arthritis can affect a number of other tissues (Hollingsworth, 1968). These extraarticular manifestations probably occur with considerable frequency, but are usually occult and of limited clinical significance. Occasionally, however, the extraarticular events dominate the clinical picture. Terms like "rheumatoid disease" and "malignant rheumatoid arthritis" have been utilized to describe this form of the disease. Extraarticular features occur, by and large, in patients whose serum contains rheumatoid factor and, in general, correlate with the severity, but not with the duration of the articular disease (Gordon *et al.*, 1973; Mongan *et al.*, 1969).

A. Vasculitis

A spectrum of vascular lesions accompanies rheumatoid arthritis. The majority are "silent" and only discovered at postmortem examination. They take many forms: capillaritis and venulitis, felt to be important in the development of rheumatoid nodules and synovitis; a bland intimal proliferation commonly affecting digital and mesenteric vessels; subacute lesions of arterioles and venules in scattered locations; and, finally, an acute, widespread, necrotizing arteritis of small- and medium-sized arteries that may, at times, be indistinguishable from polyarteritis nodosum. This most severe form of rheumatoid vasculitis, designated "rheumatoid arteritis," characteristically produces polyneuropathy, skin necrosis and ulceration, digital gangrene, and visceral infarction (Schmid *et al.*, 1961). It may present in an explosive fashion and terminate in death after a few weeks or months. Fortunately, the full blown picture is rare, but any of the above manifestations can appear insidiously, over a period of months to years, and pose little threat to life. When present, the neuropathy takes the form of an acute sensorimotor mononeuritis (mononeuritis multiplex) with foot or wrist drop and a patchy sensory loss in one or more extremities (Hart *et al.*, 1957). Ischemic skin lesions appear in crops as small brown spots, not unlike splinter hemorrhages, in the nail beds, nail folds, and digital pulp. Large ischemic ulcerations can develop in the lower extremities, particularly over the malleoli. Fatal intestinal and myocardial infarctions have been reported. Patients with the acute form of rheumatoid arteritis are commonly febrile, sometimes to 104°F or more, and polymorphonuclear leukocytosis is common. Many will have concomitant episcleritis, scleromalacia, pleuritis, myocarditis, and/or pericarditis. The prognosis for life in the fulminant form of vasculitis is exceedingly poor, and the terminal picture is usually complicated by the superimposition of malnutrition, infection, congestive heart failure, and/or gastrointestinal bleeding.

The cause of the various vascular lesions and their relationship to one another has not been defined, but a number of observations suggest that they result from injury induced by immune complexes, especially those containing antibodies to IgG. These include (1) the generally held view that patients with the largest amount of serum IgM rheumatoid factor have more systemic manifestations of the disease (Epstein and Engleman, 1959; Mongan *et al.*, 1969); (2) the correlation of depressed serum hemolytic complement activity, decreased concentration of several complement components (C4, C2), and hypercatabolism of C3 with the clinical signs of vasculitis (Franco and Schur, 1971; Mongan *et al.*, 1969; Weinstein *et al.*, 1972); and (3) immunofluorescent deposits of IgG, IgM, and complement (C3) in the vasonervorum of patients with rheumatoid neuropathy, and immunoglobulins and rheumatoid factor in vessel walls of vasculitis patients (Conn *et al.*, 1972).

Immune complexlike materials were identified in the circulation of patients with rheumatoid arthritis as early as 1957. Kunkel and his associates demonstrated, by analytical ultracentrifugation, a high molecular weight material (22 S) in the serum of rheumatoid arthritis patients. Acid or 6 *M* urea dissociation revealed 7 S and 19 S components, with the latter containing anti-Ig activity (Franklin *et al.*, 1957). Subsequently, the same workers demonstrated large amounts of unusual γ-globulin complexes with sedimentation rates ranging from 9 to 17 S in patients with advanced rheumatoid arthritis (Kunkel *et al.*, 1959). These complexes, which are readily dissociated to 7 S units, have been designated as "intermediate complexes."

A precise definition of the role of these presumed complexes in the pathogenesis of rheumatoid arthritis was not possible because of the lack of sensitive, reproducible, quantitative methods. Some of these problems have recently been obviated by the development of techniques for accurately measuring complexes, such as binding to C1q or precipitation with monoclonal rheumatoid factors (obtained from the sera of certain patients with lymphoproliferative diseases), cryoprecipitation, histamine release assays, or the use of Raji cells, a cultured human lymphoblastoid cell line with receptors for the Fc portion of human IgG, but lacking membrane bound immunoglobulin.

Winchester *et al.* (1970) first showed that monoclonal IgM rheumatoid factors can be used to demonstrate small complexes or aggregates of IgG in the serum of approximately 50% of patients with rheumatoid arthritis. This method detects aggregates that escape precipitation by polyclonal rheumatoid factors or C1q. A radioimmunoassay based on the ability of test samples to inhibit the interaction of iodinated aggregated IgG with monoclonal rheumatoid factor detected immune complexlike material in the serum of 12 of 51 (27%) rheumatoid arthritis patients examined, and correlates with more severe disease, greater functional impairment, and more advanced joint destruction. Serum C4 levels were inversely correlated with the amount of inhibiting material, but no relationship existed with rheumatoid factor titers. Three-fourths of the patients had extraarticular manifestations including Sjögren's syndrome, leg ulcers, Felty's syndrome, neuropathy, and pulmonary fibrosis (Luthra *et al.*, 1975).

A sensitive biologic assay for soluble antigen–antibody complexes was developed, based on the capacity of such complexes to liberate histamine from the perfused guinea pig lung. The histamine releasing activity found in rheumatoid arthritis serum is removed by antisera to human IgG, but not to IgA or IgM. Activity persists following reduction and alkylation, and unlike conventional complexes, are not completely dissociable at low pH. Broder *et al.* named this soluble, complexlike material rheumatoid biologically active factor (RBAF) and found it in the serum of 38 of 127 (30%) carefully studied patients with rheumatoid arthritis (Gordon *et al.*, 1969). RBAF is correlated with disease activity and impaired function, and there is an overall statistical correlation of its presence with a composite of extraarticular manifestations of rheumatoid arthritis, although no one feature (e.g., arteritis, neuropathy, etc.) is present with increased frequency in these patients. Rheumatoid factor titers and RBAF are not correlated (Gordon *et al.*, 1969, 1973).

Quantitative cryoprecipitation of sera from an unselected group of 38 patients with rheumatoid arthritis revealed that 12 (31%) had significant amounts of cryoglobulins. Two-thirds of the cryoprecipitable protein was composed of IgG and IgM, with the relative amount of IgM to IgG greater than found in serum. Complement components were detected in six precipitates and anti-nuclear antibody in seven (Weisman and Zvaifler, 1975b). Systemic vasculitis, present in 3 of the original 38 patients, was associated with the largest amount of cryoglobulin. Subsequently, five more patients with vasculitis were studied, all of whom had detectable cryoglobulins (Weisman and Zvaifler, 1975a). The cryoglobulin IgG and IgM were polyclonal. Density gradient analysis demonstrated the majority of the cryoglobulin anti-globulin activity to reside in the 19 S IgM fraction. A monoclonal rheumatoid factor did not detect 7 S–anti-IgG complexes in the cryoprecipitates, but acid eluates from some cryoglobulins absorbed with insoluble IgG revealed an anti-globulin of the IgG class. Serial studies performed on vasculitis patients treated with cyclophosphamide disclosed a close relationship between clinical evidence of vasculitis and the presence of cryoglobulins. The findings were interpreted as evidence that the widespread vascular complications of rheumatoid arthritis are mediated, at least in part, by circulating immune complexes.

Other forms of rheumatoid factor have been described in the rheumatoid vasculitis. Theofilopoulous and his associates (1974) detected IgG rheumatoid factor in 10 of 15 (67%) patients with rheumatoid vasculitis, but in only 3 of 33 without vasculitis. Eighty percent of the vasculitis patients also had 7 S IgM in their serum, whereas only 18% of the nonvasculitis patients had this unusual immunoglobulin. Stage and Mannick (1971) also found an increased frequency of 7 S IgM in vasculitis patients.

In summary, it appears that a quarter to one-third of patients with rheumatoid arthritis have circulating soluble complexes detectable by a variety of techniques. Anti-γ-globulins of the IgG and IgM classes and IgG are integral parts of these soluble complexes. The presence of these materials seems to correlate with the severity of rheumatoid arthritis and the presence of extraarticular manifestations, vasculitis in particular. Whether they are responsible for these changes, or are merely markers for severe rheumatoid disease remains a moot question.

B. Pleuropulmonary Complications

Respiratory symptoms encountered in rheumatoid patients can usually be ascribed to more common disorders. Some findings, however, seem to be intimately related to the rheumatoid process: (1) pleurisy with or without effusion; (2) nonpneumoconiotic intrapulmonary rheumatoid nodules; (3) rheumatoid pneumoconiosis (Caplan's syndrome); (4) diffuse interstitial fibrosis and pneumonitis. Considerable overlap exists among these syndromes (Hollingsworth, 1968; Martel *et al.*, 1968; Walker and Wright, 1968).

Rheumatoid pleural disease is most commonly asymptomatic, with the diagnosis being made incidentally on chest X-ray or at postmortem examination. When symptomatic pleurisy does occur, it may appear prior to, simultaneous with, or long after the onset of arthritis. There is a greater risk of involvement in middle-aged and elderly men and in seropositive patients with subcutaneous nodules. Effusions tend to be chronic and occasionally are of sufficient size to cause respiratory embarrassment. The pleural fluid is typically exudative. White blood cell counts vary greatly, but are usually less than $5000/mm^3$, with a predominance of either mononuclear or polymorphonuclear leukocytes. LDH enzyme is usually high, and glucose values tend to be low, frequently less than 25 mg/100 ml. Normal glucose levels do not exclude the diagnosis. Rheumatoid factor detection is of limited value in differential diagnosis because of high serum titers and the fact that it may also be found in some nonrheumatoid effusions (Levine *et al.*, 1968).

Total hemolytic complement, and individual complement components C3 and C4 are significantly lower in rheumatoid pleural effusions than in simultaneous serum samples or nonrheumatoid inflammatory fluids (Hunder *et al.*, 1972). No specific cause has been found for the complement reduction. The mechanism may be similar to that responsible for the low pleural fluid sugar, namely, an active inhibition of transport into the pleural space (Dodson and Hollingsworth, 1966), but it is more likely that complement components enter the pleural space and are subsequently inactivated by immunologic reactions. Pleural fluids have been shown to be strongly anticomplementary (Hunder *et al.*, 1972). Glovsky noted complement-fixing activity in pleural fluids from five of six patients with seropositive rheumatoid arthritis and in none of three with seronegative rheumatoid arthritis. In one of these fluids, the complement-fixing activity resided in sucrose density gradient fractions containing materials greater than 19 S (Glovsky *et al.*, 1977). Cytoplasmic inclusions that stain for immunoglobulins have been reported in polymorphonuclear leukocytes from rheumatoid (Carmichael and Golding, 1967) and nonrheumatoid pleural effusions (Levine *et al.*, 1968). Thus, the findings in the pleural space are similar to those in the articular cavity.

Nodular densities are occasionally seen in chest roentgenograms of patients with rheumatoid arthritis, especially those with subcutaneous nodules. Their appearance as solitary or multiple densities 0.5–3 cm in diameter at the periphery of the lung is indistinguishable radiographically from other types of coin lesions. While usually asymptomatic, they may cavitate, become infected, or rupture into the pleural space with the production of pneumothorax or pyopneumothorax. On histological examination, they are identical to rheumatoid nodules from any other location.

The presence of numerous rheumatoid nodules in the lungs of patients with a history of rheumatoid arthritis and a pneumoconiotic exposure is referred to as rheumatoid pneumoconiosis or Caplan's syndrome. First described in Welsh soft coal miners, the same phenomenon has since been observed in asbestos and ceramic workers, gold and chalk miners, and others with arthritis and an appropriate industrial exposure. Chest roentgenograms usually reveal multiple well-defined nodular opacities of 0.5–5 cm diameter widely distributed throughout the lungs, but particularly abundant in the periphery. Alternatively, large numbers of smaller nodules present a "snowstorm" appearance or nodules may coalesce into large conglomerate masses. Cavitation has been observed. Typical lesions sometimes antedate the development of rheumatoid arthritis, occassionally by years; such patients usually have positive tests for rheumatoid factor, even in the absence of arthritis. Williams (1974, p. 42) suggests that the syndrome is a manifestation of altered tissue reactivity to inhaled antigen in rheumatoid subjects, perhaps because of an adjuvant action of the pneumoconiotic particles.

Noteworthy, in this regard, was the acute appearance of high titers of serum rheumatoid factor in a group of patients who developed chronic hypersensitivity pneumonitis from mold contamination of an air conditioner. Subsequent avoidance of exposure resulted in a loss of precipitating antibodies to the offending antigen (thermophilic actinomycetes) and a reversal of all serological abnormalities (Banaszak *et al.*, 1970).

Patients with rheumatoid arthritis develop a diffuse interstitial fibrosis (DIF) that is clinically and radiographically indistinguishable from the idiopathic variety. This pulmonary complication, like the others, occurs predominantly in males and contrasts with the higher incidence of both rheumatoid arthritis and idiopathic DIF in females. Radiographic findings in the early stages are diffuse patchy infiltrates or fine reticulonodular densities most pronounced at the lung bases. Later, a diffuse mottling and interstitial fibrosis develops that progresses to an end-stage "honeycomb appearance" with bronchiolar ectasia. Such a picture may evolve rapidly or, more commonly, over 5–10 years. Symptoms are predominantly progressive dyspnea and cough productive of scanty sputum. Diffuse or basilar dry crackling rales are generally heard, and clubbing is common. Pulmonary function tests show a diminished compliance and a restrictive ventilatory pattern. Histologically, there is thickening of alveolar walls, lymphoreticular hyperplasia, and interstitial infiltration with chronic inflammatory cells (Walker and Wright, 1968).

Much indirect evidence suggests immune mechanisms are operative in interstitial pulmonary fibrosis. In many cases, lung changes occur in the absence of other diseases, but it is striking how often autoimmune disorders, such as rheumatoid arthritis, Sjögen's syndrome, systemic lupus erythematosus, scleroderma, and dermatomyositis are implicated. Equally provocative is the frequent observation of anti-nuclear antibodies or high titers of conventional (19 S) rheumatoid factor or the presence of large amounts of intermediate (11–17 S) complexes in the serum of patients without the accompanying connective tissue diseases (Turner-Warwick and Doniach, 1965). Tomasi suggested that pulmonary involvement might result from the trapping of intermediate (IgG–IgG complexes) in the pulmonary vasculature (Tomasi *et al.*, 1962). The phlogogenic properties of these complexes have been described in detail in other sections. Immunofluorescent study of rheumatoid pulmonary tissues discloses only faint IgG staining in a patchy alveolar distribution, in amounts which the authors felt were inadequate to support a major role for intermediate complexes (De Horatius *et al.*, 1972). These same workers found significant amounts of conventional IgM rheumatoid factor in pulmonary arterioles, alveolar walls, and adjacent cavitary nodules, and proposed that rheumatoid factors may aggravate immune inflammatory lesions in the lung. In support of this idea, they tested the effect of 19 S IgM rheumatoid factors on an experimental model of diffuse proliferative lung disease. Multiple, small pulmonary granulomas develop when rabbits are given intravenous complete Freund's adjuvant. These lesions were accelerated or aggravated by the simultaneous administration of isolated human IgM rheumatoid factor, but not by IgM without rheumatoid factor activity (De Horatius and Williams, 1972).

C. Cardiac Manifestations

Although a variety of cardiac lesions are demonstrable at postmortem examination, clinically detectable heart disease attributable solely to the rheumatoid process is unusual. Pericarditis is the most frequent histopathological abnormality, occurring in about 40% of autopsied patients. Less commonly seen are granulomatous lesions, histologically similar to rheumatoid nodules, involving the epicardium, myocardium, and valves; focal interstitial myocarditis; and arteritis of coronary vessels. Occassionally, valvular insufficiency or conduction abnormalities may be recognized during life, and, rarely, myocardial infarction occurs as a manifestation of coronary arteritis (Weintraub and Zvaifler, 1963).

The commonest symptomatic lesion is acute pericarditis, which appears most often in males with seropositive disease (Franco *et al.*, 1972; Kirk and Cosh, 1969). It is unrelated to the duration of arthritis and presents in the usual fashion with left-sided pleuritic chest pain, with or without an audible friction rub. An associated pleural effusion is found in a high percentage of cases. Characteristics of the pericardial fluid are remarkably similar to pleural effusions and include a low glucose concentration, increased LDH, and γ-globulin levels and lower than expected complement activity.

D. Felty's Syndrome

In 1924, A. R. Felty described a symptom complex of chronic rheumatoid arthritis associated with splenomegaly and leukopenia. Subsequently, additional features have been recognized, including skin hyperpigmentation, leg ulcers, generalized lymphadenopathy, anemia, and thrombocytopenia. The arthritis tends to be far advanced and deforming, appearing as either active or "burnt out" joint disease. Commonly, patients have high titers of rheumatoid factor and anti-nuclear antibodies, subcutaneous nodules, and manifestations of systemic rheumatoid disease or the sicca complex (Sjögren's syndrome) (Louie and Pearson, 1971; Ruderman *et al.*, 1968). The leukopenia is, in fact, a selective neutropenia and may be very profound. Total polymorphonuclear counts of less than 1000 mm^3 are frequently recorded. Marrow examination usually reveals moderate hypercellularity with a paucity of mature neutrophils, so-called maturation arrest. The importance of recognizing this variant lies in its association with recurrent infections of the skin, mucous membranes, and respiratory tract and in its poor prognosis. Common gram-positive pathogens are usually the cause of the infections, but they frequently respond poorly to antibiotics. It is interesting to note that the incidence of infection can decline following splenectomy, even when the neutropenia remains unaltered (Barnes *et al.*, 1971).

There is no single satisfactory explanation for the granulocytopenia that characterizes Felty's syndrome. Early speculations implicated hypersplenism and/or splenic sequestration of neutrophils. An inability to demonstrate trapping of radiolabeled cells in the spleen and the frequent failure of splenectomy to correct the leukopenia tends to diminish the importance of this organ in Felty's syndrome (Vincent *et al.*, 1974). Evidence of impaired production of granulocytes is lacking, since the bone marrow is typically hyperplastic. This makes the observation that serum from most Felty's patients inhibits the growth of murine marrow cells in culture less interesting (Duckham *et al.*, 1975). Indeed, although neutropenia is considered the hallmark of Felty's syndrome, recent leukokinetic studies show that two-thirds of these patients have a normal total blood neutrophil pool. Thus, their neutropenia appears to be due to an excessive margination of neutrophils, presumably into extravascular locations (Vincent *et al.*, 1974).

A number of observations suggest that circulating factors, particularly antibodies, play a pathogenetic role in Felty's patients. For instance, etiocholanolone will normally mobilize granulocytes from the bone marrow. Patients with Felty's syndrome do not respond to etiocholanolone and, in one instance, influsion of plasma from a Felty's patient blocked the granulocyte mobilizing effect of this agent (Kimball *et al.*, 1973).

In another study, circulating IgG antibody direct against white blood cells was detected in 13 out of 15 patients with Felty's syndrome (Rosenthal *et al.*, 1974). Some anti-nuclear antibodies only react with polymorphonuclear cell nuclei. Such granulocyte specific anti-nuclear factors are found in virtually all cases of Felty's syndrome, 75% of patients with rheumatoid arthritis, and 30% of patients with lupus erythematosus. The granulocyte-specific antibodies fix human complement, unlike the conventional organ nonspecific anti-nuclear factors in Felty's syndrome (Faber and Elling, 1966; Wiik and Munthe, 1974).

Immune complexes are demonstrable in the circulating white blood cells and serum of the majority of patients with Felty's syndrome. Immunofluorescent inclusions of IgG, IgM, and C3 have been observed in the cytoplasm of peripheral blood neutrophils from patients with Felty's syndrome and similar inclusions are formed when normal neutrophils are incubated with Felty's serum (Hurd *et al.*, 1974). In a recent study, seven of nine Felty's patients had significant amounts of cryoglobulins, greater than in patients with uncomplicated rheumatoid arthritis but similar to rheumatoid patients with vasculitis. The cryoglobulins contained IgG, IgM, complement components, and anti-nuclear and anti-γ-globulin antibodies. Granulocyte specific anti-nuclear antibody was selectively concentrated in the cryoglobulins of some Felty's patients (Weisman and Zvaifler, 1975c). These findings are consistent with the suggestion that complexes containing IgG granulocyte specific anti-nuclear factors, anti-γ-globulins and complement can cause neutropenia by attaching to the IgG or complement receptors or the surface of circulating neutrophils (Wiik and Faber, 1973). Cells with altered cell membrane would be rapidly removed by the reticuloendothelial system. This explanation is consistent with the observation of excessive margination of neutrophils in Felty's patients.

REFERENCES

Abrahamsen, T. G., Natvig, J. B., Fröland, S. S., and Pahle, J. (1975). *Scand. J. Rheum. Suppl.* **8,** 14 (abstr.).

Abruzzo, J. L., and Christian, C. L. (1961). *J. Exp. Med.* **114,** 791–806.

Agnello, V., Winchester, R. J., and Kunkel, H. G. (1970). *Immunology* **19,** 909–919.

Andreis, M., Stastny, P., and Ziff, M. (1974). *Arthritis Rheum.* **17,** 537–551.

Banaszak, E. G., Thiede, W. H., and Fink, J. N. (1970). *N. Engl. J. Med.* **283,** 271–276.

Barnes, C. G., Turnbull, A. L., and Vernon-Roberts, B. (1971). *Ann. Rheum. Dis.* **30,** 359–374.

Bokisch, V. A., Chiao, J. W., and Bernstein, D. (1973). *J. Exp. Med.* **137,** 1354–1368.

Britton, M. C., and Schur, P. H. (1971). *Arthritis Rheum.* **14,** 87–95.

Carmichael, D. S., and Golding, D. N. (1967). *Br. Med. J.* **2,** 814–815.

Conn, D. L., McDuffie, F. C., and Dyck, P. J. (1972). *Arthritis Rheum.* **15,** 135–143.

Cooke, T. D., Hurd, E. R., Jasin, H., Bienenstock, J., and Ziff, M. (1975). *Arthritis Rheum.* **18,** 541–551.

Cracchiolo, A., Goldberg, L. S., Barnett, E. V., and Bluestone, R. (1971). *Immunology* **20,** 1067–1077.

De Horatius, R. J., and Williams, R. C. (1972). *Arthritis Rheum.* **15,** 293–301.

De Horatius, R. J., Abruzzo, J. L., and Williams, R. C., Jr. (1972). *Arch. Intern. Med.* **129,** 441–446.

Dingle, J. T. (1971). *In* "Tissue Proteinases" (A. J. Barrett and J. T. Dingle, eds.), pp. 313–326. North-Holland Publ., Amsterdam.

Dodson, W. H., and Hollingsworth, J. W. (1966). *N. Engl. J. Med.* **275,** 1337–1342.

Duckham, D. J., Rhyne, R. L., Smith, F. E., and Williams, R. C., Jr. (1975). *Arthritis Rheum.* **18,** 323–334.

Epstein, W. V., and Engleman, E. P. (1959). *Arthritis Rheum.* **2,** 250–258.

Faber, V., and Elling, P. (1966). *Acta Med. Scand.* **179,** 257–267.

Fish, A. J., Michael, A. F., Gewurz, H., and Good, R. A. (1966). *Arthritis Rheum.* **9,** 267–280.

Franco, A. E., Schur, P. H. (1971). *Arthritis Rheum.* **14,** 231–238.

Franco, A. E., Levine, H. D., and Hall, A. P. (1972). *Ann. Intern. Med.* **77,** 837–844.

Franklin, E. C., Holman, H. R., Müller-Eberhard, H. J., and Kunkel, H. G. (1957). *J. Exp. Med.* **105,** 425–438.

Gardner, D. L. (1965). "The Pathology of the Connective Tissue Disease." Williams & Wilkins, Baltimore, Maryland.
Glovsky, M. M., Louie, J. S., Pitts, W. H., and Alenty, A. (1977). In press.
Gordon, D. A., Bell, D. A., Baumal, R., and Broder, I. (1969). *Clin. Exp. Immunol.* **5,** 57–66.
Gordon, D. A., Stein, J. L., and Broder, I. (1973). *Am. J. Med.* **54,** 445–452.
Hamerman, D., Janis, R., and Smith, C. (1967). *J. Exp. Med.* **126,** 1005–1012.
Hamerman, D., Barland, P., and Janis, R. (1969). *Biol. Basis Med.* **3,** 269–309.
Hannestad, K. (1967). *Clin. Exp. Immunol.* **2,** 511–529.
Harris, E. D., Jr., DiBona, D. R., and Krane, S. M. (1969). *J. Clin. Invest.* **48,** 2104–2113.
Harris, E. D., Jr., Parker, H. G., Radin, E. L., and Krane, S. M. (1972). *Arthritis Rheum.* **15,** 497–503.
Hart, F. D., Golding, J. R., and MacKenzie, D. H. (1957). *Ann. Rheum. Dis.* **16,** 471–480.
Hedberg, H. (1964). *Acta Rheum. Scand.* **10,** 109–127.
Hedberg, H., Lundh, B., and Laurell, A. B. (1970). *Clin. Exp. Immunol.* **6,** 707–712.
Henson, P. (1971). *J. Immunol.* **107,** 1547–1557.
Hollander, J. L., McCarty, D. J., Astorga, G., and Castro-Murillo, E. (1965). *Ann. Intern. Med.* **62,** 271–280.
Hollingsworth, J. W. (1968). "Local and Systemic Complications of Rheumatoid Arthritis." Saunders, Philadelphia, Pennsylvania.
Hunder, G. G., McDuffie, F. C., and Hepper, N. G. (1972). *Ann. Intern. Med.* **76,** 357–363.
Hurd, E. R., LoSpalluto, J., and Ziff, M. (1974). *Pan-Am. Congr. Rheum. Dis., 6th, 1974.*
Kimball, H. R., Wolff, S. M., Talal, N. Plotz, P. H., and Decker, J. L. (1973). *Arthritis Rheum.* **16,** 345–352.
Kirk, J., and Cosh, J. (1969). *Q. J. Med.* **38,** 397–423.
Kobayashi, I., and Ziff, M. (1973). *Arthritis Rheum.* **16,** 471–486.
Kobayashi, I., and Ziff, M. (1975). *Arthritis Rheum.* **18,** 475–483.
Krane, S. M. (1974). *Arthritis Rheum.* **17,** 306–312.
Kulka, J. P., Bocking, D., Ropes, M. W., and Bauer, W. (1955). *Arch. Pathol.* **59,** 129–150.
Kunkel, H. G., and Tan, E. M. (1964). *Adv. Immunol.* **4,** 351–395.
Kunkel, H. G., Franklin, E. C., and Müller-Eberhard, H. J. (1959). *J. Clin. Invest.* **38,** 424–434.
Levine, H. Szanto, M., Grieble, H. G., Bach, G. L., and Anderson, T. O. (1968). *Ann. Intern. Med.* **69,** 487–492.
Louie, J. S., and Pearson, C. M. (1971). *Semin. Hematol.* **8,** 216–220.
Luthra, H. S., McDuffie, F. C., Hunder, G. G., and Samayoa, E. A. (1975). *J. Clin. Invest.* **56,** 458–466.
Maini, R. N., Hersfall, A., Raffe, L., Hanson, J., and Dumonde, D. C. (1975). *Scand. J. Rheumatol., Suppl.* **8,** 14. (abstr.).
Marcus, R., and Townes, A. S. (1971). *J. Clin. Invest.* **50,** 282–293.

Martel, W., Abell, M. R., Mikkelsen, W. M., and Whitehouse, W. M. (1968). *Radiology* **90,** 641–653.

Medicus, R. G., Schreiber, R. D., Goetze, O., and Müller-Eberhard, H. J. (1976). *Proc. Natl. Acad. Sci. U.S.A.* **73,** 612–616.

Mongan, E. S., Cass, R. M., Jacox, R. F., and Vaughan, J. H. (1969). *Am. J. Med.* **47,** 23–35.

Müller-Eberhard, H. J. (1972). *Harvey Lect.* **66,** 75–104.

Munthe, E., and Natvig, J. B. (1972a). *Clin. Exp. Immunol.* **12,** 55–70.

Munthe, E., and Natvig, J. B. (1972b). *Scand. J. Immunol.* **1,** 217–229.

Natvig, J. B., and Munthe, E. (1975). *Ann. N.Y. Acad. Sci.* **256,** 88–95.

Oronsky, A. L., Ignarro, L., and Perper, R. J. (1973). *J. Exp. Med.* **138,** 461–472.

Pearson, C. M., Paulus, H. E., and Machleder, H. I. (1975). *Ann. N.Y. Acad. Sci.* **256,** 150–168.

Pekin, T. J., and Zvaifler, N. J. (1964). *J. Clin. Invest.* **43,** 1372–1382.

Robitaille, P., Zvaifler, N. J., and Tan, E. M. (1973). *Clin. Immunol. Immunopathol.* **1,** 385–397.

Rosenthal, F. D., Beeley, J. M., Gelsthorpe, K., and Doughty, R. W. (1974). *Q. J. Med.* **43,** 187–203.

Ruddy, S., and Austen, K. F. (1970). *Arthritis Rheum.* **13,** 713–723.

Ruddy, S., Everson, L. K., Schur, P. H., and Austen, K. F. (1971). *J. Exp. Med.* **134,** 259s–275s.

Ruddy, S., Fearon, D., Austen, K. F. (1975). *Arthritis Rheum.* **18,** 289–295.

Ruderman, M., Miller, L. M., and Pinals, R. S. (1968). *Arthritis Rheum.* **11,** 377–384.

Russell, M. L., Gordon, D. A., and Broder, I. (1974). *J. Rheumatol.* **1,** 153–158.

Sandson, J., and Hamerman, D. (1964). *J. Clin. Invest.* **43,** 1372–1382.

Schmid, F. R., Cooper, N. S., Ziff, M., and McEwen, C. (1961). *Am. J. Med.* **30,** 56–83.

Schumacher, H. R., and Kitridou, R. C. (1974). *Arthritis Rheum.* **15,** 465–485.

Sheldon, P. J., and Holborow, E. J. (1975). *Scand. J. Rheum., Suppl.* **8,** 14 (abstr.)

Short, C. L., Bauer, W., and Reynolds, W. S. (1957). "Rheumatoid Arthritis." Harvard Univ. Press, Cambridge, Massachusetts.

Sliwinski, A. J., and Zvaifler, N. J. (1970). *J. Lab. Clin. Med.* **76,** 304–310.

Smiley, J. D., Sachs, C., and Ziff, M. (1968). *J. Clin. Invest.* **47,** 624–632.

Stage, D. E., and Mannik, M. (1971). *Arthritis Rheum.* **14,** 440–450.

Stage, D. E., and Mannik, M. (1973). *Bull Rheum. Dis.* **23,** 720–725.

Stastny, P., Rosenthal, M., Andreis, M., Cooke, D., and Ziff, M. (1975a). *Ann. N.Y. Acad. Sci.* **256,** 117–131.

Stastny, P., Rosenthal, M., Andreis, M., and Ziff, M. (1975b). *Arthritis Rheum.* **18,** 237–243.

Theofilopoulos, A. N., Burtonboy, G., LoSpalluto, J. J., and Ziff, M. (1974). *Arthritis Rheum.* **17,** 272–284.

Tomasi, T. B., Fudenberg, H. H., and Finby, N. (1962). *Am. J. Med.* **33,** 243–248.

Torrigiani, G., and Roitt, I. M. (1967). *Ann. Rheum. Dis.* **26,** 334–340.

Turner-Warwick, M., and Doniach, D. (1965). *Br. Med. J.* **1,** 886–891.

Van Boxel, J. A., and Paget, S. A. (1975). *N. Engl. J. Med.* **293,** 517–520.
Vincent, P. C., Levi, J. A., and MacQueen, A. (1974). *Br. J. Haematol.* **27,** 463–475.
Walker, W. C., and Wright, V. (1968). *Medicine* (*Baltimore*) **47,** 501–520.
Wangel, A. G. and Klockars, M. (1977). *Ann. Rheum. Dis.* **36,** 176–180.
Ward, P. A., and Zvaifler, N. J. (1971). *J. Clin. Invest.* **50,** 606–616.
Weinstein, A., Peters, K., Brown, D., and Bluestone, R. (1972). *Arthritis Rheum.* **15,** 49–56.
Weintraub, A. M., and Zvaifler, N. J. (1963). *Am. J. Med.* **35,** 145–162.
Weisman, M., and Zvaifler, N. J. (1975a). *J. Clin. Invest.* **56,** 725–739.
Weisman, M., and Zvaifler, N. J. (1975b). *J. Rheumatol.* **6,** 1–8.
Weisman, M., and Zvaifler, N. J. (1975c). *Arthritis Rheum.* **19,** 103–110.
Weissman, G. (1972). *N. Engl. J. Med.* **286,** 141–147.
Wiik, A., and Faber, V. (1973). *N. Engl. J. Med.* **289,** 981–982.
Wiik, A., and Munthe, E. (1974). *Immunology* **26,** 1127–1134.
Williams, R. C. (1974). "Rheumatoid Arthritis as a Systemic Disease." Saunders, Philadelphia, Pennsylvania. p. 154–176.
Williams, R. C., and Kunkel, H. G. (1962). *J. Clin. Invest.* **41,** 666–675.
Winchester, R. J. (1975). *Ann. N.Y. Acad. Sci.* **256,** 73–81.
Winchester, R. J., Agnello, V., and Kunkel, H. G. (1970). *Clin. Exp. Immunol.* **6,** 689–706.
Zvaifler, N. J. (1965). *Arthritis Rheum.* **8,** 289–293.
Zvaifler, N. J. (1969). *J. Clin. Invest.* **48,** 1532–1542.
Zvaifler, N. J. (1973). *Adv. Immunol.* **16,** 265–336.
Zvaifler, N. J. (1974). *Arthritis Rheum.* **17,** 297–305.
Zvaifler, N. J., and Greenberg, P. D. (1977). *In* "Mechanisms of Immunopathology" (S. Cohen, R. D. McCluskey, and P. Ward, eds.), Wiley, New York (in press).

Chapter 20

Cell-Surface Receptors and Autoimmune Responses

I. R. MACKAY AND P. R. CARNEGIE

I. INTRODUCTION

Currently there is great interest in the isolation and characterization of receptors for antigens, hormones, and neurotransmitters. Immunologists have, for several years, been interested in the nature of the receptor for antigen on both B and T lymphocytes; while there is consensus that the B lymphocyte receptor is an immunoglobulin molecule of class M or D, there is no consensus on the nature of the T cell receptor. At the same time, workers in a seemingly quite unrelated field have been making considerable progress in the study of the receptors for various peptide hormones. These hormones include insulin, glucagon, adrenocorticotropin, thyrotropin, angiotensin, calcitonin, growth hormone, prolactin, follicle-stimulating hormone, luteinizing hormone, chorionic gonadotropin, oxytocin, and vasopressin and, equally well studied, are receptors for mediators of cell activity, such as acetylcholine, catecholamines, prostoglandins, and opiates (Cuatrecasas, 1974).

In most cases, there has been little attempt to exploit isolated receptor preparations in studies on disease of the endocrine system and, in particular, to diseases possibly mediated by antibodies to receptors. However, since receptors for peptide hormones are on the cell surface and accessible to hormones in the circulation, then they must also be exposed to other serum proteins, such as immunoglobulins. Lennon and Carnegie (1971) suggested that disease could occur as a result of antibody interfering with the interaction of a hormone with its receptor. This antibody could arise in several ways, e.g., as a result of an immune response to an infecting microorganism that carries a surface structure similar in shape to a hormone receptor. Alternatively, a virus could lodge in the plasma membrane at a receptor site, and an immune response to the virus could trigger a concomitant response to the modified receptor. Disease would result when lymphoid cells from the initial clone mutated to yield cells capable of producing antibody against the normal receptor. There is no evidence at present for such a progression, but, in the model disease, experimental autoimmune myasthenia gravis as induced in the rat (see below), there is an initial production of antibody to the foreign acetylcholine receptor prepared from the electric eel when it is injected, but a negligible response to the natural acetylcholine receptor of the rat. Gradually, in susceptible animals, a clone of cells builds up, which produces antibody to the rat receptor, causing the production of a chronic autoimmune disease (Lindstrom *et al.*, 1976a). In most cases of such a viral intrusion into the membrane, no disease would result, as homeostatic processes of immunologic tolerance would prevent an immune response to self-antigens; however, in individuals with a genetic predisposition to failure of immunologic tolerance, an ongoing and harmful immune response to a hormone receptor could occur.

Little is known of the detailed molecular organization of receptors in the plasma membrane. Probably the best characterized is the acetylcholine receptor isolated from the electric eel and believed to be similar to the receptor at the neuromuscular junction. In Fig. 1, a diagram illustrates the possible structure and function of the acetylcholine receptor. Acetylcholine interacts with the acetylcholine-binding site in the receptor, causing a conformational change that results in the opening of an ion channel. With other receptors, such as that for glucagon, the formation of the hormone receptor complex triggers the enzyme adenylate cyclase which, through the formation of cyclic adenosine 3′,5′-monophosphate, can stimulate a physio-

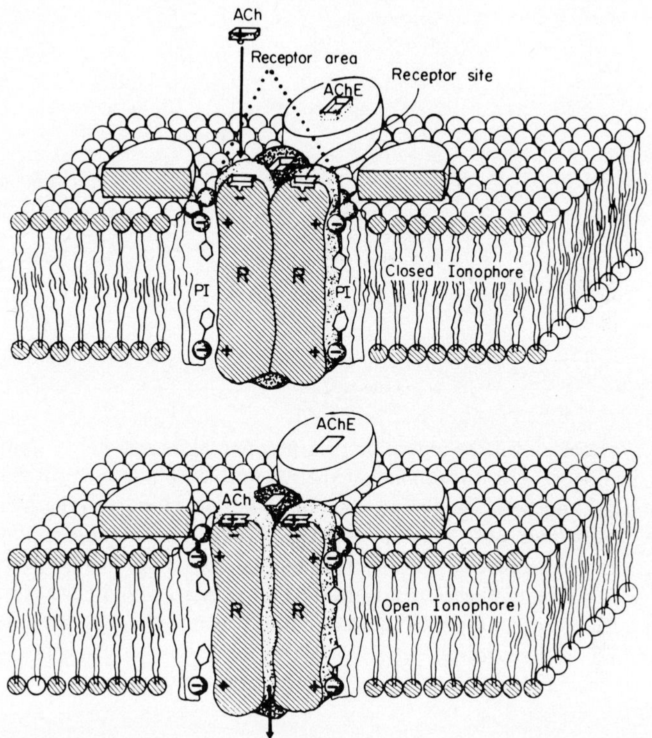

Fig. 1. Tetrameric model of a cholinergic receptor area showing the receptor protein subunits traversing the lipid matrix (intrinsic protein). Each receptor subunit shows the site of binding for acetylcholine on the outer surface of the membrane; the four parallel subunits constitute the ionophore. The presence of phosphatidylinositol (PI) attached to the receptor protein is indicated. The diagram also shows the presence of acetylcholinesterase (AChE) molecules that are peripheral to the membrane. In the upper drawing, the receptor site has not yet interacted, and the ionophore is in the closed condition. In the lower drawing, the receptor site has been occupied by acetylcholine, and this has evoked a conformational change, resulting in the opening of the ionophore. (From De Robertis, 1975, reproduced with permission of Springer-Verlag, Heidelberg.)

logical change. The use of hormones attached to solid supports, e.g., insulin–agarose, can give a different response to that of the free hormone (Cuatrecasas, 1974). Thus, we could envisage the situation where an antibody molecule, with an active site mimicking the structure of the part of a hormone which interacts with its receptor, could either block the action of the hormone or in other cases activate the receptor, but in an uncontrolled way.

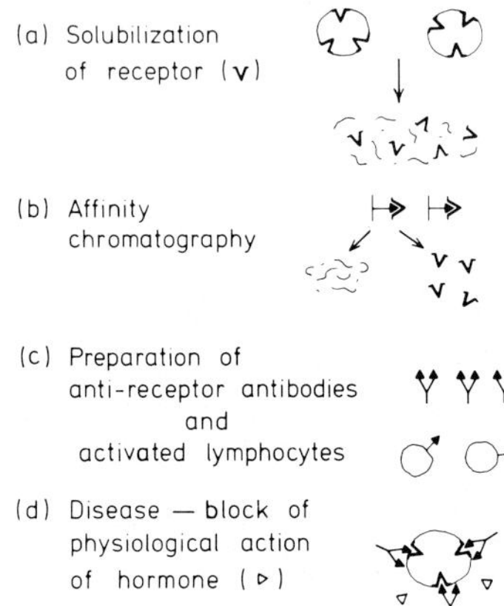

Fig. 2. Scheme for the induction of experimental anti-receptor antibody is based on the protocol used to produce experimental autoimmune myasthenia gravis. Detergents would be necessary to solubilize the receptor from the membrane, and affinity chromotography could be used to produce a fraction containing a high concentration of receptor. Because of marked variation in response of different species and differences between strains, several animals would have to be immunized with the receptor preparation. In addition to the usual immunologic tests for cellular and humoral immune responses, it would be necessary to use a physiological test system which would specifically assay receptor function.

Returning to the lymphoid system, we have the analogous system of cell surface receptors on immunocytes being activated by molecular determinants of antigen. The evidence that such receptors can themselves function as immunogens (antigens) is now so substantial that a highly plausible theory (the "network" theory) can be built up to explain "self-regulatory" functions within the system (Jerne, 1973; Hoffmann, 1975). However, as yet, there has been no attempt to examine immunopathology in the network concept.

This chapter will review the recent evidence in support of the concept that hormone and antigen receptors are vulnerable to autoimmune attack (Carnegie and Mackay, 1975). It should be possible to develop experimental models for some of the diseases discussed in this chapter, but there could be considerable difficulty in purifying sufficient quantities of the receptors, especially from human material. The general protocol is illustrated in Fig. 2 and is based on the now well-established procedure for the induction of experimental myasthenia gravis where a cellular and humoral immune response to the acetylcholine receptor is induced (see below). In assessing the immune response to receptors, we emphasize that physiological test systems would be more sensitive and specific than classical techniques such as immunofluorescence. Binding or viable cell assays developed for the study of receptors could readily be modified to detect an interference by antibody on receptor function.

II. MYASTHENIA GRAVIS

That myasthenia gravis was associated with immunologic abnormalities was recognized for 30 years, but the role of the immune response in the pathogenesis was not clear. Simpson (1960) and later Lennon and Carnegie (1971) suggested that there was an immune response to the acetylcholine receptor at the neuromuscular junction which interfered with the transmission of impulses. The recent development of an experimental model for myasthenia gravis in animals and the correlation of its features with the human disease has dramatically illustrated our general concept that receptors can be particularly vulnerable to autoimmune attack.

A. Experimental Autoimmune Myasthenia Gravis (EAMG)

In the course of work directed towards producing antibody to the nicotinic acetylcholine receptor isolated from the electric eel, it was reported by Patrick and Lindstrom (1973) that the immunized rabbits became paralyzed, and this paralysis could be reversed by anticholinesterase drugs. Their observation was rapidly confirmed in other laboratories and in other animals (Sugiyama *et al.*, 1973; Heilbronn and Mattson, 1974; Heilbronn *et al.*, 1975; Tarrab-Hazdai *et al.*, 1975; Green *et al.*, 1975). Detailed studies by Lindstrom, Lennon, and colleagues have elucidated the autoimmune pathogenesis of the experimental disease (Lennon *et al.*, 1975; 1976; Seybold *et al.*, 1976; Lindstrom *et al.*, 1976a). EAMG has now been produced in rabbits, rats, guinea pigs, monkeys, and goats.

In rats, there is both a cellular and humoral response to autologous acetylcholine receptor (Lennon *et al.*, 1975). However there are two phases in EAMG, with a typical response in a rat being shown in Fig. 3. At 8–10 days after inoculation, there is an acute and transient appearance of myasthenia, and then a second chronic phase occurs 25–30 days later. In the acute episode, there is no detectable antibody to the syngeneic receptor, but such antibody increased prior to and during the chronic phase. Animals with EAMG show striking similarities to the clinical symptoms of myasthenia gravis. At low and rapid rates of motor nerve stimulation, there is a decremental response of muscle, and rapid repetitive stimulation is followed by postactivation facilitation followed by exhaustion. Inhibitors of acetylcholine esterase repair the electrophysiological defect (Seybold *et al.*,

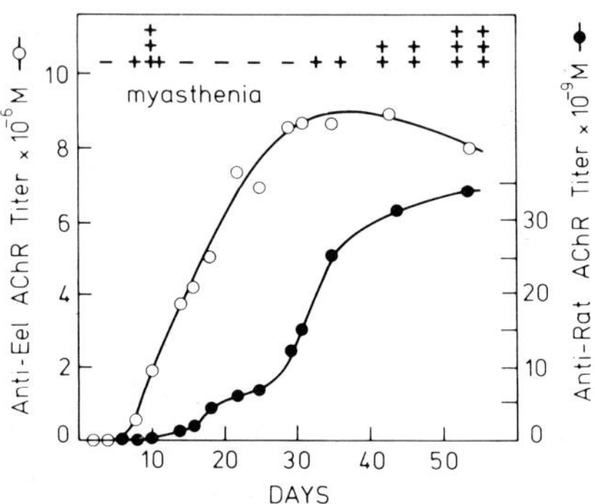

Fig. 3. Time course of humoral response in a rat immunized with eel acetylcholine receptor (AChR) at day 0. Titers are expressed in moles ^{125}I-cobra toxin binding sites precipitated per liter of serum. Antibody to syngeneic muscle AChR appeared later than antibody to the eel receptor. The rat had two severe episodes of experimental autoimmune myasthenia gravis (EAMG) (‡), transient at 8–12 days and chronic from 30 days; the latter resulted in death. Lennon *et al.* (1976) have suggested that the early symptoms are produced by inflammatory cells at the motor end-plate and the chronic myasthenia by the syngeneic antibody (modified from Lennon *et al.*, 1976, and Lindstrom *et al.*, 1976a).

1976). The amplitude of the miniature end-plate potentials is reduced, but the amount of acetylcholine released is normal (Lambert *et al.*, 1976). The lesions at motor end-plates of rats with chronic EAMG are strikingly similar to those of patients with myasthenia gravis (Engel *et al.*, 1976).

B. Human Myasthenia Gravis

Several groups have reported that patients with myasthenia gravis have an immune response against acetylcholine receptors by a variety of techniques (Almon *et al.*, 1974; Abramsky *et al.*, 1975a,b; Appel *et al.*, 1975; Bender *et al.*, 1975; Lindstrom *et al.*, 1976b). The most clear-cut results have been obtained with a preparation of human acetylcholine receptors complexed with ^{125}I-α-bungarotoxin. With this preparation, Lindstrom *et al.* (1976b) found antibody to the receptor in 87% of sera from 71 patients with myasthenia gravis, but not in any of 175 sera from normal adults or patients with neurological and autoimmune diseases other than myasthenia gravis (Fig. 4). Their simple test should be a most useful diagnostic aid. Because α-bungarotoxin forms a complex with the actual site of binding of acetylcholine within the receptor (Lindstrom *et al.*, 1976b), the antibody probably binds to components other than the site for acetylcholine.

However, using an assay in which there was a direct competition between antibody and α-bungarotoxin for the receptor, Almon *et al.* (1974) demonstrated that 30% of sera from patients with myasthenia gravis had an antibody capable of blocking the binding of this toxin; however, this does not prove the ability of antibody to interact with the binding site because an interaction with a determinant close to the binding site could interfere with the binding of the toxin (Almon and Appel, 1975). In Fig. 5, we present a diagrammatic view of the interaction that would explain the above results and the fatigability effect in EAMG and in myasthenia gravis.

The precise roles of antibody and cellular immune response to acetylcholine receptor in the pathogenesis of myasthenia gravis is still unclear, and the presence or titer of antibody did not appear to correlate with age, sex, steroid therapy, or duration of symptoms (Lindstrom *et al.*, 1976b). Possibly, the antibody causes an alteration in the synthesis and degradation of the receptor. These antibodies that cause the dysfunction of the myoneural junction in myasthenia gravis could also interfere with function at other acetylcholine receptors, e.g., in the central nervous system, provided the blood–brain barrier was breached, and this could explain psychic disturbances which occur in myasthenia gravis.

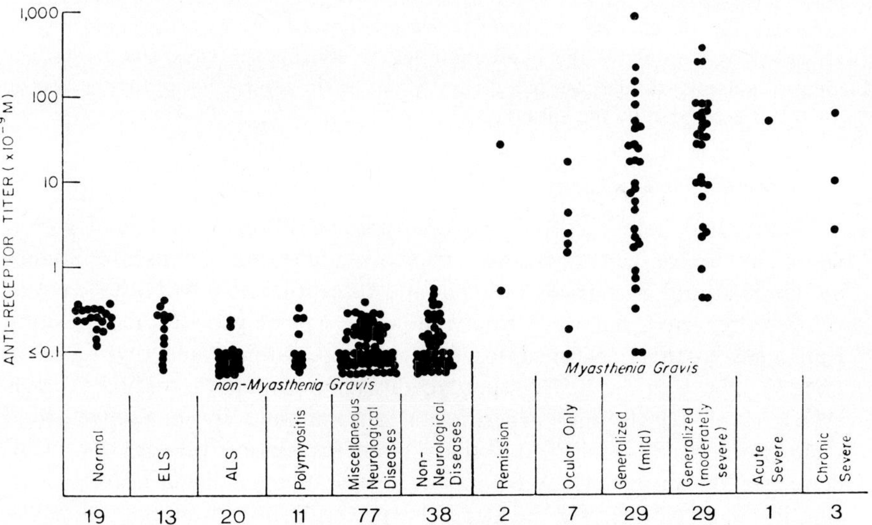

Fig. 4. Antibody to acetylcholine receptor in myasthenia gravis and various diseases. Antibody was assayed with human muscle acetylcholine receptor labeled with ^{125}I-α-bungarotoxin as test antigen (modified from Lindstrom *et al.*, 1976b). The number of patients examined in each disease is indicated. ELS and ALS are Eaton-Lambert syndrome and amyotrophic lateral sclerosis, respectively.

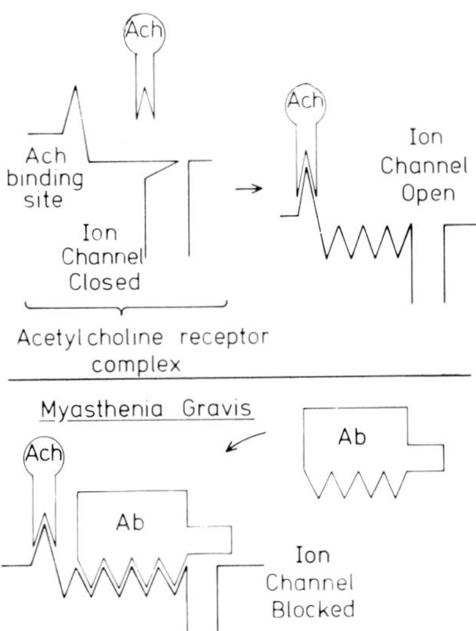

Fig. 5. A hypothetical scheme that may explain the fatigability effect in myasthenia gravis (N. R. Sims, personal communication). The majority of antibodies in patients with myasthenia gravis do not react with site in the receptor that binds acetylcholine, but with some other component in the receptor complex. It is suggested that *in vivo* the antibody preferentially interacts with the conformation presented as a result of the interaction with acetylcholine. Thus, the greater the input of nervous stimulation, the greater would be the availability of the receptor in the form recognized by the antibody.

1. Genetic Considerations

Finally, with reference to a possible predisposition to failure of immunologic tolerance, genetic factors are involved in the human disease. Studies on inbred strains of animals resistant and susceptible to EAMG have not as yet been reported, but we predict that there will be genetic predisposition equivalent to that described for experimental autoimmune thyroiditis in mice (Tomazic *et al.*, 1974), spontaneous autoimmune thyroiditis in fowls (Wick *et al.*, 1974), and experimental autoimmune encephalomyelitis in mice (Bernard, 1976). In man, there is an association between the histocompatibility antigen HLA-B8 and that type of myasthenia gravis occurring in young women who lack the characteristic myoid antibody demonstrable by immunofluorescence (Feltkamp *et al.*, 1974); however, such patients do have antibody to the acetylcholine receptor (Lindstrom *et al.*, 1976b). On the other hand, HLA-A2 is associated with the other group of myasthenic patients who are elderly, have thymoma, and have both myoid antibody and antibody to the receptor site (Fritze *et al.*, 1974; Lindstrom *et al.*, 1976b). However, despite these and other interesting associations between HLA and disease, there is yet to be demonstrated an association between a particular HLA antigen and a failure of immunologic tolerance to a particular self-antigen.

2. *Neonatal Myasthenia Gravis*

The occurrence of transient myasthenia gravis in babies from mothers with the disease was one of the factors which prompted Simpson (1960) to propose that antibody to acetylcholine receptor could be involved in pathogenesis. IgG can cross the placenta and could cause symptoms in the infant. Recently, Lindstrom *et al.* (1976b) found that twin sons with neonatal myasthenia gravis had about 25% of the level of anti-acetylcholine receptor antibody found in their mother. Scott (1976) recently reviewed the pathogenesis of neonatal myasthenia gravis and certain other diseases as model systems illustrating pathogenic effects of placentally transferred autoantibodies in saturating doses.

Experimental transfer of symptoms of myasthenia gravis from man to animals would be expected to be difficult because of the difficulty of transferring sufficient antibody and the limited cross-reactivity between human and animal acetylcholine receptors (Lindstrom *et al.*, 1976a). Nevertheless, Toyka *et al.* (1975) have demonstrated that repeated injections of immunoglobulins from patients with myasthenia gravis into mice produced myasthenic abnormalities.

3. *Thymus and Myasthenia Gravis*

There is considerable literature on the role of the thymus in myasthenia gravis. Notably, abnormalities of the thymus are usually present in this disease, and there is definite benefit from thymectomy (reviewed by Goldstein and Mackay, 1969). About 30% of patients have antibodies that react with thymic myoid cells which are antigenically similar to skeletal muscle cells. Acetylcholine receptor has been identified in the thymus, using antibody to electric eel receptor (Aharonov *et al.*, 1975). Goldstein (1974) isolated from the thymus a polypeptide that induced lymphoid stem cells to differentiate to thymocytes; this polypeptide (thymopoietin) was also claimed to have an effect on neuromuscular transmission (Goldstein, 1968; Goldstein and Schlesinger, 1975). Lennon (1975) recently assessed these studies and criticized some of the electrophysiological experiments, with a call for more data on the influence of thymopoietin on neuromuscular transmission before a role for this polypeptide can be accepted in myasthenia gravis (see addendum).

III. THYROID GLAND AND GRAVES' DISEASE

The autonomous hyperthyroidism of Graves' disease is a special example of effects of functionally important autoantibodies against receptors, with stimulatory rather than inhibitory effects. Adams and Purves (1956) identified in serum a thyroid stimulator other than thyrotropin (TSH) and, from its bioassay characteristics, called this long-acting thyroid stimulator (LATS). This was later identified as an immunoglobulin G (Kriss *et al.*, 1964) and, thus, qualified as an autoantibody. Both LATS and TSH stimulate adenylate cyclase in thyroid cells, resulting in formation of cyclic adenosine 3′,5′-monophosphate (cyclic AMP); TSH acts within minutes of its addition to thyroid slices (Kaneko *et al.*, 1970), whereas LATS acts more slowly.

Controversy developed over the pathogenic role of LATS in thyrotoxicosis because of apparent discrepancies: it was not regularly demonstrable, nor was it regularly associated with other indices of this disease. This controversy has been largely resolved by the recognition of another thyroid-stimulating immunoglobulin, which was originally detected by its ability to inhibit the absorption of LATS to thyroid microsomes; because it "protected" LATS from being absorbed it was designated "LATS protector" (Adams and Kennedy, 1967; Shishiba *et al.*, 1973). This immunoglobulin stimulates specifically human thyroid tissue *in vitro* and *in vivo* and is the "real LATS," being present in all patients with proven disease; it is now more appropriately known as human thyroid-stimulating immunoglobulin (HTSI) (Editorial, 1975a).

The receptor reactivity of HTSI is well established. There is a conventional receptor assay for TSH using thyroid membranes, and, in this assay, HTSI will inhibit or displace TSH from its binding site (Mehdi *et al.*, 1973; Manley *et al.*, 1974a,b; Smith and Hall, 1974). Thus, the stimulating immunoglobulin both competes with and mimics the action of TSH, but in an uncontrolled way, and, in immunologic terms, represents an antibody that is complementary to a receptor site as antigen.

Thus, in Graves' disease, there is an HTSI, the activity of which will correlate with other indices of hyperthyroidism, and the original LATS, which stimulates receptors of the thyroid of animals and has associations with various features of thyroid autoimmunity. We can predict that immunoglobulins from patients with Graves' disease would allow isolation of the TSH receptor by affinity chromatography. This would allow the creation of important disease models by appropriate immunization with the receptor. There is no reference in the literature to a cellular immune response to the TSH receptor but, by analogy with myasthenia gravis, this could be expected.

1. Genetic Considerations

Drawing on the review by Vanhaelst *et al.* (1972), we can cite (1) the numerous observations from family studies that there is an inherited predisposition to thyrotoxicosis, (2) the raised incidence of antibodies to thyroid components in relatives of thyrotoxic patients, and (3) the presence of LATS in euthyroid relatives of thyrotoxic patients. These observations can now be considered with those showing a raised incidence in thyrotoxicosis of the histocompatibility antigen HLA-B8 (Grumet *et al.*, 1973; Whittingham *et al.*, 1975a). There is a major paradox, however, in that, whereas associations and overlaps between thyrotoxicosis and autoimmune (Hashimoto's) thyroiditis are well recognized clinically (Vanhaelst *et al.*, 1972), there is not in Hashimoto's thyroiditis any increase in HLA phenotypes, including HLA-B8, according to two studies (Bode *et al.*, 1973; Whittingham *et al.*, 1975b), although an increase in HLA-A1 and B8 was shown in one (Farid *et al.*, 1975). If the HLA-B8 association was specific for thyrotoxicosis, the presence of this antigen could be associated with production of anti-receptor antibody.

2. Neonatal Thyrotoxicosis

Just as in myasthenia gravis, there is a natural model of transfer of anti-receptor disease in neonatal thyrotoxicosis. Hoffmann *et al.* (1966) reviewed some 20 cases of neonatal thyrotoxicosis and described 4 further instances, including a twin pair, born to 3 mothers suffering from hyperthyroidism. Raised levels of LATS were demonstrable in the three mothers, and in the four infants in whom LATS and symptoms were only transiently present. Scott (1976) comments further on neonatal thyrotoxicosis and emphasizes that LATS protector (HSTI) is transferred, as well as LATS.

IV. DIABETES MELLITUS

The juvenile onset type of diabetes has attracted considerable attention as a possible autoimmune disease by reason of the raised incidence of autoantibodies (Table I). At present, evidence for anti-receptor antibody in diabetes mellitus is slender, although assay systems involving insulin receptors are well developed.

Considering the juvenile onset type of diabetes mellitus, an assay system would use isolated β-islet cells whose receptors for glucose would be blocked by serum that contained antibodies to such cells, comparable with the pharmacologic action of somatostatin (Okamoto *et al.*, 1975), and such studies are in progress (A. Lernmark, personal communication). In the adult-onset type of diabetes mellitus, different considerations would apply:

TABLE I

Features of Major Types of Diabetes Mellitus

Characteristic	Juvenile-onset type 1	Maturity-onset type 2	References
Onset	Adolescence	Mid-adult	
Insulin dependence	Strong	Mild	
Insulin resistance	Low	High	
Insulin response to stimuli	Absent	Present, delayed	
Hereditary	Weak	Strong	Editorial (1975b); Lendrum *et al.* (1976)
Overlap with thyroid and stomach disease	Present	Rare	Whittingham *et al.* (1971)
Autoantibodies to thyrogastric antigens	Frequent	Infrequent	Ungar *et al.* (1968); Irvine *et al.* (1970)
Autoantibodies to pancreatic islet cells	Present early stages	Absent	Bottazzo *et al.* (1974); MacCuish *et al.* (1974); Lendrum *et al.* (1975); MacLaren *et al.* (1975)
Cell-mediated immunity to pancreatic islet cells	Present	Absent	Nerup *et al.* (1971); Haung and MacLaren (1976)
HLA associations	B8, B15	None	Thomsen *et al.* (1975); Lendrum *et al.* (1976); Editorial (1957b)
Postulated target for anti-receptor antibody	"Glucose" receptor	Insulin receptor	

target cells are insensitive to the action of the natural agonist insulin because receptors are either deficient in number or "blocked," and the concentration of insulin in blood rises (Cuatrecasas, 1974). As far as blocking of receptors by antibody is concerned, the only study so far available is that of Flier *et al.* (1975) who found that in three of six patients with extreme insulin resistance, there were antibodies to insulin receptors on monocytes. The competitive binding assay they used did not detect anti-receptor antibody in the more usual type of insulin-resistant diabetic; with such patients, a more sensitive assay would be the isolated fat cell or isolated insulin receptors. Fat cells respond to insulin by increasing uptake of glucose (Cuatrecasas, 1974; Lockwood *et al.*, 1975), and antibody to the insulin receptor would be expected to block this response to insulin.

1. Genetic Considerations

The complex polygenic inheritance of diabetes mellitus is beyond the scope of this chapter, and reference can be made only to current highlights. Earlier proposals relating to "major" and "minor" genes, or cumulative effects of polygenes, reviewed by Steinberg *et al.* (1970), did not take into consideration the two major types, the juvenile-onset insulin-dependent type and the maturity-onset non-insulin-dependent type. This differentiation is relevant to our thesis because maturity-onset diabetes has a strong familial tendency, but is not HLA linked (Editorial, 1975b) and is not strongly associated with organ-specific autoantibodies; in the juvenile onset type, there is weaker familial tendency, yet a close linkage to HLA phenotypes (HLA-B8 and B15) and a predisposition to organ-specific autoantibodies, including islet cell autoantibodies (see addendum).

Studies on concordant and discordant identical twins with insulin-dependent diabetes provide evidence for differing pathogeneses; HLA-B8 was increased in concordant but not in discordant pairs, whereas B15 was increased in both pairs, and islet cell antibodies were more often present in the diabetic than the nondiabetic member of discordant pairs (Lendrum *et al.*, 1976). The simplest explanation is that most insulin-dependent diabetics inherit a susceptibility to an "insulotropic" virus (dependent on HLA-B15) and some inherit a susceptibility to develop islet cell antibody and, possibly, antibody to receptors for glucose (dependent on HLA-B8).

Genetic influences could operate in those strains of mice in which there is an associated diabetes–obesity syndrome, and one such strain, NZO, is related to the frankly autoimmune strain, NZB. The usual explanation for diabetes–obesity syndromes in mice, as in maturity-onset human diabetes, is a decrement in concentration of insulin receptors on the cell surface, but an alternative possibility would be receptor blockade by anti-receptor antibody.

2. *Neonatal Diabetes Mellitus*

This condition is included in "nature's experimental system," (Scott, 1976) illustrating serum transfer, during pregnancy, of maternal disease. This transient neonatal form of diabetes mellitus has long been recognized (Cornblath and Schwartz, 1966) and could be attributed to transplacental transfer of antibody to insulin receptors. Unfortunately for this hypothesis, these mothers show no evidence of diabetes mellitus and, mostly, have no family history; Scott (1976) proposed that the mothers had, in addition, a blocking antibody which did not cross the placenta.

V. OTHER ENDOCRINOPATHIES

There are a number of diseases in which the features could be accounted for by blockage of receptor sites. These features include a failure of the target organ, progressively rising levels of the tropic hormone, but an apparent resistance to its action, and some response to the tropic hormone after its administration. The causes of defective function of receptor sites in endocrine diseases are uncertain, but, in those conditions in which there are autoantibodies demonstrable by immunofluorescence, or serum factors reactive with receptor sites as in thyrotoxicosis, an anti-receptor antibody effect can be postulated.

One obvious example is Addison's adrenal disease, in which there is adrenal failure, presence of anti-adrenal autoantibodies, and elevated serum levels of ACTH (Bresser *et al.,* 1971). Another example is pernicious anemia in which levels of gastrin, an agonist for gastric parietal cells, are highly raised (Strickland and Mackay, 1973), and this could be associated with a block of the gastrin receptor. A third example is pseudohypoparathyroidism, in which there are features of hypoparathyroidism despite normal or raised levels of parathyroid hormone in the blood (Chase *et al.*, 1969); the postulated "insensitivity" of the receptor could be due in some cases to antibody blockage. We can envisage currently available techniques being applied to the above possibilities, with the caveat that human receptors would probably be more specific and sensitive than animal receptors. Indeed, Jarrett *et al.* (1976) have demonstrated that "naturally-occurring" antibody to the human insulin receptor, linked with ^{125}I, could be used to detect anti-receptor antibody in patients with diabetes. They suggested that their protocol could be adapted to the study of other diseases where anti-receptor antibodies could be involved.

Recently, a procedure similar to that outlined in Fig. 2 was used to produce antibody to prolactin receptors in guinea pigs (Shiu and Friesen,

1976). Both binding and physiological assays were used to demonstrate a specific immune response to the receptors.

VI. MULTIPLE SCLEROSIS

The original motivation for the "immunopharmacologic block" hypothesis of Lennon and Carnegie (1971) was an attempt to explain the discrepancy between the striking functional disabilities and mild histological lesions in guinea pigs immunized with an encephalitogenic peptide from myelin basic protein. Carnegie (1971) proposed that the peptide might fulfill the requirements for the structure of a binding site for serotonin, and, hence, an immune response to this peptide would cause a block of serotonin receptors. It was later shown that serotonin could, in fact, block the interaction between myelin basic protein and lymphocytes from patients with multiple sclerosis (Carnegie *et al.*, 1972). Further, albeit limited, support for this concept came from examination of serotonin and its metabolities in brains of animals with experimental autoimmune encephalomyelitis (Lycke and Roos, 1973; Khoruzhaya and Saakov, 1975), together with studies of the accompanying neurophysiological disturbances (White *et al.*, 1973). Oligodendrocytes presumably have receptors for serotonin, as they respond to serotonin by changing their pulsation rate (Murray, 1958).

Our speculative view on the pathogenesis of multiple sclerosis is illustrated in Fig. 6. This model is consistent with the recent HLA studies (see below), the postulated transmissible agent in brain tissue from patients with multiple sclerosis (Carp *et al.*, 1972; Koldovsky *et al.*, 1975), with the frequent appearance of lesions near blood vessels (Lumsden, 1971), and with the fluctuating symptoms observed in the disease.

Parts of the model have supporting evidence. The acute fluctuating clinical symptoms characteristic of the disease would be most readily explained by a temporary immune response to a functional component in the central nervous system (Paterson, 1969). The presence in serum of factors (possibly antibodies) which block "polysynaptic" activity in tissue culture has been reported by Bornstein and Crain (1965) and Lumsden *et al.* (1975), but the site of reaction of these factors has not been identified. In the cultures used in these studies, there was selective damage to oligodendrocytes (Raine *et al.*, 1973). Patients with multiple sclerosis have no cell-mediated immune response to myelin but do exhibit a response to a "synaptic" membrane fraction (Alvord *et al.*, 1974) and to oligodendrocytes (Myers *et al.*, 1975). Plasma membranes from oligodendrocytes would probably be present in the "synaptic" membrane fraction. Three groups have reported that, in multiple sclerosis, there are somewhat abnormal

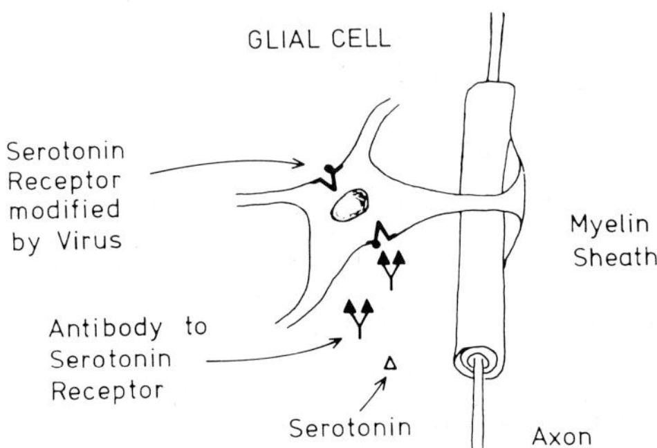

Fig. 6. Highly speculative model on the pathogenesis of multiple sclerosis. Because of deficiency in an immune response gene, a virus which would normally be eliminated is permitted to invade the central nervous system. It would lodge in dividing oligodendrocytes and alter the plasma membrane close to a receptor. Several years would elapse before there was a sufficient buildup of virus to cause an immune response. An immune response to the virus or altered receptor would interfere with the function of the receptor. Prolonged blockage could lead to death of the oligodendrocyte and demyelination due to a failure to replace metabolically active proteins in myelin (see Note Added in Print p. 619).

levels of serotonin metabolites in the cerebrospinal fluid (Sonninen *et al.*, 1973; Johansson and Roos, 1974; Calveria *et al.*, 1974). The strongest support has come from experiments by Harrer and Fischbach (1973) who used a sensitive test of optic nerve function in patients to monitor the rapid deterioration induced by mild hyperthermia. This deterioration could be prevented by raising the tryptophan concentration in the blood, a procedure known to increase brain serotonin levels. Among numerous compounds tested, tyrosine, a precursor of noradrenalin, was the only other substance able to prevent the deterioration. Recently Hyyppä *et al.* (1975) administered L-tryptophan to patients with multiple sclerosis over a short period; although there was no dramatic improvement in their condition, there was some improvement in bladder and motility disturbances.

There is a need for further work on the characterization of the antigen in multiple sclerosis which stimulates the production of abnormal levels of oligoclonal immunoglobulin in the cerebrospinal fluid; tissue culture systems need to be developed to test the physiological effects of such immunoglobulin.

Genetic Considerations

The several studies cited by Alter and Harshe (1975) show that the risk for multiple sclerosis in family members is several times greater than in the general population, but the genetic mechanisms are unclear; considerable interest, however, attaches to the well-established increase in frequency in multiple sclerosis of HLA phenotypes A3 and B7, and the lymphocyte-defined determinant 7a (Jersild *et al.*, 1975). Lamoureux *et al.* (1976) have confirmed the association of these HLA phenotypes with multiple sclerosis and have presented evidence for an altered immune response to a variety of naturally occurring antigens.

VII. LYMPHOCYTE RECEPTORS FOR ANTIGEN

The effects of anti-receptor antibody are most elegantly illustrated within the lymphoid system itself. We can begin with the immunogenic and antigenic sites on the immunoglobulin molecule, these being the Fc portion which is reactive with allotypic antibodies and rheumatoid factors (Natvig *et al.*, 1972), the hinge region which is reactive with "normal serum agglutinators" (Waller, 1973) and the specific antigen-binding sites of the variable region which elicits and is reactive with idiotypic antibodies.

By special maneuvers one can create antibodies to idiotypes (Strayer *et al.*, 1974), and these have the immunologic properties of the original antigen. Moreover, if antigen-binding receptors on immunocytes are similar to the serum antibody secreted by the cell, then idiotypic antibody would be reactive with such receptors.

The inhibitory effects of antibody to determinants of immunoglobulin expressed on the lymphoid cell surface were first shown by the phenomenon of allotype suppression, best exemplified in the rabbit. This subject is reviewed by Dray (1972); in brief, lymphoid cells with a genetic capability of expressing on their surface an immunoglobulin phenotype (allotype) can be blocked, from uterine life on, by exposure to maternal serum which contains the corresponding anti-allotype antibody.

Functional inhibitory effects of anti-idiotypic antibody were recognized by Ramseier (1973) by a rather unconventional assay, which initially attracted little attention, depending on the cutaneous inflammatory effects of a factor (product of antigenic recognition, PAR) released when antibody reacted with histocompatibility antigen. This interaction was shown to be blocked by anti-idiotypic antibody, implying that this might regulate immune responses to such antigens. From another standpoint, Strayer *et al.* (1974) reported experiments showing that tolerance to an antigen (phosphorylcholine) could be induced in neonatal mice by antibody to the idiotype reacting with phosphorylcholine.

The theoretical interest of idiotypic antibodies is considerable. First, there is mounting evidence (McKearn, 1974; Binz and Wigzell, 1975; Eichmann, 1975) that such antibodies are reactive with membrane determinants of T cells which share determinants with the variable portion of Ig molecules, pointing to the immunoglobulin nature of the T cell receptor (Marchalonis, 1975). Second, functional activity of idiotypes and anti-idiotypic antibodies at cell surfaces could have inhibitory (damping) effects on immune responses, so providing an internal self-regulatory system, the "network" concept of Jerne (1973). Third, the "balance of power" in immune responses to tumors is delicate and susceptible to subtle influences which may include anti-idiotype antibodies. In melanoma, for example, Hartman *et al.* (1974) claimed that "protective" antibody against membrane antigens may function to limit spread of the tumor. The appearance of anti-idiotypic antibody could inhibit protective antibody (or cells concerned in its production) and result in a blocking effect on tumor immunity. Fourth, autoimmune diseases show fluctuating clinical features, well exemplified by the course of systemic lupus erythematosus (SLE) and myasthenia gravis. In such diseases, clones of cells have expanded and escaped from normal controlling influences, although it is uncertain whether abnormal helper T cells (for autoantigen) have been recruited, or whether suppressor T cells (for autoreactive B or T cells) are hypofunctional. Considering SLE as a particular example, there would be cells with receptors for antigens of DNA or nucleoprotein, and this receptor should be susceptible to antibody to the idiotype of anti-DNA. According to theory, the "fault" in the patient with SLE (or other autoimmune disease) would be failure to develop or maintain a controlling antibody to a relevant cell receptor: this may be due to a general weakness of a suppressor system or to a genetic (possibly MHC related) incapability to respond to a specific receptor idiotype.

The reality of autoimmunization to antigen receptors has been shown further by Binz and Wigzell (1976) who took advantage of the presence in rat serum of idiotypic antigen-binding receptors with specificity for major histocompatibility (AgB) locus antigens. Using such lymphocyte receptors as immunogens, auto-anti-idiotypic antibodies were induced, demonstrable by selective loss of immune reactivity against the relevant histoincompatible antigens, thus demonstrating that autoimmunization to receptors can induce specific tolerance to transplantation antigens. This adds weight to the likelihood that antibody to receptors has a controlling effect over responses to autoantigens.

VIII. CONCLUSION

It must be emphasized that an autoimmune reaction to receptors will only occur where there is a failure of tolerance. While a considerable amount of information has been accumulated on the induction of tolerance to foreign antigens, these laboratory systems may not be directly relevant to the complex multistep controls which must be necessary to maintain self-tolerance. The striking association of certain HLA phenotypes with a failure of self-tolerance has been taken to indicate a possible linkage association with an immune response gene. However, these HLA moieties are cell-surface glycoproteins, and it is thus possible that they are actually involved in some regulatory mechanism. It is known that the acetylcholine receptor and insulin receptor contain glycoproteins (Cuatrecasas, 1974), and it is conceivable that certain conformations of some of these glycoproteins might prevent lymphocytes bearing the similar HLA moieties from gaining access to the receptors.

Alternatively, lymphocytes with certain HLA antigens might stick more readily to some cell-surface glycoproteins and thus enhance the chances of an autoimmune reaction occurring. There is increasing evidence that cell-surface glycoproteins together with glycosyltransferases are involved in the maintenance of contact inhibition (cf. Blanden *et al.*, 1976). Because of its free-roaming nature, the lymphocyte should have a lack of moieties involved in contact inhibition, but with certain HLA types there could be a greater chance of lymphocyte–cell-surface interaction. Such an enhanced ability to interact might explain the genetic clustering of certain types of autoimmune diseases (Mackay, 1969).

While it is established that anti-receptor antibody is responsible for myasthenia and hyperthyroidism, analogous effects on other receptor systems are still hypothetical. The immune system is one of particular interest because, here, anti-receptor antibody could be "physiological" in the sense of a normal self-regulatory process with both facilitory and inhibitory controls, as proposed by the "network" theory. Certain autoimmune diseases could represent a different type of "fault" in these being a failure of normal function of anti-receptor antibody to regulate unwanted reactions against self-components. Spontaneous remissions and exacerbations could reflect partial failures associated with a rise and fall in levels of anti-receptor antibody.

ACKNOWLEDGMENTS

Original work from our laboratories was supported by the National Health and Medical Research Council of Australia and the National Multiple Sclerosis Society, New York. This is publication No. 2240 from the Walter and Eliza Hall Institute of Medical Research.

REFERENCES

Abramsky, O., Aharonov, A., Teitelbaum, D., and Fuchs, S. (1975a). *Arch. Neurol. (Chicago)* **32,** 684.

Abramsky, O., Aharonov, A., Webb, C., and Fuchs, S. (1975b). *Clin. Exp. Immunol.* **19,** 11.

Adams, D. D., and Kennedy, T. H. (1967). *J. Clin. Endocrinol. Metab.* **27,** 173.

Adams, D. D., and Purves, H. D. (1956). *Proc. Univ. Otago Med. Sch.* **34,** 11.

Aharonov, A., Tarrab-Hazdai, R., Abramsky, O., and Fuchs, S. (1975). *Proc. Natl. Acad. Sci. U.S.A.* **72,** 1456.

Almon, R. R., and Appel, S. H. (1975). *Biochim. Biophys. Acta* **393,** 66.

Almon, R. R., Andrew, C. G., and Appel, S. H. (1974). *Science* **186,** 55.

Alter, M., and Harshe, M. (1975). *J. Neurol.* **210,** 1.

Alvord, E. C., Hsu, P. C., and Thron, R. (1974). *Arch. Neurol. (Chicago)* **30,** 296.

Appel, S. H., Almon, R. R., and Levy, N. (1975). *N. Engl. J. Med.* **293,** 760.

Bender, A. N., Ringle, S. P., Engel, W. K., Daniels, M. P., and Vogel, Z. (1975). *Lancet* **1,** 607.

Bernard, C. C. A. (1976). *J. Immunogenet.* **3,** 263.

Binz, H., and Wigzell, H. (1975). *J. Exp. Med.* **142,** 218.

Binz, H., and Wigzell, H. (1976). *J. Exp. Med.* **144,** 1438.

Blanden, R. V., Hapel, A. J., and Jackson, D. C. (1976). *Immunochemistry* **13,** 179.

Bode, H. H., Dorf, M. E., and Forbes, A. P. (1973). *J. Clin. Endocrinol. Metab.* **37,** 692.

Bornstein, M., and Crain, S. M. (1965). *Science* **148,** 1242.

Bottazzo, G. F., Florin-Christensen, A., and Doniach, D. (1974). *Lancet* **2,** 1279.

Bresser, G. M., Cullen, D. R., Irvine, W. J., Ratcliffe, J. G., and Landon, J. (1971). *Br. Med. J.* **1,** 374.

Calveria, K. E., Curzon, G., Harrison, M. J. G., and Kantamaneni, B. D. (1974). *J. Neurol., Neurosurg. Psychiatry* **37,** 715.

Carnegie, P. R. (1971). *Nature (London)* **229,** 25.

Carnegie, P. R., and Mackay, I. R. (1975). *Lancet* **2,** 684.

Carnegie, P. R., Smythies, J. R., Caspary, E. A., and Field, E. J. (1972). *Nature (London)* **240,** 561.

Carp, R. J., Licursi, P. C., Merz, P. A., and Merz, G. S. (1972). *J. Exp. Med.* **136,** 618.

Chase, L. R., Melson, L., and Aurbach, G. D. (1969). *J. Clin. Invest.* **48,** 1832.

Cornblath, M., and Schwartz, R. (1966). "Disorders of Carbohydrate Metabolism in Infancy." Saunders, Philadelphia, Pennsylvania.

Cuatrecasas, P. (1974). *Annu. Rev. Biochem.* **43,** 169.

De Robertis, E. (1975). *Ergeb. Physiol., Biol. Chem. Exp. Pharmakol.* **73,** 9.

Dray, S. (1972). *Ontog. Acquired Immun., Ciba Found. Symp., 1971* pp. 87–113.

Editorial. (1975a). *Br. Med. J.* **2,** 457.

Editorial. (1975b). *Br. Med. J.* **4,** 127.

Eichmann, K. (1975). *Eur. J. Immunol.* **5,** 511.

Engel, A. G., Tsujihata, M., Lambert, E. H., Lindstrom, J. M., and Lennon, V. A. (1976). *J. Neuropathol. Exp. Neurol.* **35,** 569.

Farid, N. R., Barnard, J., Kutas, C., Noel, E. P., and Marshall, W. H. (1975). *Int. Arch. Allergy Appl. Immunol.* **49,** 837.

Feltkamp, T. E. W., van den Berg-Loonen, P. M., Nijenhuis, L. E., Englefriet, C. P., van Rossum, A. L., van Loghem, J. J., and Oosterhuis, H. J. G. H. (1974). *Br. Med. J.* **1,** 131.

Flier, J. S., Kahn, C. R., Roth, J., and Bar, R. S. (1975). *Science* **190,** 63.

Fritze, D., Herrman, C., Naeium, F., Smith, G. S., and Walford, R. L. (1974). *Lancet* **1,** 240.

Goldstein, G. (1968). *Lancet* **2,** 119.

Goldstein, G. (1974). *Nature* (*London*) **247,** 11.

Goldstein, G., and Mackay, I. R. (1969). "The Human Thymus." Heinemann, London.

Goldstein, G., and Schlesinger, D. H. (1975). *Lancet* **2,** 256.

Green, D. P. L., Miledi, R., and Vincent, A. (1975). *Proc. R. Soc. London, Ser. B* **189,** 57.

Grumet, F. C., Konishi, J., Payne, R., and Kriss, J. P. (1973). *Clin. Res.* **21,** 493.

Harrer, G., and Fischbach, R. (1973). *J. Neural Transm.* **34,** 205.

Hartman, D., Lewis, M. G., Proctor, J. W., and Lyons, H. (1974). *Lancet* **2,** 1481.

Huang, S. W., and MacLaren, N. K. (1976). *Science* **192,** 64.

Heilbronn, E., and Mattson, C. (1974). *J. Neurochem.* **22,** 315.

Heilbronn, E., Mattson, C., Stalberg, E., and Hilton-Brown, P. (1975). *J. Neurol. Sci.* **24,** 59.

Hoffmann, G. W. (1975). *Eur. J. Immunol.* **5,** 638.

Hoffmann, M. J., Hetzel, B. S., and Manson, J. (1966). *Australas. Ann. Med.* **15,** 262.

Hyyppä, M. T., Jolma, T., Riekkinen, P., and Rinne, U. K. (1975). *J. Neural Transm.* **37,** 297.

Irvine, W. J., Clarke, B. F., Scarth, L., Cullen, D. R., and Duncan, L. J. P. (1970). *Lancet* **2,** 163.

Jarrett, D. B., Roth, J., Kahn, C. R., and Flier, J. S. (1976). *Proc. Natl. Acad. Sci. U.S.A.* **73,** 4115.

Jerne, N. K. (1973). *Sci. Am.* **229,** 52.

Jersild, C., Dupont, B., Fog, T., Platz, P. J., and Svejgaard, A. (1975). *Transplant. Rev.* **22,** 148.

Johansson, B., and Roos, B.-E. (1974). *Eur. Neurol.* **11,** 37.

Kaneko, T., Zor, U., and Field, J. B. (1970). *Metab., Clin. Exp.* **19,** 430.

Khoruzhaya, T. A., and Saakov, B. A. (1975). *Byull. Eksp. Biol. Med.* **79,** 677.

Koldovsky, U., Koldovsky, P., Henle, G., Henle, W., Ackermann, R., and Hasse, G. (1975). *Infect. Immun.* **12,** 1355.

Kriss, J. P., Pleshakov, V., and Chain, J. R. (1964). *J. Clin. Endocrinol. Metab.* **24,** 1005.

Lambert, E. H., Lindstrom, J. M., and Lennon, V. A. (1976). *Ann. N.Y. Acad. Sci.* **274,** 300.

Lamoureux, G., Giard, N., Jolicoeur, R., Toughlian, V., and DesRosiers, M. (1976). *Br. Med. J.* **1,** 183.

Lendrum, R., Walker, G., and Gamble, D. R. (1975). *Lancet* **1,** 880.

Lendrum, R., Nelson, P. G., Pyke, D. A., Walker, G., and Gamble, D. R. (1976). *Br. Med. J.* **1,** 553.
Lennon, V. A. (1975). *Nature* (*London*) **258,** 11.
Lennon, V. A., and Carnegie, P. R. (1971). *Lancet* **1,** 630.
Lennon, V. A., Lindstrom, J. M., and Seybold, M. E. (1975). *J. Exp. Med.* **141,** 1365.
Lennon, V. A., Lindstrom, J. M., and Seybold, M. E. (1976). *Ann. N.Y. Acad. Sci.* **274,** 283.
Lindstrom, J. M., Lennon, V. A., Seybold, M. E., and Whittingham, S. (1976a). *Ann. N.Y. Acad. Sci.* **274,** 254.
Lindstrom, J. M., Seybold, M. E., Lennon, V. A., Whittingham, S., and Duane, D. D. (1976b). *Neurology* **26,** 1054.
Lockwood, D. H., Livingston, J. N., and Amatruda, J. M. (1975). *Fed. Proc., Fed. Am. Soc. Exp. Biol.* **34,** 1564.
Lumsden, C. E. (1971). *Brain Res.* **28,** 365.
Lumsden, C. E., Howard, L., Aparicio, S. R., and Bradbury, M. (1975). *Brain Res.* **93,** 283.
Lycke, E., and Roos, B.-E. (1973). *Int. Arch. Allergy Appl. Immunol.* **45,** 341.
MacCuish, A. C., Barnes, E. W., Irvine, W. J., and Duncan, L. J. P. (1974). *Lancet* **2,** 1529.
Mackay, I. R. (1969). *Med. J. Aust.* **1,** 696.
McKearn, T. J. (1974). *Science* **183,** 94.
MacLaren, N. K., Huang, S. W., and Fogh, J.A. (1975). *Lancet* **1,** 997.
Manley, S. W., Bourke, J. R., and Hawker, R. W. (1974a). *J. Endocrinol.* **61,** 419.
Manley, S. W., Bourke, J. R., and Hawker, R. W. (1974b). *J. Endocrinol.* **61,** 437.
Marchalonis, J. J. (1975). *Science* **190,** 20.
Mehdi, S. Q., Nussey, S. S., Gibbons, C. P., and El Kabir, D. J. (1973). *Biochem. Soc. Trans.* **1,** 1005.
Murray, M. R. (1958). *In* "Biology of Neuroglia" (W. F. Windle, ed.), pp. 176–190 Thomas, Springfield, Ill.
Myers, L. W., Ellison, G. W., Fewster, M. E., and Wolfgram, F. (1975). *Arch. Neurol.* (*Chicago*) **32,** 354.
Natvig, J. B., Gaarder, P. I., and Turner, M. W. (1972). *Clin. Exp. Immunol.* **12,** 177.
Nerup, J., Andersen, O. O., Bendixen, G., Egeberg, J., and Poulsen, J. E. (1971). *Diabetes* **20,** 424.
Okamoto, H., Noto, Y., Miyamoto, S., Mabuchi, H., and Takeda, R. (1975). *FEBS Lett.* **54,** 103.
Paterson, P. Y. (1969). *Annu. Rev. Med.* **20,** 75.
Patrick, J., and Lindstrom, J. M. (1973). *Science* **180,** 871.
Raine, C. S., Hummelgard, A., Swanson, E., and Bornstein, M. B. (1973). *J. Neurol. Sci.* **20,** 127.
Ramseier, H. (1973). *Curr. Top. Microbiol. Immunol.* **60,** 31.
Scott, J. S. (1976). *Lancet* **1,** 78.
Seybold, M. E., Lambert, E. H., Lennon, V. A., and Lindstrom, J. M. (1976). *Ann. N.Y. Acad. Sci.* **274,** 275.

Shishiba, Y., Shimizu, T., Yoshimura, S., and Shizume, K. (1973). *J. Clin. Endocrinol. Metab.* **36,** 517.

Shiu, R. P. C., and Friesen, H. G. (1976). *Science* **192,** 259.

Simpson, J. A. (1960). *Scott. Med. J.* **5,** 419.

Smith, B. R., and Hall, R. (1974). *Lancet* **2,** 427.

Sonninen, V., Riekkinen, R., and Rinne, U. K. (1973). *Neurology* **23,** 760.

Steinberg, A. G., Rushforth, N. B., Bennett, P. H., Burch, T. A., and Miller, M. (1970). *Pathog. Diabetes Mellitus, Proc., Nobel Symp., 13th, 1969* p. 237.

Strayer, D. S., Cosenza, H., Lee, W. M. F., Rowley, D. A., and Kohler, H. (1974). *Science* **186,** 640.

Strickland, R. G., and Mackay, I. R. (1973). *Am. J. Dig. Dis.* **18,** 426.

Sugiyama, H., Benda, P., Meunier, J.-C., and Changeux, J.-P. (1973). *FEBS Lett.* **35,** 124.

Tarrab-Hazdai, R., Aharonov, A., Silman, I., Fuchs, S., and Abramsky, O. (1975). *Nature* (*London*) **256,** 128.

Thomsen, M., Platz, P., Andersen, O. O., Christy, M., Lyngsoe, J., Nerup, J., Rasmussen, K., Ryder, L. P., Nielsen, L., and Svejgaard, A. (1975). *Transplant. Rev.* **22,** 125.

Tomazic, V., Rose, N. R., and Shreffler, D. C. (1974). *J. Immunol.* **112,** 965.

Toyka, K. V., Dracham, D. B., Pestronk, A., and Kao, I. (1975). *Science* **190,** 397.

Ungar, B., Stocks, A. E., Martin, F. I. R., Whittingham, S., and Mackay, I. R. (1968). *Lancet* **2,** 415.

Vanhaelst, L., Bonnyns, M., Ermans, A. M., and Bastenie, P. A. (1972). *In* "Thyroiditis and Thyroid Function" (P. A. Bastenie and A. M. Ermans, eds.), pp. 303–315. Pergamon, Oxford.

Waller, M. (1973). *Am. J. Med.* **54,** 731.

White, S. R., White, F. P., Barnes, C. D., and Albright, J. F. (1973). *Brain Res.* **52,** 251.

Whittingham, S., Mathews, J. D., Mackay I. R., Stocks, A. E., Ungar, B., and Martin, F. I. R. (1971). *Lancet* **1,** 763.

Whittingham, S., Morris, P. J., and Martin, F. I. R. (1975a). *Tissue Antigens* **6,** 23.

Whittingham, S., Youngchaiyud, U., Mackay, I. R., Buckley, J. D., and Morris, P. J. (1975b). *Clin. Exp. Immunol.* **19,** 289.

Wick, G., Sundick, R. S., and Albini, B. (1974). *Clin. Immunol. Immunopathol.* **3,** 272.

NOTE ADDED IN PRINT

We draw attention to the following recently published papers relevant to this Chapter. Engel et al (1977, *Lancet* **1,** 1310) describe the presence of acetyl choline receptor on human thymic epithelial cells. Irvine (1977, *Lancet* **1,** 638) introduces a new classification of diabetes, Type 1 (with subtypes a-c) for the former juvenile-onset type and Type 2 for the former maturity-onset type. Weinstock et al (1977), *Brain*

Res. **125,** 192) report that, in guinea pigs with EAE, neuronal receptors for serotonin in the ileum show evidence of block, and Schauf et al (1976, *J. Neurol. Neurosurg. Psychiat.* **39,** 680) find the sera from animals with EAE and patients with multiple sclerosis produce a significant decrease in the ventral root response in preparations of isolated spinal cord.

Chapter 21

Autoantibodies to the Thyrotropin (TSH) Receptors on Thyroid Epithelium and Other Tissues

DEBORAH DONIACH AND
NICHOLAS J. MARSHALL

I. INTRODUCTION

Thyrotoxicosis is the first example of a "primary" autoimmune disorder where antibodies appear to be directed against a specific hormone receptor, activate cell metabolism and cause the symptoms and signs of the disease (Adams, 1976). It is generally accepted that thyroid-stimulating antibodies

(TSAb) closely mimic TSH and, after binding to the cell surface, initiate the molecular events that lead to stimulation of adenyl cyclase and synthesis of the second metabolic messenger cAMP. However, recent studies suggest that there is considerable diversity in the mode of interaction between immunoglobulins and the hormone receptor, such that the characteristics of binding need not be directly related to stimulation of adenyl cyclase and hormone production. This might be expected due to the extensive range of antibody species produced in polyclonal immune responses, and it probably explains why some TSH receptor antibodies are human specific, while others cross-react with other species, and also why some interact preferentially with TSH-sensitive sites on tissues outside the thyroid gland itself.

II. CLINICAL BACKGROUND

A. Definition of Autoimmune Thyroid Disease

Graves' disease should be considered with the other two syndromes involved in thyroid autoimmunity, i.e., Hashimoto's thyroiditis and primary myxedema, despite their very different clinical presentations. Briefly, Hashimoto's disease may be defined as a diffuse destructive inflammatory lesion with enlargement of the thyroid gland, due to simultaneous loss and regeneration of thyroid epithelium, resulting in high titers of antibodies to microsomal, thyroglobulin, and other thyroid-specific antigens (Doniach and Roitt, 1975). In primary myxedema, these antibodies can be detected in low titers, and the gland is similarly infiltrated with immunocytes, but the stimulus to formation of new acini is lacking, and the gland atrophies. In time, both conditions lead to gradual hormonal failure.

In Graves' disease, there are always traces of the microsomal antibodies typical of autoimmune thyroiditis, which are cytotoxic to thyroid cells in monolayer cultures in the presence of complement (Mori and Kriss, 1971), and foci of lymphocytic thyroiditis are seen in most glands removed at operation. However, the main feature is a diffuse hyperplasia and overgrowth of the acinar tissue and marked overproduction of the thyroid hormones, L-thyroxine (T_4) and L-triiodothyronine (T_3). These features are now considered to be due to the presence of thyroid-stimulating antibodies, which interact specifically with receptors for TSH, as mentioned above, and reproduce more or less closely the actions of this pituitary hormone. The two main extra thyroidal manifestations of Graves' disease, endocrine exophthalmos and pretibial myxedema, are probably due to related but distinct antibodies that interact with TSH receptors in retroorbital or subcutaneous tissues.

B. Overlap between the Three Thyroid Autoimmume Syndromes

The three thyroid autoimmune diseases are closely interlinked in that they occur in the same families (Hall and Stanbury, 1967; Hall *et al.*, 1972), one or other may be seen in identical twins (Doniach *et al.*, 1967), and the conditions may develop concurrently or sequentially in the same individual. These intricate relationships are understandable in terms of intermittent activation and subjugation of related abnormal clones directed against a variety of thyroid components. The most common transition is from a Hashimoto goiter to thyroid atrophy. Over half these goiters disappear completely under T_4 replacement or rarely, spontaneously, and the gland is then functionally and structurally indistinguishable from that of primary myxedema. In other words, the stimulus to thyroid epithelial regeneration appears to diminish with time in these patients, though it is not attributable to a raised TSH.

In Graves' disease, hyperthyroidism progresses to myxedema spontaneously after some years in about 10% of cases. This can be deduced from the follow-up of patients before the advent of specific therapy in the form of thyroidectomy, radioiodine ablation, or anti-thyroid drug treatment. More rarely, thyrotoxicosis and a diffuse goitrous thyroiditis coexist (Doniach *et al.*, 1960), and the condition is inelegantly referred to as "hashitoxicosis" (Buchanan *et al.*, 1962). Less frequently still, a patient with a classical euthyroid Hashimoto goiter may develop unequivocal Graves' disease with exophthalmos, requiring several therapeutic doses of ^{131}I to attain remission. Cases of severe endocrine exophthalmos (ophthalmic Graves') are not infrequently seen in combination with a Hashimoto goiter or with thyroid atrophy, although more often exophthalmic patients have had an episode of thyroid overactivity in the past. The rarest sequence in a single individual is the transition from primary myxedema to thyrotoxicosis. Although in the past this would have been unexpected, there are now several authentic instances on record (Bremner and Griep, 1976).

Spontaneous exacerbations and remissions are a classical feature of thyrotoxicosis, and prolonged follow-up of Hashimoto goiters suggests a similar tendency, as judged by large fluctuations in the titers of microsomal antibodies found in some cases on repeated testing over a period of years. Permanent remissions of hyperthyroidism are observed in over half the thyrotoxic patients given one or more courses of anti-thryoid drugs

(McLarty *et al.*, 1971; Alexander *et al.*, 1973). It seems that clones that synthesize TSAb reacting with a cell-surface antigen are subdued more easily than those reacting with intracellular components such as thyroglobulin or thyroid microsomes.

If Jerne's (1973) network theory of the immune responses can be substantiated, it will be easier to understand the spontaneous fluctuations in the clinical activity and in TSAb's in Graves' disease. This theory suggests that forbidden clones of lymphocytes making antibodies against self-antigens are constantly attacked by other clones with anti-idiotypic specificity.

III. PATHOGENESIS OF THYROTOXICOSIS

A. Thyroid-Stimulating Antibodies: Action *In Vivo*

Until recently, TSH receptor antibodies were detected by bioassays, each of which measured different parameters and may have detected separate species of antibodies. The bioassays reflected both binding to the receptor and the molecular events leading to hormone secretion. Now that specific attachment to thyroid membranes can be detected by displacement of TSH and distinguished from activation of adenyl cyclase and intermediary metabolism, such as ^{32}P incorporation into phospholipids or eventual hormone synthesis, it is evident that some antibodies bind to the receptor but do not activate the cell, and, furthermore, some bind only to human cells, while others cross-react with animal cells. The study of antibodies that block adenyl cyclase has only just begun and already promises to reveal different points of blockade. The fact that the same serum may contain all these species of antibodies concurrently or sequentially is a further complication. Published work was frequently done with selected high titer sera that were more likely to contain an array of distinct antibodies with differing biologic effects.

Thyroid-stimulating antibodies will be discussed as two groups: (1) those which appear to act solely on the human thyroid, termed human thyroid stimulators (HTS), LATS protectors (LATS-P) (Adams and Kennedy, 1967, 1971), and human thyroid adenyl cyclase stimulators (HTACS) (Orgiazzi *et al.*, 1976) and (2) those which react with other species, and are termed mouse thyroid stimulators (MTS), since they are measured in a mouse bioassay and probably belong to the group of antibodies referred to previously as long-acting thyroid stimulators (LATS). This division is an oversimplification, and future work will undoubtedly show that a more graduated classification is required (see McKenzie and Zakarija, 1976).

1. *Human Thyroid-Stimulating Antibodies* (HTS, LATS-P, or HTACS)

The presence of TSAb specific for the human thyroid was first suggested by the observations that (1) only 20–40% of thyrotoxic sera could be demonstrated to stimulate thyroid activity in mouse bioassay systems, and (2) mouse thyroid-stimulating activity could be absorbed out by incubation with human thyroid homogenate, but if the homogenate was first incubated with an MTS-negative thyrotoxic serum, MTS activity remained undiminished. This phenomenon was explained as due to binding of HTS to the human tissue, which resulted in "protection" of MTS against absorption, i.e., blocking of the antigenic site, and, consequently, the HTS was initially named "LATS protector" (LATS-P), the method forming the basis of assay for its presence in a given serum.

HTS has been reported present in approaching 100% of thyrotoxic patients (Adams *et al.*, 1974a), and we will discuss later in depth the evidence that HTS interacts with the TSH receptor in human thyroid cells and mimics TSH in the stimulation of thyroid activity *in vitro*.

The "protection" offered by a given thyrotoxic serum against absorption of MTS activity in the "protector assay" correlated with parameters of hyperthyroidism, such as the 20-minute ^{131}I uptake, or the 1-hour plasma clearance rate in thyrotoxic patients (Adams *et al.*, 1974a). Moreover, when injected into euthyroid volunteers (Adams *et al.*, 1974b), a discharge of iodinated proteins into the circulation, similar to the mouse response to LATS, was observed. Further evidence for the bioactivity of HTS is the occurrence of neonatal thyrotoxicosis. This is due to transplacental passage of HTS, such that babies born of mothers with high levels of TSAb, as estimated in the "protector assay" may show the features of Graves' disease (Dirmikis *et al.*, 1974; Dirmikis and Munro, 1975). The duration of the symptoms (4–6 weeks) is consistent with the half-life of the immunoglobulins.

Immunoglobulins prepared from thyrotoxic sera have been reported to displace TSH bound to partially purified preparations of plasma membranes from guinea pig (Manley *et al.*, 1974) and human (Smith and Hall, 1974) thyroid tissue. This phenomenon forms the basis of a detection system for such immunoglobulins frequently referred to as the radioligand assay, which will be discussed in greater detail later. Since specificity for interaction between human, as opposed to beef, mouse, or guinea pig thyroid, can be demonstrated in this system (Hall *et al.*, 1975), and, since there is evidence that a response in this assay may be associated with thyroid stimulation (Clague *et al.*, 1976), the relationship between Ig's that displace bound TSH and those measured as human-specific TSAb in the protector assay is currently a subject of close investigation. The radioligand test with membranes from human thyroid should prove a convenient *in vitro* assay suitable for large-scale screening studies. Another *in vitro* detection system for HTS, the stimulation of colloid droplets in human thyroid slices, has been described (Shishiba *et al.*, 1973; Onaya *et al.*, 1973) and will be discussed later.

2. *Mouse Thyroid-Stimulating Antibodies* (MTS or LATS)

Using a guinea pig bioassay for TSH, Adams and Purves (1956) noted that thyrotoxic sera provoked a delayed and prolonged response (the release of ^{131}I from the prelabeled guinea pig thyroid compared with TSH). The stimulator present in thyrotoxic sera was termed long-acting thyroid stimulator (LATS).

This assay, with several modifications (Chopra *et al.*, 1970), remains in use today, and is, in brief, as follows: IgG is injected intravenously into mice that have been pretreated with T_4 and ^{131}I, and plasma radioactivity is measured after specific time intervals—for example 2, 7, and 24 hours. Normal Ig, like saline, produces no significant increase in plasma ^{131}I, but, after bovine TSH, this response peaks at 2–3 hours, declining to control values by 7 hours. However, some thyrotoxic Ig preparations result in prolonged stimulation, blood radioactivity rising at 7 hours with no sign of decline at 24 hours. Considerable variation in the magnitude of the response is observed, ranging from sera requiring concentration before a response is obtained to those which induce a 20-fold increase, necessitating predilution for accurate determinations.

The frequency of detection of LATS in thyrotoxicosis (generally about 40%, but rising to 60–80% after 12-fold Ig concentration) tends to vary with the strain of mice used and the preinjection regimen, certain strains giving more consistent and reproducible results. It has been commonly reported that highest levels are seen in patients with progressive exophthalmos and pretibial myxedema, who may require thyroid ablation by surgery and several doses of radioiodine to achieve remission.

In vitro procedures, such as those based on stimulation of colloid droplet formation (Shishiba *et al.*, 1970, 1973) or displacement of bound TSH (Hall *et al.*, 1975) may be used to detect immunoglobulins that interact with the mouse thyroid, but as with HTS, the exact nature of the relationship between Ig's provoking responses in these assays has yet to be determined (see, for example, Schleusener *et al.*, 1976).

LATS was found to be an IgG soon after its initial discovery (Kriss *et al.*, 1964) and it has been shown to be synthesized in lymph nodes and blood lymphocytes cultured in the presence of phytohemagglutinin (Wall *et al.*, 1973). LATS–IgG is polyclonal, as are other anti-thyroid antibodies. However, Lonergan *et al.* (1973) claimed a certain degree of homogeneity following an isoelectric-focusing procedure. Papain digestion of LATS–IgG into Fab and Fc fragments showed the biologic activity to reside in the Fab portion and to produce a short-acting response similar to TSH in the bioassay (Dorrington *et al.*, 1966; Burke, 1969a). Molecular dissection into H and L chains (Meek *et al.*, 1964; Smith, 1969) demonstrated the main antigen-binding site to be associated with the H chain, since reconstitution of the latter with L chains derived from control IgG produced a bioactive antibody. LATS bioactivity was neutralized with anti-IgG, but anti-TSH was without effect, suggesting that LATS–IgG does not require to be bound to TSH to exert thyroid stimulation (see McKenzie, 1974; Beall *et al.*, 1973).

As mentioned previously, LATS activity can be absorbed out or "neutralized" with subcellular fractions enriched in plasma membranes prepared from the thyroid (Beall *et al.*, 1969a), and, interestingly, on a tissue weight basis, the human thyroid appears to be more effective in this respect than the mouse (Shishiba *et al.*, 1972). After absorption, LATS can be eluted using either low pH or high salt concentrations, and several groups have attempted LATS purification by this means. However, although 10 to 20-fold concentration of LATS activity was achieved, persistent contamination with anti-thyroglobulin and anti-microsomal IgG's thwarted attempts to develop a radioligand assay, using iodinated purified LATS, toegether with thyroid membrane preparations, as the binding agent (Wong and Litman, 1969; Pinchera *et al.*, 1970).

Evidence that some LATS–IgG's do not stimulate the human thyroid has been slow to accumulate, particularly since LATS-P is invariably present in LATS-positive sera take from hyperthyroid cases, and LATS itself binds to human thyroid tissue. However, LATS has been detected in euthyroid relatives of thyrotoxic cases (Wall *et al.*, 1969) and in some patients with exophthalmos who have T_3-suppressible iodine uptakes (Chopra and Solomon, 1970). These authors cited a case with a high LATS response for several years while euthyroid, but who later became thyrotoxic. Also, recent work has shown that parameters of hyperactivity do not correlate with LATS levels (Adams, 1976) and that patients may go into prolonged remissions despite a strongly positive mouse bioassay (Henneman *et al.*, 1975). Moreover, temporal changes in antibody specificity occur, and McKenzie cites examples of patients who presented with LATS-positive thyrotoxicosis but, subsequently, changed to LATS negative in the face of continued hyperthyroidism (McKenzie, 1972). The positive correlation between human adenyl cyclase stimulation and LATS responses found by

Orgiazzi *et al.* (1976) in 11 treated thyrotoxics could have been due to the simultaneous presence of HTS and MTS in the sera.

B. Thyroid-Stimulating Antibodies: Action *In Vitro*

1. Interaction with Membrane Receptor/Adenyl Cyclase Systems

From these observations on TSAb activation of the gland *in vivo*, it is clearly pertinent to question the mechanisms of action of these antibodies as studied in *in vitro* systems and, in particular, to compare immunoglobulin stimulation with that obtained by TSH.

Since the first report of a thyroidal adenyl cyclase system responsive to TSH (Klainer *et al.*, 1962), much evidence has accumulated that stimulation of thyroid cell metabolism and thyroid hormone production, in particular, is mediated via a hormone receptor/adenyl cyclase system (for reviews, see Schell-Frederick and Dumont, 1970; Dumont, 1971). TSH has been demonstrated to bind to receptors located on the surface of the cell, and the binding has been related to subsequent stimulation of adenyl cyclase (Lissitzky *et al.*, 1975; Tate *et al.*, 1975a,b; Winand and Kohn, 1975b; Goldfine *et al.*, 1976; for review, see Marshall, 1976). Binding is reversible, specific, and of high affinity, consistent with the suggestion that interaction between the hormone and its physiological receptor is being observed. At present, detailed kinetic parameters are subject to dispute, but we anticipate that future studies will reveal that the conflicts stem mainly from the different methodologies employed and do not necessarily invalidate the physiological relevance of the observations reported.

Technical difficulties, at present, preclude the direct demonstration of TSAb binding to receptors located on the surface of the thyroid, and binding is inferred from the observation that Ig's derived from LATS-positive sera displace bound TSH. Manley *et al.* (1974) reported displacement of TSH bound to membranes prepared from the guinea pig thyroid, and, subsequently, others (Mehdi *et al.*, 1974; Smith and Hall, 1974; Mehdi and Nussey, 1975; Mehdi, 1975; Mukhtar *et al.*, 1975; Hall *et al.*, 1975; Marshall *et al.*, 1976) demonstrated displacement from membranes and solubilized receptor preparations obtained from human thyroids. Hall *et al.* (1975) claim a frequency of detection of immunoglobulins that displace TSH bound to human membranes approaching 100% in active Graves' disease. Moreover, studies with nonhuman thyroid tissue indicate that immunoglobulins show considerable species specificity in this respect. However, Mehdi and Nussey (1975) found several Graves' sera, which were both LATS negative and failed to significantly displace TSH bound to human thyroid membranes, and, more recently, Schleusener *et al.* (1976) reported LATS-positive sera which were negative in the displacement assay. Bryson *et al.* (1976) detected greater than normal TSH displacement by immunoglobulin fractions from 21 of 45 Graves' sera. Thus, further work is necessary before the frequency in Graves' sera of immunoglobulins that displace bound TSH may be regarded as established.

As discussed above, displacement of TSH bound to human thyroid membranes is currently used in several laboratories as a clinical assay to detect immunoglobulins directed against a component associated with the TSH receptor. However, such displacement cannot be correlated with overall activation of the gland without testing at the same time for stimulation of some intermediate metabolic process, such as adenyl cyclase activation. The latter has been demonstrated by several groups in both human and nonhuman thyroid tissue preparations, although, once again, estimates of the frequency of detection have varied greatly (for review, see Marshall, 1976; Orgiazzi *et al.*, 1976; McKenzie and Zakarija, 1976; Smith, 1976). Restricting observations to immunoglobulins prepared from one thyrotoxic serum, Manley *et al.* (1974) reported stimulation of enzymatic activity in guinea pig thyroid which correlated with displacement of bound TSH. More recently Hall *et al.* (1975) reported correlation between displacement of TSH from human thyroid tissue and stimulation of adenyl cyclase for a series of Graves' sera.

The relationship between receptor/adenyl cyclase systems in the thyroid plasma membrane, responsive to TSH and TSAb, is at present uncertain. One must clearly question whether the antibody is directed against the TSH receptor or against another membrane component remote from this receptor, which subsequently interacts with it and results in displacement of bound hormone. Yamashita and Field (1972) reported a particular TSAb that inhibited the response of adenyl cyclase to TSH. The apparently noncompetitive nature of this inhibition would appear to argue against a simple model whereby the antibody binds reversibly to the hormone receptor, but it is possible that a relatively slow dissociation rate of the antibody from the receptor necessitated more detailed kinetic analysis to reveal competitive inhibition. It should also be remembered that stimulation of adenyl cyclase is a multistep process, and it is possible that competitive inhibition of binding might be masked by noncompetitive inhibition of the transduction process. The failure of Manley *et al.* (1974) to detect an antibody–TSH-receptor triple complex, following chromatographic analysis of solubilized receptor preparations which revealed hormone receptor and antibody receptor complexes, suggests that a model whereby the antibody binds to a site on the receptor remote from TSH, resulting in conformational changes of the complex that lead to displacement of TSH, does not apply. This, of course, assumes that any triple complex which might have formed was not degraded during the chromatographic analysis.

Orgiazzi *et al.* (1976) studied the relationship between the effect of TSH and TSAb on adenyl cyclase stimulation in crude human thyroid membranes and found great heterogeneity in the behavior of different thyrotoxic IgG's. Some gave dose-response curves parallel to TSH, and the only difference was a slight delay in the onset of adenyl cyclase stimulation with the antibodies and a more prolonged effect. When submaximal amounts of TSH were used, the effect of the antibodies was additive, though no further stimulation occurred when TSH stimulation reached its plateau. These features suggest that the antibodies react with the TSH receptor itself. However, two IgG's inhibited the adenyl cyclase stimulation produced by another TSAb, and one, obtained from the same LATS-positive patient studied by Yamashita and Field (1972) and discussed above, in addition, inhibited the adenyl cyclase stimulation produced by TSH. Such blocking antibodies could account for the negative results obtained with some Ig's from untreated thyrotoxics as suggested by Orgiazzi *et al.* (1976).

Thus, it now looks as if the TSAb's interact directly with the TSH receptor, and the heterogeneity of responses in either the radioligand assay or adenyl cyclase stimulation is consistent with interactions with different epitopic sites. If this model is valid, it should be possible to produce TSAb's experimentally *in vivo* by injecting animals with a purified preparation of solubilized TSH receptors, and to obtain thyrotoxic animals. Previous attempts to induce thyrotoxicosis were inconclusive, as injection of crude microsomal fractions gave rise to autoimmune thyroiditis in the rabbit (Beall and Solomon, 1968; Solomon and Beall, 1968; McKenzie, 1968; Beall *et al.*, 1969a,b). More recently, Ong *et al.* (1976) immunized rabbits with purified bovine thyroid plasma membranes and obtained an IgG capable of stimulating adenyl cyclase *in vitro* in these membranes. TSAb production *in vitro* has also been reported, following the culture of circulating lymphocytes from patients with Graves' disease, in the presence of normal human thyroid tissue homogenates (Knox *et al.*, 1976).

2. *Kinetics of Responses to TSAb Versus TSH*

As mentioned previously, stimulation of the thyroid *in vivo* by TSAb shows a delayed peak response compared with TSH. If this is not due to differences in kinetics of delivery or peripheral degradation, one would expect to detect different kinetics of activation in *in vitro* experiments. Moreover, should both agonists act via adenyl cyclase, evidence for delayed activation of this step by TSAb might be expected. At present, delayed responses to TSAb compared with TSH have been reported following experiments with dog thyroid slices (Kaneko *et al.*, 1970), intact mouse thyroid lobes (Kendall-Taylor, 1972), and crude human plasma membrane preparations (Orgiazzi *et al.*, 1976). However, caution is advised in interpretation of such kinetic experiments, since the rate of stimulation would also be expected to vary with dose of agonist applied (Shishiba *et al.*, 1970), and rates should only be compared between what may be considered equivalent doses of each agonist. When potencies of agonists have been determined in response systems remote from the one undergoing investigation, however, "dose equivalence" can be difficult to determine (Ekins, 1976).

Delayed activation by TSAb compared with TSH has also been reported for other intermediate metabolic parameters, such as glucose oxidation and ^{32}P incorporation into phospholipids in sheep and and dog thyroid slices (Scott *et al.*, 1966; Field *et al.*, 1968). Significant stimulation by LATS was generally detected only after 4–5 hours incubation, compared with periods of 2 hours or less for TSH. Moreover, maximum responses seen with increasing doses of the two agonists were always greater for TSH than LATS. Low doses of TSH have been reported to inhibit, rather than stimulate, glucose oxidation in beef thyroid slices (Merlevede *et al.*, 1963), and it is interesting that Field *et al.* (1968) reported that this effect was also observed with LATS. However, besides other temporal distinctions between LATS and TSH action, Scott *et al.* (1966) also reported that, whereas LATS stimulated ^{32}P incorporation into both phosphatidylcholine and phosphatidylinositol, TSH increased incorporation into the latter compound preferentially.

The two reports described above estimated TSH and LATS stimulation of [1-^{14}C]-glucose oxidation 45 minutes after the addition of the agonists. Shishiba *et al.* (1970), using an ionization chamber method to record glucose oxidation, reported significant stimulation by equivalent doses of LATS and TSH after 9 minutes and 12.7 minutes, respectively, i.e., the latent period for LATS was slightly less than that for TSH. Moreover, similar kinetics were reported in this study when stimulation of colloid droplet formation was followed. Burke (1968, 1969b), working with sheep thyroid slices, studying both phospholipogenesis and glucose oxidation, also found no delayed effect of LATS. Further evidence that the *in vitro* effects of LATS are not delayed, compared with TSH, was reported in studies describing stimulation of the release of ^{131}I from prelabeled mouse thyroid lobes maintained under organ culture conditions (Brown and Munro, 1967; Enser *et al.*, 1971). However, using a highly sensitive cytochemical bioassay for TSH, Bitensky *et al.* (1974) and Petersen *et al.* (1975) reported marked delay in response to LATS compared with TSH.

Thus, many of the processes which can be stimulated *in vitro* by TSH can be demonstrated to respond to TSAb, but the relative kinetics of response remains an open question. The specificity of the stimulator can be demonstrated by selective inhibition with anti-TSH or anti-IgG, respectively (Burke, 1969a). As yet, however, the precise relationship between the response to these two agonists is undetermined. Clearly, the effects upon the surface receptors will have to be analyzed for the different types of TSAb, and these will specify the later metabolic events.

It should be mentioned that not all thyroid surface-reacting antibodies appear to be directed against TSH receptors. The antibodies, which Fagraeus and Jonsson (1970) detected by immunofluorescece on suspensions of living thyroid cells or by mixed hemadsorption on monolayer cultures, are found equally in myxedema, Hashimoto's disease, and Graves' disease, and their presence could not be correlated with LATS (Fagraeus *et al.*, 1970). Probably owing to the small number of TSH receptors per cell (estimated at 500), it is unlikely that antibodies to them will be visible by insensitive methods, and, indeed, some sera with extremely high LATS or HTS values show no thyroid cell immunofluorescence staining.

C. TSH Receptor Antibodies in Autoimmune Thyroiditis

There is no difficulty in accepting the coexistence of thyrotoxicosis and thyroiditis. The destruction of some thyroid acini would tend to minimize the overall rise in metabolism produced by TSAb's in patients with the two diseases, but one or the other process may predominate. In ophthalmic Graves' disease, by definition, the patient has the eye signs of thyrotoxicosis but remains euthyroid. If thyroid function is completely normal, the McKenzie assay is usually negative, and results of the radioligand test are not yet available. When the patient is euthyroid but has a flat TRH curve, i.e., the pituitary thyrotrophs are inhibited by a borderline high output of thyroid hormone and the ^{131}I uptake is not suppressible by T_3, the LATS test may be positive. In some ophthalmic cases, there is an associated Hashimoto goiter or a thyroid atrophy with high titers of microsomal and thyroglobulin antibodies, but with positive LATS or a positive radioligand test. It is possible that the degree of cell destruction prevents the expression of the TSAb. Alternatively, the LATS in these cases might be capable of binding to the human TSH receptor without stimulating cell metabolism, as in the euthyroid LATS-positive relatives.

In classical Hashimoto's disease, there is little data on the incidence of LATS. D. J. El Kabir (unpublished) performed the McKenzie test on 12- to 15-fold Ig concentrates in three cases to investigate the cause of the large goiter, but results remained negative. The only positive was in the

Hashimoto twin of a Graves' patient. Hall *et al.* (1975) report 17% of positive radioligand assays in Hashimoto patients, and our experience is similar. Marked displacement of TSH was found in a patient with no hint of present or past toxicity, whose histologically proven Hashimoto goiter responded poorly to T_4 replacement, but who had overactive pituitary thyrotrophs and myxedema when T_4 was stopped.

D. Extrathyroidal Effects of TSAb or Associated Antibodies

TSH has been reported to stimulate metabolic activity in tissues other than the thyroid, namely, adipose and retroorbital tissue (White and Engel, 1958; Freinkel, 1961; Rudman *et al.*, 1963; Kendall-Taylor and Munro, 1971; Hart and McKenzie, 1971; Gospodarowicz, 1973; Kohn and Winand, 1971; Winand and Kohn, 1972, 1975a; Bolonkin *et al.*, 1975). It is clearly pertinent to question whether immunoglobulins that stimulate thyroid function also interact with these extrathyroidal tissues.

Immunoglobulins prepared from sera of patients with Graves' disease have been shown to stimulate lipolysis in isolated rat fat cells (Kendall-Taylor and Munro, 1971) and slices of guinea pig epididymal tissue (Hart and McKenzie, 1971) and to displace TSH bound to crude membrane fractions prepared from guinea pig epididymal fat (Teng *et al.*, 1975). The immunoglobulin stimulation of lipolysis appeared to parallel that due to TSH in many respects, e.g., potentiation by theophylline and T_3 and inhibition by prostaglandin E_1 (Kendall-Taylor and Munro, 1971). Moreover, in one of these studies (Hart and McKenzie, 1971), immunoglobulin stimulation of lipolysis was inhibited after preincubation with a thyroid microsomal preparation, suggesting that the antibodies interacting with TSH receptors on adipose and thyroid tissue were derived from the same population. In this context, it is of interest that Karlberg *et al.* (1974) found a twofold increase in cAMP content in muscle and adipose tissue biopsies taken from thyrotoxic patients. It remains to be determined whether the increased fat mobilization observed in thyrotoxic patients, raised plasma glycerol (Laurel and Tibbling, 1968), and plasma nonesterified fatty acids (Rich *et al.*, 1959) is a direct consequence of the presence of these immunoglobulins. This is perhaps unlikely in view of the reported insensitivity of human adipose tissue to TSH compared with the guinea pig (Raben, 1959; Mosinger *et al.*, 1965) although this has recently been contested (Mullin *et al.*, 1976a). Future studies may have to differentiate between white and brown adipose tissue (BAT), since the latter is now known to be an important thermogenic organ (see Doniach, 1976).

Correlation between reversible and specific binding of TSH to guinea pig harderian gland tissue, and stimulation of adenyl cyclase activity in this retroorbital tissue has been claimed (Winand and Kohn, 1975a). Similar effects were also reported for a pepsin-digested fragment of TSH, referred to as the exophthalmos-producing factor (EPF), which is inactive in the thyroid but capable of producing experimental exophthalmos (Kohn and Winand, 1971, 1975). Immunoglobulins prepared from Graves' sera, when the patient showed no clinical exophthalmos, neither stimulated the retroorbital tissue nor displaced bound TSH or EPF (Winand and Kohn, 1972, 1975a). However, immunoglobulins prepared from patients with exophthalmopathy were shown to increase the binding of TSH and EPF to retroorbital tissue membranes (Winand and Kohn, 1972; Bolonkin *et al.*, 1975; Mullin *et al.*, 1976a), suggesting the presence of exophthalmos-producing antibodies (EPAbs). These were shown to be without stimulating effect on thryoid tissue and are, therefore, considered to be independent from TSAb, which is consistent with clinical observations of eye changes independent of hyperthyroidism. Their mode of action has been suggested to be mainly due to an increase in the number and affinities of receptors on retroorbital tissue responsive to TSH and EPF, and sensitization of the tissue to these polypeptides (Winand and Kohn, 1975a).

Severe endocrine exophthalmos cannot be explained by an single theory that can be formulated in the present state of our knowledge (see Doniach and Florin-Christensen, 1975). Its usual association with Graves' disease or with autoimmune thyroiditis and its irregular exacerbations and remissions are in favor of an autoimmune pathogenesis. The disease has several components varying independently of each other which could be triggered by separate mechanisms. Immunologic phenomena have been put forward to explain two important aspects. One is the myositis involving the periocular muscles, and the other is the increased bulk of retroorbital tissue. These separate phenomena both contribute to the proptosis and raised orbital pressure. Secondary vascular changes play an important role, but will not be discussed.

Myositis of a slight degree apparently exists in most cases of Graves' disease, and lesions sufficient to cause diplopia are not rare. In extreme cases, the muscle fibers are fragmented, there are lymphorrhages and edema between fibers, and the muscle bulk is greatly increased, sometimes leading to rigid immobility of the eye. Kriss *et al.* (1975) believe that this myositis is caused by immune complexes formed between thyroglobulin and thyroglobulin antibodies, which have been shown to have an increased affinity for ocular muscle membranes. Undegraded thyroglobulin is known to be released into the lymphatics in increased amounts from the thyrotoxic gland, especially at thyroidectomy and following radioiodine therapy, and drains upwards during recumbency to a deep preauricular node into which the eye lymphatics drain as well.

Pretibial myxedema and progressive exophthalmos are seen in about 1% of thyrotoxics, although benign eye signs are present in about 50%, and subclinical changes in the periorbital muscles can be demonstrated in almost all cases by ultrasonography (Werner *et al.*, 1974). Patients with dermopathy nearly always show high values in the LATS assay, although many cases may be cited of LATS activity without pretibial myxedema. It is, therefore, likely that stimulation of subcutaneous tissues to produce increased mucopolysaccharide synthesis, and edema is due to a separate Ig which happens to occur in the more severe chronic cases of Graves' disease where LATS is commonly found. Skin biopsies from these lesions have not shown any deposits of immune complexes and could not be stained in the immunofluorescence test with FITC-conjugated LATS–IgG (personal observation). However, we must bear in mind that afinity for LATS and other TSAb's likewise cannot be demonstrated by this method on thyrotoxic thyroid sections or on the surface of isolated living thyroid cells, probably because of the relatively small number of TSH receptor molecules per cell.

There are some interesting experimental results which suggest that LATS–IgG stimulates the mouse adrenal cortex (El Kabir and Hockaday, 1969; El Kabir *et al.*, 1971) and even increases the permeability of *Escherichia coli* membranes (Mehdi *et al.*, 1971). The heterogeneity of autoantibodies to the same or closely related receptor molecules is such that the same serum may contain, not only LATS and HTS, but also EPAb's, dermotrophic Ab's, and other unidentified species of stimulating IgG which cannot be separated except by correlating all these metabolic parameters on a large number of sera. The work on the adrenal cortex is particularly interesting because the degree of stimulation was proportional to the LATS levels, and TSH itself had no effect on the mouse adrenal, suggesting the existence of chemical similarities between TSH and ACTH receptors detected by these autoantibodies.

E. Hypothetical TSAb

In the foregoing sections, we have discussed the substantial *in vivo* and *in vitro* evidence for immunoglobulins which stimulate thyroid hormone production. We would also like to discuss evidence for extending the concept to include those which stimulate thyroid growth, rather than hormone synthesis [thyroid growth antibodies (TGAb)]. At present, we can cite mainly clinical observations in support of this hypothesis.

As already mentioned, the significant difference between goitrous and atrophic autoimmune thyroiditis is the continuous regeneration of thyroid tissue in the goitrous variants. HTS and LATS are only rarely detected in

Hashimoto's disease. Pituitary TSH cannot explain the goitrogenesis, since the level rises only after the onset of hypothyroidism (El Kabir *et al.*, 1963). Treatment with T_4 usually leads to reduction in goiter size, and this happens more quickly in hypothyroid cases through suppression of pituitary TSH. Some proven Hashimoto goiters remain large after high dosage T_4 replacement with undetectable TSH, and some of these could have TGAb's.

In Graves' disease, it is possible that the presence of TGAb, where levels may vary independently from TSAb, explains the frequently observed lack of correlation between thyroid size and thyroid function. For example, it is common knowledge that 2–10% of thyrotoxics have no goiter, yet may have a high output of thyroid hormones, and, conversely, other cases develop a large goiter with only slight or moderate toxicity (Adams *et al.*, 1974a). Moreover, recently we have described a new variant of euthyroid Graves' disease, which may well be explicable in terms of TGAb's (Doniach *et al.*, 1977). We have observed five women who had close relatives with autoimmune thyroid disease who developed a diffuse goiter in adolescence which was nonresponsive to T_4. Iodine uptake levels were high, but suppressible with T_3 and TSH was both low and did not rise in response to TRH. The radioligand test was negative. These cases have been followed for up to 12 years and, throughout, have remained with T_3 and T_4 values lying in the normal range, and minimal physical signs reminiscent of thyrotoxicosis, such as staring gaze or a tendency to sweating. Such cases of euthyroid goiter might be caused by TGAb. In patients with endocrine exophthalmos, the TRH test has allowed distinction of subclinical hyperthyroidism, and cases with goiters behaving as in the five patients described might exist in association with eye signs.

At present, there is no *in vitro* evidence for TGAb's, but differentiation between TSH stimulation of thyroid growth and function has been observed (Tata, 1976). Winand and Kohn (1975b) reported that TSH could be observed to have a trophic effect on thyroid cells seeded to grow as a nonconfluent culture, without accompanying stimulation of structural or functional differentiation, but, since the timing of the presence of bioactive TSH in confluent cultures is critical to commitment to cell differentiation, this observation with nonconfluent cultures could be explained as due to lack of bioactive TSH when confluence is finally achieved, because of degradation during the prolonged period of culture. Moreover, TSH is thought to control metabolic processes such as ^{32}P incorporation into phospholipids in a manner which is independent of changes in intracellular cAMP, providing alternative response systems such as modulation via calcium ions and/or cGMP (Van Sande *et al.*, 1975) which could be linked to cell growth, rather than to hormone production. In this context, it may be relevant that several groups (e.g., Moore and Wolf, 1974; Kotani *et al.*, 1975) have interpreted the results of TSH-binding studies to indicate the presence of two species of TSH receptor. Future *in vitro* studies with immunoglobulins derived from the variant of euthyroid Graves' disease described above are clearly necessary to test what at present can only be considered a hypothesis.

IV. CONCLUSIONS

It is now generally accepted that, in patients with autoimmune thyroid disease, there is a family of autoantibodies reacting with a thyroid cell-surface component identical or closely associated with the TSH receptor. These can be stimulating, i.e., TSAb, when they can be either human specific or cross-reactive with other species and, at times, closely mimic TSH. The exact epitope within the TSH receptor site will determine characteristics of action of a given antibody, such as its binding affinity, the potency for subsequent stimulation of adenyl cyclase, whether the antibodies react preferentially with receptors located in membranes derived from thyroid gland, adipose cells, or retroorbital tissues, and whether species specificity is observed. If the antibodies are able to initiate the transduction process which culminates in stimulation of adenyl cyclase, the end result will lead to increased thyroid hormone production, but, as discussed, a given antibody might stimulate anabolic events including cell growth, rather than hormone secretion, independently of cAMP mediation. It is now obvious that several biologic parameters must be measured in order to distinguish between various antibodies occurring together in the serum and to perfect membrane and tissue culture assays.

Prior to solving the detailed molecular mechanisms operating between TSAb and TSH receptors, it will be useful to obtain more detailed knowledge of those acting between the receptor and TSH. Recent studies emphasize the importance of TSH–ganglioside interaction, analogous to those observed with choleratoxin, and suggest that gangliosidelike structures form a component of what may be regarded as the TSH receptor, isolated in a solubilized form (Mullin *et al.*, 1976b,c). However, TSH interaction with membranes also depends on the lipid environment of the receptor, as shown by studies with fluorescence probes (Bashford *et al.*, 1975). Since hormone binding is a discrete process that can be distinguished from subsequent cellular activation, it might be anticipated that antibodies blocking the binding process could be more frequently observed than those such as TSAb, which both interact at receptor level and cause subsequent stimulation. In this context, the antibodies which block the acetylcholine receptors in neuromuscular junctions in myasthenia gravis are of special interest (see Mittag *et al.*, 1976). Another example is the antibodies which block the insulin receptor on peripheral cells in rare cases of insulin-resistant diabetes mellitus (Kahn *et al.*, 1976). Interestingly, this disease is associated with acanthosis nigricans, which represents an overgrowth of some layers in stratified epithelium and could possibly turn out to be due to epithelial growth antibodies mimicking the epithelial growth factor. Moreover, Flier *et al.* (1976) have recently described anti-insulin-receptor antisera which mimicked insulin stimulation of glucose oxidation on rat adipocytes. The next era in the study of autoimmune disorders will be, therefore, more clearly directed towards the study of interactions between membrane antigens and antibodies than in the past, revealing as yet unrecognized cell-stimulating Ig's, as well as those producing "immunopharmacologic blockade" (Lennon and Carnegie, 1971) as discussed by Carnegie and Mackay (1975). The latter postulate that membrane components should prove more autoantigenic, since they are readily available to unrepressed lymphocytes. On the other hand, as discussed recently (Singer, 1974; Raff, 1976), detailed analysis of lymphoid cell interactions will undoubtedly contribute to knowledge regarding autoantibodies to hormone receptors.

Thus, the interaction between TSAb and the TSH receptor present an excellent example of hormone/receptor/immunoglobulin interactions from which we hope to gain further insight into the molecular basis of autoimmunity and, conversely, the mechanisms of hormonal stimulation of target cells.

REFERENCES

Adams, D. D. (1976). *In* "Immunology in Medicine" (J. Holborow and W. G. Reeves, eds.), Chapter 12. Academic Press (in press).

Adams, D. D., and Kennedy, T. H. (1967). *J. Clin. Endocrinol. Metab.* **27,** 173–177.

Adams, D. D., and Kennedy, T. H. (1971). *J. Clin. Endocrinol. Metab.* **33,** 47–51.

Adams, D. D., and Purves, H. D. (1956). *Proc. Univ. Otago Med. Sch.* **34,** 11–12.

Adams, D. D., Kennedy, T. H., and Stewart, R. D. H. (1974a). *Br. Med. J.* **2,** 193–201.

Adams, D. D., Fastier, F. N., Howie, J. B., Kennedy, T. H. Kilpatrick, J. A., and Stewart, R. D. H. (1974b). *J. Clin. Endocrinol. Metab.* **39,** 826–832.

Alexander, W. D., McLarty, D. G., and Horten, P. (1973). *Clin. Endocrinol.* (*Oxford*) **2,** 43–50.

Bashford, C. L., Harrison, S. J., Radda, G. K., and Mehdi, Q. (1975). *Biochem. J.* **146,** 473–479.

Beall, G. N., and Solomon, D. H. (1968). *J. Clin. Endocrinol. Metab.* **28,** 503–510.

Beall, G. N., Doniach, D., Roitt, I. M., and El Kabir, D. J. (1969a). *J. Lab. Clin. Med.* **73,** 988–999.

Beall, G. N., Daniel, P. M., Pratt, O. E., and Solomon, D. H. (1969b). *J. Clin. Endocrinol. Metab.*, **29,** 1460–1469.

Beall, G. N., Chopra, I. J., Solomon, D. H., Pierce, J. G., and Cornell, J. S. (1973). *J. Clin. Invest.* **52,** 2979–2985.

Bitensky, L., Alaghband-Zadeh, D., and Chayen, J. (1974). *Clin. Endocrinol.* (*Oxford*) **3,** 363–374.

Bolonkin, D., Tate, R. L., Luber, J. H., Kohn, L. D., and Winand, R. J. (1975). *J. Biol. Chem.* **250,** 6516–6521.

Bremner, W. J., and Griep, R. J. (1976). *J. Am. Med. Assoc.* **235,** 1361–1362.

Brown, J. and Munro, D. S. (1967). *J. Endocrinol.* **38,** 439–449.

Bryson, J. M., Joasoo, A., and Turtle, J. R. (1976). *Acta Endocrinol.* **83,** 528–538.

Buchanan, W. W., Koutras, D. A., Crooks, J., Alexander, W. D., Brass, W., Anderson, J. K., Goudie, R. B., and Gray, K. G. (1962). *J. Endocrinol.* **24,** 115–125.

Burke, G. (1968). *Endocrinology* **83,** 1210–1216.

Burke, G. (1969a). *Endocrinology* **84,** 1063–1070.

Burke, G. (1969b). *Metab., Clin. Exp.* **18,** 132–140.

Carnegie, P. R., and MacKay, I. R. (1975). *Lancet* **2,** 684–687.

Chopra, J. I., and Solomon, D. H. (1970). *Ann. Intern. Med.* **73,** 985–990.

Chopra, J. I., Solomon, D. H., and Lindberg, N. P. (1970). *J. Clin. Endocrinol. Metab.* **31,** 382–390.

Claugue, R., Mukhtar, E. D., Pyle, G. A., Nutt, J., Clark, F., Scott, M., Evered, D., Rees-Smith, B., and Hall, R. (1976). *J. Clin. Endocrinol.* **43,** 550–556.

Dirmikis, S. M., and Munro, D. S. (1975). *Br. Med. J.* **2,** 665–666.

Dirmikis, S. M., Munro, D. J., Hiller, E. J., Crawford, M. J., Wynne, J., and Purcell, M. (1974). *Lancet* **2,** 1579–1580.

Doniach, D. (1976). *Biochem. Basis Thyroid Stimulation Thyroid Horm. Action, Celle Symp.,* (A. V. Z. Mühler, H. Schleusener, and G. Thieme, eds), 1976, pp. 24–34.

Doniach, D., and Florin-Christensen, A. (1975). *Clin. Endocrinol. Metab.* **4,** 341–350.

Doniach, D., and Roitt, I. M. (1975). *In* "Clinical Aspects of Immunology" (P. Gell, R. R. A. Coombs, and P. J. Lachman, eds.), 3rd ed., pp. 1355–1386. Blackwell, Oxford.

Doniach, D., Hudson, R. V., and Roitt, I. M. (1960). *Br. Med. J.* **1,** 365–373.

Doniach, D., Roitt, I. M., Benhamou-Glynn, N., Jayson, M. I. V., and El Kabir, D. J. (1967). *In* "Thyrotoxicosis" (W. J. Irvine, ed.), pp. 76–84. Livingstone, Edinburgh.

Doniach, D., Ball, P. A. J., and Bottazzo, G. F. (1977) *Clin. Endocrinol* (in press).

Dorrington, R. J., Carneiro, L., and Munro, D. S. (1966). *Biochem. J.* **98,** 858–861.

Dumont, J. E. (1971). *Vitam. Horm.* (*N.Y.*) **29,** 287–412.

Ekins, R. P. (1976). *In* "Hormone Assays and their Clinical Application" (J. A. Loraine and E. T. Bell, eds.), 4th ed., pp. 1–49. Livingstone, Edinburgh.

El Kabir, D. J., and Hockaday, T. D. R. (1969). *Nature* (*London*) **224,** 608–609.

El Kabir, D. J., Doniach, D., and Turner-Warwick, R. (1963). *J. Clin. Endocrinol. Metab.* **23,** 510–520.

El Kabir, D. J., Hockaday, T. D. R., Richards, M. R., Dandona, P., and Naftolin, F. (1971). *Proc. R. Soc. Med.* **64,** 154–155.

Enser, J., Kendall-Taylor, P., Munro, D. S., and Smith, B. R. (1971). *J. Endocrinol.* **49,** 487–492.

Fagraeus, A., and Jonsson, J. (1970). *Immunology* **18,** 413–416.

Fagraeus, A., and Jonsson, J., and El Kabir, D. J. (1970). *J. Clin. Endocrinol. Metab.* **31,** 445–446.

Flier, J. S., Kahn, C. R., Janett, D. B., and Roth, J. (1976). *Immunol. Commun.* **5,** (5), 361–373.

Field, J. B., Remer, A., Bloom, G., and Kriss, J. P. (1968). *J. Clin. Invest.* **47,** 1553–1560.

Freinkel, N. (1961). *J. Clin. Invest.* **40,** 476–484.

Goldfine, I. D., Amer, S. M., Ingbar, S. H., and Tucker, G. (1976). *Biochim. Biophys. Acta.* **448,** 45–56.

Gospodarowicz, D. (1973). *J. Biol. Chem.* **248,** 1314–1317.

Hall, R., and Stanbury, J. B. (1967). *Clin. Exp. Immunol.* **2,** 719–725.

Hall, R., Dingle, P. R., and Roberts, D. F. (1972). *Clin. Genet.* **3,** 319–324.

Hall, R., Smith, B. R., and Mukhtar, E. D. (1975). *Clin. Endocrinol.* (*Oxford*) **4,** 213–230.

Hart, I. R., and McKenzie, J. M. (1971). *Endocrinology* **88,** 26–30.

Henneman, G., Dolman, A., Docter, R., De Rens, A., and Van Zijl, J. (1975). *J. Clin. Endocrinol. Metab.* **40,** 935–941.

Jerne, N. (1973). *Sc. Am.* **229,** (No. 1), 52–60.

Kahn, C. R., Flier, J. S. Archer, J. A., Gorden, P., Martin, M. M., and Roth, J. (1976). *N. Engl. J. Med.* **294,** 739–746.

Kaneko, T., Zor, U., and Field, S. B. (1970). *Metab., Clin. Exp.* **19,** 430–438.

Karlberg, B. E., Henrikson, K. G., and Andersson, R. G. G. (1974). *J. Clin. Endocrinol. Metab.* **39,** 96–101.

Kendall-Taylor, P. L. (1972). *J. Endocrinol.* **52,** 533–540.

Kendall-Taylor, P. L., and Munro, D. S. (1971). *Biochim. Biophys. Acta* **231,** 314–319.

Klainer, L. M., Chi, Y. M., Friedberg, S. L., Rall, T. W., and Sutherland, E. W. (1962). *J. Biol. Chem.* **237,** 1239–1343.

Knox, A. J. S., von Westarp, C., Row, V. V., and Volpé, R. (1976). *J. Clin. Endocrinol. Metab.* **43,** 330–337.

Kohn, L. D., and Winand, R. J. (1971). *J. Biol. Chem.* **246,** 6570–6575.

Kohn, L. D., and Winand, R. J. (1975). *J. Biol. Chem.* **250,** 6503–6508.

Kotani, M., Kariya, T., and Field, J. B. (1975). *Metab., Clin. Exp.* **24,** 959–971.

Kriss, J. B., Pleshakov, V., and Chien, J. R. (1964). *J. Clin. Endocrinol. Metab.* **24,** 1005–1028.

Kriss, J. P., Konishi, J., and Herman, M. (1975). *Recent Prog. Horm. Res.* **31,** 533–566.

Laurel, S., and Tibbling, G. (1968). *Clin. Chim. Acta* **21,** 127–132.

Lennon, V. A., and Carnegie, P. R. (1971). *Lancet* **1,** 630–633.

Lissitzky, S., Fayet, G., and Verrier, B. (1975). *Adv. Cyclic Nucleotide Res.* **5,** 133–152.

Lonergan, C., Babiarz, D., and Burke, G. (1973). *J. Clin. Endocrinol. Metab.* **36,** 439–444.

McKenzie, J. M. (1968). *J. Clin. Endocrinol. Metab.* **28**, 596–602.

McKenzie, J. M. (1972). *Metab., Clin. Exp.* **21**, 883–894.

McKenzie, J. M. (1974). *Hand. Physiol., Sect. 7: Endocrinol.*, **3**, 285–301.

McKenzie, J. M., and Zakarija, M. (1976). *J. Clin. Endocrinol. Metab.* **42**, 778–780.

McLarty, D. G., Alexander, W. D., Harden, R. McG., and Robertson, J. W. K. (1971). *Lancet* **1**, 6–9.

Manley, S. W., Bourke, J. R., and Hawker, R. W. (1974). *J. Endocrinol.* **61**, 419–436.

Marshall, N. J. (1976). *In* "Eukaryotic Cell Function and Growth" (J. E. Dumont, B. L. Brown, and N. J. Marshall, eds.). Plenum, New York (in press).

Marshall, N. J., Florin-Christensen, A., and von Borcke, S. (1976). *Biochem. Soc. Trans.* **4**, 149–151.

Meek, J. C., Jones, A. E., Lewis, U. J., and Vanderlaan, W. P. (1964). *Proc. Natl. Acad. Sci. U.S.A.* **52**, 342–349.

Mehdi, S. Q. (1975). *In* "Radioimmunoassay in Clinical Biochemistry" (C. A. Pasternak, ed.), pp. 213–224. Hayden and Sons, Ltd.

Mehdi, S. Q., Hockaday, T. D. R., Newlands, E., and El Kabir, D. J. (1971). *Proc. R. Soc. Med.* **64**, 1268–1269.

Mehdi, S. Q. and Nussey, S. S. (1975) *Biochem. J.*, **145**, 105–111.

Mehdi, S. Q., Nussey, S. S., Simpson, R. D., and Adlkofer, F. (1974). *Endocrinol. Exp.* **8**, 163–164.

Merlevede, W., Weaver, G., and Landau, B. R. (1963). *J. Clin. Invest.* **42**, 1160–1171.

Mittag, T., Kornfeld, P., Tormay, A., and Woo, C. (1976). *N. Engl. J. Med.* **294**, 691–693.

Moore, W. V., and Wolf, J. (1974). *J. Biol. Chem.* **249**, 6255–6263.

Mori, T., and Kriss, J. P. (1971). *J. Clin. Endocrinol. Metab.*, **33**, 688–695.

Mosinger, B., Kuhn, E., and Kujalova, V. (1965). *J. Lab. Clin. Med.* **66**, 380–389.

Mukhtar, R. D., Smith, B. R., Pyle, G. A., Hall, R., and Vice, P. (1975). *Lancet* **1**, 713–715.

Mullin, B. R., Lee, G., Ledley, F. D., Winand, J., and Kohn, L. D. (1976a). *Biochem. Biophys. Res. Commun.* **69** (No. 1), 55–62.

Mullin, B. R., Fishman, P. H., Lee, G., Aloj, S. M., Ledley, F. D., Winand, R. J., Kohn, L. D., and Brady, R. D. (1976b). *Proc. Natl. Acad. Sci. U.S.A.* **73**, 842–846.

Mullin, B. R., Aloj, S. M., Fishman, P. H., Lee, G., Kohn, L. D., and Brady, R. O. (1976c). *Proc. Natl. Acad. Sci. U.S.A.* **73**, 1679–1683.

Onaya, T., Kotani, M., Yamada, T., and Ochi, Y. (1973). *J. Clin. Endocrinol. Metab.* **36**, 859–866.

Ong, M., Malkin, D., Tay, S. K., and Malkin, A. (1976). *Endocrinology* **98**, 880–885.

Orgiazzi, J., Williams, D. E., Chopra, I. J., and Solomon, D. H. (1976). *J. Clin. Endocrinol. Metab.* **42**, 341–355.

Petersen, V., Smith, B. R., and Hall, R. (1975). *J. Clin. Endocrinol. Metab.* **41**, 199–202.

Pinchera, A., Rovis, L., Grasso, L., Liberti, P., Martino, E., Fenzi, G. F., and Baschieri L., (1970). *Endocrinology* **87,** 217–225.

Raben, M. S. (1959). *Recent Prog. Horm. Res.* **15,** 71–83.

Raff, M. (1976). *Sci. Am.* **234,** 30–36.

Rich, C., Bierman, E. I., and Schwartz, I. L. (1959). *J. Clin. Invest.* **38,** 275–278.

Rudman, D., Brown, S. J., and Malkin, M. F. (1963). *Endocrinology* **72,** 527–543.

Schell-Frederick, E., and Dumont, J. E. (1970). *In* "Biochemical Actions of Hormones" (G. Litwack, ed.), Vol. 1, pp. 415–459. Academic Press, New York.

Schleusener, H., Kotulla, P., Kruck, I., and Geissler, D. (1976). *Thyroid Res., Proc. Int. Thyroid Conf., 7th, 1975 Abstract 140.*

Scott, T. W., Good, B. F., and Ferguson, K. A. (1966). *Endocrinology* **79,** 949–954.

Shishiba, Y., Solomon, D. H., and Davidson, W. D. (1970). *Endocrinology* **86,** 183–190.

Shishiba, Y., Shimizu, T., Yoshimura, S., and Shizume, K. (1972). *J. Clin. Endocrinol. Metab.* **34,** 7–12.

Shishiba, Y., Shimizu, T., Yoshimura, S., and Shizume, K. (1973). *J. Clin. Endocrinol. Metab.* **36,** 517–521.

Singer, S. J. (1974). *Annu. Rev. Biochem.* **43,** 805–833.

Smith, B. R. (1969). *Biochim. Biophys. Acta* **188,** 89–100.

Smith, B. R. (1976). *Immunol. Commun.* **5** (5), 345–360.

Smith, B. R., and Hall, R. (1974). *Lancet* **2,** 427–431.

Solomon, D. H., and Beall, G. N. (1968). *J. Clin. Endocrinol. Metab.* **28,** 1496–1502.

Tata, R. J. (1976). *Polypep. Horm.: Mol. Cell. Aspects, Ciba Found. Symp., 1976* Ciba Found. Symp. No. 41, pp. 297–312.

Tate, R. L., Schwartz, H. I., Holmes, J. M., Kohn, L. D., and Winand, R. J. (1975a). *J. Biol. Chem.* **250,** 6509–6526.

Tate, R. L., Holmes, J. M., Kohn, L. D., and Winand, R. J. (1975b). *J. Biol. Chem.* **250,** 6527–6533.

Teng, C. S., Rees-Smith, B., Anderson, J., and Hall, R. (1975). *Biochem. Biophys. Res. Commun.* **66,** 836–841.

Van Sande, J., Decoster, C., and Dumont, J. E. (1975). *Arch. Int. Physiol. Biochim.* **83,** 416.

Wall, J. R., Good, B. F., and Hetzel, B. S. (1969). *Lancet* **2,** 1024–1028.

Wall, J. R., Good, B. F., Forbes, I. J., and Hetzel, B. S. (1973). *Clin. Exp. Immunol.* **14,** 555–561.

Werner, S. C., Coleman, D. J., and Franzen, L. A. (1974). *N. Engl. J. Med.* **290,** 1447–1450.

White, J. E., and Engel, F. L. (1958). *J. Clin. Invest.* **37,** 1556–1563.

Winand, R. J., and Kohn, L. D. (1972). *Proc. Natl. Acad. Sci. U.S.A.* **69,** 1711–1715.

Winand, R. J., and Kohn, L. D. (1975a). *J. Biol. Chem.* **250,** 6522–6526.

Winand, R. J., and Kohn, L. D. (1975b). *J. Biol. Chem.* **250,** 6534–6540.

Wong, E. T., and Litman, G. W. (1969). *J. Clin. Endocrinol. Metab.* **29,** 72–78.

Yamashita, K., and Field, J. B. (1972). *J. Clin. Invest.* **51,** 463–472.

Chapter 22

Autoimmune Neurological Disease: Experimental Animal Systems and Implications for Multiple Sclerosis

PHILIP Y. PATERSON

I. INTRODUCTION*

The seeds for thinking that nervous tissue has unique antigenic constituents, and the autoimmune responses to such antigens in one's own brain, spinal cord, or peripheral nerve tissues may cause neurological disease were sown almost 100 years ago. The notion that virus infections may "trigger" immune responses injurious to nervous tissues can be traced to observations made 50 years ago. What is relatively new and a by-product of the explosive growth of immunology and virology during the past 25 years is the concept that both immune reactivity to "self" and infection by a virus, probably acting synergistically, are important determinants of autoimmune neurological disease.

From a historical standpoint, the nervous system has been the vanguard organ for discoveries concerning "self-reactivity" and mechanisms of autoimmunity. Organ-specific tissue antigens calling forth specific antibodies were first described utilizing nervous tissues. The finding that injections of brain and spinal cord can induce a striking neurological disease in animals, called experimental allergic encephalomyelitis (EAE), provided the first laboratory autoimmune disease model system and underlined the stark reality that immune responses to one's own tissue antigens can cause immunologic disease. And it has been especially studies of virus infections of the nervous system that have shown the important role of persistent virus infection in initiating and augmenting self-reactivity, culminating in a variety of different types of autoimmune tissue injury.

This chapter will focus on three aspects of immunologically mediated neurological disease. First, major immunologic and virus-related events spanning close to a century will be briefly summarized. This will give a historic backdrop for much of the current lines of thinking about neuroallergy, neurovirology, and neurological disease of animals and man. A specific effort will be made to show how interdigitations of immunologic discoveries, on the one hand, and key virological findings, on the other hand, have led to immunovirological mechanisms being the most likely explanation for certain neurological diseases of man. This is certainly the case for the important demyelinating disease of man, multiple sclerosis (MS).

* Abbreviations used are as follows: B-cells, bone marrow derived lymphocytes; C, complement; CFA, complete Freund's adjuvant; CNS, central nervous system; Cop1, random polymer of alanine, glutamic acid, lysine, and tyrosine; CSF, cerebrospinal fluid; DH, delayed hypersensitivity; EAE, experimental allergic encephalomyelitis; EAN, experimental allergic neuritis; FA, incomplete Freund's adjuvant; Ir, immune response (gene); LNC, lymph node cells; MBP, myelin basic protein; MIF, migration inhibitory factor; MS, multiple sclerosis; MSAA, multiple sclerosis associated agent; PLL, poly-L-lysine; PNS, peripheral nervous system; T cells, thymic-derived lymphocyte.

Secondly, EAE will be discussed in detail as the cornerstone for thinking about autoimmune reactivity to nervous tissues. The focus will be on key immunopathogenetic determinants in this prototypic autoimmune disease which have emerged from relatively recent work. A variety of monographs and review articles are available to the interested reader who wishes access to more detailed and inclusive discussions (Paterson, 1966, 1971, 1976a; Alvord, 1970).

Finally, since one objective of most basic research is securing greater insight into human disease, EAE as an immunologic disease of animals will be examined with an eye as to how well it serves as an experimental counterpart of MS in man. Special pains will be taken to highlight both concordance and discordance of immunologic data in both diseases and to identify clues suggesting where a virus may play a role in the MS process. For readers wishing a more detailed discussion of this topic and more information about MS per se, a number of recently published books, monographs, and symposia proceedings are available (McAlpine *et al.*, 1972; Wolfgram *et al.*, 1972).

Because of limitations of space, this chapter will deal solely with immunologic disease of the central nervous system (CNS). It should be stressed that virtually everything discussed here with respect to the CNS appears to be directly applicable to immunologic disorders affecting the peripheral nervous system (PNS). Knowledge concerning PNS immunologic diseases, including experimental allergic neuritis (EAN) as a model disease system in animals and its clinical counterpart in man, i.e., the Guillain-Barré-Strohl syndrome, has accumulated at a rapid rate in the past 30 years, spearheaded by immunovirological studies of CNS disease. Several excellent reviews and chapters in books recently published can be consulted for details (Waksman and Adams, 1955; Asbury *et al.*, 1969; Arnason, 1975; Paterson, 1976b).

II. EMERGING CONCEPTS OF NEUROALLERGY AND AUTOIMMUNE CNS DISEASE AND NEUROIMMUNOVIROLOGICAL MECHANISMS IMPLICATED IN MS

Major immunologic observations and virus-related events providing the matrix of current thinking concerning autoimmune reactivity and CNS tissue injury, in general, and with specific reference to MS, are listed chronologically in Table I. By way of introduction, Charcot first described the clinical manifestations of the chronic disease now known as multiple sclerosis in 1868. In 1884, Marie formally proposed that MS might have an

TABLE I

Major Historical Events Establishing Neuroantigen Autoreactivity as Basis for Immunologic Central Nervous System (CNS) Disease and Implicating Neuroimmunovirological Mechanisms in Multiple Sclerosis (MS)

1868, MS described as a CNS disease (Charcot); 1884, infectious etiology of MS espoused	
	A. Immunobiologic events
1885–1888	Pasteur rabies vaccine introduced; acute encephalomyelitis associated with injections of rabies vaccine reported
1919–1927	Introduction of Semple phenol-treated rabies vaccine; continued occurrence of postrabies vaccinal encephalomyelitis
1928–1933	Organic-specific antigenic constituents of nervous tissue described
1933–1935	Production of acute disseminated encephalomyelitis in monkeys receiving multiple injections of CNS tissue
1947–1953	Production of an accelerated form of acute encephalomyelitis in monkeys and other species of laboratory animals after one injection of CNS tissue combined with Freund's adjuvant; experimental allergic encephalomyelitis (EAE) characterized as a model system of immunologically mediated CNS disease
1952–1963	Histopathological similarities of EAE and MS described and EAE accepted as a promising means for study of the MS process
1960–1962	Transfer of EAE in outbred and inbred rats by means of dissociated lymph node cells described and confirmed in other species of animals
1961–1963	Complement-dependent cytotoxic demyelinating antibodies in the sera of both animals with EAE and patients with MS reported
1965–1966	Myelin basic protein (MBP) established as a major encephalitogenic (EAE-inducing) antigen of CNS tissue
1965	*In vivo* and *in vitro* correlation of delayed-type hypersensitivity to CNS tissue or MBP with occurrence of EAE described
1969	Drug-induced complete remission in EAE reported; feasibility of reversing disease with therapeutic regimens established
1971	Peripheral blood lymphocytes of MS patients reported to exhibit hypersensitivity to MBP
1972	Reversal of EAE by injections of MBP into monkeys and other animal species with advanced EAE described
1973	Specific immunogenetic determinants of histocompatibility antigens shown to influence susceptibility to EAE, as well as be associated with occurrence of MS

Table I (*Continued*)

(Marie); 1888, nervous tissue-derived vaccine induces CNS disease	
	B. Viral infection and virus-related events
1926–1930	Acute encephalitis reported to occur in close temporal relationship to smallpox vaccination. Concepts of post-infectious encephalitides defined
1942–1947	Recovery of measles virus from patients with post-measles encephalitis
1954	Sigurrdson's thesis concerning "slow virus infections" in animals described, with implications for disease of man
1964	First report of elevated titers of measles antibody in sera and cerebrospinal fluids of patients with MS
1966–1971	Viral etiology or transmissible nature of four chronic neurological diseases of man established: kuru, Creutzfeldt-Jacob disease, subacute sclerosing panencephalitis, and progressive multifocal leucoencephalopathy
1970	Increasing evidence presented for an environmental factor(s) influencing occurrence of MS
1970–1972	Diminished cellular immunity to measles virus reported to occur in patients with MS
1972	Recovery of defective measles virus from brain of patient with post-measles encephalitis
1972	Reported isolation of parainfluenza virus from MS brain specimens; transmissible agent associated with MS reported to replicate in mice and continuous cell culture line

infectious basis. Just a few years later, occurrence of acute encephalitis or myelitis was observed in some patients receiving injections of a rabies vaccine prepared from infected brain tissue by Pasteur. Whether these post-rabies vaccine "neuroparalytic accidents" were caused by the virus in the vaccine or resulted from some type of allergic response to injected brain was uncertain. Thus, just about 100 years ago, lines of thinking already had been drawn implicating immunologic and virological mechanisms in acute and chronic forms of CNS disease.

A. Immunobiologic Events

In 1885, Pasteur introduced his vaccine for prevention of rabies. This vaccine consisted of brain infected with a strain of rabies virus that had been attenuated or "fixed" by repeated passage in rabbits. Patients bitten by dogs suspected of having rabies received repeated injections of the vaccine in efforts to induce active immunity to virulent or "street" rabies virus. Acute neurological disease developed in occasional subjects receiving a course of vaccine prophylaxis. By 1888, it was clear that these "neuroparalytic complications" represented an acute inflammatory process of the CNS, i.e., encephalitis, myelitis, or encephalomyelitis. There was initial concern that the attenuated rabies virus in the vaccine might be the cause. Since the majority of patients with post-vaccinal encephalomyelitis survived and the histopathological changes in the CNS of those that succumbed differed materially from those characterizing rabies virus infection, factors other than the virus soon were suspected. The question was raised as to whether the nervous tissue in the vaccine per se was evoking an abnormal host response, which led to acute inflammation of the brain and spinal cord. Further development of this idea was delayed as a result of Paul Ehrlich's dictum *horror autotoxicus* enunciated at the turn of the century. Ehrlich considered immunologic reactivity to one's own tissues to be a biologic impossibility.

The Semple phenol-treated rabies vaccine was introduced in 1919. Continued occurrence of cases of post vaccinal encephalomyelitis, using this killed vaccine excluded rabies virus as an etiologic factor and riveted attention on immunologic responses to nervous tissue. Increasing suspicion during the 1920's that post-rabies vaccinal encephalomyelitis was an allergic reaction to nervous tissue antigens accelerated studies in experimental animals related to the immunogenic potential of mammalian tissues. By 1928 (Witebsky and Steinfeld, 1928), brain tissue was shown to contain specific antigenic constituents which stimulated antibodies specifically reactive with CNS tissue.

It remained for Rivers and his associates (1933; Rivers and Schwentker, 1935) in the early 1930's to discover that an acute disseminated encephalomyelitis could be produced in monkeys receiving repeated injections of nervous tissue extracts or emulsions over a period of many weeks or months. The acute encephalomyelitis induced in these monkeys by nervous tissue immunization bore a striking resemblance to post-rabies vaccinal encephalomyelitis. It also resembled closely the recently described occurrence of acute encephalitis in association with smallpox vaccination (Turnbull and McIntosh, 1926). Rivers *et al.* (1933; Rivers and Schwentker, 1935) were impressed with the degree of demyelination present in their monkeys, noting that immunologic responses to nervous tissue antigens conceivably might be related to the profound degrees of myelin injury characterizing MS.

During the early 1940's, Freund and his associates were developing what was to become known as Freund's adjuvant, a mixture of paraffin oil with suspended killed mycobacteria and emulsifying agent, with a remarkable capacity to augment antibody and cell-mediated immune responses of animals to a variety of antigenic stimuli. In 1947, Freund *et al.* (1947), Morgan (1947), Kabat *et al.* (1947), and Morrison (1947) simultaneously reported that a single injection of nervous tissue emulsified in complete Freund's adjuvant (CFA), i.e., containing mycobacteria, regularly induced an accelerated and extremely severe form of disseminated encephalomyelitis in guinea pigs, monkeys, and rabbits within a matter of 2 or 3 weeks time. This disease, soon to be known as experimental allergic encephalomyelitis (EAE), was characterized by a variety of clinical paralytic signs and histopathological changes consisting of focal areas of intense perivascular cellular infiltration with varying degrees of demyelination within the brain and spinal cord.

The fact that monkeys developed EAE following sensitization with their own brain, i.e., autologous tissue (Kabat *et al.*, 1949), provided a powerful argument for excluding sensitization to isoantigens or an infectious agent as etiologic determinants. Occurrence of delayed-type hypersensitivity (DH) cutaneous reactivity to nervous tissue in parallel with development of EAE (Freund *et al.*, 1947; Waksman and Morrison, 1951; Alvord *et al.*, 1975), in contrast to the poor correlation with titers of circulating brain antibodies (Thomas *et al.*, 1950; Lumsden *et al.*, 1950) and inability to transfer the disease to normal animals with immune serum (see review of Chase, 1959), provided increasing support that pathogenetic mechanisms responsible for EAE involved intact "immune cells," rather than antibody.

A number of comparative neuropathological studies of EAE published during the period from 1952 to 1963 emphasized the many similarities between the histopathological hallmarks of the experimental animal disease and those characterizing MS in man (Adams, 1959; Wolf, 1963). This was especially true in those forms of the human disease that were characterized by an acute or subacute course leading to death in a comparatively short period of time. These studies collectively reinforced the view that EAE is a meaningful laboratory model for MS and that immune responses to autologous CNS tissue might well play a role in both diseases.

Transfer of EAE during the 1960's, first in rats (Paterson, 1960, 1962, 1963; Paterson and Didakow, 1961) and later in guinea pigs (Stone, 1961) and rabbits (Astrom and Waksman, 1962), using suspensions of dissociated sensitized lymph node cells (LNC), provided the essential evidence that EAE has an immunologic mechanism. The fact that EAE could now be transferred by means of sensitized LNC, together with innumerable unsuccessful attempts to transfer the disease with immune serum (reviewed by Chase, 1959), provided compelling evidence that cell-mediated immune responses analogous to DH were of major immunopathological significance. It should also be emphasized that the EAE–cellular transfer system provided a completely new means for dissecting the complex multiplicity of events, starting with antigen-stimulation of host lymphoid tissue and culminating in immunologic injury of the sensitized animal's CNS target tissue.

In 1961, complement-dependent cytotoxic demyelinating antibodies were described in the sera of animals with EAE (Bornstein and Appel, 1961), using myelinated organotypic mammalian brain explant cultures as targets. Essentially identical demyelinating antibodies were soon reported in the sera of patients with MS (Bornstein and Appel, 1965; see review of Bornstein, 1973). These observations, more than any other, provided compelling evidence that EAE in animals and MS in man have in common at least one immunologic response directed specifically against nervous tissue antigens. These findings reinforced the view that insights into the enigma of MS might well be secured from studies of EAE. These reports momentarily shifted thinking away from cellular immunity and toward antibody-mediated immune responses as being of potential significance in autoimmune forms of neurological disease, but not for long.

During the 1960's, the work of many laboratories, but especially those of Kies and her collaborators and Einstein and her associates (see reviews by Einstein and Chao, 1970; Rauch and Einstein, 1974; Kies, 1975), was vital in identifying a basic protein of white matter myelin as a major encephalitogenic (EAE-inducing) antigen of CNS tissue. The availability of myelin basic protein (MBP) as a completely soluble neuroantigen of defined molecular weight and amino acid composition (see Section III,A) opened the door for a crescendo of incisive studies of specific immunopathological mechanisms responsible for EAE. Immunologic studies during the present decade have implicated thymus-derived (T) lymphoid cells as essential for development of EAE and also as playing a role in MS. A strong direct correlation between occurrence of EAE and DH cutaneous reactivity to MBP has been established (see review by Alvord *et al.*, 1975). *In vitro* assays for DH such as production of migration inhibitory factor (MIF), first applied to EAE by David and Paterson (1965), using whole nervous tissue as antigen, and, subsequently, by other workers, employing MBP (Brockman *et al.*, 1968; Rauch *et al.*, 1969), together with studies of cultured lymphocyte proliferative responses to MBP (Dau and Peterson, 1969; Warnatz *et al.*, 1970), have continued to build an ever stronger case for sensitized T cells in the pathogenesis of the disease. Finally, extension of these studies concerning EAE to patients with MS, utilizing peripheral blood lymphocyte cultures, have suggested that some patients have demonstrable T cell hypersensitivity to MBP and, moreover, that the expression of this type of immune response may be related to the clinical status of their disease (Bartfeld and Atoynatan, 1970; Rocklin *et al.*, 1971; Sheremata *et al.*, 1974, 1976; Webb *et al.*, 1974).

With increasing availability, during the 1950's and 1960's, of therapeutic reagents with increasingly more potent antiinflammatory or/and immunosuppressive properties, it was natural for attention to be directed toward finding a means of rapidly reversing the manifestations of EAE. Such efforts were in no small way stimulated by pressures from the clinical neurological arena to devise some type of efficacious therapeutic strategy for MS patients. Reversal of all clinical and histopathological hallmarks of EAE in rats given a 10-day course of cyclophosphamide, such therapy first beginning after the animals exhibited severe clinical signs of disease, was reported in 1969 (Paterson and Drobish, 1969). This finding underlined the feasibility of inducing complete remissions in autoimmune disease processes by altering ongoing immunologic reactions of the host through drugs or other therapeutic reagents, including specific tissue antigen(s). Earlier studies had shown that EAE could be suppressed by injections of whole nervous tissue or MBP into animals before or soon after they were sensitized to neuroantigen (see reviews by Alvord, 1970; Paterson, 1971). With these findings as a guideline, efforts were directed toward treating animals with advanced EAE by injections of MBP. Striking reversal of EAE in monkeys, followed by long-lasting clinical remission of disease, by injecting large amounts of MBP combined with Freund's incomplete adjuvant (IFA) lacking mycobacteria was reported in 1972 (Eylar *et al.*, 1972). Soon thereafter, other investigators found that remissions of EAE also could be induced in guinea pigs and rats by injections of MBP–IFA (S. Levine *et al.*, 1972; Driscoll *et al.*, 1974b). More recent work has suggested that certain amino acid sequences of the MBP molecule, which are totally lacking in encephalitogenic activity and which can be prepared as synthetic peptides, are effective in inducing remissions of EAE in guinea pigs (Hashim, 1975; Hashim *et al.*, 1976). One of the most exciting revelations of contemporary immunobiology has been the finding that genes closely associated with those genes coding for histocompatibility antigens have an important modulating influence on immunologic responsiveness of animals and man (McDevitt and Benacerraf, 1969; Benacerraf and McDevitt, 1972; B. Levine *et al.*, 1972). Immunogenetic factors have been shown to be important in susceptibility of rats, guinea pigs, and mice to EAE (see Section III, C). Especially noteworthy is the fact that certain histocompatibility antigens specified by three different genetic loci have been found to have an unusually high incidence in patients with MS or their first-degree relatives (see review of McFarlin and McFarland, 1976). Since the genes coding for histocompatibility antigens are so closely associated with immune response genes in animals, they serve as potential markers for subtle aberrations in underlying immune responsiveness, which, in turn, might be of etiologic importance in the development of MS.

B. Viral Infection and Virus-Related Events

As a quick glance at Table I will indicate, evidence for viruses and virus-initiated host responses leading to immunologic CNS disease began to accumulate only 50 years ago. Observations implicating specific viruses as etiologic factors in MS have been described only in recent years.

The description in 1926 of several cases of acute encephalitis temporarily associated with small pox vaccination (Turnbull and McIntosh, 1926) indicated that a virus, in these cases an attenuated one, can in some way trigger acute inflammatory disease of the CNS. Within the next few years, an identical form of acute encephalitis was observed to be temporarily associated with rare cases of spontaneously occurring virus infections, e.g., measles, chickenpox, and rubella. By 1930, the concept of acute post-infectious encephalitides had been established as a clinical entity. The essential features of this syndrome included (1) onset of neurological signs of disease a matter of days after antecedent virus infection, (2) histopathological changes involving the brain, particularly, but also the spinal cord, characterized by perivascular cellular infiltrates and accompanied by variable degrees of perivascular demyelination, together with minimal evidence of the neuronal degenerative changes expected with neurotropic virus infections per se, and (3) inability to demonstrate evidence of the associated viral agent in CNS tissues. The sequence of virus infection followed by CNS manifestations several days later, and the similarity of the histopathological changes to those already known to be associated with post-rabies vaccinal encephalomyelitis, suggested that the antecedent virus infection initiated immunologic responses injurious to CNS tissue.

Isolation of measles virus in 1942 and 1947 from brain tissue of patients dying of post-measles encephalitis strengthened the view that the acute neurological inflammation was related to the antecedent measles virus infection (Shaffer *et al.*, 1942; Fernandez *et al.*, 1947). Retrospectively, these reports can now be seen as important clues pointing to unusual persistence of virus in nervous tissues as a factor in development of the post-infectious encephalitides.

Sigurrdson's concept of slow virus infections, outlined in 1954 and seemingly remote from the MS process, was a key factor in development of new perspectives of CNS virus infection. Based on experience with unusual diseases of animals, Sigurrdson (1954) postulated that certain viral agents can initiate diseases characterized by exceptionally long latent periods, measured in months or years, with a relentless and progressive course leading to death after clinical manifestations first appear. Demyelination was a major histopathological characteristic in one of the animal diseases described by Sigurrdson. It is important to note that, between 1966 and 1971, Sigurrdson's views concerning slow virus infections were shown to be directly applicable to man. During this period specific viruses, e.g., a defective form of measles and a papovavirus and a new class of atypical infectious agents, have been etiologically linked to four chronic degenerative neurological diseases of man. These diseases are kuru, subacute sclerosing panencephalitis, Creutzfeldt-Jacob disease, and progressive multifocal leukoencephalopathy (see reveiw articles and monographs by Lampert *et al.*, 1972; Fucillo *et al.*, 1974; Zeman and Lennette, 1974). These findings served to consolidate thinking that MS might be another chronic neurological disease caused by a "slow virus" or by a defective virus, such as measles. This line of thinking was materially reinforced by observations during the 1960's (Alter *et al.*, 1966, and Dean, 1967, 1970), which implicated an environmental factor as operating in the development of MS, probably exerting its effect before 15 years of age (see review of Dean, 1970). Viruses obviously were the most likely candidate as "environmental factor."

In recent years, a search for a specific role of measles virus in the MS process has been the major objective of many laboratories (see review of Black, 1975). The extraordinary amount of investigative activity devoted to this virus is the direct result of four observations. First, in 1962 Adams and Imagawa reported that elevated measles antibody titers are demonstrable in a high proportion of sera and cerebrospinal fluid (CSF) specimens of patients with MS. This finding has been subsequently confirmed by more than two dozen laboratories around the world. Second, the discovery (Baublis and Payne, 1968; Horta-Barbosa *et al.*, 1969) that defective measles virus was the cause of subacute sclerosing panencephalitis provided a strong impetus for seeing if this or other strains of defective measles virus might be implicated in other chronic neurological disease such as MS. Third, recovery of defective measles virus from a patient dying of post-measles encephalitis (terMeulen *et al.*, 1972a) indicated that defective forms of this agent might have a special propensity to initiate immune responses against nervous tissue of importance in MS. Fourth, increasing evidence for an abnormality in cell-mediated immune responses of MS patients to paramyxoviruses, in general, and measles virus, in particular, provided a particularly strong stimulus for searching for additional clues that this class of viruses might be closely associated with the MS process (Ciongoli *et al.*, 1973; Utermohlen and Zabriskie, 1973).

In 1972, electron microscopic studies suggested existence of myxovirus nucleocapsids in MS brain material (Prineas, 1972). In the same year, parainfluenza virus was reportedly isolated from brain specimens from two patients with MS (terMeulen *et al.*, 1972b). In 1972, defective measles virus was successfully isolated from a patient with post-measles encephalitis dying several weeks following onset of disease (terMeullen *et al.*, 1972a). This finding suggested that defective virions might be especially prone to persist in a host's CNS and have a special propensity for causing chronic, progressive neurological disease of man. Finally, in this same year, an agent associated with MS patients and present in brain tissue and peripheral blood was reported to replicate in mice and a continuous cell culture (Carp *et al.*, 1972, 1975). Very recently, support for the existence of this multiple sclerosis associated agent (MSAA) has been reported by other investigators (Koldovsky *et al.*, 1975).

III. IMMUNOPATHOGENESIS OF EAE

Attempts to devise a "black-and-white" explanation as to how aberrant discrimination between self and nonself leads to immune injury of the CNS cannot be anything more than an empty exercise in view of presently limited insight into the intricacies of the immunologic system. Moreover, such attempts, by necessity, would need to suppress conflicting data, which often are important clues to better understanding. This discussion of the key determinants of EAE as set out in Table II, therefore, is drawn so as to include minority viewpoints and controversial issues.

A. Myelin Basic Protein

The discovery that MBP is responsible for a major portion of the encephalitogenic activity of CNS tissue opened the flood gates for an incredible amount of research on this antigenic constituent. No other antigenic component of mammalian tissue implicated in autoimmune disease, has been so extensively studied from a biochemical and immunologic standpoint. MBP has been completely characterized down to the last amino acid residue, the biologic activity specified by specific sequences of amino acids determined, and critical sequences synthesized in the laboratory so as to provide peptides with EAE-inducing activity (Eylar and Hashim, 1968; Eylar *et al.*, 1970; see reviews by Rauch and Einstein, 1974; Kies, 1975;

TABLE II

Key Immunopathogenetic Determinants in EAE

A.	Myelin basic protein (MBP): a major encephalitogenic (EAE-inducing) antigen of nervous tissue
B.	Neuroantigen autoreactivity: defective clonal elimination or somatic mutation versus aberrant immunoregulation
C.	Immunogenetic factors: immune responses to immunogenetic determinants of neuroantigens and their interaction with determinants in target tissues
D.	Immunologic adjuvants: prerequisites for immunopotentiation
E.	Primary role of T cells and T cell-mediated immune responses
F.	Evidence implicating B cell immune responses

Paterson, 1976a). These studies reflect the labors of a large number of investigators and collectively represent a monumental accomplishment in molecular immunopathology with enormous implications for the field of autoimmunity and autoimmune disease (see review of Carnegie *et al.*, 1973).

MBP represents approximately one-third of the total protein content of myelin and about 1% of the weight of whole nervous tissue. It is readily extracted from delipidated mammalian brain or spinal cord at acid pH ranges of 1.0–2.5, and can be easily purified by various combinations of resin–gel chromatography (Rauch and Einstein, 1974; Kies, 1975). Even the most "pure" MBP preparations, however, reveal varying degrees of microheterogeneity (Chou *et al.*, 1976). This microheterogeneity may well account for differences in specific activity of MBP preparations reported by different laboratories. MBP is a heat-stable, acid-resistant, relatively flat molecule with a molecular weight (MW) in the range of 18,000–22,000 daltons (Rauch and Einstein, 1974; Kies, 1975). Amino acid sequencing reveals about 170 residues for all MBP preparations derived from nervous tissue of all mammalian species, except in the case of the rat. The rat has, in addition to a 170-residue molecule, a smaller molecular weight species MBP lacking a 40-amino acid sequence comprising the carboxyl terminal position of the parent molecule (Martenson *et al.*, 1972).

A number of defined peptides prepared by pepsin or trypsin digestion of MBP, together with a limited number of synthetic peptides, have been used to map amino acid sequences corresponding to specific antigenic determinant regions of the whole molecule. This work has focused primarily on identifying determinants responsible for encephalitogenic activity, and only secondarily on determinants engendering cell-mediated immune responses and antibody production. A surprising finding is that different amino acid sequences of a given MBP molecule are recognized as the major encephalitogenic determinant by different species of animals. As illustrated in Fig. 1, residues 116–122 containing the only tryptophan residue in the whole molecule represents a major encephalitogenic region for the guinea pig, but it has little or no activity in rabbits, rats, and monkeys (Chao and Einstein, 1970; Swanborg, 1970). Treatment of MBP with 2-hydroxyl-5-nitrobenzyl bromide blocks the tryptophan residue, causing the molecule to lose most of its encephalitogenic activity for guinea pigs (Swanborg, 1970; Eylar *et al.*, 1972), but not other species of animals. Residues 44–89, more specifically 66–75, appear to be the major encephalitogenic determinant for the rabbit (Shapira *et al.*, 1971). Amino acid residues adjacent to those comprising the 64–75 sequence appear to be crucial for activity in the rat (McFarlin *et al.*, 1973).

The reason for such striking species specificity of the EAE determinant is unclear. Increasing evidence that phenotypic expressions of immunologic

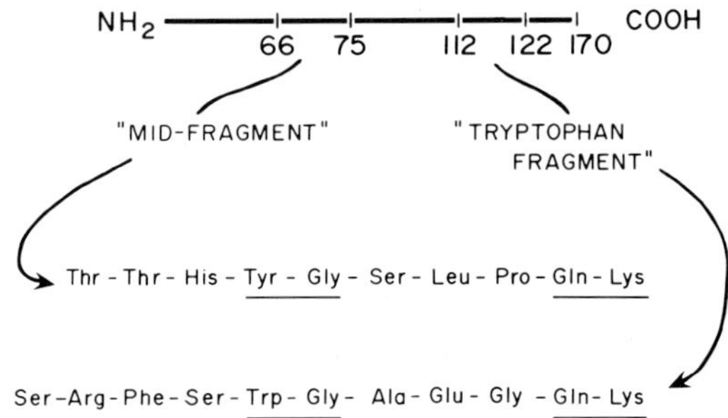

Fig. 1. Myelin basic protein of bovine origin. The "tryptophan fragment" represents amino acid residues 116–122 and contains the only tryptophan residue in the whole MBP molecule. Amino acids Trp-Gly and Gln-Lys appear to be critical residues comprising the major EAE-inducing determinant for guinea pigs. The "mid-fragment" shown here as representing amino acid residues 66–75 is a major EAE-inducing determinant for rabbits. The amino acids Tyr-Gly and Gln-Lys appear to be critical residues comprising this determinant. Note the similarity of this determinant to that of the tryptophan fragment determinant.

responsiveness reflect gene-dictated activities, and the fact that susceptibility to EAE exhibited by different species is under genetic control (see Section III,C) suggests that recognition of a specific sequence of amino acids as an encephalitogenic determinant might well be controlled by immune response genes. Another possibility, however, is that every host sensitized to MBP responds immunologically to many different amino acid sequences, each comprising different encephalitogenic determinants. Which immune response causes EAE, of the several responses to different determinants made by a host, might be decided by how accessible a particular amino acid sequence may be as it exists in that host's target tissue, i.e., intact brain and spinal cord. In other words, the way in which MBP is synthesized and inserted into the matrix of lipids and lipoproteins that make up the myelin in the guinea pig might result in tryptophan and adjacent residues being more available to bind sensitized cells or/and antibodies. This sequence of amino acids, thus, becomes the target determinant for point injury essential for initiating the sequence of immunopathological events causing full-blown CNS injury. This explanation is still dependent on genetic factors, but the genes in question are registering their effect at the very end of the immune response arc, i.e., where effector cells or antibodies bind to CNS target antigenic determinants.

At least eight different loci for inducing DH to MBP have been identified, and at least three different loci concerned with antibody production have been described (Bergstrand, 1973). As might be expected, many of these specific determinants represent regions of the MBP molecule or peptides shown to be devoid of encephalitogenic activity. What is a surprise is the uncertainty that still prevails as to whether the major encephalitogenic determinant for any given species of animal does or does not represent a determinant for T cell responses versus bone marrow derived lymphocyte (B cell) responses. The most definitive data has been derived from studies in guinea pigs, a species particularly favorable for detecting and quantitating DH responses *in vivo* and *in vitro*. These studies have utilized the nonapeptide synthetic fragment known to be encephalitogenic for this species of animal (Fig. 1). It is clear that the tryptophan residue in this fragment is essential for EAE-activity (Swanborg, 1970), and that the Gly-Gln-Lys residues are crucial for DH (Hashim and Sharpe, 1974). This sequence does not contain determinants for antibody production; these are found in larger fragments embracing residues 90–116 and 117–170, respectively (Driscoll *et al.*, 1974a). Lennon and Carnegie (1974) found that a synthetic peptide representing residues 112–122 had almost as much encephalitogenic activity in guinea pigs as whole MBP, and that the peptide induced excellent DH responses in this host, as assessed by MIF production by peritoneal exudate cells and proliferative responses of cultured splenocytes. Looking at these data, there is a very close association of encephalitogenic activity and T cell responsiveness confined to just a few amino acid residues represented in this peptide.

However, other data, which completely dissociate EAE-inducing activity and DH activity, can be cited. For example, Spitler and her associates (1972) found that a larger synthetic peptide identical to the nonapeptide, but containing the additional residues Ser and Arg on the N-terminal end of the fragment, has the capacity to induce EAE in guinea pigs without eliciting any demonstrable DH reactivity to MBP. MBP treated so as to block the tryptophan induced both *in vivo* and *in vitro* manifestations of DH, but was totally lacking in encephalitogenic activity. Obviously, more work is needed before one can say exactly what type of T cell subpopulation becomes activated by the tryptophan-containing encephalitogenic peptide in the guinea pig.

The specific antigenic activity of MBP preparations, in terms of dry weight, invariably falls short of that characterizing whole brain or spinal cord. One explanation for this discrepancy in EAE activities may be that MBP has a far greater immunogenetic potential as it exists in intact nervous tissue in physical–chemical linkage to lipids and lipoproteins, in contrast to its more limited antigenic activity when extracted from delipidated nerve tissue. Another explanation, however, may be that other antigenic constituents of CNS have a role in the pathogenesis of EAE. There are some clues suggesting that such may be the case. Although guinea pigs sensitized to MBP in adjuvant develop clinical paralytic signs and perivascular cellular infiltrates essentially indistinguishable from those observed in animals sensitized to whole spinal cord–adjuvant, they do not develop the degree of demyelination that characteristically occurs in association with the cellular infiltrates following sensitization with spinal cord–adjuvant (Hoffman *et al.*, 1973). This is even more true of the type of disease induced by sensitization with one of the synthetic EAE peptides (Hoffman *et al.*, 1973). Hand-in-hand with these observations is the finding that complement-dependent cytotoxic antibodies causing glial cell alterations and demyelination in organotypic brain cultures and appearing regularly in the sera of rabbits and other animals sensitized to whole nervous tissue adjuvant are not present in sera of animals sensitized to MBP-adjuvant (Seil *et al.*, 1968). Two groups of workers, however, have found sera of rabbits immunized with cerebroside to contain anti-glial and demyelinating antibodies (Dubois-Dalcq *et al.*, 1970; Fry *et al.*, 1974). In biochemical studies of sulfatide and cerebroside content of nervous tissue of animals with EAE induced by whole nervous tissue–adjuvant, only sulfatide abnormalities are demonstrable after sensitization with MBP–adjuvant (Maggio and Cumar, 1975). Sensitization with MBP plus adjuvant, together with a mixture of cerebrosides, however, elicit the sulfatide and cerebroside changes observed after whole nervous tissue–adjuvant. More attention needs to be paid to the role of CNS cerebrosides, not only in production of EAE, but with respect to their capacity to induce demyelinating antibodies. It is the occurrence of myelin injury per se, more than any other histopathological change characterizing EAE, that marks this disease as a promising model system for studies of the MS process.

B. Neuroantigen Autoreactivity

Key questions regarding the development of autoreactivity to neuroantigen in EAE and MS are no different from those concerning all forms of self-reactivity and autoimmune disease. Do the overwhelming majority of individuals remain clinically free of autoimmune neurological disease because of the absence of potential clones of immunocytes reactive with MBP, such clones having been deleted by exposure to this antigen during embryogenesis and early maturation? According to Burnet (1972), presence of MBP-reactive clones might occur under exceptional circumstances: (1) clones might fail to be eliminated because MBP is sequestered in the host's CNS, and a critical amount of this autoantigen is never able to impinge on the central and peripheral lymphoid tissues of the host, or (2) lymphocytes with receptors for MBP and potential reactivity for autologous MBP might arise through mutations. Contrary to Burnetian thinking and more in line with recent developments in cellular immunology, perhaps all individuals possess clones of MBP-reactive lymphoid cells in numbers potentially capable of causing CNS autoimmune disease, but they are restrained from causing CNS injury by various immunoregulatory factors, e.g., circulating MBP or MBP–antibody complexes; "blocking" antibody or T suppressor cell products (see Chapter 9 by I. R. Cohen and H. Wekerle) or thymus hormone factor (Small and Trainin, 1975).

The idea that MBP is unable to delete reactive clones of lymphoid cells because it is sequestered within the CNS is hard to accept in the light of recent information. Under normal conditions, the turnover rate of myelin constituents, including MBP, is relatively rapid (see review by Norton, 1975). Using a sensitive radioimmunoinhibition assay, McPherson *et al.* (1972) have obtained evidence that MBP is detectable in the CSF of patients with MS or other neurological diseases. Thomas (1975) has reported that relatively large amounts of neuroantigen are demonstrable in the systemic circulation a few days after severe head trauma. On the basis of this limited evidence, it seems very likely that, in normal subjects, minute amounts of CNS antigenic constituents, including MBP in all probability, periodically enter the CSF or/and systemic circulation and impinge upon peripheral lymphoid tissues.

Direct evidence for the existence of MBP-reactive lymphoid cells in animals and man has been reported by several laboratories using isotopically labeled MBP and autoradiographic technique. Coates and Lennon (1973) found appreciable binding of ^{125}I-MBP by normal guinea pig splenocytes, but little or no such binding by lymph node cells (LNC). Yung *et al.* (1973) reported human peripheral blood lymphocytes and both human and guinea pig LNC to bind ^{125}I-MBP. Several questions immediately arise. To what class of lymphoid cells is the labeled MBP binding, i.e., T cells or B cells? What specific immunogenic determinant is being bound by the lymphoid cell receptors? Yung *et al.* (1973) showed that if lymphoid cells were incubated with rabbit anti-human IgG in the cold for 30 minutes, subsequent binding of ^{125}I-MBP was reduced by about 80%, suggesting that the majority of the cells were B cells. Since there is compelling evidence from studies in guinea pigs that those antigenic determinants of MBP which elicit antibody production lie outside the 114–122 amino acid sequence encephalitogenic region, most of the MBP binding lymphoid cells reported by Coates and Lennon (1973) and Yung *et al.* (1973) may well involve antigenic determinants not directly concerned with production of EAE.

Lamoureux *et al.* (1967) showed that lightly ^{125}I-iodinated MBP, of the order of 35 μCi per microgram of protein, retains its encephalitogenic activity for guinea pigs. On this basis, it can be assumed that the ^{125}I-labeled MBP preparations used by Coates and Lennon (1973) and Yung *et al.*

(1973) contained intact encephalitogenic regions. A small percentage of the MBP-binding cells, of the order of about 20% (judging from the data of Yung *et al.*, 1973), therefore, might well be T cells with receptor sites for EAE-inducing immunogenic determinants.

The importance of taking the precaution to bioassay MBP preparations into which markers or labels have been inserted by chemical means is clearly evident in the study of Gonatas *et al.* (1974). They found the encephalitogenic activity of ^{125}I-MBP for Lewis rats to be no different from noniodinated MBP, thereby confirming the findings of Lamoureux *et al.* (1967) in guinea pigs. But Gonatas *et al.* (1974) went on to show that MBP following conjugation to horseradish peroxidase is virtually devoid of activity. Binding of horseradish peroxidase–MBP conjugates by sensitized rat lymphoid cells, as described by Gonatas *et al.* (1974), therefore, must involve an immunogenic determinant(s) on the molecule other than that responsible for EAE.

Orgad and Cohen (1974) reported that thymocytes of normal Lewis rats added to syngeneic fibroblast monolayers and allowed to incubate with CNS tissue for suitable periods had the capacity to transfer EAE into normal Lewis recipient rats. Noteworthy is the fact that the thymocytes were exposed to neuroantigen in the absence of normal rat serum. This work dramatically emphasizes the fact that cells clearly exist in normal lymphoid tissues having the potential for recognizing encephalitogenic determinants of MBP. The findings of these workers also underline the immense biologic importance of factors in normal serum, and presumably whole blood, which restrict such MBP reactive cells from being activated and proliferating to a degree which culminates in EAE under ordinary circumstances.

Ortiz-Ortiz and Weigle (1976) recently have provided pointed evidence that T cells and B cells of Lewis rats bind MBP and that it is the interaction of MBP with T cells that is the critical event with respect to EAE. They prepared monospecific antibodies reactive with B cell immunoglobulin surface receptors and monospecific immune serum against T cells. By determining to what extent these antibodies were able to reduce the binding of syngeneic ^{125}I-MBP by lymphoid tissues, these workers secured convincing data that both T cells and B cells with MBP-binding capacity exist in the thymus and spleen of Lewis rats. They then went on to take advantage of the "cell suicide" technique, namely, using radioiodinated MBP of very high specific activity capable of irreversibly injuring those lymphoid cells to which the labeled neuroantigen specifically binds. Thymectomized and irradiated Lewis rats reconstituted with normal bone marrow as a source of immunocompetent B cells, together with "suicided T cells," were unable to develop EAE when subsequently sensitized with unlabeled syngeneic MBP–CFA.

One explanation for lymphoid cells bearing receptors for the encephalitogenic determinant of MBP, in addition to those already mentioned above, is the sharing of MBP immunogenic determinants by unrelated antigens. Exposure to such cross-reacting antigens might well expand MBP-reacting clones to numbers easily detectable. Cross-reactivity between MBP and purified protein derivative (PPD), as well as cancer tissue demonstrable by both *in vivo* and *in vitro* assay systems for assessing DH, has been reported by several investigators (Goldstone *et al.*, 1973; McDermott *et al.*, 1974; Coates and Carnegie, 1975; Vandenbark *et al.*, 1975). Most unexpected are the findings of Teitelbaum *et al.* (1972) and Webb *et al.* (1973a). These investigators found that a random linear basic copolymer of alanine, glutamic acid, lysine, and tyrosine, designated as Cop 1, although completely lacking encephalitogenic activity, can suppress development of EAE in guinea pigs. The synthetic polymer must be injected intravenously in relatively large doses 5, 10, and 15 days after sensitization of animals with MBP–CFA. Webb *et al.* (1973a) showed that Cop 1 shares one or more immunogenic determinants responsible for DH with MBP, but had only limited cross-reactivity with respect to antibody production. Chelmicka-Szorc and Arnason (1975) have reported that poly-L-lysine (PLL) has a marked suppressive effect on development of EAE in outbred guinea pigs when administered daily via the subcutaneous route. Treatment could be started as late as 8 days after sensitization to neuroantigen and still be effective. Noteworthy is the fact that, in rats, Chelmicka-Szorc and Arnason (1975) found that PLL not only does not suppress EAE but actually potentiated the disease in this species of animals. This observation is reminiscent of observations reported by Kornguth *et al.* (1962) in rabbits treated with PLL. From these observations and those of Webb *et al.* (1973a), it seems likely that the EAE-suppressive effect of these synthetic polymers, and, conceivably, the EAE-potentiating effect as well, is due to cross-reactivity with MBP. The specific EAE-inhibiting activity of Cop 1 and species-specific inhibitory or suppressive effect of PLL, suggest that the cross-reactivity of these polymers must involve very restricted amino acid sequences on the MBP molecule.

Finally, polyadenylic acid [poly(A)], a synthetic polyribonucleotide homopolymer, in IFA lacking mycobacteria, has the capacity to induce histopathological changes indistinguishable from those of EAE in guinea pigs (Paterson, 1976c). The reason for believing that induction of disease resulted from cross-reactivity between poly(A) and MBP, in contrast to this synthetic polyribonucleotide acting merely as a clone-expanding adjuvant is the earlier observation indicating that poly(A) has no EAE adjuvanticity, which is a striking property of polyuridylic acid [poly(U)] (Paterson and Drobish, 1974).

C. Immunogenetic Factors

For many years, it was known that different strains of guinea pigs, mice, and rats differed in their susceptibility to EAE (see review of Paterson, 1976a). More recent data have shown that genes segregating in close association with those coding for specific histocompatibility antigens exert an important influence on EAE susceptibility. Gasser *et al.* (1973), in studies using Lewis and DA inbred strains of rats, known to be highly susceptible to EAE, and the EAE-resistant BN inbred strain of rats, found that susceptibility to the disease was controlled by a single gene effect closely linked to but not identical to the Ag-C major histocompatibility locus. Williams and Moore (1973), in more detailed immunogenetic studies of Lewis and BN rats, including elaborate backcrossing, concluded that an autosomal dominant gene linked to the histocompatibility locus determines susceptibility to EAE by acting as an immune response (Ir) gene. In the preceding studies, rats were sensitized either with whole guinea pig spinal cord–CFA or MBP combined with CFA. Levine and Sowinski (1975) have uncovered the important fact that the resistance of the BN rat strain is not absolute. BN rats sensitized with rat or guinea pig spinal cord, using carbonyl iron as a different immunologic adjuvant, clearly have the capacity to develop EAE. Levine and Sowinski (1975) made the suggestion that the gene influencing susceptibility to EAE may be exerting its effect more in terms of how well rats respond to immunologic adjuvants, i.e., expansion of MBP-reactive clones by adjuvants. McFarlin *et al.* (1975a,b), again working with the Lewis and BN inbred strains of rats and intact MBP or an encephalitogenic MBP fragment (amino acid residues 45–86) containing the EAE determinant for this species of animal, have provided very strong evidence that an Ir gene(s) not only determines susceptibility to EAE, but all other immune responses to this molecule or antigenic fragment; these were monitored in parallel with development of the disease, namely, lymphocyte proliferation, DH and MBP antibody production (as measured by radioimmunoassay). Lewis rats showed excellent proliferation of lymphocytes and intense DH- and MBP-binding activity in concert with EAE; BN rats had virtually no capacity to exhibit any of these four parameters of immunologic responsiveness.

The most pointed observation comes from the work of Ortiz-Ortiz and Weigle (1976). These workers showed that the BN rat essentially has no demonstrable T-cells with MBP receptors in thymic tissue or spleen. One is left with the dilemma of explaining the occurrence of EAE in BN rats sensitized to spinal cord as reported by Levine and Sowinski (1975) if it is assumed that T cells bear the major, if not sole, responsibility for development of disease. It should be noted that there is no reason to believe that a single T cell response is all that is necessary for EAE. All of the studies of Ortiz-Ortiz and Weigle (1976) utilized MBP as the neuroantigen. Conceivably, other antigenic constituents in whole spinal cord might be important for the production of EAE in the BN rat. It is also conceivable that the use of carbonyl iron as an EAE adjuvant employed by Levine and Sowinski (1975) causes expansion of very few potential T-cell clones in normal BN rat lymphoid tissues which escape detection using the method of Ortiz-Ortiz and Weigle (1976).

Levine and Sowinski (1973, 1974) and Bernard (1976), using a variety of isohistogeneic and congenic strains of mice, have secured definitive evidence that susceptibility to EAE is controlled by genes closely associated with genes comprising the H-2 alleles coding for histocompatibility antigens. Since the most susceptible strains of mice had different H-2 alleles, it seems likely that susceptibility to EAE is inherited as a dominant, polygenic trait and, thus, is not dictated by a single Ir gene. Bernard (1976) has been able to pinpoint the locus of gene control of disease susceptibility as being on the K end of the histocompatibility gene complex, and he has shown that this same locus also controls cell-mediated immune responsiveness to MBP, as reflected by MIF production.

A major question concerning immunogenetic influences over susceptibility of a given species of animal to EAE is whether the gene determinant influences immune responsiveness to the encephalitogenic determiant per se, or, alternatively, materially influences other immunologic responses to other immunogenic determinants on the molecule, which may diminish or enhance the expression of the immune response to the EAE determinant. It may be added also, as already discussed (see Section III,A), that gene effects may be expressed at the target site in terms of the possible accessibility antigenic determinants in intact nervous tissue regarding their capacity to bind sensitized cells or antibodies. It should be noted that in the studies of Webb *et al.* (1973b), although strain 2 guinea pigs have very little capacity to develop EAE, they exhibit no appreciable impairment in other responses to neuroantigens. For example, strain 2 guinea pigs develop DH and antibodies reactive with MBP just as well as outbred or strain 13 guinea pigs, both of which are highly susceptible to EAE. In fact, strain 2 guinea pigs appear to have a much greater capacity to produce antibody to MBP than the other two strains, and Webb *et al.* (1973b) suggest that this may account, at least in part, for their EAE resistance. Such antibody may be acting as blocking antibody and interfering with other immune responses directly concerned with pathogenesis of disease.

D. Immunopotentiation Prerequisites

The availability of EAE as a model disease in its present form is a reflection of the development of immunologic adjuvants that could potentiate the inherently weak immunogenic activity of CNS antigens. Early studies of EAE adjuvanticity showed that different immunologic adjuvants differed strikingly in their capacity to augment immune responses to neuroantigen in different species of animals, or even within different strains of animals of a given species. For example, Freund and Stone (1959) found that EAE cannot be produced in the guinea pig unless the neuroantigen is incorporated in CFA, i.e., paraffin oil containing killed mycobacteria or other microorganisms which usually have less adjuvanticity. In contrast, rats were found to develop excellent EAE following sensitization to spinal cord incorporated into IFA lacking mycobacteria (Bell and Paterson, 1960; Paterson and Bell, 1962). On the other hand, a suspension of *Bordetella pertussis* (pertussis vaccine), although having a dramatic accelerating and intensifying effect on production of EAE in Lewis rats, has no potentiating activity for EAE production in the guinea pig and, in fact, may actually interfere with production of the disease in this species of animal (Paterson, 1973a).

Adjuvants probably act as immunopotentiating agents by providing a second signal to a lymphoid cell bearing specific receptor surface configurations for one or more antigenic determinants, as illustrated in Fig. 2.

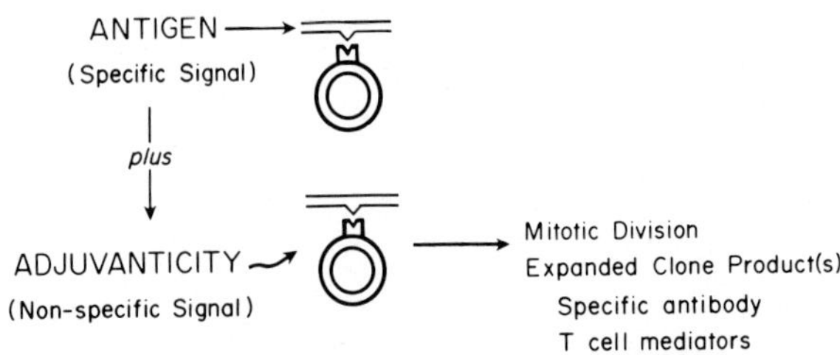

Fig. 2. Double-signal triggering of T or B lymphocytes. Interaction of specific antigenic determinants and nonspecific adjuvant moiety with their respective receptor sites on the same lymphoid cell is depicted as essential for maximum clonal expansion and output of immune cell products.

Interaction of the adjuvant moiety upon the lymphoid cell surface causes activation of the cell if it has already bound specific antigen. Activation of the cell leads to clonal expansion and a marked increase in the total output of whatever immunologic products the cell may be destined to make, as determined by its genetic status. Based on recent evidence, different immunologic adjuvants would appear to have selectivity, if not specificity, for different classes of cells acting singly or in collaboration in the immune response (Allison, 1973). That is, some immunologic adjuvants, such as *B. pertussis*, may act as T cell expanders in contrast to gram-negative bacterial lipopolysaccharide, which is a polyclonal B cell expander. More recently, evidence suggests that the locus of action of some other adjuvants is at the site of the macrophage. Referring to Fig. 2, one can visualize that different specific adjuvants have different stereospecific receptor areas on specific lymphocyte populations or lymphoid cell subsets, and in order for maximum adjuvanticity to occur, a given adjuvant must impact upon a lymphocyte which has a receptor site for the antigen (injected with the adjuvant) against which the immune response is to be immunopotentiated. In terms of EAE, the adjuvant receptor, therefore, must be on a lymphocyte, possibly a T cell, which also bears MBP receptors in order to generate a critical mass of immune effectors (sensitized T or antibody-producing B cells) sufficient to exceed the threshold for development and recognition of disease.

One implication of this MBP–adjuvant double signal cell activation concept (Fig. 2) needs to be emphasized at this point. Suppression of EAE might be accomplished by saturation of adjuvant receptors on lymphoid cells which also bear MBP receptor areas. That is, exposure of such cells to excessive amounts of the EAE–adjuvant alone, resulting in saturation of all adjuvant receptor sites, might render such MBP-reactive lymphoid cells incapable of being activated by the neuroantigen. Phenotypically, the host would appear to be tolerant of MBP. Lisak and Zweiman (1974) have reported that EAE is significantly suppressed in guinea pigs receiving an injection of CFA several days or weeks before sensitization of nervous tissue or MBP–CFA. Detailed immunologic studies of such animals has shown that suppression of disease correlated directly with diminished cell-mediated immune responses to the neuroantigen. Undiminished responsiveness of the CFA-pretreated guinea pigs to *in vitro* mitogenic stimulation with the plant lectin, phytohemagglutinin, together with augmented PPD cutaneous reactivity in such animals, provided evidence that the adjuvant-induced suppression of EAE was specific for MBP. It is unlikely that the CFA suppression of EAE is due to the antigenic sharing between PPD and MBP (McDermott *et al.*, 1974; Vandenbark *et al.*, 1975) already referred to, since PPD has little or no adjuvant activity for EAE production. furthermore, the quantity of PPD represented by the relatively small amount (100 μg) of mycobacteria (in oil), which sufficed to elicit suppression of disease was well below that required for demonstrating cross-reactivity with MBP. Conceivably, the mechanism of inducing tolerance to an autoantigen as outlined here might be especially useful in situations where giving the autoantigen itself would be considered hazardous.

E. Primary Role of T Cells and Cell-Mediated Immune Responses

The lines of evidence for T cells engendering DH to MBP playing a major role in the pathogenesis of EAE may be summarized as follows.

First, many studies in outbred or inbred species of animals susceptible to EAE have described a direct correlation between the presence of DH to MBP and occurrence of disease (see review of Alvord *et al.*, 1975). In some of these studies, no such correlation could be discerned with respect to presence or titer of MBP antibody.

Second, prevention of EAE by injections of MBP in IFA either before or after sensitization to whole CNS tissue or MBP or other preparations, e.g., CFA or Cop 1, invariably has been accompanied by marked diminution or absence of *in vivo* or/and *in vitro* correlates of DH in protected animals without any corresponding suppression of antibody production.

Third, cell transfer of EAE with sensitized lymphoid cells, in the face of no substantial evidence for reproducible transfer of disease with immune serum, has provided the most telling evidence supportive of a cell-mediated immune mechanism. Several reservations should be kept in mind, however, concerning this line of thinking. Transfer of any immunologic process may be due to antibody-producing B cells, and not necessarily the result of sensitized T cells. The precise type of cell in suspensions of sensitized donor LNC with EAE transfer activity has not been identified with certainty. Transfer of EAE with immune serum has been reported (see Section III,F). Based on transfer of other autoimmune diseases with immune serum, the essential conditions for passive transfer of EAE with antibody may so far not have been considered. Finally, both sensitized T cells and antibody-shedding B cells may be required for transfer of EAE having all the clinical and immunohistopathological features characterizing that form of the disease observed in actively sensitized animals.

Fourth, early studies of EAE implicated T cell participation in the development of the disease. Only recently, however, has evidence been secured that T cells are essential for induction of disease and that the specific T cell subpopulation involved is one distinct from that possessing "helper" function for B cells, and, thus, is not linked to antibody production in any way.

It is useful to examine some of the studies related to T cell function in the pathogenesis of EAE. Arnason *et al.* (1962) showed that neonatally thymectomized rats had a markedly reduced capacity to develop EAE. This finding was difficult to interpret because such animals also were compromised with respect to production of antibody. A singular report (Blaw *et al.*, 1967) that EAE occurs in chickens rendered hypo- or aggamaglobulinemic by prior extirpation of the bursa of Fabricius is difficult to interpret because of the small number of birds that were truly agammaglobulinemic.

Gonatas and Howard (1974) were the first to secure definitive evidence that T cells are a prerequisite for development of EAE in rats. Adult Lewis rats were thymectomized, subjected to total body irradiation, and reconstituted with bone marrow cells from thymectomized, thoracic duct-drained donors, thereby assuring that no T cells were represented in the bone marrow suspension. Such rats were totally lacking in their capacity to develop EAE following sensitization to guinea pig spinal cord or MBP–CFA. Absence of MBP-binding antibody indicated that the rats were deficient in T cells collaborating with antibody-producing B cells. The absence of helper T cells provided indirect evidence that the rats were being truly depleted of all T cell subpopulations, but left open the question of whether antibody might have a role in the disease.

The studies of Ortiz-Ortiz and Weigle (1976) and Ortiz-Ortiz *et al.* (1976) have provided compelling evidence that a specific T cell subpopulation causes EAE. Neonatally thymectomized and irradiated Lewis rats, when reconstituted with LNC and splenocytes of normal syngeneic donors, developed EAE after sensitization to MBP–CFA. If such immunocompromised rats, however, were reconstituted with donor lymphoid cells which had been treated with rabbit immune serum specific for T cells, plus complement, the animals did not develop EAE. LNC and splenocytes collected from donors 9 days after sensitization to MBP–CFA transferred EAE and MBP antibody production to immunocompromised recipients. Recipients of sensitized lymphoid cells, which has been treated with antithymocyte serum plus complement, however, had demonstrable levels of circulating MBP antibody, but virtually no evidence of EAE.

Further evidence for the primary function of T cells in EAE was provided by the suicide experiments of Ortiz-Ortiz and Weigle (1976) already mentioned (see Section III,B). That is, using ^{125}I-MBP of very high specific activity, these workers showed that when a mixture of normal T cells, together with suicided B cells, was used to reconstitute immunocompromised Lewis recipient rats and the animals were subsequently challenged with MBP–CFA, the rats developed typical EAE unaccompanied by MBP antibody production. Recipients reconstituted with normal B cells plus suicided T cells and challenged with MBP–CFA developed neither EAE nor demonstrable MBP antibody production.

From the foregoing experiments, Ortiz-Ortiz and his associates concluded that (1) T cells other than "helper cells" are a prerequisite for production of EAE, (2) Lewis rats can develop EAE without evidence of MBP antibody production, and, (3) presence of MBP antibody by itself is not sufficient to result in disease. What is yet to be determined is whether the pattern of EAE elicited in these rats by MBP–CFA had all the features of this autoimmune disease which characteristically occur in normal unmanipulated rats actively sensitized to MBP–CFA or to whole CNS tissue combined with CFA.

F. Observations Suggesting a Role for B Cells and Antibody

Reference already has been made to studies (see Section III,A) showing that (1) CNS constituents other than MBP may well induce cytotoxic antibodies which demyelinate organotypic brain culture targets, (2) such antibodies do not appear in animals sensitized to MBP–CFA, and (3) the pattern of EAE in such animals does not have the degree of demyelination characteristically associated with that form of EAE induced by whole nervous tissue. On balance, these findings suggest that antibodies reactive with antigens other than MBP may contribute to myelin injury, which most workers view as an essential histopathological features of the disease. Since Wolfgram and Duquette (1976) found that purified myelin had very little capacity to absorb demyelinating antibodies, in contrast to the residual myelin pellet left behind following isolation of myelin from brain white matter, it is clear that the antigenic constituents against which the demyelinating antibody is directed may well not be myelin per se.

Earlier studies from the author's laboratory (Paterson and Harwin, 1963) showed that if immune serum was collected from Wistar rats following recovery from EAE and given daily or every other day to other Wistar rats sensitized to spinal cord–CFA, the serum treatment had a marked inhibitory effect on development of EAE. EAE-inhibitory activity of the immune serum appeared to be directly related to the presence, but not the titer, of antibodies fixing complement with lipid extracts of brain. It was argued that if immune serum can transfer inhibition of EAE in actively sensitized rats, then antibodies must play some role in the disease. These findings were confirmed by Hughes (1974), using the same treatment regimen but a different strain of rat. Hughes and Leibowitz (1975) subsequently showed that the EAE-inhibitory activity of immune serum did not reside in antibodies directed against galactocerebroside.

Simon and Simon (1975) recently reported mild clinical neurological signs and electroencephalographic abnormalities in rabbits following a single injection of a relatively small volume of rabbit anti-brain immune serum either into the ventricle or into the suboccipital subarachnoid space (cerebellum–pontine cistern). Histopathological changes, consisting of focal perivascular accumulations of inflammatory cells localized largely to subpial and subependymal areas of brain tissue and occasionally accompanied by significant myelin injury, were present in the majority of the animals (all of which were killed 35 days after injection of immune serum). These workers took the trouble to demonstrate by means of appropriate fluoresceinated antibody that the injected immune immunoglobulin spread from the subarachnoid space and ventricular system into and for considerable distances along perivascular spaces of the brain and actually penetrated the neuropil. Rabbits similarly injected with normal rabbit serum remained clinically well. Mild and transitory electroencephalographic changes were observed following injection of one of the three normal sera. Except for small areas of what was interpreted to be perivascular edema, these control animals had no demonstrable inflammatory reactions or demyelinative changes suggestive of EAE. This study is important for several reasons. It is the only real confirmation of an earlier report of Janković *et al.* (1965) describing histopathological changes resembling EAE in guinea pigs after multiple intraventricular injections of brain immune serum. The experiments of Simon and Simon (1975) carries greater weight because (1) the rabbits received only a single injection of immune serum, (2) the animals exhibited clinical as well as electroencephalographic abnormalities, (3) histopathological changes indistinguishable from EAE were found at least 1 month after injection of immune serum, and (4) binding of IgG (presumably specific brain antibody) to brain tissue, not only was demonstrated, but was shown to occur at exactly those anatomic sites where inflammatory changes and myelin injury subsequently occurred. On balance, the studies of Janković *et al.* (1965) and Simon and Simon (1975) suggest that antibody against CNS tissue antigen(s) may play a role in the pathogenesis of EAE. These studies can also be looked at as supporting the idea previously outlined by the author (Paterson, 1966,1976a) that the blood–cerebrospinal fluid–brain vascular barriers, known to restrict passive diffusion of macromolecules the size of immunoglobulins from the vascular compartment into CNS neuropil, undoubtedly represent a formidable physiological obstacle for successful passive transfer of EAE with immune serum. Indeed, it could be this unique feature of the CNS vasculature that accounts for the enormous difficulty in securing evidence of transfer of EAE with serum, in contrast to the successful passive transfers of other autoimmune experimental diseases with immune serum.

One ancillary role for antibody, specifically IgE antibody, might be through increasing the permeability of the CSF–brain–blood vascular barriers so that sensitized T cells, IgG-synthesizing B cells, and/or circulating free antibody itself might have a greater opportunity to enter the CNS. For example, IgE antibody reactive with MBP conceivably might bind to mast cells or basophils residing within or circulating through nervous tissue. If the bound IgE then reacted with MBP, it could cause the release of vasoactive pharmacologic mediators, thereby serving as an "anaphylactic trigger" to increase vascular permeability. Such a role for IgE antibody has been shown by Benveniste *et al.* (1972) with respect to increasing deposition of circulating immune complexes in vessels of rabbits developing serum sickness.

IgE most likely would be a candidate for assuming an ancillary role in the accelerated, hyperacute form of EAE induced in Lewis rats sensitized to nervous tissue of MBP combined with *B. pertussis* as a supplemental immunologic adjuvant (see review of Levine, 1974). Rats immunized to a variety of different antigens, together with pertussis vaccine, have a striking propensity to produce so-called homocytotrophic antibody, i.e., reaginic or IgE antibody responses (Tada and Okumura, 1971). Moore *et al.* (1974a) have demonstrated that a proportion of Lewis rats sensitized to spinal cord–CFA plus pertussis vaccine produce low titers of IgE antibody reactive with MBP, based on serum assays using passive cutaneous anaphylaxis (PCA). There was no correlation between the presence of serum PCA activity or PCA titer and the pattern of EAE in individual rats. In a companion study, Moore *et al.* (1974b) reported that treatment with cyproheptadine or/and methyseride maleate, which block the pharmacologic action of serotonin and histamine, did not alter the pattern of hyperacute EAE in Lewis rats. For these reasons, these authors believed it unlikely that IgE has a role in the disease in rats. These authors noted, however, that in the rat slow-reacting substance A (SRS-A), in addition to histamine and serotonin, may be a mediator for IgE-elicited reactions. It was suggested that additional studies need to be undertaken, using a drug which blocks SRS-A. One additional reservation about the study of Moore *et al.* (1974b) might be mentioned. Mast cells have been reported to occur in the CNS of rats (Kruger, 1974), although not in anything like the numbers seen in the connective tissues of PNS. IgE-elicited release of histamine or/and serotonin from mast cells within the CNS might not be blocked by parenterally administrated drugs unless given in doses sufficient to penetrate the restrictive CSF–brain–blood vascular barriers and reach whatever critical concentrations are required within the central neuraxis for pharmacologic blockade.

Johnson *et al.* (1971) and Lennon *et al.* (1972) have shown that occasional cells reactive with MBP can be detected among the inflammatory cells comprising the focal CNS perivascular cellular infiltrates of rabbits and guinea pigs with EAE induced by MBP–CFA. In the electron microscopic study of Johnson *et al.* (1971), horseradish peroxidase–MBP conjugate was used as a marker for those inflammatory cells binding MBP. The cells binding the conjugate had the morphological features of plasmacytoid–plasma cells. The findings suggested that such cells might be antibody-producing cells, raising the question of local or *in situ* release of MBP antibody by B cells within target tissues.

As has already been discussed (see Section III,B), the process of conjugating MBP to horseradish peroxidase causes enough alteration of the 44–89 residue sequence to render this major encephalitogenic determinant for rats totally inactive in this species of animal (Gonatas *et al.*, 1974). Since this region of MBP also contains the major encephalitogenic determinant for rabbits (Fig. 1), one might well assume that horseradish peroxidase–MBP conjugates would be nonencephalitogenic for this species of animal. Therefore, the lymphoid cells binding horseradish peroxidase–MBP within the cellular infiltrates described by Johnson *et al.* (1971) probably were B cells with specificity for immunogenic determinants of MBP distinct from that endowing the molecule with encephalitogenic activity. In this light, such immunocytes and their putative antibody product would not be likely to play a primary role in development of the disease.

Lennon *et al.* (1972) used an ingenious technique to show that antibody reactive with MBP is released by cells within the CNS perivascular cellular infiltrates of guinea pigs. Cryostat sections of CNS tissue were air dried and dipped in a gel menstruum containing sheep red blood cells (SRBC) coated with Fab fragments of rabbit anti-SRBC IgG to which MBP was conjugated by means of glutaraldeyde. After addition of complement, incubation at 37°C, fixation, and staining, clear plaques corresponding to areas of SRBC lysis were observed and found to be localized to focal cellular infiltrates within the tissue sections. Not all focal perivascular cellular infiltrates had such evidence of MBP antibody having been shed into the gel menstruum.

Although Lennon *et al.* (1972) did not determine whether conjugating MBP to the FAB–SRBC indicator system seriously altered the tryptophan region of MBP, the encephalitogenic determinant for guinea pigs (Fig. 1), two observations indirectly suggest that such was not the case. First, antibody synthesized and released by cells within the CNS infiltrates was reactive with native MBP, as shown by inhibition of hemolytic plaques when an excess of free MBP was added to the gel menstruum. Second, essentially identical patterns of hemolytic plaques occurred in CNS sections of guinea pigs following sensitization with a synthetic peptide containing the enceph-alitogenic tryptophan determinant.

Taken together, the studies summarized in this and the preceding section can be interpreted as clues that antibody to CNS antigen(s) or B cells with receptors for such antigen(s) may participate to some degree in the development of EAE. This seems especially likely if one considers EAE with all of its varied manifestations and, particularly, the occurrence of demyelination.

It is worthwhile considering the role of antibody-producing B cells, as opposed to free circulating antibody, as immune effectors in EAE, especially the role they may play in terms of antibody production within the target. Werdelin and McCluskey (1971), in their study of cellular transfer of EAE in Lewis rats, used donor LNC, labeled *in vitro* with ^{3}H-thymidine, ^{3}H-adenosine, or ^{3}H-uridine. Labeled donor cells could be located within the CNS cellular infiltrates of the recipient rats, using conventional autoradiographic methods. Werdelin and McCluskey (1971) showed that peripheral lymphoid cells of sensitized rats are demonstrable in areas of CNS injury characterizing EAE in the recipients. Donor cells represented only 10% or less, usually less, of the inflammatory cells in any given perivascular cellular infiltrate. The donor cells had no evident preferential propensity for localizing to the CNS infiltrates, based on their presence in comparable numbers in the infiltrates of a control organ, e.g., the adrenal gland of recipients previously actively sensitized to adrenal tissue and developing adrenalitis.

The studies of Johnson *et al.* (1971) and Lennon *et al.* (1972), extend the finding of Werdelin and McCluskey (1971) by showing that sensitized B cells specifically reactive with MBP, at least, are present in the CNS cellular infiltrates. One can visualize such antibody-producing lymphocytes entering an area of immune CNS injury, perhaps initially caused by the interaction of sensitized T lymphocytes with MBP in the target. Once within the neuropil and stimulated by MBP, the B cells might well shed large amounts of antibody *in situ*. The amount of antibody would be expected to exceed concentrations which could be attained by antibody penetrating the neuraxis by passive diffusion. This sequence of immunologic events has been proposed and discussed in greater detail by the author in a previous review article (Paterson, 1966). This postulated mode of participation of antibody in the EAE process would require intact B cells to enter the CNS target, thereby appearing consistent with the prevailing view that EAE is a cell-mediated type of immune response. This thesis would readily explain why EAE cannot be transferred with parenterally injected free antibody, unless it is deposited directly within the target, as it was in the studies of Janković *et al.* (1965) and Simon and Simon (1975).

IV. EAE AS AN EXPERIMENTAL MODEL SYSTEM FOR MS

Ever since its discovery, EAE has been subjected to critical examination as to how well it serves as an experimental counterpart of MS (Paterson, 1972, 1973b; Mackay *et al.*, 1973). It is useful to compare the major immunologic events associated with both diseases, keeping two points in mind. On the one hand, concordance of immunologic responses in EAE and MS provides the core evidence that autoreactivity to neuroantigen plays a role in the human disease. Discordance of immunologic events, on the other hand, serves as a clue that nonimmunologic determinants, such as viruses, may be important in the MS process.

Comparative immunologic responses in EAE and MS are listed in Table III. Within the CNS target tissue, conspicuous amounts of γ-globulin appears to be selectively deposited within the peripheral margins of the plaques of demyelination and gliosis characterizing MS (Tourtellotte,

TABLE III

Comparative Immunologic Responses in EAE and MS

Immunologic event	EAE	MS
CNS lesions		
IgG deposits	±	+
Complement deposits	± or 0	0
CSF compartment		
Elevated IgG	+	+
Oligoclonal IgG	ND[a]	+
Altered κ/λ ratio of IgG	ND	+
Ig-secreting mononuclear cells	ND	+
Vascular compartment		
Gel-ppt or C-fix antibodies	+	0
Antiglial-demyelinating antibodies	+	+
Cutaneous reactivity (DH)	+	0
MIF production	+	+ or 0

[a] ND, Not determined.

1971). There is some evidence that IgG extracted from MS plaque lesions may cause C-dependent demyelination of organotypic brain cultures, but more work along this line is needed before the observations can be accepted as fact. At the very least, the C-dependent cytotoxic demyelinating antibodies demonstrable in a high proportion of EAE and MS sera (see Section III,F) may well be of pathogenetic significance in human demyelinating disease. In contrast, deposits of IgG within or in juxtaposition to the perivascular cellular infiltrates of EAE have been noted in only a small proportion of animals (Oldstone and Dixon, 1968). No attempts to extract IgG from EAE lesions and to determine whether it exhibits demyelinating activity for brain cultures have been reported. Conceivably, C-dependent demyelinating antibody may accumulate very slowly at sites of CNS injury, and require much longer periods of time before significant deposits of IgG are detectable. This would explain the infrequency of such deposits in animals usually examined during initial episodes of acute EAE occurring only 2 or 3 weeks after sensitization to CNS tissue. It would be of interest to search for CNS deposits of IgG in rats and guinea pigs with the recurrent or chronic progressive forms of EAE that have been recently described (McFarlin *et al.*, 1974; Snyder *et al.*, 1975). In neither EAE nor MS had deposition of C been shown to occur with regularity in CNS lesions. Furthermore, occurrence of characteristic EAE in rats depleted of serum C, to a degree insufficient for development of renal injury after injection of nephrotoxic immune serum, would appear to exclude a role for the C cascade in the pathogenesis of this autoimmune disease (Levine *et al.*, 1971).

The CSF of animals with EAE and a high proportion of patients with clinically active MS shows a selective increase in immunoglobulin content, usually IgG (Kabat *et al.*, 1951; Tourtellotte, 1971). The IgG in MS–CSF specimens is oligoclonal, i.e., of restricted heterogeneity, and has an altered κ–λ ratio compared to the serum IgG of the same individual (see reviews by Paterson, 1972, 1973b). Cultures of cells in the CSF of MS patients are known to synthesize and shed immunoglobulins (Cohen and Bannister, 1967). These observations indicate that the increased amounts of IgG in MS–CSF samples reflect synthesis and secretion of immunoglobulin by B cells within the neuraxis. There are no comparable data concerning the nature and origin of the elevated IgG in CSF of animals with EAE. A key question of paramount importance in both the animal and human diseases is the specificity of the CSF–Ig. EAE–CSF on rare occasions has been tested for C-dependent demyelinating activity and found to be positive (Appel and Bornstein, 1964), suggesting that the IgG may be directed against oligodendroglial cells (see Section III,G). MS–CSF has been reported by several laboratories to cause demyelination or/and glial cell toxicity in brain cultures, but the specificity of this effect for MS was often not clear-cut. It is clear that the CSF–IgG in neither EAE nor MS reacts specifically with MBP (see review by Paterson, 1969, 1971).

Turning to the systemic circulation, antibodies reactive with a variety of CNS constituents, including MBP, are demonstrable in the sera of animals with EAE using conventional gel-precipitating or C-fixation tests, or by sensitive methods such as radioimmunoassay (Day and Pitts, 1974). Circulating antibodies specifically reactive with MBP or other CNS components and restricted to patients with MS have not been detected in studies where control groups of patients have been included and studied in double-blind fashion. In contrast, and as already stressed (see Section III,G), the sera of animals with EAE and patients with MS very often contain C-dependent cytotoxic immunoglobulins, which cause essentially identical glial cell toxicity and dissolution of myelin in organotypic myelinating brain cultures (see reviews of Bornstein, 1973; Paterson, 1971). This finding, at the very least, indicates that EAE and MS have in common an immune response to CNS and one which may well be implicated in the occurrence of demyelination in both diseases. Production of seemingly identical cytotoxic antibodies by animals with EAE and patients with MS is the strongest available evidence that immunopathogenetic determinants play an important role in the development of each disease.

Lebar *et al.* (1976) have shown that, in guinea pigs with EAE, the C-dependent demyelinating antibodies have the characteristics of IgG2 class immunoglobulins and that they are directed against CNS antigenic constituents distinct from MBP and cerebroside. Based on the observations of Wolfgram and Duquette (1976), it is likely that these cytotoxic antibodies produced by animals with EAE and as well as patients with MS are specifically directed against oligodendroglia. These glial cells in CNS tissue are responsible for the synthesis and maintenance of myelin. Injury of oligodendroglial cell membranes resulting from binding of antibody and activation of the C cascade is a plausible explanation for the dramatic alternations in integrity of myelinated nerve fibers so evident in brain cultures exposed to EAE and MS sera. It is important to note that these injurious effects are reversible; replacement of serum with fresh tissue culture maintenance fluid is followed by evidence of remyelination within a matter of hours (see review of Bornstein, 1973).

With respect to cell-mediated immune responses, innumerable studies have shown a direct correlation between occurrence of DH as reflected by cutaneous reactivity to CNS tissue antigens, especially MBP, and development of EAE (see review of Alvord *et al.*, 1975). Less extensive investigation, using *in vitro* assay systems for detection of cell-mediated immunity, best exemplified by production of MIF, also has revealed a close association with development of EAE. In contrast, the few studies that have been conducted with MS patients have failed to demonstrate any significant cutaneous reactivity to nervous tissue. Since skin testing with any neuroantigenic preparation, in theory, might increase the intensity of preexisting cell-mediated immune responses to nervous tissue and represent a potential hazard for MS patients, it is not surprising that relatively few patients have been studied and that virtually no information is available concerning reactivity to MBP, as opposed to extracts of whole nervous tissue.

Using *in vitro* correlates of DH, such as MIF production, which bypass the need for skin testing patients, the evidence for participation of cell-mediated immune responses in the MS process is impressive.

Two different laboratories (Bartfeld and Atoynatan, 1970; Bartfeld *et al.*, 1972; Rocklin *et al.*, 1971; Sheremata *et al.*, 1974, 1976) have secured strong evidence that peripheral blood lymphocyte cultures derived from a variable proportion of MS patients produce MIF when stimulated by whole CNS tissue extracts of MBP. Sheremata *et al.* (1976), in a prospective study of MS patients, have clearly shown that MBP-induced production of MIF is demonstrable a few days before occurrence of an acute exacerbation of disease and is most likely to be found in those patients studied 4 weeks or less after onset of an acute relapse. These findings are important because they suggest that cell-mediated immune reactions against MBP, as reflected by MIF production, may be causally related to the development of the intermittent acute clinical relapses characterizing the MS process. A third laboratory (Behan *et al.*, 1972), however, was unable to confirm these findings using the same basic assay technique for MIF production and the same preparation of MBP antigen as employed by Rocklin *et al.* (1971). Perhaps the reason for the failure of Behan *et al.* (1972) to demonstrate MIF production lies in their not including sufficient numbers of MS patients who were studied very soon after appearance of acute exacerbations of disease, i.e., within 3 or 4 weeks or less.

It should be stressed that MIF production in response to MBP is not a specific *in vitro* response limited to MS. Bartfeld *et al.* (1972) reported MIF production by some patients with amyotropic lateral sclerosis, which is not considered to represent a primary demyelinative disorder. Rocklin *et al.* (1971) and Sheremata *et al.* (1976) observed MIF production by a fairly high proportion of patients with acute cerebrovascular accidents and by occasional patients with various CNS disorders other than MS. It is noteworthy that Sheremata *et al.* (1976) found MIF production associated with acute cerebral infarctions to be demonstrable only in those patients studied 3 or more weeks after onset of the cerebrovascular accident. This finding would imply that this *in vitro* correlate of cell-mediated immunity reflects a *de novo* immune response called forth by CNS injury, possibly due to altered MBP being released into the systemic circulation and impinging upon peripheral lymphoid tissues.

On balance, the pattern of immune responses in EAE and MS (Table III) may reflect, in fact, radical differences in how neuroantigen is presented to the animal or human host. In the induction of EAE, the neuroantigen is emulsified in adjuvant and injected parenterally in a manner designed to maximally sensitize peripheral lymphoid tissues. It is in such peripheral lymphoid tissues that all immune responses implicated in the pathogenesis of EAE must be generated. From these sites, the products of these immune responses must travel via the blood stream to interact with their target and cause CNS injury. There should be no difficulty, therefore, in detecting sensitized lymphocytes and antibodies directed against MBP or other neuroantigens in the blood of animals developing EAE. In MS, on the other hand, there is no compelling reason to believe that immune responses to neuroantigen, which occur in parallel with the disease, are made to a large degree, or even at all, in the peripheral lymphoid tissues. Conceivably, the trigger mechanisms for such immune responses may be a persistent virus infection of the CNS (see Section V). The virus might incite production of immune responses to neuroantigen by immunocompetent lymphoid cells which have nonspecifically been attracted to the CNS in response to ongoing injury caused by the persistent virus in that organ. In other words, the sequences of immune responses specific for neuroantigen, either native or altered by the virus, would begin and end within the CNS itself. The situation as envisioned would account for a number of observations: local production of IgG within the CNS, deposition of IgG in large amounts around and in the lesions characterizing MS, the rarity of circulating antibody detected by conventional serological testing, and the apparent sparse numbers of sensitized lymphocytes in the systemic circulation. Antibody found in the circulation conceivably may represent "spillover" from that made locally within the CNS and will require a highly sensitive means of detection, such as that offered by myelinating brain cultures as targets. It might also be added that, if the major immune attack upon the CNS in MS is confined to the neuraxis, it would explain the relative lack of success of immunosuppressive drug regimens that act primarily on peripheral lymphoid tissues. Such drugs would not be expected to enter the CNS and impinge effectively on lymphoid cells actively engaging in ongoing immune responses to neuroantigens.

V. IMMUNOVIROLOGICAL MECHANISMS IN MS

A. General Aspects

Foregoing sections of this essay have considered the following topics: (1) immunologic and immunogenetic determinants which appear to be of major pathogenetic importance in EAE and MS (see Sections II and III, Tables I and II), (2) evidence implicating virus infection as an etiologic factor in the MS process (see Section II and Table I), and (3) well-substantiated immunologic responses closely associated with the development of EAE and the occurrence of MS (see Section IV and Table III). From this core information several concepts emerge, and certain generalizations can be made. These are summarized here as a preamble for the remaining section.

MBP is a relatively weak antigen (see Fig. 1). In order for its greatest immunogenic potential to be realized, it must impinge upon the host's immunocompetent lymphoid tissue simultaneously with an immunologic adjuvant. The purpose of the adjuvant or immunopotentiating agent is to provide a second signal essential for activating and expanding those clones of lymphoid cells bearing receptors for and interacting with MBP antigen (see Fig. 2). The degree of clonal expansion will depend on the inherent immunogenicity of MBP, the properties of the adjuvant, and especially its capacity to bypass or override immunoregulatory mechanisms, which collectively serve to suppress proliferation of MBP-reactive (autoreactive) cells. In the final outcome, whether immunologic injury to the CNS occurs or not, is a reflection of (1) the degree of proliferation of MBP clones which, in turn, determines the net number of sensitized lymphocytes or net output of products that can serve as immune effector reagents, and (2) their capacity to penetrate the CNS and bind to neuroantigenic determinants in the hosts' nervous tissues.

There are several immunologic responses or events that are common to EAE and MS (Table III). While the relative importance of each one in the pathogenesis of each disease remains to be determined, there is no *a priori* reason to presently exclude any of them as a pathogenetic factor in the development of autoimmune neurological disease. On balance, it would appear that the immunologic responses causing EAE are initiated in peripheral lymphoid tissues. These responses give rise to immune effectors that enter the vascular compartment and circulate. These effectors cause CNS immune injury to whatever extent they are able to leave the circulation, enter the host's neuraxis, and specifically interact with antigenic determinants in the target tissue. In MS, however, there is much less evidence for circulating immune effectors and a strong case can be made for ongoing immunologic responses made by immunocompetent lymphoid cells residing in the CNS. It would seem that the sequence of immunologic events which participate in the development of MS are initiated within, and thereafter are confined to the host's nervous tissues.

Although there are notable exceptions, EAE characteristically is a monophasic and transitory disease. The host develops acute neurological disease, recovery ensues, and subsequent spontaneous relapses of the disease are the exception. It would appear that the neuroantigen, in combination with a suitable immunologic adjuvant, causes a burst of immunologic activity which is intense, capable of injuring the host's CNS for a period of time, and then subsides, possibly due to metabolic degradation and elimination of the antigen and adjuvant moieties within systemic lymphoreticular tissues. In contrast, MS is a chronic, progressive, waxing and waning, neurologic disease characterized by clinical relapses and remissions of varying degree and duration. Similarly, the immunologic events associated with the disease are more localized and persistent.

One cannot help but conclude that the initiating stimulus for the train of events underlying the MS process is a durable and everpresent one. The characteristic features of this initiating persistent stimulus might be most readily fulfilled by a chronic, persistent CNS viral infection. In a very real sense, the putative persistent virus might well be serving as the biologic equivalent of Freund's adjuvant, thereby augmenting host responses to neuroantigen. The persistent virus would differ from traditional EAE-adjuvants in at least two ways: (1) by confining most, if not all, of its immunopathological activity to the target tissue, and (2) because of its capacity to replicate and its propensity for long persistence, exert an immunopotentiating impact on the host for a prolonged or even infinite period of time. Viewed in this light, the degree of persistence of the neurotropic virus becomes a key determinant for the degree, extent, and chronicity of the CNS injury that ensues. Some strains of virus endowed with limited capacity to persist might initiate an intense but short-lived immunologic attack upon the hosts' nervous tissue before its persistence is terminated and immunologic consequences of its presence are dissipated. This type of virus and this sequence of events might be responsible for the occurrence of acute and usually transitory attacks of encephalitis or encephalomyelitis intimately associated with antecedent virus infections, i.e., the postinfectious encephalitides (see Section II and Table I). These CNS disorders in many ways simulate the clinical and immunohistopathological characteristics of EAE. Other strains of virus with the capacity for much longer or even indefinite persistence within the CNS would fulfill the prerequisite for an everpresent stimulus perpetually driving sequences of immunologic events and, thereby, account for the chronicity and remittency of the MS process.

The questions to be examined briefly now are as follows. What is the core evidence for viruses causing MS? Is the disease caused by a single virus or group of viruses? Or is the disease a syndrome caused by many different kinds of viral agents? Finally, by what means does a virus persistently infecting the nervous system serve as a trigger for unleashing immune responses directed against self-antigens which are capable of participating in ongoing immunologic injury to the host's own CNS? It is this last question, bearing on the synergy of virus infection and host immune responses, that is occupying center stage in current thinking about autoimmune processes in man.

B. Specific Viruses Implicated in MS

1. Measles Virus

The reason so many neurovirological studies have focused on this specific paramyxovirus already have been mentioned (see Section II,B) and have been discussed in recent reviews (Black, 1975; Johnson, 1975). Briefly, serological surveys have shown that unusually high titers of serum antibody against measles virus and higher ratios of CSF antibody:serum antibody reactive with this virus occur in at least 50% of MS patients (Adams and Imagawa, 1962; Brown *et al.*, 1971; Norrby *et al.*, 1974a,b). As pointed out by Black (1975), measles is a ubiquitous disease and MS is not. Therefore, patients with the neurological disease may well represent a special subpopulation with a propensity for producing higher titers of measles antibody for reasons having nothing directly to do with the MS process. Strong clues that this may indeed be the case have emerged from recent immunogenetic studies of MS patients (see Section II and reviewed by McFarlin and McFarland, 1976). These studies suggest that specific histocompatibility antigens occurring with unusual frequency in MS patients are closely associated with other genes, simulating immune response genes, which direct excessive production of antibody against measles virus (Arnason *et al.*, Paty *et al.*, 1976). This observation has special impact concerning the interpretation of the results of past measles antibody surveys of MS patients and the experimental design of future studies along similar lines. That is, the critical group(s) of control subjects should be matched for specific histocompatibility antigens to the degree that they are represented in MS patients.

Occurrence of measles at a very early age, specifically before 2 years of age, is considered important in subacute sclerosing panencephalitis (see review of Fucillo *et al.*, 1974; also monograph edited by Zeman and Lennette, 1974). Following this clue, Black (1975) has gathered data concerning age-specific measles attack rates and prevalence of MS. The figures suggest that in Northern Europe and North America at least 5–10% of MS patients acquire measles during the second decade of life. In these regions, there is an intriguing parallel relationship between the percentage of the population experiencing rubeola between the ages of 10 to 19, and MS prevalence rates. Specific attempts to incriminate measles virus in MS, however, have been unsuccessful. For example, studies have shown that MS nervous tissue specimens have no demonstrable measles virus antigen and that only an insignificant percent of the elevated CSF–IgG in MS subjects is reactive with measles virus (Dubois-Dalcq *et al.*, 1975; Norrby and Vandik, 1975).

There is increasing evidence from several quarters for aberrant antibody synthesis against measles virus (Haire *et al.*, 1973), suppression of cell-mediated immunity for measles virus (Utermohlen and Zabriskie, 1973), and abnormalities concerning receptor sites for measles virus on the lymphocytes of MS patients (Levy *et al.*, 1976). These varied observations tally with other studies revealing alterations in numbers of circulating T cells and B cells in MS subjects (Lisak *et al.*, 1975; Oger *et al.*, 1975). Whether the suppression of cellular immunity in MS patients, as assessed by altered *in vitro* migration responses of peripheral blood leukocytes, is specific for measles virus (as reported by Utermohlen and Zabriskie, 1973), or extends to other paramyxoviruses (Cunningham-Rundles *et al.*, 1975), the finding can be interpreted as evidence for the persistence of measles virus. Nonspecific loss of DH cutaneous reactivity during the course of uncomplicated rubeola is a long-known immunologic concomitant of measles virus infection (von Pirquet, 1908). Indeed, these reported abnormalities in T cell-mediated immune responses already have led some investigators to utilize transfer factor as a therapeutic modality in MS. The hope has been that this form of immunologic reconstitution might reinforce cellular immunity, terminate a persistent myxovirus infection, and exert a beneficial effect on the course of disease. Preliminary reports of therapeutic trials with transfer factor have indicated varying success (Fog *et al.*, 1975; Behan *et al.*, 1976).

These recent developments implicating measles virus and/or aberrant immunologic responses to the virus are tantalizing clues to the enigma of MS. The task that lies ahead is determining whether these observations represent primary abnormalities in host immunity favoring and promoting persistence of measles virus, secondary manifestation of persistent infection with much less etiologic significance, or completely unrelated consequences of immunogenetic determinants having nothing directly to do with MS per se. It should be remembered that measles virus is implicated in only about half of the patients with MS, leaving open the possibility that other viruses may be of etiologic significance.

2. *Other Viruses*

Kempe and his associates (Kempe *et al.*, 1973; Miyamoto *et al.*, 1976) have reported a significantly higher frequency of antibody to vaccinia in the CSF of MS patients. Antibody was quantitated using complement-fixation tests or the sensitive plaque-reduction assay for neutralizing antibody. The highest incidence of such antibodies was found in those patients with chronic, unremitting progressive forms of the disease. These workers suggest that the failure of Brown *et al.* (1973) to confirm their initial findings might be due to the fact that the CSF specimens tested by Brown *et al.* (1973) were collected from patients with acute exacerbations of MS. It should also be noted that all of the patients studies by Kempe and Miyamoto and their associates were Americans, whereas all the subjects providing the CSF specimens tested by Brown and his collaborators were French. It is hard to see how differences in national smallpox vaccination practices would account for the striking disparity in results reported by these two groups of investigators. Genetic differences influencing immune responsiveness to vaccinia virus of American versus French MS patients might be a more plausible explanation.

The report of terMuelen *et al.* (1972b) describing the recovery of parainfluenza type 1 virus from brain tissue of two patients with MS using two different cell fusion "rescue" techniques focused intense activity on this particular paramyxovirus. Unhappily, no additional recoveries of a similar or identical virus have been reported by this group and many other groups of investigators, despite intensive and extensive efforts to secure confirmation.

It is too early to assess the recent reports of Carp *et al.* (1972) and Koldovsky *et al.* (1975) of MS-associated agent (MSAA) in MS brain and blood samples which replicates in mice. One of the distressing aspects of this work is the necessity for detecting the presence and replication of the MSAA by its capacity to significantly lower the absolute number of circulating polymorphonuclear (PMN) cells in the injected mice. PMN counts vary frequently and widely in normal mice, in part due to intercurrent laboratory infections of one type or another. This problem makes it very difficult to know if reduced PMN counts are or are not due to the putative MSAA (Brown and Gajdusek, 1974).

C. Virus–Host Immune Response Interactions

There is an extensive literature concerning the many different ways that viruses may "trigger" immunopathological responses of infected mammalian hosts leading to immunologically mediated disease of the CNS or other organ systems. Superb reviews have been prepared by several authors (Harter and Choppin, 1971; Notkins, 1971; Oldstone, 1975; Hirsch and Proffitt, 1975). There are a few points that need emphasis in considering immunovirological mechanisms that might be important in the MS process.

Major attention has been focused on the paramyxoviruses. This is not only because of the substantial evidence pointing to measles virus, but also because this class of viruses has the capacity to insert virus-specified "foreign" antigenic constituents into the membranes of infected host cells. In other words, a host infected with a persistent neutrotropic paramyxovirus would have cells in his CNS representing "self plus virus." The virus component of this altered-self complex would be expected to induce an immune response. In the course of responding to the antigenic stimulus of the virus, sensitized cells and antibody produced by the host might well interact with virus membrane constituents in infected cells of the CNS. Interaction of host immune responses with such "self plus virus targets would lead to injury and neurological disease. The important point to stress in this type of injury is that the specific target antigen is not self but nonself;" that is, the virus antigenic component responsible for both initiating and interacting with specific immune responses made by the infected host. The CNS disease that results from this immunovirological mechanism, therefore, is not truely "autoimmune" in nature. The type of injury that occurs might best be labeled "self-induced immunologically mediated disease."

A lot of interest has been generated in the possibility that virus infections may cause subtle alterations in self-antigens, which nevertheless are sufficient to render them foreign. The theory as frequently outlined by various authors would see the host make immune responses to altered self; these are capable of cross-reacting with and causing injury to native, noninfected host cells. The key question is whether viruses clearly can alter mammalian nervous tissue antigens in this fashion. Recent experiments conducted at Northwestern University (Massanari *et al.*, 1977) were designed to examine this question. Neonatal or weanling hamsters were injected by intracerebral injection with hamster-adapted strains of measles virus which caused an acute encephalitis of varying severity and mortality. Brains from moribund measles-infected hamsters and normal hamster littermates were lyophilized, reconstituted in suitable suspending medium, mixed with CFA, and bioassayed for EAE-inducing activity in groups of normal rats, guinea pigs, and hamsters. Encephalitogenic activity was calculated and expressed in terms of the dose of brain, in milligrams dry weight, required to induce EAE in exactly 50% of sensitized animals, i.e., the EAE $dose_{50}$. Based on comparative $EAED_{50}$'s, measles-infected hamster brain was no more and no less encephalitogenic than normal uninfected hamster brain. Within the limitations of this bioassay system, the strains of measles virus employed for our work did not demonstrably alter brain tissue insofar as its inherent encephalitogenic activity was concerned.

Recent attempts to incorporate persistent virus infections of one type or another into the EAE model system appear especially relevant, since they simulate the conditions and sequences of events that may be envisioned to occur in the MS process. At Northwestern University, Massanari *et al.* (1975) have shown that weanling hamsters persistently infected by intracerebral injection of a defective strain of measles virus, isolated from a patient with subacute sclerosing panencephalitis, and, showing no clinical neurological signs of illness during adult life, exhibit a striking increase in their susceptibility to EAE following sensitization to neuroantigen–CFA. Whether the persistent virus in the brain merely increases the permeability of the CSF–brain–blood barrier so that more sensitized cells or antibody reactive with MBP can enter target tissues or whether the virus causes antigenic determinants in the CNS to become more accessible for binding immune effectors elaborated by the sensitized host are questions currently under intensive study. The availability of this type of model system, and similar ones being developed in other laboratories by other workers, provides a promising means for investigating the subtleties of *in vivo* interactions between persistent CNS virus infections and host immune responses directed against neuroantigen. These model systems hopefully will be able to better define basic immunovirological mechanisms responsible for neurological disease of animals and man, including the MS process.

ACKNOWLEDGMENTS

Research performed by the author and referred to in this essay was supported in part or totally by USPHS Research Grant NS-06262 from the National Institute of Neurologic and Communicative Disorders and Stroke, Training Grant AM-05069 from the National Institute of Arthritis, Metabolic and Digestive Disorders and the James C. Hemphill Grant for research on multiple sclerosis (811-A-1) from the National Multiple Sclerosis Society.

REFERENCES

Adams, J. M., and Imagawa, D. T. (1962). *Proc. Soc. Exp. Biol. Med.* **111**, 562–566.

Adams, R. D. (1959). *In* "Allergic Encephalomyelitis" (M. W. Kies and E. C. Alvord, Jr., eds.), pp. 183–209. Thomas, Springfield, Illinois.

Allison, A. C. (1973). *Immunopotentiation, Ciba Found. Symp., 1973* Ciba Found. Symp. No. 18, pp. 73–94.

Alter, M., Leibowitz, U., and Speer, J. (1966). *Arch. Neurol.* (*Chicago*) **15,** 234–237.

Alvord, E. C., Jr. (1970). *Hand. Clin. Neurol.* **9,** 500–571.

Alvord, E. C., Jr., Shaw, C.-M., Hruby, S., Peterson, R., and Harvey, F. H. (1975). *Nerv. Syst.* **1,** 647–653.

Appel, S. H., and Bornstein, M. B. (1964). *J. Exp.Med.* **119,** 303–312.

Arnason, B. G., Janković, B. D., Waksman, B. H., and Wennersten, C. (1962). *J. Exp. Med.* **116,** 177–186.

Arnason, B. G. W. (1975). In "Peripheral Neuropathy" (P. J. Dyck, P. K. Thomas, and E. H. Lambert, eds.), pp. 1110–1148. Saunders, Philadelphia, Pennsylvania.

Arnason, B. G. W., Fuller, T. C., Lehrich, J. R., and Wray, S. H. (1974). *J. Neurol. Sci.* **22,** 419–428.

Asbury, A. K., Arnason, B. G., and Adams, R. D. (1969). *Medicine* (*Baltimore*) **48,** 173–215.

Astrom, K., and Waksman, B. H. (1962). *J. Pathol. Bacteriol.* **83,** 89–106.

Bartfeld, H., and Atoynatan, T. (1970). *Int. Arch. Allergy Appl. Immunol.* **39,** 361–367.

Bartfeld, H., Atoynatan, T., and Donnenfeld, H. (1972). *In* "Multiple Sclerosis" (F. Wolfgram *et al.*, eds.), pp. 333–351. Academic Press, New York.

Baublis, J. V., and Payne, F. E. (1968). *Proc. Soc. Exp. Biol. Med.* **129,** 593–597.

Behan, P. O., Behan, W. M. H., Feldman, R. G., and Kies, M. W. (1972). *Arch. Neurol.* (*Chicago*) **27,** 145–152.

Behan, P. O., Melville, I. D., Durward, W. F., McGeorge, A. P., and Behan, W. M. H. (1976). *Lancet* **1,** 988–990.

Bell, J., and Paterson, P. Y. (1960). *Science* **131,** 1448.

Benacerraf, B., and McDevitt, H. O. (1972). *Science* **175,** 273–279.

Benveniste, J., Henson, P. M., and Cochrane, C. G. (1972). *J. Exp. Med.* **136,** 1356–1377.

Bergstrand, H. (1973). *Immunochemistry* **10,** 611–620.

Bernard, C. C. A. (1976). *J. Immunogenet.* **3,** 263–274.

Black, F. L. (1975). *Prog. Med. Virol.* **21,** 158–164.

Blaw, M., Cooper, M. D., and Good, R. A. (1967). *Science* **158,** 1198–1200.

Bornstein, M. B. (1973). *Prog. Neuropathol.* **II,** 69–90.

Bornstein, M. B., and Appel, S. H. (1961). *J. Neuropathol. Exp. Neurol.* **20,** 141–157.

Bornstein, M. B., and Appel, S. H. (1965). *Ann. N.Y. Acad. Sci.* **122,**280–286.

Brockman, J. A., Stiffey, A. V., and Tesar, W. C. (1968). *J. Immunol.* **100,** 1230–1236.

Brown, P., and Gajdusek, D. C. (1974). *Nature* (*London*) **247,** 217–218.

Brown, P., Cathala, F., Gajdusek, D. C., and Gibbs, C. J., Jr., (1971). *Proc. Soc. Exp. Biol. Med.* **137,** 956–961.

Brown, P., Cathala, F., and Gajdusek, D. C. (1973). *Proc. Soc. Exp. Biol. Med.* **143,** 828–829.

Burnet, M. (1972). "Auto-immunity and Autoimmune Disease." MTP (Medical and Technical Publishing), Lancaster.

Carnegie, P. R., MacKay, I. R. and Coates, A. S., "Aetiology and Pathogenesis of the Demyelinating Diseases", (Shiraki, H., Yonezawa, T., and Kuriowa, Y., eds.) Japanese Society of Neuropathology, 1976, pp. 275–283.

Carp, R. I., Licursi, P. C., Merz, P. A., and Merz, G. S. (1972). *J. Exp. Med.* **136,** 618–629.

Carp, R. I., Licursi, P. C., and Merz, G. S. (1975). *Infect. Immun.* **11,** 737–741.

Chao, L.-P., and Einstein, E. R. (1970). *J. Biol. Chem.* **245,** 6397–6403.

Chase, M. W. (1959). *In* "Allergic Encephalomyelitis" (M. W. Kies and E. C. Alvord, Jr., eds.), pp. 348–374. Thomas, Springfield, Illinois.

Chelmicka-Szorc, E., and Arnason, B. (1975). *Clin. Exp. Immunol.* **22,** 539–545.

Chou, F. C.-H., Jen Chou, C.-H., Shapira, R., and Kibler, R. F. (1976). *J. Biol. Chem.* **251,** 2671–2679.

Ciongoli, A. K., Platz, P., Dupont, B., Svejgaard, A., Fog, T., and Jersild, C. (1973). *Lancet* **2,** 1147.

Coates, A. S., and Carnegie, P. R. (1975). *Clin. Exp. Immunol.* **22,** 16–21.

Coates, A. S., and Lennon, V. A. (1973). *Immunology* **24,** 425–434.

Cohen, S., and Bannister, R. (1967). Lancet **1,** 366–367, 1967.

Cunningham-Rundles, S., Dupont, B., Posner, J. B., Hansen, J. A., and Good, R. A. (1975). *Lancet* **2,** 1204.

Dau, P. C., and Peterson, R. D. A. (1969). *Int. Arch. Allergy Appl. Immunol.* **35,** 353–368.

David, J. R., and Paterson, P. Y. (1965). *J. Exp. Med.* **122,** 1161–1171.

Day, E. D., and Pitts, O. M. (1974). *Immunochemistry* **11,** 651–659.

Dean, G. (1967). *Br. Med. J.* **2,** 724–730.

Dean, G. (1970). *Sci. Am.* **233,** 40–46.

Driscoll, B. F., Kramer, A. J., and Kies, M. W. (1974a). *Science* **184,** 73–75.

Driscoll, B. F., Kies, M. W., and Alvord, E. C., Jr. (1974b). *J. Immunol.* **112,** 392–397.

Dubois-Dalcq, M., Niedieck, B., and Buyse, M. (1970). *Pathol. Eur.* **5,** 331–347.

Dubois-Dalcq, M., Schumacher, G., and Worthington, E. K. (1975). *Neurology* **25,** 496 (abstr.).

Einstein, E. R., and Chao, L.-P. (1970). *In* Protein Metabolism of the Nervous System," pp. 643–657. Plenum, New York.

Eylar, E. H., and Hashim, G. A. (1968). *Proc. Natl. Acad. Sci. U.S.A.* **61,** 644–650.

Eylar, E. H., Caccam, J., and Jackson, J. J. (1970). *Science* **168,** 1220–1223.

Eylar, E. H., Jackson, J., Rothenberg, B., and Brostoff, S. W. (1972). *Nature* (*London*) **236,** 74–76.

Fernandez, F. L., Sora, E. P., and Corria, F. R. (1947). *Rev. Med. Cir. Habana* **52,** 385–396.

Fog, T., Jersild, C., Dupont, B., Platz, P. J., Svejgaard, A., Thomsen, M., Midholm, S., Raun, N. E., and Grob, P. (1975). *Neurology* **25,** 489–490, (abstr.).

Freund, J., and Stone, S. H. (1959). *J. Immunol.* **82,** 560–567.

Freund, J., Stern, E. R., and Pisani, T. M. (1947). *J. Immunol.* **57,** 179–194.

Fry, J. M., Weissbarth, S., and Lehrer, G. M. (1974). *Science* **183,** 540–542.

Fuccillo, D. A., Kurert, J. E., and Sever, J. L. (1974). *Annu. Rev. Microbiol.* **28,** 231–264.

Gasser, D. L., Newlin, C. M., Palm, J., and Gonatas, N. K. (1973). *Science* **181,** 872–873.

Goldstone, A. H., Kerr, L., and Irvine, W. J. (1973). *Clin. Exp. Immunol.* **14,** 469–472.

Gonatas, N. K., and Howard, J. C. (1974). *Science* **186,** 839–841.

Gonatas, N. K., Gonatas, J. O., Stieber, A., Lisak, R., Suzuki, K., and Martenson, R. E. (1974). *Am. J. Pathol.* **76,** 529–548.

Haire, M., Fraser, K. B., and Millar, J. H. D. (1973). *Clin. Exp. Immunol.* **14,** 409–416.

Harter, D. H., and Choppin, P. W. (1971). *Res. Publ., Assoc. Res. Nerv. Ment. Dis.* **49,** 342–354.

Hashim, G. A. (1975). *Nature (London)* **256,** 593–595.

Hashim, G. A., and Sharpe, R. D. (1974). *Immunochemistry* **11,** 633–640.

Hashim, G. A., Sharpe, R. D., Carvalho, E. F., and Stevens, L. E. (1976). *J. Immunol.* **116,** 126–130.

Hirsch, M. S., and Proffitt, M. R. (1975). *In* "Viral Immunology and Immunopathology" (A. L. Notkins, ed.), pp. 419–434. Academic Press, New York.

Hoffman, P. M., Gaston, D. D., and Spitler, L. E. (1973). *Clin. Immunol. Immunopathol.* **1,** 364–371.

Horta-Barbosa, L., Fuccillo, D. A., Sever, J. L., and Zeman, W. (1969). *Nature (London)* **221,** 974.

Hughes, R. A. C. (1974). *Immunology* **26,** 703–711.

Hughes, R. A. C., and Leibowitz, S. (1975). *Immunology* **28,** 213–218.

Janković, D., Draskoci, M., and Janjić, M. (1965). *Nature (London)* **207,** 428–429.

Johnson, A. B., Wisniewski, H. M., Raine, C. S., Eylar, E. H., and Terry, R. D. (1971). *Proc. Natl. Acad. Sci. U.S.A.* **68,** 2694–2698.

Johnson, R. T. (1975). *Adv. Neurol.* **13,** 1–46.

Kabat, E. A., Wolf, A., and Bezer, A. E. (1947). *J. Exp. Med.* **85,** 117–129.

Kabat, E. A., Wolf, A., and Bezer, A. E. (1949). *J. Exp. Med.* **89,** 395–398.

Kabat, E. A., Wolf, A., Bezer, A. E., and Murray, J. P. (1951). *J. Exp. Med.* **93,** 615–633.

Kempe, C. H., Takabayashi, K., Miyamoto, H., McIntosh, K., Tourtellotte, W. W., and Adams, J. M. (1973). *Arch. Neurol. (Chicago)* **28,** 278–279.

Kies, M. W. (1975). *Nerv. Syst.* **1,** 637–646.

Koldovsky, U., Koldovsky, P., Henle, G., Henle, W., Ackerman, R., and Haase, G. (1975). *Infect. Immun.* **12,** 1355–1366.

Kornguth, S. E., Bennett, D. R., Thompson, H. G., Zurhein, G. M., and Stahmann, M. A. (1962). *Nature (London)* **193,** 1081.

Kruger, P. G. (1974). *Experientia* **30,** 810–811.

Lamoureux, G., Carnegie, T. R., and McPherson, T. A. (1967). *Immunochemistry* **4,** 273–281.

Lampert, P. W., Gajdusek, D. C., and Gibbs, C. J., Jr. (1972). *Am. J. Pathol. 68,* 626–652.

Lebar, R., Boutry, J.-M., Vincent, C., Robineaux, R., and Voisin, G. A. (1976). *J. Immunol.* **116,** 1439–1446.

Lennon, V. A., and Carnegie, P. R. (1974). *Eur. J. Immunol.* **4,** 60–62.

Lennon, V. A., Feldmann, M., and Crawford, M. (1972). *Int. Arch. Allergy Appl. Immunol.* **43,** 749–758.

Levine, B. B., Stember, R. H., and Fotino, M. (1972). *Science* **178,** 1201–1203.

Levine, S. (1974). *Acta Neuropathol.* **28,** 179–189.

Levine, S., and Sowinski, R. (1973). *J. Immunol.* **110,** 139–143.

Levine, S., and Sowinski, R. (1974). *Immunogenetics* **1,** 352–356.

Levine, S., and Sowinski, R. (1975). *J. Immunol.* **114,** 597–601.

Levine, S., Cochrane, C. G., Carpenter, C. B., and Behan, P. O. (1971). *Proc. Soc. Exp. Biol. Med.* **138,** 285–289.

Levine, S., Sowinski, R., and Kies, M. W. (1972). *Proc. Soc. Exp. Biol. Med.* **139,** 506–510.

Levy, N. L., Auerbach, P. S., and Hayes, E. C. (1976). *N. Engl. J. Med.* **294,** 1423–1427.

Lisak, R. P., and Zweiman, B. (1974). *Cell. Immunol.* **14,** 242–254.

Lisak, R. P., Levinson, A. I., Zweiman, B., and Abdou, N. I. (1975). *Clin. Exp. Immunol.* **22,** 30–34.

Lumsden, C. E., Kabat, E. A., Wolf, A., and Bezer, A. E. (1950). *J. Exp. Med.* **92,** 253–270.

McAlpine, D., Lumsden, C. E., and Acheson, E. D. (1972). *In* "Multiple Sclerosis: A Reappraisal," 2nd ed., Livingstone, Edinburgh.

McDermott, J. R., Caspary, E. A., and Dickinson, J. P. (1974). *Clin. Exp. Immunol.* **17,** 103–111.

McDevitt, H. O., and Benacerraf, B. (1969). *Adv. Immunol.* **11,** 31–74.

McFarlin, D. E., and McFarland, H. F. (1976). *Arch. Neurol.* (*Chicago*) **33,** 395–398.

McFarlin, D. E., Blank, S. E., Kibler, R. F., McKneally, S., and Shapira, R. (1973). *Science* **179,** 478–480.

McFarlin, D. E., Blank, S. E., and Kibler, R. F. (1974). *J. Immunol.* **113,** 712–715.

McFarlin, D. E., Hsu, S. C.-L., Slemenda, S. B., Chou, F. C.-H., and Kibler, R. F. (1975a). *J. Exp. Med.* **141,** 72–81.

McFarlin, D. E., Hsu, S. C.-L., Slemanda, S. B., Chou, S. C.-H., and Kibler, R. F. (1975b). *J. Immunol.* **115,** 1456–1458.

Mackay, I. R., Carnegie, P. R., and Coates, A. S. (1973). *Clin. Exp. Immunol.* **15,** 471–482.

McPherson, T. A., Gilpin, A., and Seland, T. P. (1972). *Can. Med. Assoc. J.* **107,** 856–859.

Maggio, B., and Cumar, F. A. (1975). *Nature* (*London*) **253,** 364–365.

Martensen, R. E., Deibler, G. E., Kies, M. W., McKneally, S. S., Shapira, R., and Kibler, R. F. (1972). *Biochim. Biophys. Acta* **263,** 193–203.

Massanari, R. M., Lipton, H. L., and Paterson, P. Y. (1975). *Am. Soc. Microbiol., Abstr.* p. 71.

Massanari, R. M., Paterson, P. Y., and Lipton, H. L. (1977). Unpublished observations.

Miyamoto, H., Walker, J. E., Ginsberg, A. H., Burks, J. S., McIntosh, K., and Kempe, C. H. (1976). *Arch. Neurol.* (*Chicago*) **33,** 414–417.

Moore, M. J., Behan, P. O., Kies, M. W., and Matthews, J. M. (1974a). *Res. Commun. Chem. Pathol. Pharmacol.* **9,** 119–132.

Moore, M. J., Mathews, J. M., Matthews, T. K., Behan, P. O., and Kies, M. W. (1974b). *Res. Commun. Chem. Pathol. Pharmacol.* **9,** 133–144.

Morgan, I. (1947). *J. Exp. Med.* **85,** 131–140.

Morrison, L. R. (1947). *Arch. Neurol. Psychiatry* **58,** 391–416.

Norrby, E., and Vandvik, B. (1975). *Neurology* **25,** 493 (abstr.).

Norrby, E., Link, H., and Olsson, J.-E. (1974a). *Arch. Neurol.* (*Chicago*) **30,** 285–292.

Norrby, E., Link, H., Olsson, J.-E., Panelius, M., Salmi, A., and Vandvik, B. (1974b). *Infect. Immun.* **10,** 688–694.

Norton, W. T. (1975). *Nerv. Syst.* **1,** 467–481.

Notkins, A. L. (1971). *Prog. Immunol.* **1,** 180–186.

Oger, J. F., Arnason, B. G. W., Wray, S. H., and Kistler, J. P. (1975). *Neurology* **25,** 444–447.

Oldstone, M. B. A. (1975). *Nerv. Syst.* **1,** 631–636.

Oldstone, M. B. A., and Dixon, F. J. (1968). *Am. J. Pathol.* **52,** 251–263.

Orgad, S., and Cohen, I. R. (1974). *Science* **183,** 1083–1085.

Ortiz-Ortiz, L., and Weigle, W. O. (1976). *J. Exp. Med.* **144,** 604–616.

Ortiz-Ortiz, L., Nakamura, R. M., and Weigle, W. O. (1976). *J. Immunol.* **117,** 576–579.

Paterson, P. Y. (1960). *J. Exp. Med.* **111,** 119–136.

Paterson, P. Y. (1962). *In* "Mechanism of Cell and Tissue Damage Produced by Immune Reactions" (P. Grabar and P. A. Miescher, eds.), pp. 184–192. Schwabe, Basel.

Paterson, P. Y. (1963). *In* "Cell-bound Antibodies" (B. Amos and H. Koprowski, eds.), pp. 101–105. Wistar Inst. Press, Philadelphia, Pennsylvania.

Paterson, P. Y. (1966). *Adv. Immunol.* **5,** 131–208.

Paterson, P. Y. (1969). *Annu. Rev. Med.* **20,** 75–100.

Paterson, P. Y. (1971). *In* "Immunological Diseases" (M. Samter, ed.), 2nd ed., pp. 1269–1299. Little, Brown, Boston, Massachusetts.

Paterson, P. Y. (1972). *In* "Multiple Sclerosis" (F. Wolfgram *et al.*, eds.), pp. 539–563. Academic Press, New York.

Paterson, P. Y. (1973a). *J. Reticulendothel. Soc.* **14,** 426–440.

Paterson, P. Y. (1973b). *J. Chronic Dis.* **26,** 119–126.

Paterson, P. Y. (1976a). *In* "Textbook of Immunopathology" (P. A. Miescher and H. J. Müller-Eberhard, eds.), 2nd ed., pp. 179–213. Grune & Stratton, New York.

Paterson, P. Y. (1976b). *In* "Introduction to Clinical Immunology" (W. J. Irvine, ed.). Blackwell, Oxford (in press).

Paterson, P. Y. (1976c). *Cell. Immunol.* **21,** 48–55.

Paterson, P. Y., and Bell, J. (1962). *J. Immunol.* **89,** 72–79.

Paterson, P. Y., and Didakow, N. C. (1961). *Proc. Soc. Exp. Biol. Med.* **108,** 768–771.

Paterson, P. Y., and Drobish, D. G. (1969). *Science* **165,** 191–192.
Paterson, P. Y., and Drobish, D. G. (1974). *J. Immunol.* **113,** 1942–1946.
Paterson, P. Y., and Harwin, S. M. (1963). *J. Exp. Med.* **117,** 755–774.
Paty, D. W., Furesz, J., Boucher, D. W., Rand, C. G., and Stiller, C. R. (1976). *Neurology* **26,** 651–655.
Prineas, J. (1972). *Science* **178,** 760–763.
Rauch, H. C., and Einstein, E. R. (1974). *Rev. Neurosci.* **7,** 283–343.
Rauch, H. C., Ferraresi, R. W., Raffel, S., and Roboz-Einstein, E. (1969). *J. Immunol.* **102,** 1431–1436.
Rivers, T. M., and Schwentker, F. F. (1935). *J. Exp. Med.* **61,** 689–702.
Rivers, T. M., Sprunt, D. H., and Berry, G. P. (1933). *J. Exp. Med.* **58,** 39–54.
Rocklin, R. E., Sheremata, W. A., Feldman, R. G., Kies, M. W., and David, J. R. (1971). *N. Engl. J. Med.* **284,** 803–808.
Seil, F. J., Falk, C. A., Kies, M. W., and Alvord, E. C., Jr., (1968). *Exp. Neurol.* **22,** 545–555.
Shaffer, M. F., Rake, G., and Hodes, H. L. (1942). *Am. J. Dis. Child.* **64,** 815–819.
Shapira, R., McKneally, S. S., Chou, F., and Kibler, R. F. (1971). *J. Biol. Chem.* **246,** 4630–4640.
Sheremata, W., Cosgrove, J. B. R., and Eylar, E. H. (1974). *N. Engl. J. Med.* **291,** 14–17.
Sheremata, W., Cosgrove, J. B. R., and Eylar, E. H. (1976). *J. Neurol. Sci.* **27,** 413–425.
Sigurdsson, B. (1954). *Br. Vet. J.* **110,** 341–354.
Simon, J., and Simon, O. (1975). *Exp. Neurol.* **47,** 523–534.
Small, M., and Trainin, N. (1975). *Cell. Immunol.* **20,** 1–11.
Snyder, D. H., Valsamis, M. P., Stone, S. H., and Raine, C. S. (1975). *J. Neuropathol. Exp. Neurol.* **34,** 209–221.
Spitler, L. E., von Müller, C. M., Fudenberg, H. H., and Eylar, E. H. (1972). *J. Exp. Med.* **136,** 156–174.
Stone, S. H. (1961). *Science* **134,** 619–620.
Swanborg, R. H. (1970). *J. Immunol.* **105,** 865–871.
Tada, T., and Okumura, K. (1971). *J. Immunol.* **107,** 1137–1145.
Teitelbaum, D., Webb, C., Meshorer, A., Arnon, R., and Sela, M. (1972). *Nature* (*London*) **240,** 564–566.
terMeulen, V., Müller, D., Käckell, Y., Katz, M., and Meyermann, R. (1972a). *Lancet* **1,** 1172–1175.
terMeulen, V., Koprowski, H., Iwasaki, Y., Käckell, Y. M., and Müller, D. (1972b). *Lancet* **2,** 1–5.
Thomas, D. G. T. (1975). *IRCS Libr. Compend.* **3,** 26.
Thomas, L., Paterson, P. Y., and Smithwick, B. (1950). *J. Exp. Med.* **92,** 133–152.
Tourtellotte, W. W. (1971). *Res. Publ., Assoc. Res. Nerv. Ment. Dis.* **49,** 112–147.
Turnbull, H. M., and McIntosh, J. (1926). *Br. J. Exp. Pathol.* **7,** 181–222.
Utermohlen, V., and Zabriskie, J. B. (1973). *J. Exp. Med.* **138,** 1591–1596.
Vandenbark, A. A., Burger, D. R., and Vetto, R. M. (1975). *Proc. Soc. Exp. Biol. Med.* **148,** 1233–1236.
von Pirquet, C. (1908). *Dtsch. Med. Wochenschr.* **34,** 1297–1300.

Waksman, B. H., and Adams, R. D. (1955). *J. Exp. Med.* **102,** 213–236.

Waksman, B. H., and Morrison, L. R. (1951). *J. Immunol.* **66,** 421–444.

Warnatz, H., Scheiffarth, F., and Kuntz, H. (1970). *J. Neuropathol. Exp. Neurol.* **29,** 575–582.

Webb, C., Teitelbaum, D., Arnon, R., and Sela, M. (1973a). *Eur. J. Immunol.* **3,** 279–286.

Webb, C., Teitelbaum, D., Arnon, R., and Sela, M. (1973b). *Immunol. Commun.* **2,** 185–192.

Webb, C., Teitelbaum, D., Abramsky, O., Arnon, R., and Sela, M. (1974). *Lancet* **2,** 66–68.

Werdelin, O., and McCluskey, R. T. (1971). *J. Exp. Med.* **133,** 1242–1263.

Williams, R. M., and Moore, M. J. (1973). *J. Exp. Med.* **138,** 775–783.

Witebsky, E., and Steinfeld, J. (1928). *Z. Immunitaetsforsch. Exp. Ther.* **58,** 271–296.

Wolf, A. (1963). *In* "Symposium on Demyelinating Diseases and Allergic Encephalomyelitis" (A. P. Rose, ed.), pp. 72–92. McGraw Hill, N.Y.

Wolfgram, F., and Duquette, P. (1976). *Neurology, Suppl.* **26,** 68–69.

Wolfgram, F., Ellison, G. W., Stevens, J. G., and Andrews, J. M., eds. (1972). "Multiple Sclerosis." Academic Press, New York.

Yung, L. L. L., Diener, E., McPherson, T. A., Barton, M. A., and Hyde, H. A. (1973). *J. Immunol.* **110,** 1383–1387.

Zeman, W., and Lennette, E. H., eds. (1974). "Slow Virus Diseases." Williams & Wilkins, Baltimore, Maryland.

NOTE ADDED IN PROOF:

There is mounting interest in and support for oligodendrocytes being the key target cell under immunologic attack in MS. This glial cell population subset is of paramount importance for synthesis and maintenance of CNS myelin [reviewed by R. P. Bunge (1968), *Physiol. Rev.* **48,** 197]. The margins of MS plaques of demyelination, believed to be the locus of ongoing tissue injury, are known to be selectively depleted of oligodendroglia (see monograph, already cited, by McAlpine, Lumsden and Acheson, 1972). Using the leukocyte migration inhibition test as an in vitro reflection of cell-mediated immune activity, L. W. Myers, G. W. Ellison, M. E. Fewster, and F. Wolfgram [(1975), *Arch. Neurol.* **32,** 354] found that the peripheral blood leukocytes (PBL) of 11 of 21 MS patients exhibited varying degrees of sensitivity to oligodendroglia whereas none of 22 patients showed significant evidence of hypersensitivity to purified myelin. M. E. Fewster, G. W. Ellison, L. W. Myers, and E. Y. Kurashige [(1975), *Neurology* **25,** 735] using ^{51}Cr-labeled isolated oligodendrocytes as immune targets found that admixed sera and PBL from MS patients, gave a different pattern of cytotoxicity, as evidenced by released ^{51}Cr, than observed with sera and PBL of clinically well subjects. As already noted (See Section III, F), Wolfgram and Duquette (1976) found that if sera from MS patients with complement-dependent glial cell toxicity and demyelinating activity for myelinated organotypic brain cultures were absorbed with purified white matter myelin, there was little or no decrease in glial cell–myelin cytotoxicity. In contrast, absorption with the nonmyelin containing and oligodendroglia-rich pellet, left behind in the process of preparing purified myelin, was able to completely absorb all glial cell–myelin toxic activity. These workers suggested that the glial cell–myelin cytotoxicity of MS sera most likely was due to antibody directed specifically against oligodendroglia or oligodendroglial plasma membranes. Since injection of suspensions of olidodendroglia, "practically free" of myelin, in combination with complete Freund's adjuvant has been reported by H. M. Wisniewski, C. F. Raine, R. Iqbal, I. Grundke-Iqbal, J. McDermott, and W. T. Norton [(1975), *J. Neuropath. Exp. Neurol.* **35,** 328] to induce an EAE-like disease in experimental animals, one can surmize that olidodendroglia may well turn out to be an important cell type eliciting immune responses implicated in the pathogenesis of EAE—the experimental animal counterpart of MS in human beings. It is obvious that a great deal of work lies ahead in determining whether persistent viral infection of olidodendroglia by itself or in concert with host immune responses triggered by virally altered olidodendrocytes is a pathogenetic event of major significance in the MS process. It is also clear that a lot of additional research is needed to ultimately assess the relative importance of olidodendroglia, myelin basic protein, and other CNS constituents as antigens engendering host immune responses in both EAE and MS.

Chapter 23

Positive Autoimmunity

HANS WIGZELL

I. INTRODUCTION

The danger of autoimmunity, or *horror autotoxicus*, has left an impressive impact on many people working in the field of human medicine. The present article will describe findings indicating that major parts of normal immune reactions may take place via specific reactions in an autoimmune manner. It will also deal with the possibilities of using autoimmune reactions in a controlled manner to obtain immune reactions directed against self-constituents where the consequences will be of benefit to the individual. It should be understood that many problems must be solved before one can use such an approach in the clinical situation. However, as will be discussed, a variety of highly precise immune processes against self-constituents may be provoked in an individual and, thus far, no negative side effects have been noted. Such reactions include antibody production against hormones involved in pregnancy, and induction of autoantibodies (normally never occurring) against such tumor-associated molecules as α-feto-protein (AFP) and carcinoembryonic antigen (CEA). They also include autoimmunization against an individual's receptors for certain antigens which can lead to specific tolerance against these antigens. The article will try to convince the reader that autoimmunity can be used as a powerful tool in a positive way for the individual. Only the future will tell whether this approach will develop into a clinically fruitful area.

II. "ANTI-SELF" REACTIVITY MAY BE A NORMAL FEATURE OF ALL IMMUNOCOMPETENT T LYMPHOCYTES

In this section, attention will be drawn to the startling fact that immunocompetent thymus-dependent lymphocytes seem to carry receptors with specificity for self-antigens, particularly for structures coded for by the major histocompatibility antigen-determining (MHC) genes. It seems likely that immunocompetent T lymphocytes become induced during immunization, in part via specific interaction with self-MHC structures present on other cells, and in part via an equally specific reaction to the foreign antigenic determinant. Neither reaction alone (to either self-MHC or to the "conventional" antigen) would seem to lead to T cell immune activation. The vices and virtues of such an arrangement will be discussed later, but let us first examine the evidence for this concept.

Inbred mice immunized against live viruses such as lymphocytic choriomeningitis develop specific killer T lymphocytes (Zinkernagel and Doherty, 1974). When such cells are analyzed for specific immune cytolytic ability, they only kill target cells carrying two minimimal but essential markers: (1) an antigenic marker typical for cells infected by the particular virus used for immunization, and (2) MHC antigen(s) of the same SD type (in the mouse H-2 antigens of the K or D region) that are present on the killer T cells (Zinkernagel and Doherty, 1975). This concept of a necessary identity (at least in part) between SD antigens of killer T and target cells (for generation of virus-specific killer T cells after *in vivo* immunization with live virus) has subsequently been shown valid in a variety of virus target killer T cell systems.

Experiments using syngeneic virus-infected teratoma cells lacking SD antigens on the surface have further emphasized the requirements for self-

SD (or SD structures in general) structures on the virus-infected target cell to make the cell sensitive to lysis (Zinkernagel and Oldstone, 1976). Another approach has involved chemical modification of cells via attachment of haptenic groups to the cell surface. Use of these modified cells as immunogens have revealed requirements for T cell killing identical to those found when using virus-infected cells as target cells. Following immunization with hapten-modified self-cells, the emerging immune T cells only kill if the target cell subsequently used also has specific hapten on its surface as well as at least one SD region shared with the effector cells (Shearer *et al.*, 1975). Experiments that interfere with the expression of self-H-2 structures on the target cells (without interfering with the haptenic groups) demonstrate the essential role of SD structures on the target cells in order for lysis to occur (Schmitt-Verhulst *et al.*, 1976).

Experiments with F_1 hybrid mice formed between strains differing at H-2 have studied the response to male antigen. Killer T cells for male antigen produced by immunizing F_1 responder females belong to two major groups: both groups react with the male antigen, but one will only react with male cells from one parental strain, and the other with male cells from the second parental strain (Gordon *et al.*, 1976).

Thus, T cells functioning as killer cells express a dual specificity requirement for target cell structures: one for the MHC structures of SD type and one for the "conventional" antigenic determinant. It should be stressed, however, that the present concept so far is based entirely on experiments performed in mice and requires confirmation in other species.

Cellular immune reactions of mixed leukocyte type predominantly involve T lymphocytes belonging to a subgroup different from the killer T lymphocytes (Cantor and Boyse, 1975). A similar requirement for self-MHC structures seems to prevail in these systems. Here, the responding T lymphocytes require reactivity against self-MHC components (of the Ia type and not the SD type), plus reactivity against some other structure behaving like a conventional antigen. Normal T cells of one inbred strain of mice can react with an MLC response against M locus structures *in vitro* [M locus products determine a strong MLC-inducing system when the M locus genes are located on a chromosome different from that containing the MHC-determining genes (Festenstein, 1973)]. When using responder and stimulator cells of the same MHC background in a primary response, such activated T cells can be tested for their ability to respond in a secondary manner to the same M locus determinants on the same or a different MHC background. They will only react in this second set if the responder and stimulator cells share Ia-region determinants (Peck *et al.*, 1977b). Restimulation with M locus on an entirely Ia-different background in the second set experiments fails to activate the anti-M locus specific, primed T cells. Data in other MLC systems support this finding (Peck *et al.*, 1977a). Thus, MLC-reactive T cells also seem to express a dual immune reactivity, this time with the specific reaction of "autoimmune" type being directed against self-MHC structures of Ia type.

In a third pattern of T cell reactivity (in which T cells help B cells produce antibodies against T dependent antigens), a similar anti-self-MHC requirement for T cell function prevails. In order for immune T cells to express efficient specific help for B cells, sharing of MHC (in particular Ia regions) between T and B cells is required (Katz *et al.*, 1975). Interestingly enough, however, T cells can be "trained" to help B cells of a given, foreign MHC genotype. This will occur if the T cells are allowed to reside (differentiate) together with the B cells for some time *in vivo* before immunization (von Boehmer *et al.*, 1975). The fact that T cells can adapt themselves to extend their anti-self MHC reactivity to MHC determinants other than those coded for by their own genotype shows that anti-self MHC restriction of T cells is a nonrigid feature that is governed by environmental factors. A detailed hypothetical discussion of how such adaptation can occur is presented elsewhere (Janeway *et al.*, 1976).

This is probably also true but not yet clearly shown for suppressor T cells. Thus, immunocompetent T cells may always carry clonally distributed receptors with specificity for self-MHC structures. These receptors would play an essential part in the triggering process of T lymphocytes to any kind of antigen. No clear-cut evidence exists as yet to tell whether such anti-self-reactive T cell receptors may under certain circumstances become triggered into "true" autoimmune activation against self-MHC without the concomitant presence of "foreign" antigen. Some experimental systems (where T cells are being activated *in vitro* under mitogenic conditions) suggest, however, that this possibility must be considered as a potential disease-provoking process (Peck *et al.*, 1977a).

According to certain theories on the generation of diversified, immunocompetent T cells (Jerne, 1971; Janeway *et al.*, 1976), anti-self-MHC reactivity is a driving force for the actual generation of discriminatory antigen-recognizing T lymphocytes during the various stages of differentiation. Presumably, the most immature T lymphocytes on the verge of becoming immunologically reactive should be the most dangerous cells with regard to "true" autoimmune reactivity. According to this hypothesis, strong reactivity against self-MHC structures (e.g., reactivity to allogeneic MHC determinants) would naturally appear on some T lymphocytes during their differentiation. Such cells would be eliminated, however, leaving as mature T cells only lymphocytes with low affinity receptors for self-MHC structures. If, however, this normal, eliminatory step should malfunction, true strong autoimmune reactivity leading to disease may appear.

Although the details of T cell reactivity towards self-MHC are poorly understood, it is clear that this controlled autoimmune reactivity behaves like an essential part of the immune cognitive ability of immunocompetent T lymphocytes. It is not known whether the whole diversity of antigen recognition by lymphocytes has evolved through this anti-self-reactivity (Jerne, 1971), or whether this selective autoimmune ability has coevolved in parallel to the "true" antigen-binding receptors in order to catalyze specific triggering to foreign structures. The behavior of this anti-self MHC reactivity with regard to find specificity and clonal distribution pattern suggests, however, that the receptors against self-MHC are constructed in a similar or identical manner to the receptors recognizing conventional antigens (Janeway *et al.*, 1976). The lesson to learn from the above reasoning would be that T cell reactivity leading to immunity of any kind may as an essential part always involve a controlled, autoimmune reaction.

III. POSITIVE CONSEQUENCES OF INDUCED AUTOIMMUNITY: A DISCUSSION AS TO POSSIBLE FUTURE APPLICATIONS

Most mammalian macromolecules accessible to the immune system would seem to be T dependent antigens. Present evidence suggests that tolerance at the helper T cell level for autologous determinants is a primary reason why autoimmunity against self-molecules and autoimmune disease are comparatively rare events. Excluding "privileged site" structures such as the eye proteins, autoimmunity would occur only when self-reactive T lymphocytes in sufficient numbers become activated into high-rate antibody synthesis. Although this activation may proceed via several pathways, the most efficient would require the existence of specific helper T lymphocytes reactive against macromolecules or particles that carry the relevant self-determinant(s). The systems discussed in the present article, using induced autoimmunization of potential beneficial value for the individual ("positive autoimmunity"), are mostly based on a requirement for helper T cells. The data obtained so far in these systems suggest that the underlying principle is valid. It should be stressed, however, that immune T cells against native determinants may become induced even if such self-structures normally occur in the form of low molecular weight molecules or in low molar concentrations. A complete immune response (involving both T and B lymphocytes) against such self-structures may be produced if the self-moiety is presented in a polymerized form, or linked up to a larger carrier molecule, or presented in a high local concentration. Detailed analysis of the parameters involved in the breaking of "tolerance" to self-structures is, outside the scope of the present chapter, and is discussed elsewhere in this volume.

What might be the benefits of having an ongoing autoimmune reaction in the body? An attractive part of the immune system is its extreme specificity (hard to come by, by other means, in most systems). The exquisite selectivity of the immune system, when used in a directed manner, may serve in a most refined way to eliminate a certain group of cells or their product(s) without interfering with other parameters. Let us discuss some systems where controlled induction of autoimmunity seems feasible, and where the outcome of such reactions might be of potential value to the individual being immunized.

IV. CONVERSION OF TUMOR-ASSOCIATED PROTEINS INTO SELF-IMMUNOGENS

The first system to be discussed deals with the possibility of inducing autoimmune reactions to tumor-associated molecules that are normally nonimmunogenic for the individual. The preliminary results already obtained may serve to illustrate the principle; it is likely that many more tumor-associated molecules will be shown to belong to the same category once they have been properly isolated. In the human tumor systems, a few tumor-associated proteins have been isolated and subsequently well defined. Two such proteins are α-feto-protein (AFP) and carcinoembryonic antigen (CEA). Both are present in the body in comparatively high concentrations during fetal life (AFP in the circulation, CEA mostly localized), and both are still present, but in very low concentrations, in normal, adult individuals. Certain tumors of distinct organ type (hepatomas or teratocarcinomas for AFP, and mostly tumors of the gastrointestinal tract for CEA) contain and produce high amounts of AFP or CEA. The sera of individuals bearing such tumors frequently exhibit increased levels of the respective proteins. AFP and CEA are both considered nonimmunogenic in the species of origin, and antibodies against them normally have to be raised by immunization across species barriers. CEA is known to be expressed at the cell surface of CEA-positive tumor cells, sometimes at concentrations higher than HLA. It seems possible that AFP may also be expressed at the surface of AFP-producing cells. It has been shown that AFP-producing hepatoma cells are killed by anti-AFP antibodies and complement *in vitro*. Similar results have been obtained using anti-CEA antibodies and CEA-positive tumor cells (Tsukada *et al*., 1974; S. Hammarström, personal communication). These proteins may serve as target antigens for an immune attack, should such an immune reaction take place in the tumor-bearing individual. Is it possible, then, to induce autoimmunity in man against these naturally occurring proteins? The answer is unknown, but is most likely yes based on experiments on animals, particularly monkeys (Ruoslahti and Wigzell, 1975; Ruoslahti *et al.*, 1976). Using either heterologous AFP (or CEA) as immunogen or chemically changed "native" protein as immunogen, it was possible to induce high-titered anti-AFP or anti-CEA antibodies in immunized monkeys with exquisite specificity for autologous AFP or CEA (Ruoslahti and Wigzell, 1975; Ruoslahti *et al.*, 1976). For instance, adult monkeys displaying a certain level of circulating AFP in serum were immunized using conventional adjuvant methodology rabbit AFP (structurally very similar yet distinct from the monkey or human AFP). The immunized monkeys developed a rapid drop in the serum AFP levels, followed by the appearance of specific antibodies reacting with monkey or human AFP in *in vitro* tests. In a similar manner, monkeys immunized with human CEA produced antibodies with high specificity for monkey CEA-like or human CEA molecules.

No negative side effects for the immunized subjects have been seen so far. When the anti-CEA antibodies were tested for ability to react with known CEA-positive tumor cells *in vitro*, strong reactions were noted. The monkey-anti-human CEA serum (in principle, equivalent to a human anti-human CEA serum) also induced a strong antibody-dependent, cell-mediated cytolysis against CEA-positive tumor cells *in vitro* when using normal human lymphocytes as effector cells (S. Hammarström, personal communication). Destruction of AFP-producing cells *in vivo* was indicated by finding definite degenerative changes in the synthesizing cells of the liver from rat fetuses immunized with AFP (Nishi *et al.*, 1973). Animals immunized against AFP may also behave in a protected manner against hepatoma outgrowth, although results are still preliminary and somewhat inconclusive (Goussev and Yasofa, 1974; Mizejewski and Allen, 1974). Thus, in patients, one would attempt to produce autoimmunity against molecules present partly in some normal cells (that seemingly can be dispensed of with no harm to the individual?), but also expressed on a cellular population potentially lethal to the individual, the tumor cells. Cellular immune reactions mediated by killer T cells are normally considered the most efficient in provoking graft rejection (in this instance, tumor rejection). Thus far, however, there is no evidence that autoimmune T killer cells appear following immunization against AFP or CEA, but such an appearance might take a comparatively longer time and require recruitment from virgin T lymphocytes just differentiating into fresh, immunocompetent cells.

Be that as it may, humoral antibodies as such and the antibody-induced, cell-mediated cytolytic reactions can at least be shown to function *in vitro*, and may possibly also function with regard to tumor growth retardation *in vivo*. The lesson of the present reasoning is that normally occurring macromolecules of nonvital type and normally nonimmunogenic may be changed into immunogens. As a consequence, the immune reaction may become directed against the cells producing these molecules, sometimes with a lytic effect on the target cells if the target molecules are present on their outer surfaces. When malignant cells are targets, such autoimmune potential would destroy target cells and would surely be of benefit. Obviously, this reasoning is based on preliminary results which establish the validity of the theoretical principles involved but which are considered hypothetical with regard to practical outcome.

V. REGULATION OF ENDOCRINE FUNCTIONS VIA AUTO-ANTI-HORMONE ANTIBODIES

Most hormones are small molecules, by themselves poorly or nonimmunogenic. They can be made immunogenic via coupling to larger, carrier antigens. By such procedures, it is possible to obtain antibodies against a variety of autologous hormones. The effects and possibilities of such autoimmunization procedures on pregnancy will be taken as a good example of how auto-anti-hormone immunity may be used in a positive sense for the individual. Chorionic gonadotrophin (CG) is a protein hormone essential for the establishment of pregnancy. Its biochemical composition is, in part, identical to or cross-reacting with other hormones, and, in part, is unique for this protein. Experiments in rats producing auto-anti-CG antibodies using impure preparations from placenta caused infertility but, as a complicating side effect, also caused immune complex renal disease. The investigators then used pure preparations of CG and, in particular, only unique parts of the CG hormone for immunization (Talwar *et al.*, 1976).

Thus, using the β-subunit of human CG coupled to the carrier tetanus toxoid, it now seems possible to overcome the negative side effects while achieving a specific, long-lasting anti-HCG antibody response in both animals and man. There was no evidence of any negative side effects, either at the level of possible immune complex disease or at the level of other endocrine functions, even over prolonged periods of time. Autopsy analysis of monkeys immunized with the HCG preparations and making anti-CG antibodies reacting with autologous CG, demonstrated completely normal pituitary glands and ovaries (Nath *et al.*, 1976). Human females immunized with the β-unit of HCG coupled to tetanus toxoid had entirely normal laboratory findings and showed no evidence of disturbed menstrual cycles

(Kumar *et al.*, 1976). The anti-HCG antibodies could be shown to block the biologic activity of HCG in several tests (Das *et al.*, 1976). In view of the results in female animals immunized with CG and developing auto-anti-CG immunity and subsequent infertility, it would seem likely that human females immunized with their "own" HCG in the same manner will be infertile.

Infertility via autoimmunization has been attempted for a long time, using such approaches as immunization against sperm (Tyler and Bishop, 1963). The results obtained with these "anti-organ" approaches to date seem far less promising than the anti-HCG approach. Reversibility of the anti-HCG immunity remains an unknown factor, however, although it is already known that the humoral anti-HCG titers decrease with increasing time after immunization. Furthermore, there is no evidence that "native" HCG can serve as an internal booster of the anti-HCG immunity. Additional support that HCG on its own is not immunogenic in HCG-immunized individuals is the failure to elicit delayed hypersensitivity using native hormone. This result indicates that immune T cells against HCG may not be present in these individuals (Nath *et al.*, 1976). It is, thus, likely that after varying time periods, perhaps 1 year or more after a single immunization, some women may again revert to a fertile stage.

Therefore, if care is taken to exclude cross-reacting determinants in the immunogen (by using only the unique parts of any given hormone as antigenic determinants coupled to a carrier immunogen), autoimmune reactions against hormones may constitute a powerful and highly specific way to regulate the activity of the endocrine system with regard to a variety of hormones.

VI. SPECIFIC AUTOIMMUNITY AGAINST ANTIGEN-BINDING RECEPTORS ON LYMPHOCYTES: A WAY TO INDUCE SPECIFIC IMMUNOLOGICAL TOLERANCE IN B AS WELL AS T LYMPHOCYTES

Immunoglobulin molecules with antigen-binding specificity have long been known to express this specificity via their antigen-combining sites. The peptide chains making up these antigen-binding areas have sequences that vary widely between individual immunoglobulin molecules. It is possible to make antibodies against such antigen-binding areas or their surroundings; such antibodies are called anti-idiotypic antibodies (Oudin and Michel, 1969). In the search for the T cell receptors for antigen, a most successful approach has been to use anti-idiotypic antibodies, hoping to find similar or identical idiotypes on the elusive T cell receptors as have been found on B cell-derived antibodies (Binz and Wigzell, 1977). Here, working within several distinct antigenic systems, evidence has accumulated to suggest that the T cell receptor for antigen is expressing idiotypic determinants. This result signifies an immunologically specific reactivity of the receptor-carrying lymphocyte against a given antigen (Eichmann and Rajewsky, 1975; Binz and Wigzell, 1975a). Furthermore, in the fine analysis of idiotypic specificities found on B and T cell receptors from the same individual reacting with the same antigenic determinants, it now seems clear that the two groups of receptors indeed share several of these idiotypes (Binz and Wigzell, 1977). Biochemical analysis, as well as studies on the T cell idiotype inheritance pattern, strongly suggests that this shared identitiy exists at the level of the heavy chain variable Ig genes (Binz and Wigzell, 1977). There is no data yet to suggest participation of conventional light chains in the creation of T cell receptors.

Anti-idiotypic antibodies in the presence of complement can be directly lytic for the B or T cells expressing these idiotypes on their surface, and could, thus, serve as powerful eliminators of the relevant clones of cells *in vitro* or *in vivo* (Binz and Wigzell, 1975a). Working with idiotypic receptors with specificity for the major histocompatibility antigens, it was possible to show that T lymphocyte populations treated with the proper anti-idiotypic antiserum and complement were selectively devoid of immune reactivity against the relevant transplantation antigens, yet perfectly normal in activity against third-party antigens (Binz and Wigzell, 1975a,b).

It is possible to induce anti-idiotypic antibodies against autologous idiotypic determinants (Rodkey, 1974). Successful induction of auto-anti-idiotypic immunity in a system such as the one described above could lead to specific unresponsiveness against a select group of transplantation antigens. Attempts were made to achieve such results. Using anti-idiotypic immunoabsorbants, it was possible to isolate from normal serum of adult rats naturally shed T cell receptors with specificity for a given transplantation antigen. In a typical example, serum from unimmunized Lewis rats was passed over an immunoabsorbant made up of anti-idiotypic antibodies with specificity anti-Lewis–anti-DA antibodies (Binz and Wigzell, 1976). Lewis and DA are inbred rat strains that differ with regard to their major histocompatibility antigens. From a large volume of normal Lewis rat serum it was possible via this immunoabsorbant technique to extract in a "pure" form small amounts of naturally occurring Lewis–anti-DA receptor molecules. Such molecules were then polymerized, using glutaraldehyde to make new antigenic determinants for helper T cells, and then injected back into normal Lewis rats using Freund's complete adjuvant (Binz and Wigzell, 1976).

The outcome was quite clear-cut: within a matter of a few weeks one could demonstrate a specific significant reduction in the MLC reactivity of lymphocytes from such "autoimmunized" Lewis rats when tested against DA, whereas reactivity against BN, a third strain, was left unimpaired. Furthermore, auto-anti-idiotypic antibodies could be detected in several sera from these rats with specificity for anti-DA receptors. Direct radioimmunoassays looking for the presence of idiotypic anti-DA lymphocytes [which are normally detectable in comparatively high numbers in normal rats (Binz and Wigzell, 1975b) in such receptor-immunized Lewis rats indicated that these cells were no longer present. Finally, when skin grafts from DA and BN rats were placed on Lewis rats immunized with such "anti-DA" receptors, prolongation of survival of DA skin was noted (extending in some rats to above three times the normal survival time). BN skin grafts were, however, rejected in a normal way. It is, thus, possible, via auto-anti-idiotypic immunizations, to produce a state of at least partial specific immune tolerance in adult immunocompetent individuals without having to evoke any other nonspecific immunosuppressive measures. The fact that the DA skin grafts were not accepted permanently we deemed quite natural in view of the fact that Lewis and DA rats differ not only with regard to major histocompatibility locus antigens but also for many minor loci.

The above experiments thus indicated the feasibility of using auto-anti-idiotypic immunity in a positive sense to achieve specific transplantation tolerance. No negative side effects were noted, even after prolonged immunizations. If one would consider trying the present approach in clinical practice, however, such autoimmunization procedures would have to be carried out without having accessible anti-idiotypic antibodies for the purification of the receptors. Therefore, a new approach was developed based on the following rationale (Andersson *et al.*, 1976): lymphocytes carry on their surface idiotypic, antigen-binding receptors signifying their potential immune reactivity. Two purification steps were employed to obtain the particular subpopulation of cells carrying receptors with a specificity for a given antigen in a pure form. Normal T lymphocytes were first purified using anti-Ig bead column fractionation. These cells were subsequently confronted with the relevant foreign cells, using a mixed leukocyte culture system. The specific cells do now respond with proliferation, allowing these cells to be purified from the smaller, nonresponding cells via 1-*g* velocity sedimentation. Such purified T lymphoblasts can be shown to carry select reactivity only against the relevant antigens and to represent, when presented locally, an "abnormally" high concentration of the relevant idiotypes. This increase in local concentration in itself may be enough to induce auto-anti-idiotypic receptors, but, to further increase immunogenicity, the cells were emulsified in Freund's adjuvant before adminstration. The latter procedure should also kill the cells.

The attempts to induce auto-anti-idiotypic immunity using autologous, *in vitro* activated, purified T lymphoblasts as immunogen have been quite successful. The results obtained so far are as follows: repeated immunization with 10–20 × 10^6 autologous immune blasts (produced in mixed leukocyte culture reactions against major histocompatibility complex antigens) caused many animals to produce detectable amounts of auto-anti-idiotypic antibodies (Andersson *et al.*, 1976). The fact that in several animals no significant amounts of anti-idiotypic antibodies were detected does not mean, however, that these individuals have failed to produce such antibodies, as the techniques used would only detect high concentrations of anti-idiotypic antibodies (Binz and Wigzell, 1975). In almost all individuals, however, both in rat or mouse strain combinations, one could show that lymphocytes from blast immunized animals were specifically unresponsive in mixed leukocyte cultures toward the relevant histocompatibility antigens, while displaying normal reactivity against third-party antigens. Immunization against autologous immune blasts could be shown to lead to long-lasting unresponsiveness against the defined antigens. In this system, the constant recruitment of virgin, idiotype-carrying lymphocytes may serve as an internal booster to maintain this tolerance for a very long time, perhaps permanently. Subsequent experiments have shown that lymphocytes from auto-blast-immunized individuals also express specifically reduced ability to react in graft versus host reactions. As to induction of specific transplantation tolerance by blast immunization, no case of complete tolerance has as yet occurred, but, in many individuals, prolongation of graft survival extending to more than three times the normal has been observed (Andersson *et al.*, 1977). Again, since the strain combinations studied differ at many weak histocompatibility loci in addition to the strong ones (with the weak ones being poor inducers of blasts *in vitro*), we are not surprised at this. Attempts to produce complete tolerance using strain combinations that differ only with regard to a single transplantation antigen are in progress. However, even at this stage it seems clear that the rationale behind this approach has proved valid. It is possible to induce a state of specific unresponsiveness via selective autoimmunization against a relevant group of idiotypic receptors.

The attempts described here are of a preliminary, but still highly promising, nature. Additional experimental systems should be tested for the auto-anti-idiotypic approach. Experiments are currently underway to analyze whether manipulation of delayed hypersensitivity can be achieved in a similar select manner using the blast immunization procedure. Certain autoimmune diseases may lend themselves to a similar approach, particularly if the causative antibodies are comparatively restricted in heterogenetity. The latter will increase the likelihood of getting an efficient eliminatory anti-idiotypic reaction. Here, one can speculate that lupus erythematosus may be a disease to try. Experiments are being planned, using autologous purified anti-DNA antibodies as immunogen. Another group of interest in this regard are the malignant tumors of lymphoid origin, in which the tumor cells are still producing and displaying specific immunoglobulin molecules. A particularly promising tumor type from the theoretical point of view is the B lymphomas of either chronic lymphatic leukemia type or Burkitt lymphoma type. Here, little secretion of immunoglobulin molecules occurs, but the tumor cells, in many cases, express a high concentration on the surface. It is known that such surface immunoglobulin markers on these tumor cells can serve as efficient targets for the cytolytic activity of anti-immunoglobulin antibodies in the presence of complement (Klein *et al.*, 1968). Thus, *in vivo* model experiments using animal B lymphomas would be of great value here, and promising results already exist (I. Green, personal communication).

In conclusion, positive autoimmunity within the immune system itself may turn out to be a field where beneficial effects for the individual may be achieved using the auto-anti-idiotype approach. Only time will tell whether the present promising results in this area will hold up to further testing and for possible introduction into human medicine.

VII. CONCLUDING REMARKS

Concepts of extreme or dogmatic nature concerning complex biologic phenomena are usually erroneous. Thus, it has been a major intention of the present article to change the commonly held view that autoimmune reactions by necessity are harmful, or at best neutral, for the individual. Examples have been selected from a comparatively small group of results where, under defined conditions, autoimmune reactions can be shown to have a decidedly positive value for the individual.

ACKNOWLEDGMENTS

This work was supported by the Swedish Cancer Society and NIH Grant AI 13485-01.

REFERENCES

Andersson, L. C., Binz, H., and Wigzell, H. (1976). *Nature* (*London*) **264,** 778–779.

Andersson, L. C., Binz, H., Soots, A., and Wigzell, H. (1977). To be published.

Binz, H., and Wigzell, H. (1975a). *J. Exp. Med.* **142,** 197–211.

Binz, H., and Wigzell, H. (1975b). *J. Exp. Med.* **142,** 1218–1230.

Binz, H., and Wigzell, H. (1976). *J. Exp. Med.* **144,** 1438–1450.

Binz, H., and Wigzell, H. (1977). *Contemp. Top. Immunobiol.* **7,** 111–175.

Cantor, H., and Boyse, E. A. (1975). *J. Exp. Med.* **141,** 1376–1389.

Das, C., Salahuddin, M., and Talwar, G. P. (1976). *Contraception* **13,** 171–182.

Eichmann, K., and Rajewsky, K. (1975). *Eur. J. Immunol.* **5,** 661–666.

Festenstein, H. (1973). *Transplant. Rev.* **15,** 62–90.

Gordon, R. D., Mathieson, B. J., Samelson, L. E., Boyse, C. A., and Simpson, E. (1976). *J. Exp. Med.* **144,** 810–820.

Goussev, A., and Yasofa, A. (1974). *In* "Colloques L' INSERM l' Alpha-foétoprotéine" (R. Massayeff, ed.), pp. 255–270. Inserm, Paris.

Janeway, C. A., Wigzell, H., and Binz, H. (1976). *Scand. J. Immunol.* **5,** 993–1001.

Katz, D. H., Graves, M., Dorf, M. E., Dimuzio, H., and Benacerraf, B. (1975). *J. Exp. Med.* **141,** 263–268.

Klein, E., Klein, G., Nadkarni, J. S., Nadkarni, J. J., Wigzell, H., and Clifford, P. (1968). *Cancer Res.* **28,** 1300–1310.

Kumar, S., Sharma, N. C., Bajaj, J. S., Talwar, G. P., and Hiugorami, V. (1976). *Contraception.* **13,** 253–268.

Mizejewski, G., and Allen, R. P. (1974). *Nature* (*London*) **250,** 50–52.

Nath, I., Gupta, P. D., Bhuyan, U. N., and Talwar, G. P. (1976). *Contraception* **13,** 213–224.

Nishi, S., Watabe, H., and Hirai, H. (1973). *Tumor Res.* **8,** 17–22.

Oudin, J., and Michel, M. (1969). *J. Exp. Med.* **130,** 595–617.

Peck, A. B., Andersson, L. C., and Wigzell, H. (1977a). *J. Exp. Med.* (in press).

Peck, A. B., Janeway, C., and Wigzell, H. (1977b). To be published.

Rodkey, L. L. (1974). *J. Exp. Med.* **139,** 713–724.

Ruoslahti, E., and Wigzell, H. (1975). *Nature* (*London*) **255,** 716–717.

Ruoslahti, E., Engvall, E., Vuento, M., and Wigzell, H. (1976). *Int. J. Cancer* **17,** 358–361.

Schmitt-Verhulst, A. M., Sachs, D. H., and Shearer, G. M. (1976). *J. Exp. Med.* **143,** 211–217.

Shearer, G. M., Rehn, T. G., and Garbarino, C. A. (1975). *J. Exp. Med.* **141,** 1348–1364.

Talwar, G. P., Sharma, N. C., Dubey, S. K., Salahuddin, M., Shastri, N., and Ramakrishnan, S. (1976). *Contraception* **13,** 131–140.

Tsukada, Y., Mikuni, M., Watabe, M., Nishi, S., and Hirai, H. (1974). *Int. J. Cancer* **13,** 187–195.

Tyler, A., and Bishop, D. (1963). *In* "Mechanisms Concerned with Conception" (C. G. Hartman, ed.), pp. 397–482. Macmillan, New York.

von Boehmer, H., Hudson, L., and Sprent, J. (1975). *J. Exp. Med.* **142,** 989–997.
Zinkernagel, R., and Doherty, P. (1974). *Nature* (*London*) **248,** 701–702.
Zinkernagel, R., and Doherty, P. (1975). *J. Exp. Med.* **141,** 1427–1436.
Zinkernagel, R., and Oldstone, M. (1976). *Proc. Natl. Acad. Sci. U.S.A.* **73,** 3666–3670.

Index

B

I

M

N

O

P

U